The Dental Reference Manual

Geraldine M. Weinstein • Mitchell T. Zientz
Editors

The Dental Reference Manual

A Daily Guide for Students and Practitioners

Springer

Editors
Geraldine M. Weinstein
University of Connecticut
School of Dental Medicine
Farmington
CT
USA

Mitchell T. Zientz
Wellspring Dental
Brooklyn
New York
USA

ISBN 978-3-319-39728-3 ISBN 978-3-319-39730-6 (eBook)
DOI 10.1007/978-3-319-39730-6

Library of Congress Control Number: 2016958298

Printed on acid-free paper

This Springer imprint is published by Springer Nature
The registered company is Springer International Publishing AG Switzerland

Preface

What Are the Benefits for the Student and/or Practitioner?

This is a succinct and truncated reference manual for the young dentist.

It will serve as an accessible means to quickly find answers to common dental questions.

It is a reference aid with an educational delivery designed for the student (both in school and in practice).

The aim is for the student to keep it handy.

It is a study guide of sorts including the particulars that should be second nature for every dentist.

It allows the new student to look ahead at the big picture and begin familiarizing with topics to come.

It allows the practicing dentist a daily reference of common and important materials/topics/techniques/conditions.

In academia, inspiration can come from the very students who you work with on a daily basis. The idea for this book was born from a dental student, Mitch Zientz, who wanted to capture the most important aspects of his clinical education. His original idea was to author each chapter on his own. A herculean task that I ultimately discouraged. Instead, we developed the idea and searched for experts in the field, mostly educators to document their evidence-based teachings. The chapters are a collective work from authors across different disciplines. The dental reference manual exhibits the necessities for the practice of general dentistry. It exemplifies answers to the most haunting questions that we stumble upon on a daily basis. We hope that it is a useful tool for all our young dental practitioners.

Our deepest gratitude to all the authors in this book who helped make the dream a reality! We hope with this collection of works to inspire the new practitioner to learn, grow, and most importantly do what is right for their patients. Dentistry is a lifelong journey of learning; never cease to ask questions!

Farmington, CT, USA Geraldine M. Weinstein
Brooklyn, NY, USA Mitchell T. Zientz

Contents

Part II The Specialties in General Dentistry

Part III References for Everyday Practice

Part IV Pathways of a Dental Career

Part I

Essentials of Dental Practice

Comprehensive Head and Neck Exam

1

Rosalia Rey, Nereyda Clark, and Pamela Sandow

Contents

Abstract

An exam of the head and neck region is essential for every patient that we encounter as dentists. When done in a systematic and efficient way, it should only take a few minutes of time. The key to performing this exam is noting asymmetries and determining if pathology is involved.

1.1 The Interview of the Patient Is Critical to Identify High Risk Factors

- *Smoking history* – Document the pack-years; multiply the number of packs of cigarettes smoked per day by the number of years the patient has smoked (National Cancer Institute).

R. Rey, DMD • N. Clark, DMD
Restorative Dental Sciences, University of Florida, College of Dentistry, Gainesville, FL, USA

P. Sandow, DMD (✉)
Oral Medicine, University of Florida, College of Dentistry, Gainesville, FL, USA
e-mail: PSANDOW@dental.ufl.edu

G.M. Weinstein, M.T. Zientz (eds.), *The Dental Reference Manual*,
DOI 10.1007/978-3-319-39730-6_1

- *Other tobacco use.*
- *Alcohol and drug use* – Document amount of use (National Institute on Alcohol Abuse and Alcoholism).
- *Poor diet.*
- *Human papillomavirus (HPV) history* – See Chap. 14, for more information. (Oral Cancer Foundation).
- *Sun exposure.*
- *Reported changes in the voice, skin, or mouth.*

1.2 Extraoral Exam

- *Head, neck, face, skin, and hairline* (Fig. 1.1)
  - Standing in front of the patient, visually inspect the face.
  - Look for symmetry; color, pigmentation, contour, consistency, and function.
- *Forehead and eyes*
  - Palpate the forehead. Look for nodules, swellings, and masses (Fig. 1.2).
- *Cranial nerves and facial muscles*

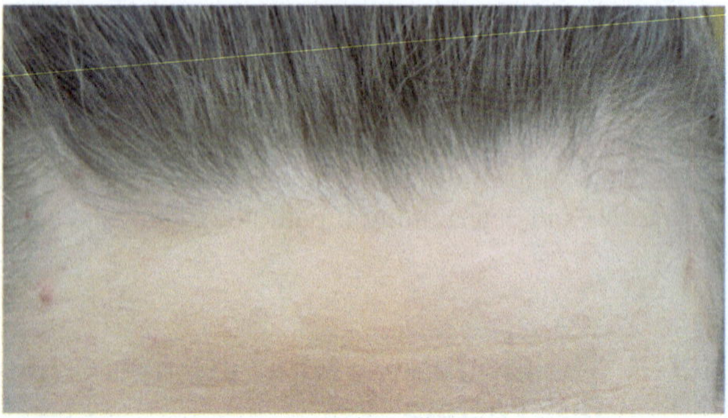

Fig. 1.1 Forehead and hairline (Photos courtesy of Anna Christine Napoli and Dr. Karin Schey)

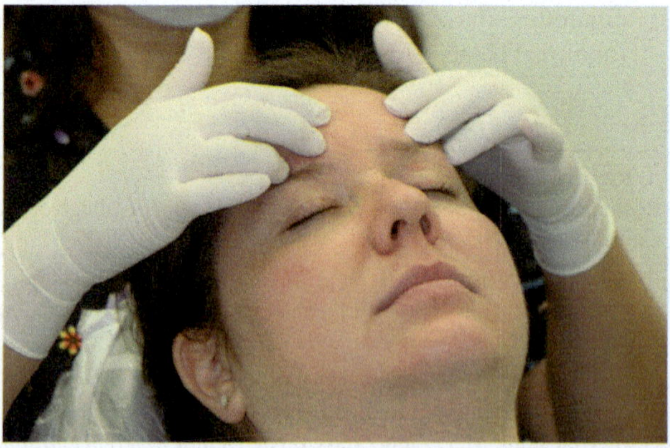

Fig. 1.2 Palpation is a quick way to examine a patient for asymmetries

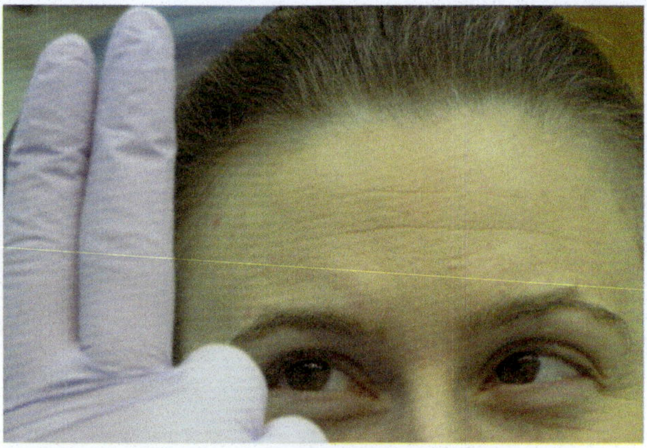

Fig. 1.3 The patient should follow finger movements with the eyes, while not moving the head. Movement of the eye is controlled by the oculomotor, trochlear, and abducens nerves

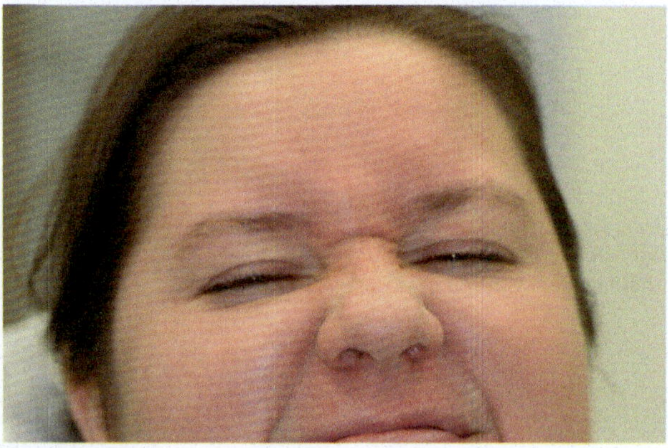

Fig. 1.4 Squinting may detect facial nerve symmetry (normal finding) or asymmetry (abnormal finding)

  - Have patient follow your fingers in an H pattern. Assess possible deficiency in facial nerve function (Fig. 1.3).
  - Have patient squint, look for symmetry. Asymmetry during squinting could indicate facial muscle deficiency (Fig. 1.4).
- *Ears*
  - Inspect and palpate all visible portions of the ear (Fig. 1.5).
  - Look for color, pigmentation, contour, consistency, and function.
- *Eyes*
  - Inspect the eyes (Fig. 1.6).
  - Look for white sclera, absence of swelling, or drainage.
  - Yellow sclera may suggest jaundice.
  - Hematoma could indicate a bleeding disorder or injury.
- *Nose*
  - Look up the nares (nostrils) and palpate the nose (Fig. 1.7).
  - Look for nodules, swellings, and masses.
- *TMJ*
  - Sitting or standing behind the patient, visually inspect the face. Look for symmetry in function. Note any abnormal deviation of the mandible.

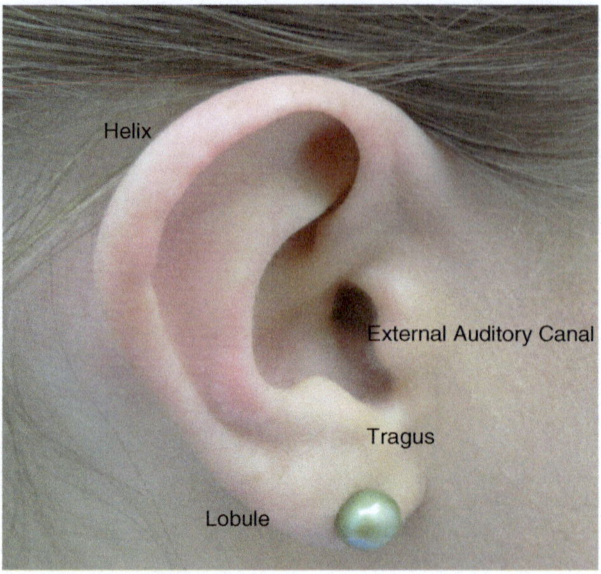

Fig. 1.5 Outer ear

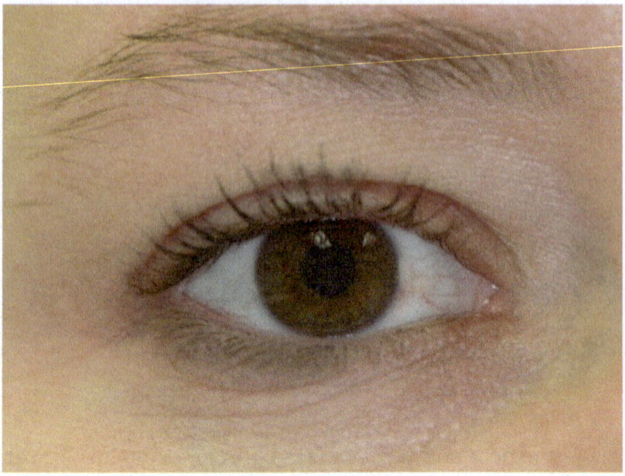

Fig. 1.6 Check the eyes for sclera coloring, drainage, or swelling

  - Palpate the temporomandibular joint (TMJ) while having patient open and close with fingers placed over the condyles, bilaterally. Note clicking, popping, and discomfort/pain (Fig.1.8).
  - Look for nodules, swellings, and/or masses.
- *Parotid gland and preauricular nodes*
  - Feel the parotid bilaterally and the preauricular nodes (Fig.1.9).
  - Compare for symmetry, identify nodes by size and if they are hard or soft, painful or painless, and freely movable or fixed.
  - Possible findings: Lymph nodes may have nodules, swelling, and/or masses.

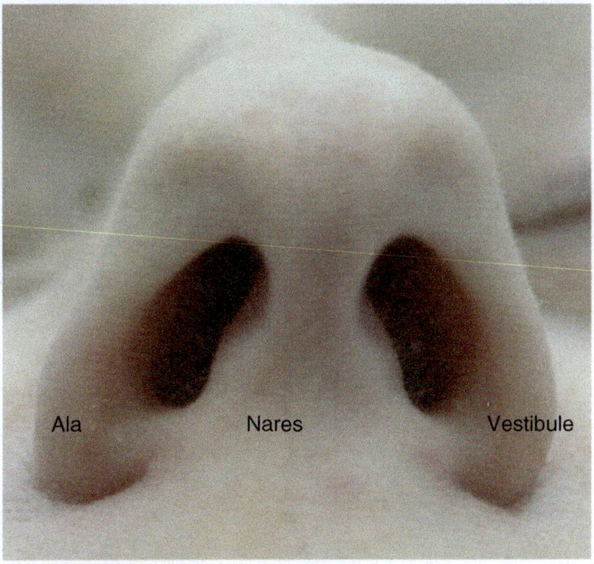

Fig. 1.7 Lack of symmetry of the nose should be noted when performing esthetic dental procedures as it may be critical when determining facial midlines

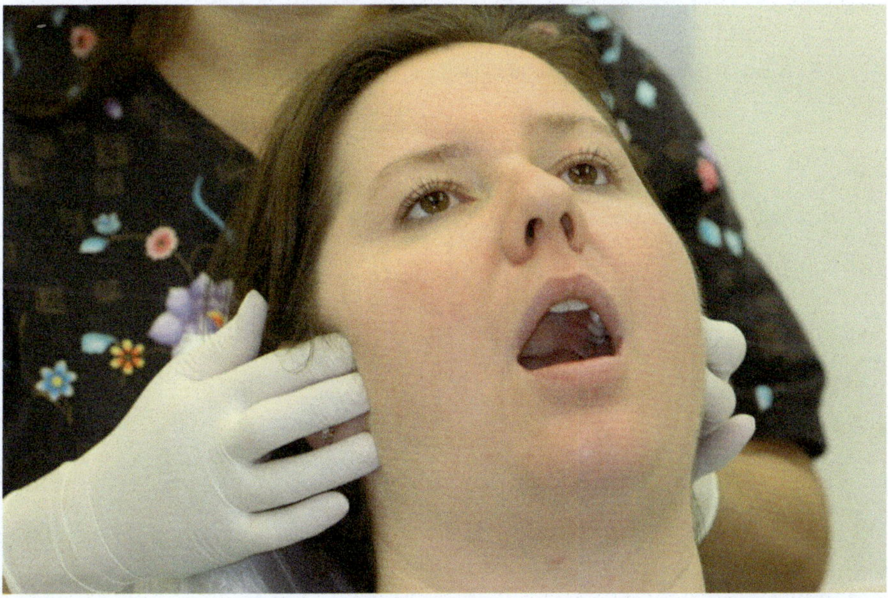

Fig. 1.8 If TMJ symptoms are present, a more extensive evaluation will be necessary

- *Posterior neck nodes*
  - To palpate the posterior auricular and occipital nodes, drop head forward to enhance access to these areas.
  - Palpate over the trapezius muscle for the spinal accessory and posterior cervical nodes (Fig. 1.10a, b).

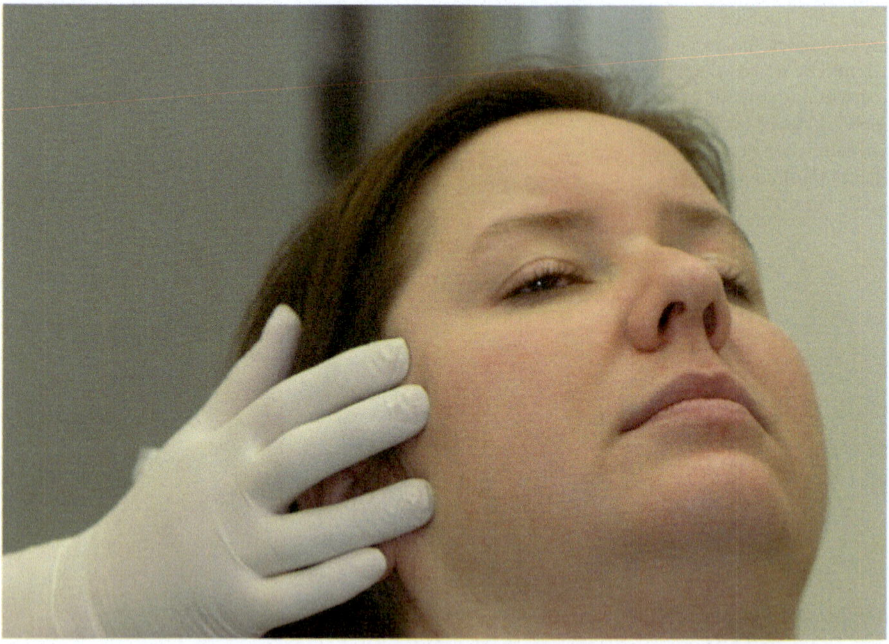

Fig. 1.9 Bilateral palpation of the parotid gland and preauricular area

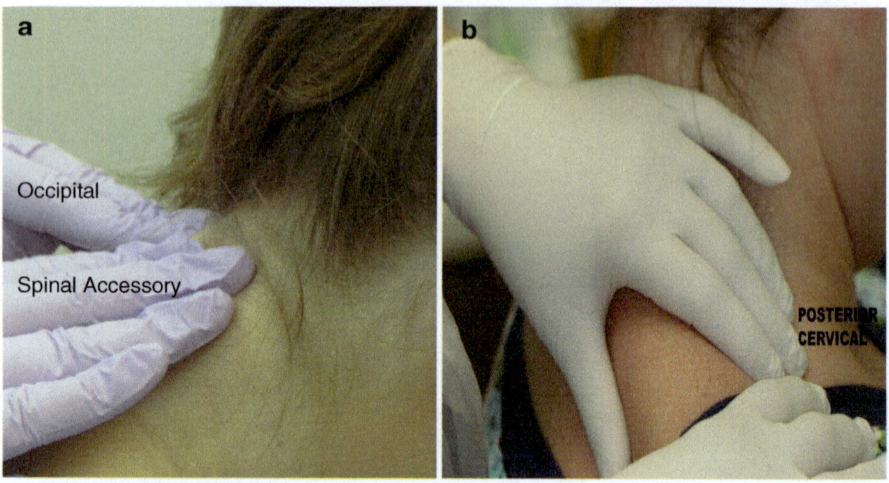

Fig. 1.10 (**a**, **b**) Tenderness to palpation should also be noted

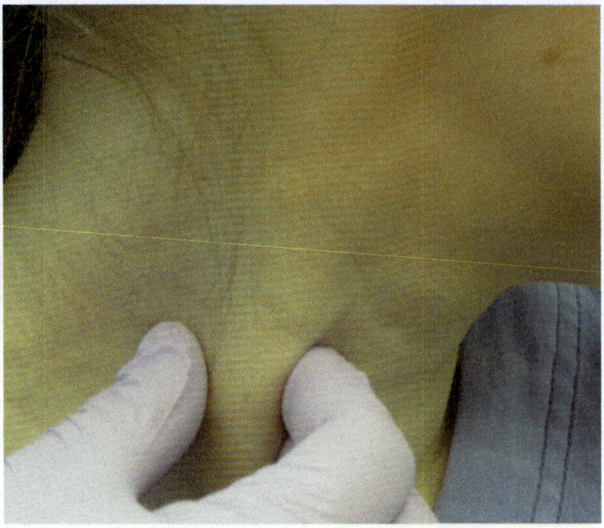

Fig. 1.11 Jugular lymph node enlargement along the sternocleidomastoid is common in patients experiencing the common cold or with head and neck cancer (Photo Courtesy of Dr. Eugenia Monaghan)

- Compare for symmetry and identify nodes for size, consistency (hard or soft), level of pain, or if freely movable or fixed.

- *Anterior neck nodes*
  - Palpate the jugular chain, deep and superficial cervical nodes, by placing fingers firmly on both sides of the sternocleidomastoid muscle from its origin at the clavicle to its insertion at the mastoid process behind the ear (Fig. 1.11).
  - Palpate the supraclavicular, anterior scalene, and delphian nodes above the clavicles and near the inferior midline of the neck.
  - Compare for symmetry and identify nodes for size, consistency (hard or soft), level of pain, or if freely movable or fixed.
- *Thyroid gland and larynx*
  - Visually inspect and bimanually palpate the thyroid. Compare both lobes for symmetry.
  - Normally, the thyroid gland is difficult to palpate.
  - Palpate the larynx while the patient swallows (Fig. 1.12).
  - Inspect for enlargement or mobility. Listen for hoarseness.
- *Submandibular neck nodes*
  - To palpate the submandibular and submental nodes have the patient lower the chin and manually palpate directly underneath the chin and the medial side of the mandible (Fig.1.13).
  - Grasp and roll the tissue over the bony edge of the mandible, anteriorly and bilaterally.

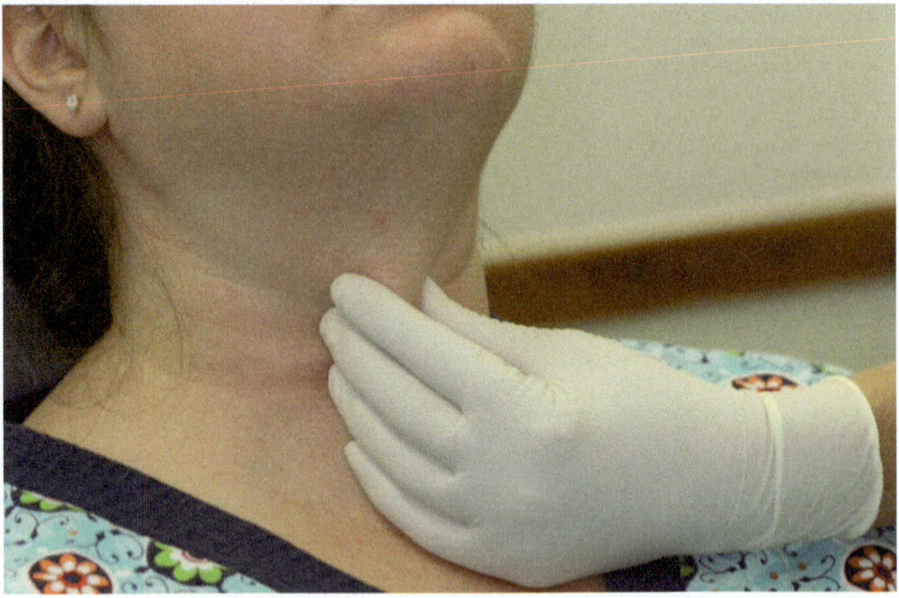

Fig. 1.12 Inquire if patient has any difficulty swallowing

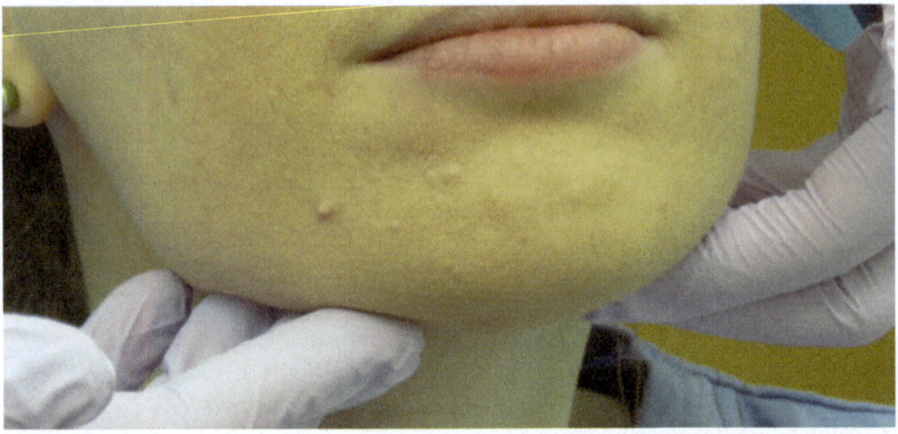

Fig. 1.13 Insure that palpation of soft tissue is done against the hard, bony surface of the mandible

1.3 Intraoral Exam

- *Gloves*
  - Remove soiled gloves and replace with clean latex-free gloves.
- *Lips*
  - Evaluate closed and open.
  - Visualize vermilion border, commissures, and mucosa. The border should be uniform and pink with no cracking or ulcerations at the commissures (Fig. 1.14).
  - Palpate bilaterally and bi-digitally between the thumb and fingers from one commissure to the other in the lower lip (Fig. 1.15a).
  - Use the same technique for the upper lip (Fig. 1.15b).
  - Submucosal lumps (minor salivary glands) should be small and uniform in size.

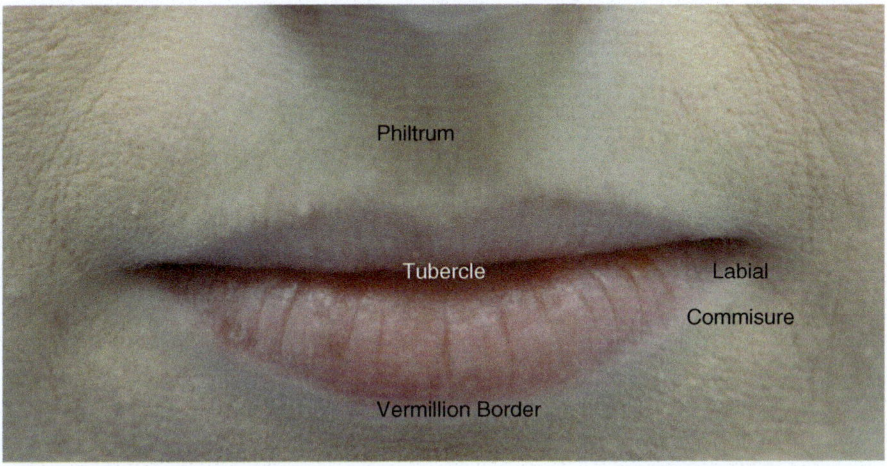

Fig. 1.14 The vermilion border

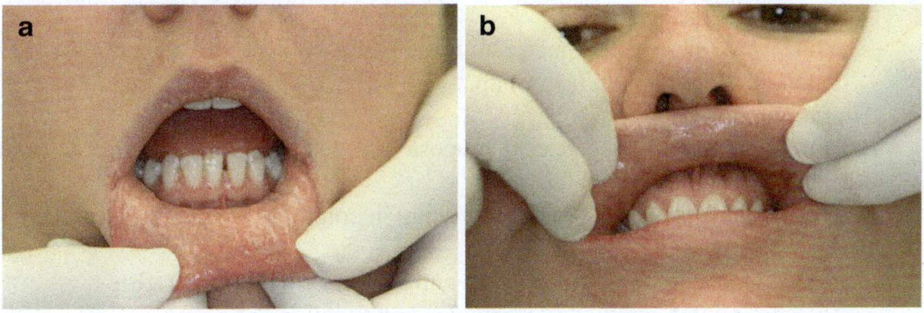

Fig. 1.15 (**a**, **b**) Palpating and visualizing the lips

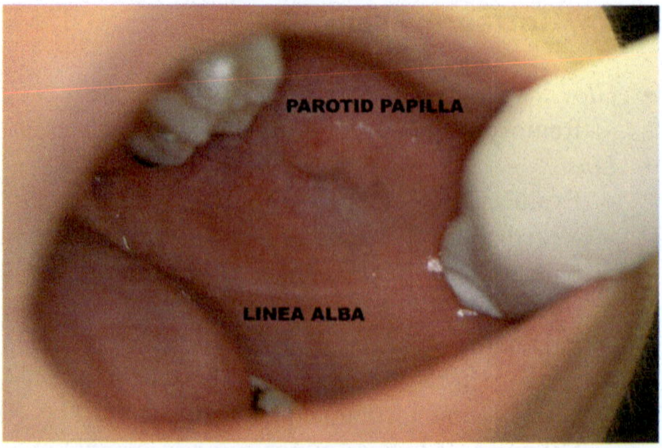

Fig. 1.16 The linea alba may be more pronounced in pigmented gingiva or people who chew their cheeks

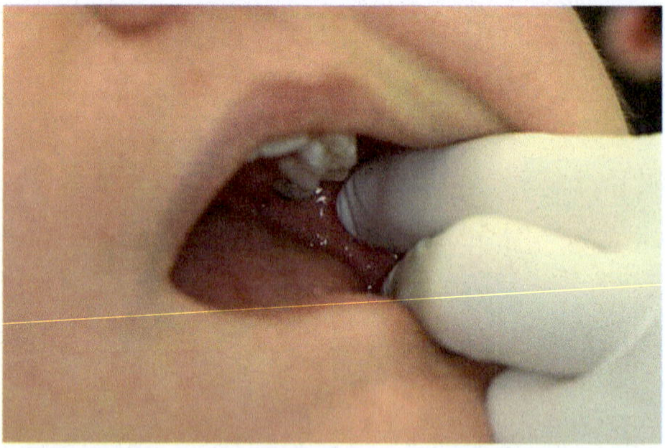

Fig. 1.17 Thorough medical history review will help determine if lesions are traumatic or pathologic

- *Buccal mucosa*
  - Retract the buccal mucosal tissue and visualize, while the mouth is in a relaxed open position.
  - Linea alba (white line) at the mid-buccal mucosa is a normal finding (Fig.1.16).
  - If the tissue appears white and disappears when stretched, it may indicate leukoedema (see Chap. 14).
  - White lacy lines on the buccal mucosa could be a sign of lichen planus or lichenoid drug reaction (see Chap. 14).
- *Parotid gland*
  - Bi-digitally palpate the buccal mucosa and parotid gland, comparing both sides for symmetry (Fig.1.17).
  - A malignancy is usually red or red/white in color and indurated (hard).
- *Alveolar ridges*
  - Visually inspect the vestibular area and alveolar ridges (Fig. 1.18).
  - Assess the color, contour, consistency, and function.
- *Buccal gingiva*
  - With an index finger, palpate the buccal and labial surfaces of the alveolar ridges and vestibules (Fig. 1.19).

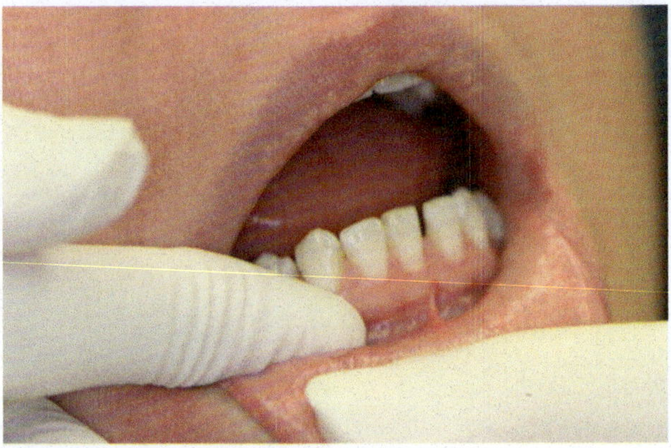

Fig. 1.18 When a lesion is found along the alveolar ridges, endodontic testing and radiographs will help determine if the lesion may be due to tooth pathology as opposed to a soft tissue lesion. (see Chaps. 12 and 14)

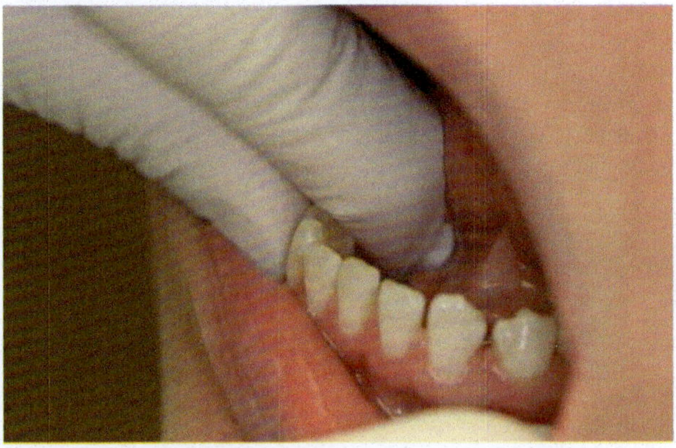

Fig. 1.19 Note tori, if present, as this may impact future restorative treatment

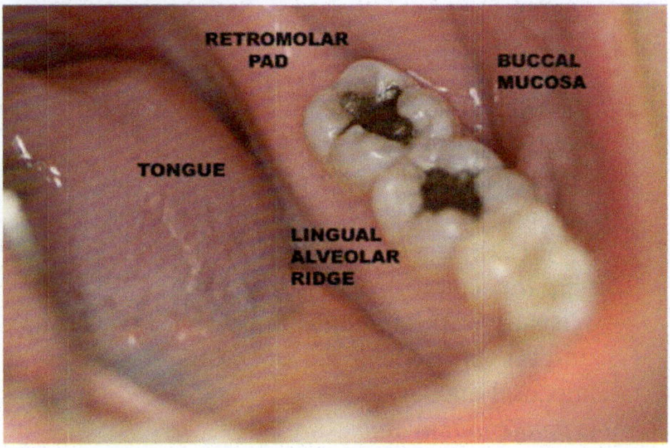

Fig. 1.20 It is important to perform a quick visual inspection of the patient at every dental visit

- *Lingual gingiva*
  - Inspect and palpate the lingual surfaces of the mandible.
  - Amalgam tattoos are common findings found near large fillings or root canals, even after teeth are extracted.

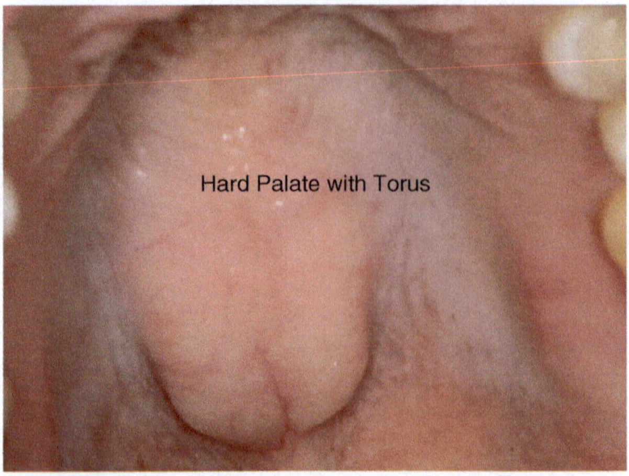

Fig. 1.21 Note palatal torus as this may impact future restorative treatment

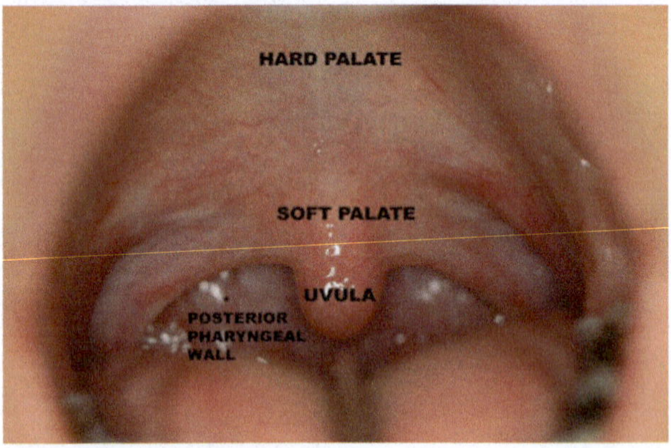

Fig. 1.22 The oropharyngeal area should be inspected as part of the head and neck exam

   - Inspect for bone loss/mobility associated with one tooth that is not consistent with the rest of the oral cavity as it could indicate underlying pathology or malignancy.
   - Inspect for unilateral enlargement of the bone as this may be a sign of an odontogenic cyst or tumor, as opposed to tori which are usually bilateral (Fig.1.20).
- *Hard palate*
   - Visually inspect and palpate the hard palate (Fig.1.21).
   - Inspect for irregularities in coloration, ulcerations, and/or asymmetrical submucosal masses.
- *Soft palate and uvula*
   - Have the patient open wide and visually inspect the soft palate and uvula.
   - Inspect for discolorations, changes in mucosal texture, swelling, asymmetrical enlargement of tonsils, ulcerations, growths, masses, bleeding, and/or pain.
- *Tonsillar pillars*
   - With gentle pressure place the mouth mirror on the middle of the tongue and ask the patient to say "ahhhh" while relaxing the tongue (Fig.1.22).

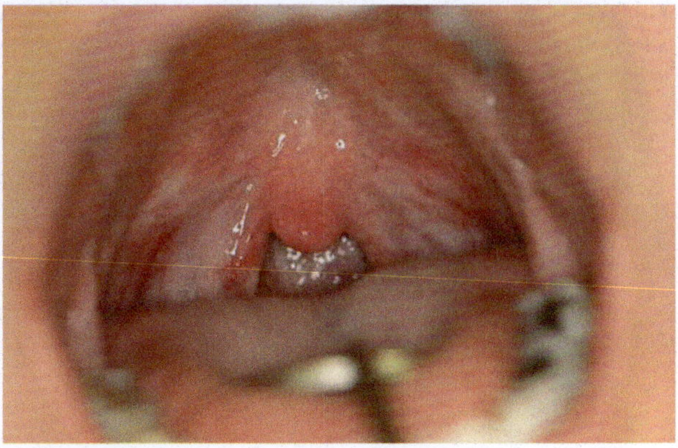

Fig. 1.23 Symmetric mobility of the uvula should be observed when a patient says "ahh"

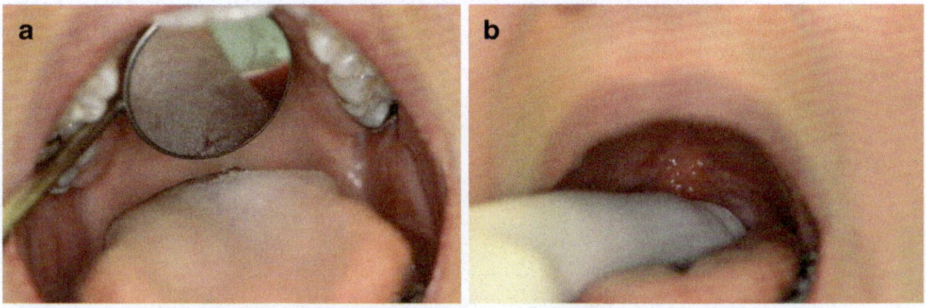

Fig. 1.24 (**a**, **b**) Visualize and palpate the tongue posterior to the circumvallate papillae

  - A unilateral earache can be a sign of oropharyngeal carcinoma or lymphoma (American Cancer Society).
- *Pharynx and portions of the oropharynx*
  - Visually inspect the uvula and the visible portions of the pharynx including the tonsils (Fig. 1.23).
- *Posterior tongue*
  - Protrude the tongue and visualize the posterior tongue, posterior to the circumvallate papillae, with the mouth mirror (Fig. 1.24a, b).
  - Also, if possible, palpate posterior to the circumvallate papillae with a sweep of the finger.
  - Inspect for discolorations, changes in mucosal texture, swelling, asymmetrical enlargement of tonsils, ulcerations, growths, masses, bleeding, and/or pain.
  - Upon protrusion observe if the tongue is symmetrical or deviates to one side.
- *Lateral surface of the tongue*
  - Have the patient gently extend the tongue and wrap a gauze square around the anterior third of the tongue in order to obtain a firm grasp (Fig. 1.25).
  - Inspect for discolorations, changes in mucosal texture, swelling, asymmetrical enlargement of tonsils, ulcerations, growths, masses, bleeding, and/or pain.
  - Turn the tongue slightly on its side.

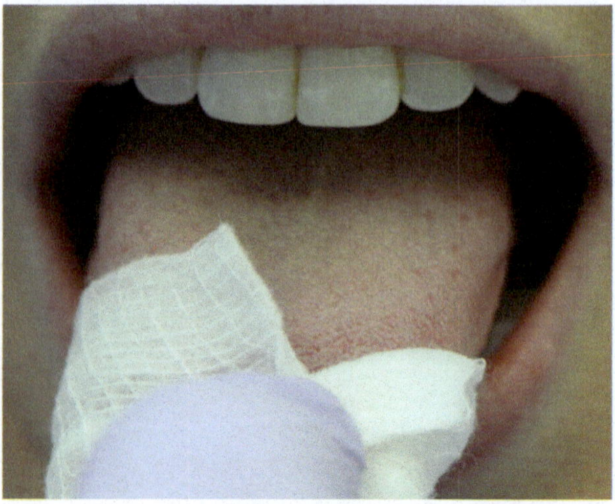

Fig. 1.25 Use of gauze allows the tongue to be examined without slipping

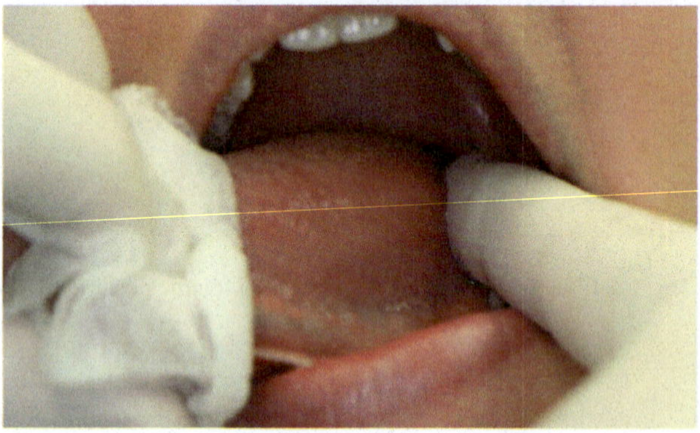

Fig. 1.26 Visualize and palpate the lateral surfaces of the tongue

   - Visually inspect and digitally palpate its base and lateral borders (Fig.1.26).
- *Dorsal tongue*
   - Bi-digitally palpate the dorsal surface (Fig.1.27).
   - Foliate papillae are a normal finding along the posterior lateral border of the tongue, bilaterally.
   - Inspect for asymmetry and palpate for masses.
- *Ventral tongue and floor of the mouth*
   - While the patient lifts the tongue to the palate, visually inspect the mucosa of the ventral tongue and floor of the mouth (Fig.1.28).
   - Use the mouth mirror to assist in lighting.
- *Submandibular and sublingual salivary glands*
   - Palpate the sublingual region by placing one index finger intraorally and the fingertips of the opposite hand under the chin, compressing the tissue between the fingers (Fig.1.29).
   - Check for symmetry.

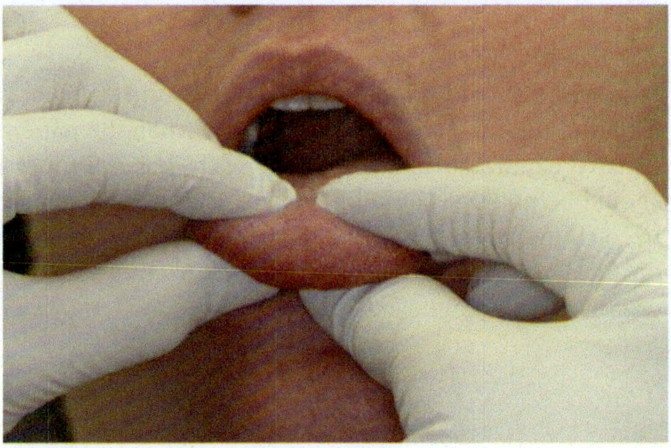

Fig. 1.27 Use fingers on both sides of the tongue to detect masses

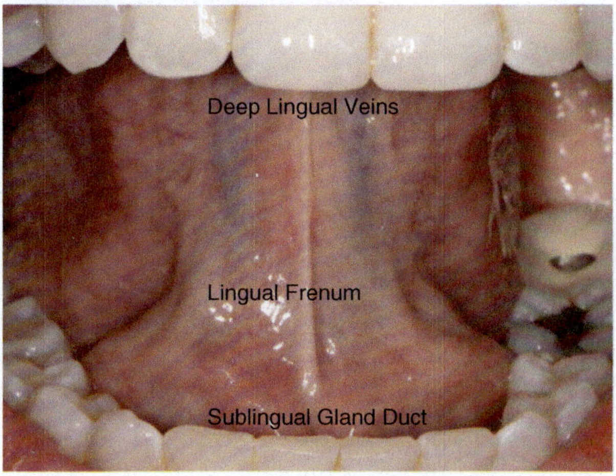

Fig. 1.28 Inspect the floor of the mouth. Normal findings like tori or unusual lingual frenum attachments should be noted as it may affect future restorative decisions

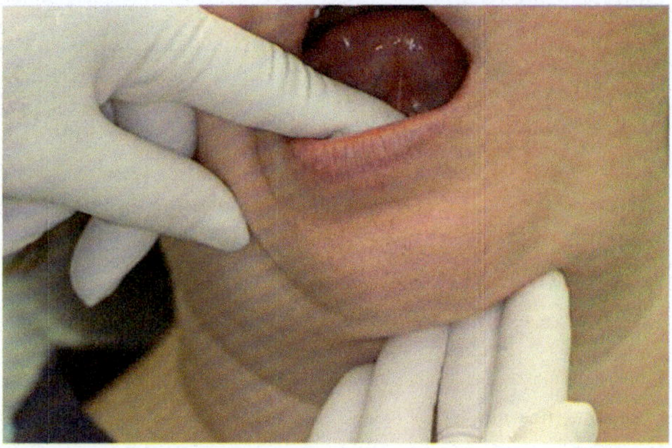

Fig. 1.29 Palpate using index fingers intraorally and in the submental region. Use the hard surface of the mandible to assist in compressing the tissue

1.4 How to Record Findings

A practice should have a standardized form to record all head and neck findings. This should be done at the initial visit when the patient first presents for a comprehensive exam and updated on a yearly basis. Proper referrals to other specialists should be noted if pathology exists. Below is an example of a form that can be utilized (Figs. 1.30a, b and 1.31). More details on oral cancer screenings can be found on the Oral Cancer Foundation website, ISSN: http://www.oralcancerfoundation.org/discovery-diagnosis/screening.php.

a

Head and Neck Screening Exam Finding Control #__________

First Name__________ Last Name__________ DOB___/___/___ SCREENING EXAM: by__________

Site	Normal	Abnor	Pho	Descriptors: Color, # of lesions, Size	Shape, Surface, Growth, Attachment	Consistency, Length of Time, Pain	Diagram
Forahead							
Eyes							
Nose							
Lower Face							
Facial Muscles							
Cranial Nerves							
TMJ							
Auricular/Parotid Nodes							
External Ears							
Post Neck Nodes							
Ant Neck Nodes							
Thyroid Larynx							
Submandibular/Mental Nodes							
Lips							

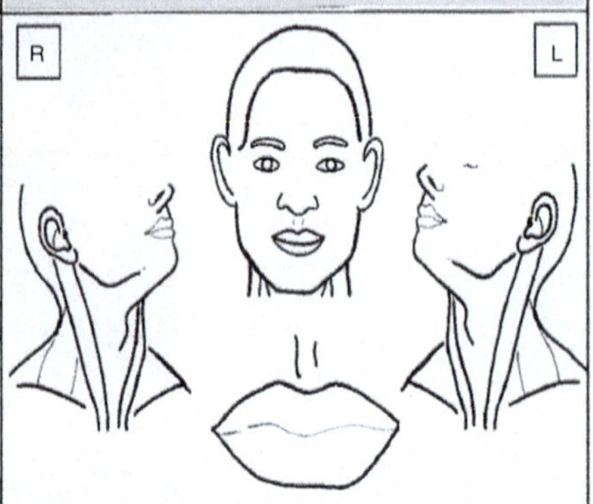

Location: Anatomical location and Symmetry
Unilateral, Bilateral, Symmetrical, Midline, Right, Left

# of lesions: Single Few Multiple, Generalize

Size: in millimeters

Color: White, Red, Red and White, Fluid Filled Vesicle, Blue, Black, Pigmented

Overall Configuration: Raised (nodular) Flat (macular)

Shape: Round, Oval, Irregular Borders, Assymentrical

Surface: Smooth, Rough, Ulcerated, Hyperkeratotic, Scaly, Crusty, Oozing, Bleeding, Dry

Attachment: Sessile/broad - Fixed Base Pedunculated-narrow stalk

Consistency: Hard Soft indurated Non-indurated (esp if ulcerated)

Growth: Endophytic, Exophytic, Compressible Blanches, Swelling

Length of time: not aware.
aware < 2 weeks aware 3 months, aware > 3 months
Has it happened before? Trauma Recurrent Medication
Has it changed?

Pain: On palpation? Unprovoked? yes no

TMJ: crepitus, popping, limited opening (<3 finger widths), abnormal translation (right, left, irregular), pain

Nodes:
Size
Hard or soft
Painful or painless
Moveable or fixed

Fig. 1.30 (**a**, **b**) Screening forms insure that a proper exam is done for each patient

b

Head and Neck Screening Exam Finding Control #____________

First Name____________ Last Name____________ DOB___/___/___ SCREENING EXAM: by____________

Site	Normal	Abnorma	Photogra	Descriptors: Color, # of lesions, Size	Shape, Surface, Growth, Attachment	Consistency, Length of Time, Pain	Diagram
Labial Mucosa							
Buccal Mucosa							
Parotid Gland							
Max Gingiva B & L							
Mand Gingiva B & L							
Hard Palate							
Soft Palate							
Tonsils							
Oropharynx							
Tongue Dorsal							
Lateral Border							
Ventral							
Floor of Mouth							
Sublingual Gland							

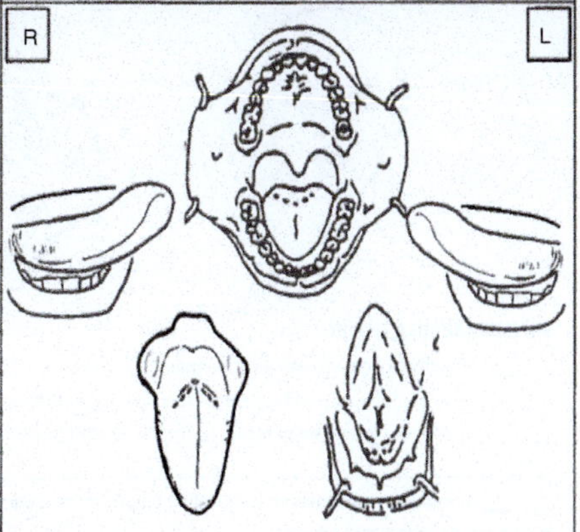

Location: Anatomical location and Symmetry
Unilateral, Bilateral, Symmetrical, Midline, Right, Left

# of lesions: Single Few Multiple, Generalize

Size: in millimeters

Color: White, Red, Red and White, Fluid Filled Vesicle, Blue, Black, Pigmented

Overall Configuration: Raised (nodular) Flat (macular)

Shape/margins: Round, Oval, Irregular Borders, Assymentrical, Stripes/papules Wicken Striae

Surface: Keratinized, Nonkeratinized, Smooth, Rough, Pebbly, Hyperplastic, Papillary/Verrucous, Ulcerated, Hyperkeratotic, Inflamed, Pseudoembranous, Scaly, Crusty, Oozing, Exudate, Bleeding, Dry

Attachment: Sessile/broad - Fixed Base Pedunculated-narrow stalk

Consistency: Hard Soft Erythematous, Petechiae
Indurated Non-indurated (esp if ulcerated)

Growth: Endophytic, Exophytic, Compressible Blanches Swelling

Length of time: not aware.
aware < 2 weeks aware 3 months, aware > 3 months
Has it happened before? Trauma Recurrent Medication
Has it changed?

Pain: On palpation? Unprovoked? yes no

Tongue: Ankyloglossia, Macroglossia, Hairy, Fissured, Scrotal, Geographic, Papilla missing

Fig. 1.30 (continued)

Head and Neck Screening Exam Finding Control #________________

First Name______________Last Name________________DOB____/____/____SCREENING EXAM: by______________________

______I participated in the oral cancer self examination

______I participated in the smoking cessation presentation

Please indicate location of abnormal finding or diagram(s) below.

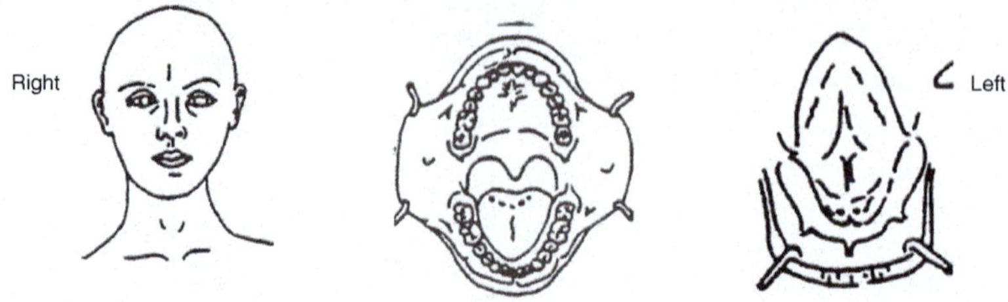

RECOMMENDATIONS:

______ Routine follow-up with your dentist.

______ Routine follow-up with primary care physician (medical doctor).

______ If problem identified persists, further head and neck evaluation id necessary with your dentist ❑ or medical doctor ❑

____

______ Immediate evaluation and possible biopsy (tissue sampling) for suspected tumor id strongly advised.

REFERRAL INFORMATION

______ Follow-up with: ________________________________ to set up an immediate appointment.

______ Appointment date and time in the ______________ Clinic on Date ____________ Time ____________

Signature of Person receiving the exam, ________________________________ Date_____/_____/_____

Fig. 1.31 This is a form that is completed and given to a patient with an unusual finding. The bottom half includes a provider that the patient needs to see for follow-up care or biopsy

References

American Cancer Society. ISSN register: http://www.cancer.org/cancer/oralcavityandoropharyngealcancer/detailedguide/oral-cavity-and-oropharyngeal-cancer-signs-symptoms. Accessed on 11 Mar 2016.

National Cancer Institute. ISSN register: http://www.cancer.gov/publications/dictionaries/cancer-terms?cdrid=306510. Accessed: 11 Mar 2016.

National Institute of Abuse and Alcoholism. ISSN register: http://pubs.niaaa.nih.gov/publications/aa65/AA65.htm. Accessed on 11 Mar 2016.

Oral Cancer Foundation. Cancer Screening Protocols. 2016. ISSN register: http://www.oralcancerfoundation.org/discovery-diagnosis/screening.php Accessed on 11 Mar 2016.

The Oral Cancer Foundation. ISSN register: http://www.oralcancerfoundation.org/hpv/. Accessed on 11 Mar 2016.

Dental Radiology

2

Rujuta Katkar

Contents

Abstract

This chapter focusses on the very basic concepts in dental radiology that a general dental practitioner should be aware of, including radiation safety and protection, current ADA imaging guidelines, radiographic exposure from common radiographic exams, normal radiographic anatomy, radiographic interpretation, radiographic features of common disease categories, and advanced imaging techniques.

2.1 Radiation Safety and Protection

- Check with local state board of dentistry for rules and regulations regarding use of radiation.
- Register all new x-ray equipment with the local state agency for radiation control.

R. Katkar, BDS, MDS, MS
University of Texas Health Science Center in San Antonio, San Antonio, TX, USA
e-mail: rujukatkar@gmail.com

G.M. Weinstein, M.T. Zientz (eds.), *The Dental Reference Manual*,
DOI 10.1007/978-3-319-39730-6_2

Table 2.1 Effective dose from radiographic examinations and equivalent background exposure (White and Pharoah 2014)

Examination	Effective dose (μSv)	Equivalent background exposure (days)
Intraoral		
Rectangular collimation		
Posterior bitewings: PSP or F- speed film	5	0.6
Full-mouth: PSP or F-speed film	35	4
Full-mouth: CCD sensor (estimated)	17	2
Round collimation		
Full-mouth: D-speed film	388	46
Full-mouth: PSP or F-speed film	171	20
Full-mouth: CCD sensor (estimated)	85	10
Extraoral		
Panoramic	9–24	1–3
Cephalometric	2–6	0.3–0.7
Cone-beam CT		
Large field of view	68–1073	8–126
Medium field of view	45–860	5–101
Small field of view	19–652	2–77
Multi-slice CT		
Head: conventional protocol	860–1500	101–177
Head: low-dose protocol	180–534	21–63
Abdomen	5300	624
Chest	5800	682
Plain films		
Skull	70	8
Chest	20	2
Barium enema	7200	847

CCD charge-coupled device, *PSP* photostimulable phosphor

- Do clinical examination and justify the need for each radiograph before ordering it. Refer to ADA/FDA selection criteria for prescribing radiographs (http://www.fda.gov/RadiationEmittingProducts/RadiationEmittingProductsandProcedures/MedicalImaging/MedicalX-Rays/ucm116503.htm).
- Follow 'ALARA' principle (As Low As Reasonably Achievable) for optimizing radiation dose based on specific diagnostic tasks.
- Use fastest speed films (F-speed)/photostimulable phosphor (PSP) plates/digital receptors.
- Rectangular collimation reduces patient dose by five times compared to round collimation.
- Use protective aprons and thyroid collars when appropriate.
- Develop a radiographic quality assurance program and document the steps taken to follow it. For digital radiography, periodically check the sensors for any physical damage, resolution, contrast, and density by comparing to good reference radiographs. Calibrate monitors periodically.
- See table 2.1 for effective radiation dose from common radiographic procedures and equivalent background radiation.

2.2 **Normal Radiographic Anatomy** (Fig. 2.1)

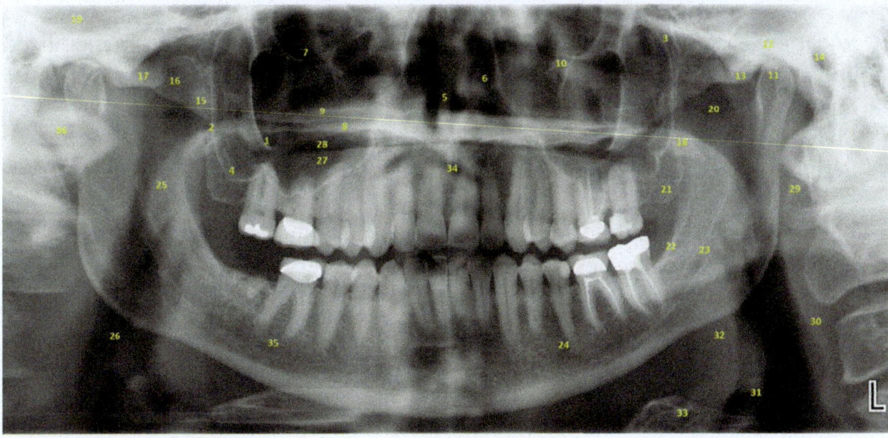

Fig. 2.1 Panoramic radiograph showing normal anatomical structures. Use the numbers in the radiograph to correspond to the key
Key: *1* zygomatic process of the maxilla, *2* posterior wall of the maxillary sinus, *3* pterygomaxillary fissure, *4* floor of the maxillary sinus, *5* nasal septum, *6* inferior nasal concha, *7* inferior orbital rim, *8* hard palate, *9* ghost image of opposite hard palate, *10* infraorbital canal, *11* mandibular condyle, *12* glenoid fossa, *13* articular eminence, *14* external auditory meatus, *15* coronoid process of the mandible, *16* zygomatico-temporal suture, *17* zygomatic arch, *18* pterygoid plate, *19* middle cranial fossa, *20* sigmoid notch, *21* maxillary tuberosity, *22* external oblique ridge, *23* mandibular canal, *24* mental foramen, *25* soft palate, *26* pharyngeal airway, *27* dorsal surface of tongue, *28* palatoglossal airway, *29* styloid process, *30* posterior pharyngeal wall, *31* epiglottis, *32* base of tongue, *33* hyoid bone, *34* intervertebral disk space between C1 and C2, *35* submandibular salivary gland fossa, *36* anterior arch of C1

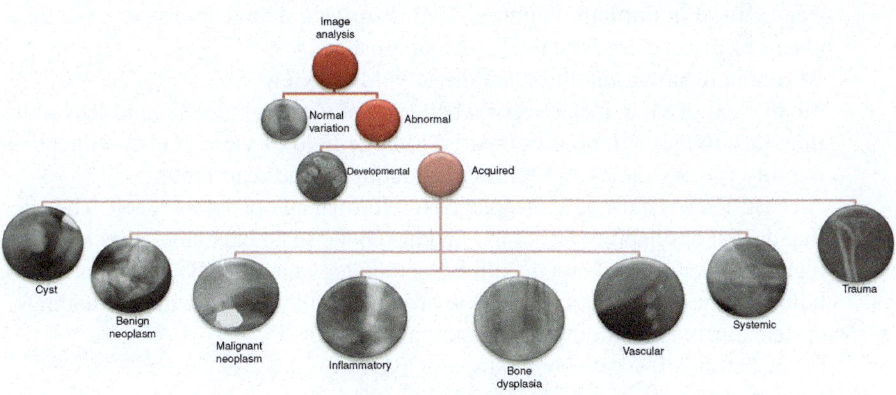

Fig 2.2 Radiographic image analysis algorithm representing the diagnostic process

2.3 Radiographic Interpretation (Fig. 2.2)

Considerations when a lesion is noted on a radiograph:

- Location: in relation to teeth, inferior alveolar canal; localized vs. generalized, unilateral vs. bilateral, single vs. multifocal
- Shape: regular vs. irregular, hydraulic
- Size: extension
- Periphery: well-defined, moderately well-defined or poorly defined
  - Corticated vs. noncorticated
- Internal structure: radiolucent, mixed, radiopaque, unilocular vs. multilocular
- See table 2.2 for characteristic radiographic features of common disease categories effect on surrounding structures: root resorption/displacement, cortical bone expansion/resorption, inferior alveolar nerve (IAN) canal, maxillary sinus floor

Radiographs showing a variety of radiolucent, mixed and radiopaque lesions. (Figs. 2.3, 2.4, 2.5, 2.6, 2.7, 2.8, 2.9, 2.10, 2.11, 2.12, 2.13, 2.14, 2.15, 2.16, 2.17, 2.18, 2.19, 2.20, 2.21, 2.22, 2.23, 2.24, 2.25, 2.26, 2.27, and 2.28)

For more examples, refer to chapter "Oral Pathology" on section "Radiopaque and Radiolucent Lesions."

2.4 Advanced Imaging

When three-dimensional information is necessary to provide direct benefit in patient's diagnosis and treatment, advanced imaging procedures may be used. This should be considered on a case by case basis. When a lesion is detected on conventional radiographs, an oral and maxillofacial radiologist may be consulted to seek advice on further investigations and management of the lesion.

- Cone-beam computed tomography (CBCT)
  - Can be used in implant planning, TMJ disorders, dental anomalies, fractures, extent of disease, and craniofacial relationships.
  - Available in small, medium, and large fields of view.
  - Small field of view usually gives better resolution, less noise, and less radiation dose to the patient as compared to large field of view. It also reduces the liability for any incidental findings by reducing the scan volume.
  - All CBCT scans must be accompanied by a formal interpretation report. The referring dentist has liability for all the findings in the scan, including areas not in the region of interest. Oral and maxillofacial radiology interpretation services may be utilized if the dentist does not want to take the liability for radiographic findings.
- Multidetector/medical computed tomography (MDCT)
  - Gives better soft tissue contrast than CBCT.
  - Radiation dose is usually higher than CBCT.
  - Used when both soft tissue and bone details are needed, e.g., extent of craniofacial disease, malignancies, aggressive benign lesions, and fractures.

Table 2.2 Radiographic features of lesions by categories

	Location	Shape	Periphery	Internal structure	Effect on adjacent roots	Effects on adjacent bone
Cysts	Odontogenic: teeth-bearing areas. Dentigerous: around crown. Radicular: periapical or lateral. Lateral periodontal: lateral to root Non-odontogenic: fissural, e.g., nasopalatine canal cyst	Regular, round/ hydraulic	Well-defined, corticated (May lose cortication or cause sclerotic borders if infected)	Radiolucent	Displacement Can cause resorption if long standing	Expansion
Benign neoplasms	Odontogenic: superior to the IAN Non-odontogenic: inferior to the IAN	Regular +/− irregular; scalloped	Well-defined, corticated, or noncorticated; may show soft tissue capsule	Unilocular or multilocular Completely radiolucent/radiopaque/ mixed; may show internal septations or calcifications	Horizontal/directional root resorption and/or displacement	Expansion: can perforate if aggressive or long standing
Malignant neoplasms	Specific to tissue of origin Could be generalized/ multifocal in hematogenic malignancies/ metastasis	Irregular; Regular in multiple myeloma (MM)	Poorly defined, invasive, ragged Punched out in MM No peripheral sclerosis unless secondarily infected	Completely radiolucent/ radiopaque/mixed	May cause vertical root resorption, irregular widening of PDL space, coronal displacement of developing teeth in leukemia, lymphoma, Langerhans' cell histiocytosis	Destruction/perforation; can cause speculated/ sunray-type periosteal reaction

(continued)

Table 2.2 (continued)

	Location	Shape	Periphery	Internal structure	Effect on adjacent roots	Effects on adjacent bone
Inflammatory lesions	Periapical or lateral to the root; involves basal bone in osteomyelitis	Irregular	Poorly defined with a zone of peripheral reactive sclerosis	Radiolucent Radiopaque in sclerosing osteitis and sclerosing osteomyelitis	Loss of lamina dura; may cause resorption if chronic	May perforate cortex, sinus tract, periosteal reaction in chronic cases
Vascular lesions	More common in mandible	Regular or irregular	Well-defined or poorly defined	Radiolucent or mixed	Root resorption, displacement, advanced development/eruption on the affected side	May enhance bone development on affected side, course trabecular pattern; may cause sunray periosteal reaction, irregular widening (serpiginous) of IAN
Endocrine/ metabolic disorders	Multifocal/generalized: maybe syndromic			May cause generalized increased or decreased bone density, altered trabecular pattern	May cause generalized widening of PDL space (systemic sclerosis), generalized loss of lamina dura (hyperparathyroidism)	May cause increased or decreased rate of bone development in endocrine disorders

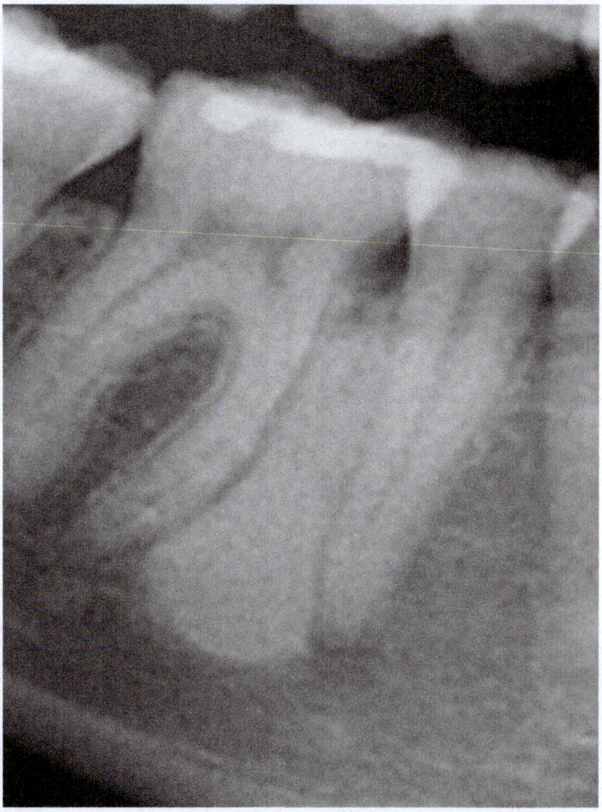

Fig 2.3 Idiopathic osteosclerosis. Note radiopaque area between the roots of #29 and 30

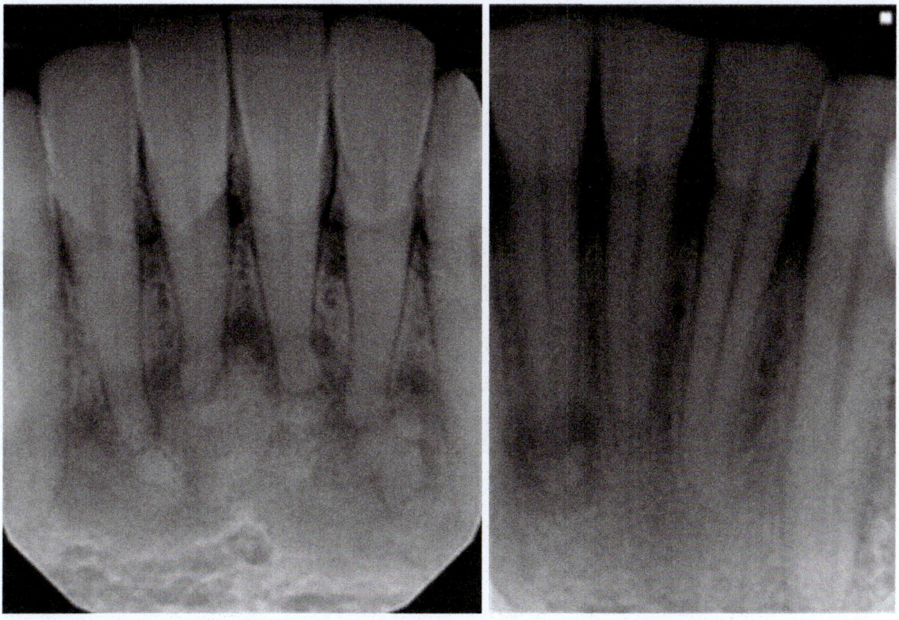

Fig 2.4 Periapical cemento-osseous dysplasia. Note mixed density lesions associated with the roots of mandibular incisors

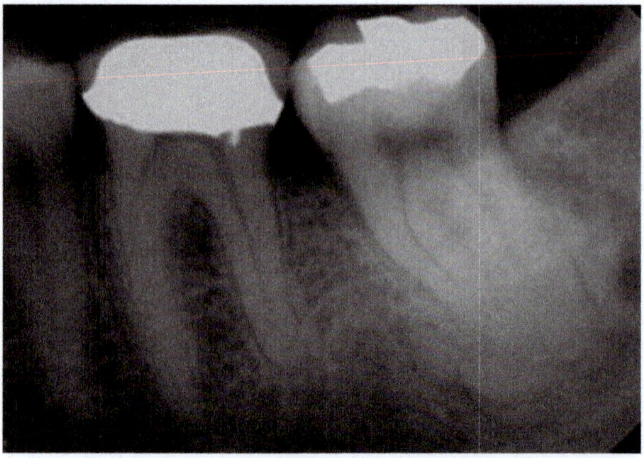

Fig 2.5 Cementoblastoma associated with #18. Note radiopaque lesion continuous with the roots and surrounded by radiolucent rim

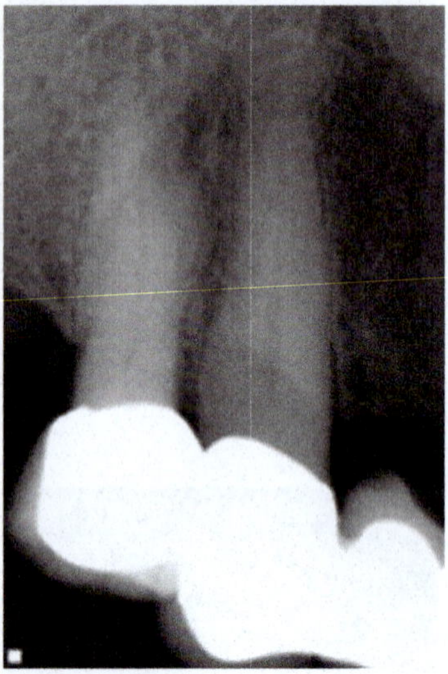

Fig. 2.6 Hypercementosis with #5 and 6

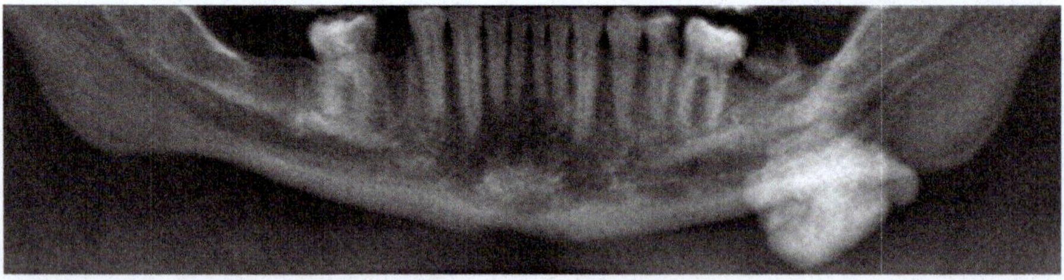

Fig. 2.7 Osteoma arising from left body of the mandible

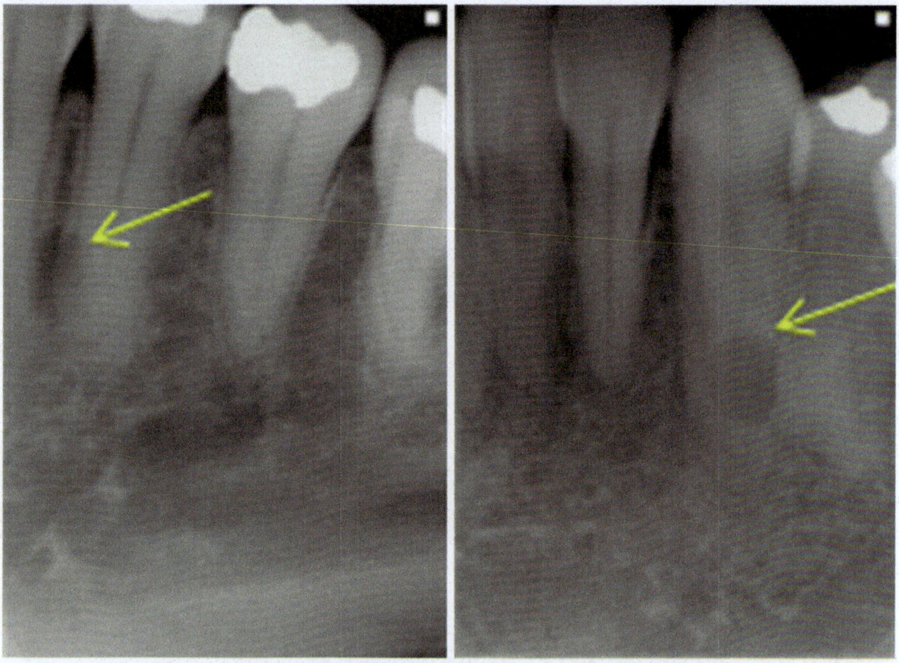

Fig. 2.8 Lateral periodontal cyst. *Arrows* denoting a well-defined corticated radiolucent lesion between the roots of mandibular canine and first premolar

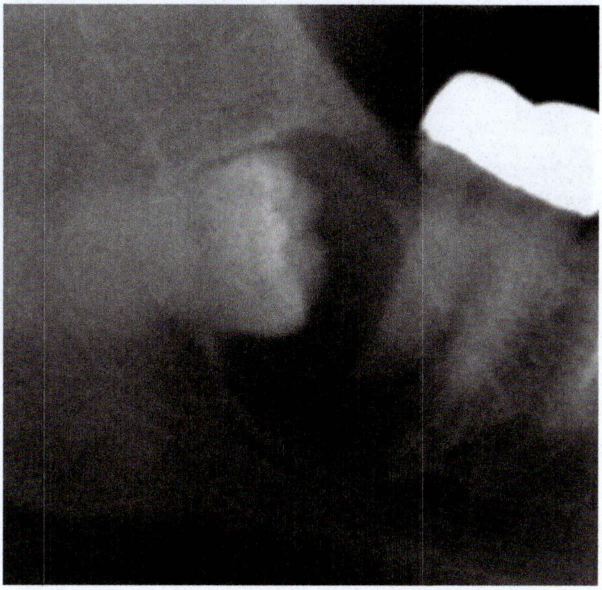

Fig. 2.9 Dentigerous cyst associated with impacted #32. Note pericoronal radiolucent area displacing the inferior alveolar canal

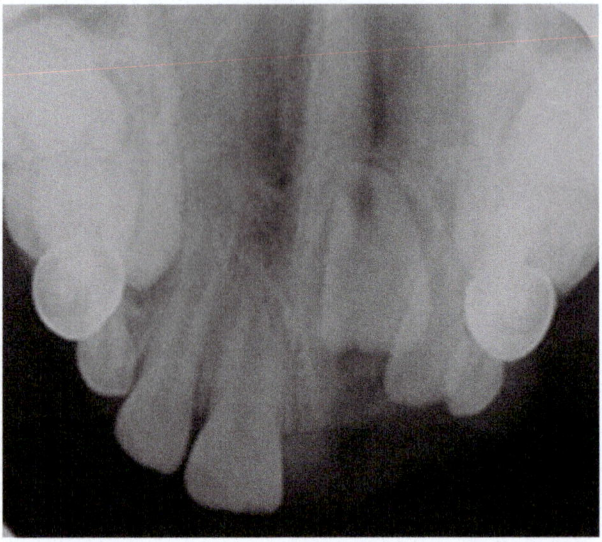

Fig. 2.10 Ameloblastic fibro-odontoma with impacted #9

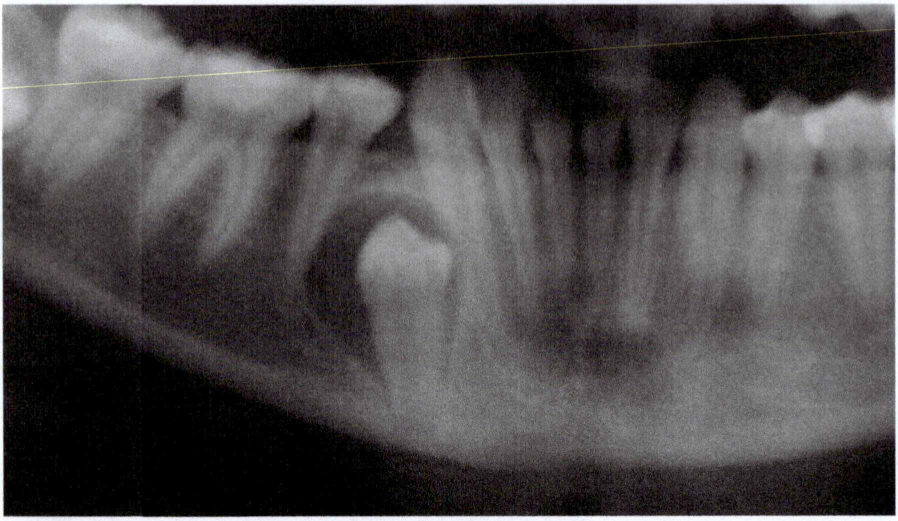

Fig. 2.11 Adenomatoid odontogenic tumor with impacted #27

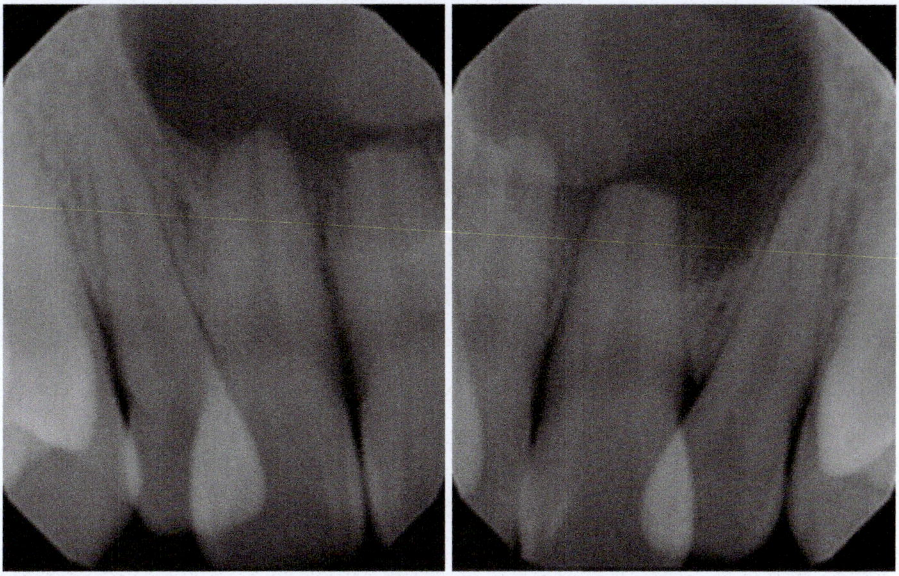

Fig. 2.12 Radicular cyst with #8 and 9 with evidence of root resorption

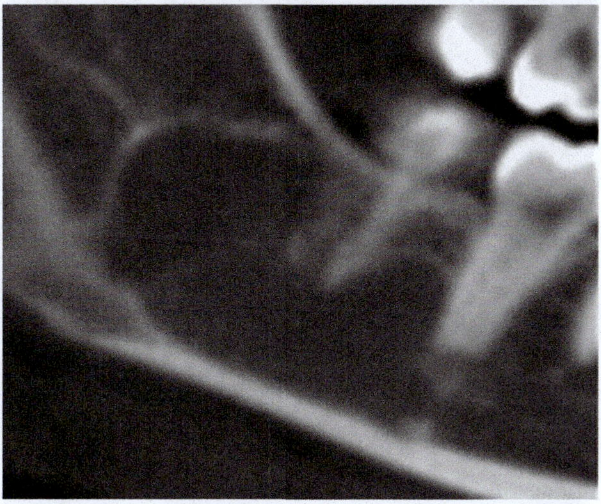

Fig. 2.13 Simple bone cyst in right mandibular molar region. Note scalloping between the molar roots

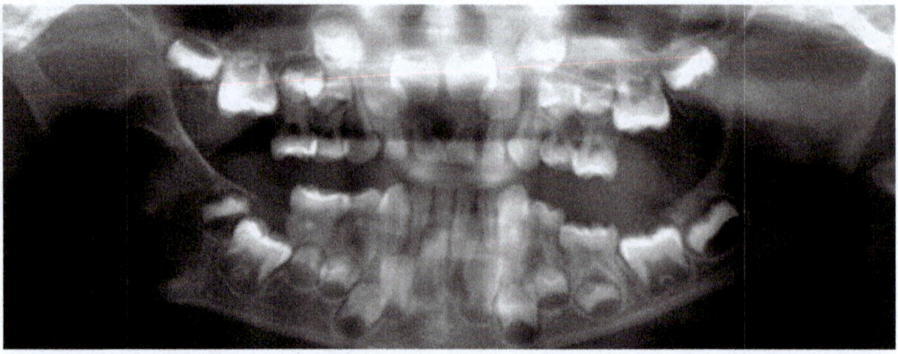

Fig. 2.14 Neurofibroma right posterior mandible. Note expansile radiolucent lesion causing displacement of unerupted tooth buds

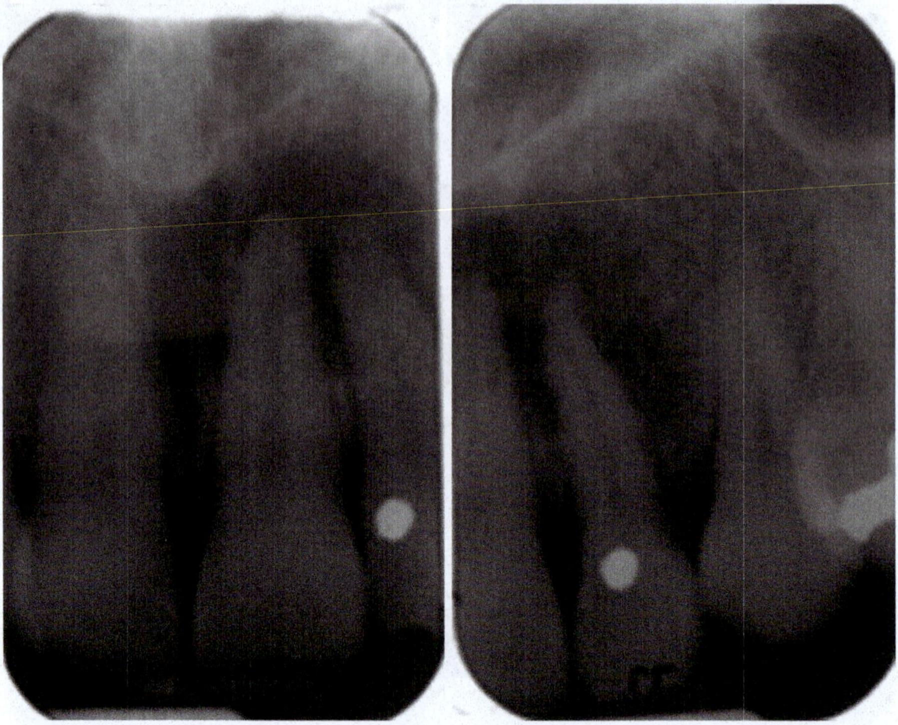

Fig. 2.15 Langerhans cell histiocytosis. Note ill-defined radiolucent lesion surrounding the roots of #s 7–8

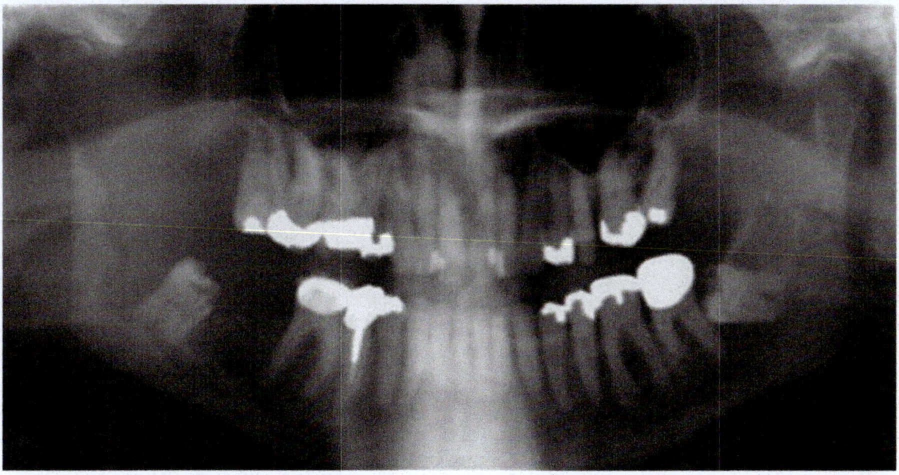

Fig. 2.16 Squamous cell carcinoma right mandible. Note extensive irregular bone destruction with pathological fracture of right condylar neck

- Magnetic resonance imaging (MRI)
  - Best for soft tissue detail.
  - Used to determine soft tissue extent of lesions, malignant involvement of lymph nodes, perineural spread of malignant neoplasms, salivary gland lesions, articular disk derangement in TMJ, articular disk, and surrounding soft tissue disorders in TMJ.
- Ultrasonography
  - Can be used for evaluation of neoplasms in thyroid, parathyroid, salivary glands, lymph nodes, sialoliths, and atherosclerotic plaques in carotid arteries.
- Nuclear medicine
  - Used to assess physiological change such as functions of the brain, thyroid, heart, and lungs and for diagnosis and follow-up of metastatic disease, bone tumors, and infection.
  - Involves use of radionuclides with gamma camera or advanced imaging such as SPECT, PET, PET/CT, and PET/MRI.

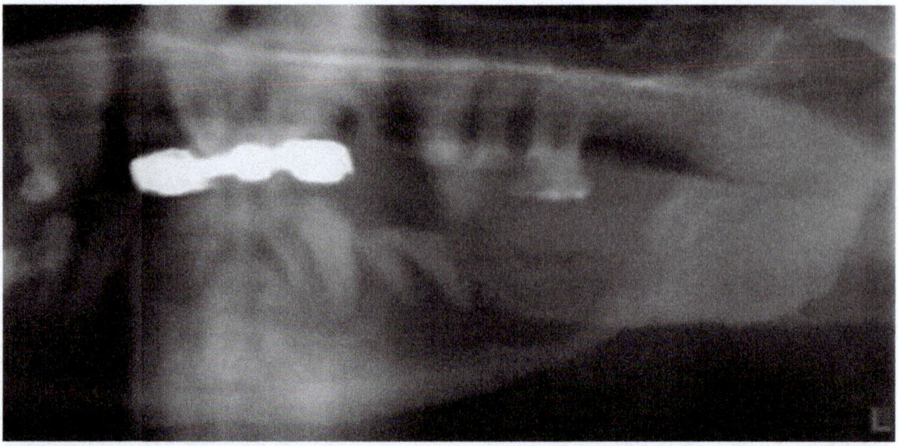

Fig. 2.17 Squamous cell carcinoma left mandible. Note irregular ill-defined bone destruction with floating teeth appearance

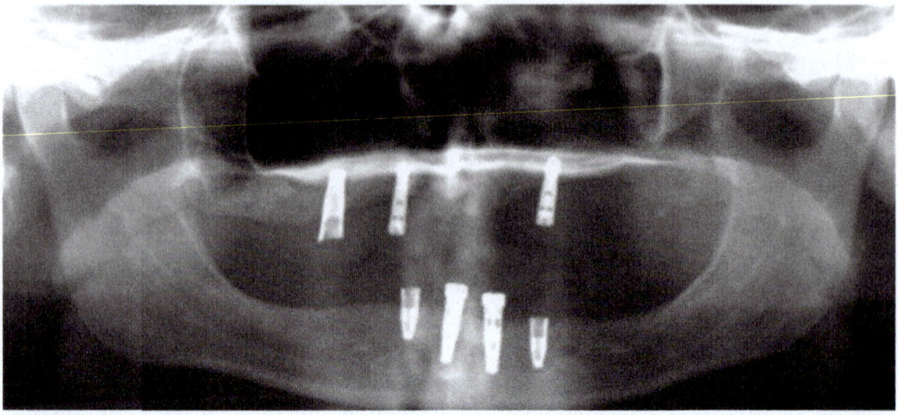

Fig. 2.18 Squamous cell carcinoma left maxilla. Note loss of cortical borders of left maxilla and maxillary sinus

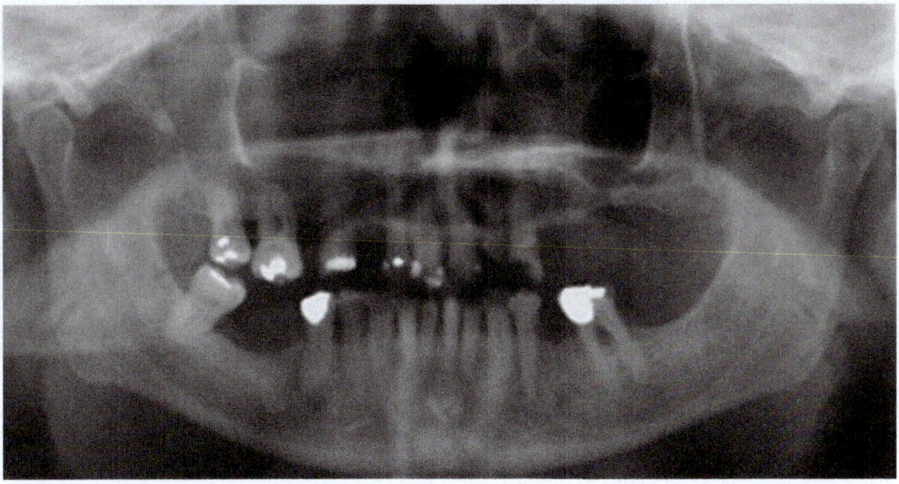

Fig. 2.19 Meningioma right maxillary sinus. Note destruction of the posterior wall of the sinus with soft tissue opacification in the sinus

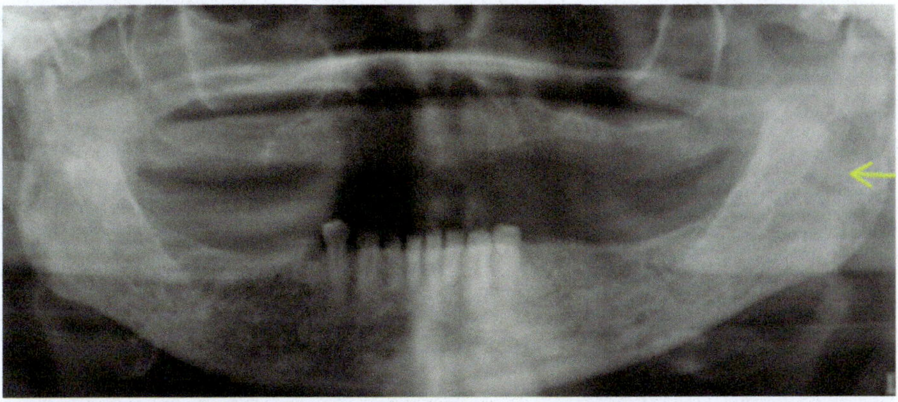

Fig. 2.20 Multiple myeloma. Generalized punched out radiolucent lesions in mandible. Note involvement of the left inferior alveolar canal (*arrow*)

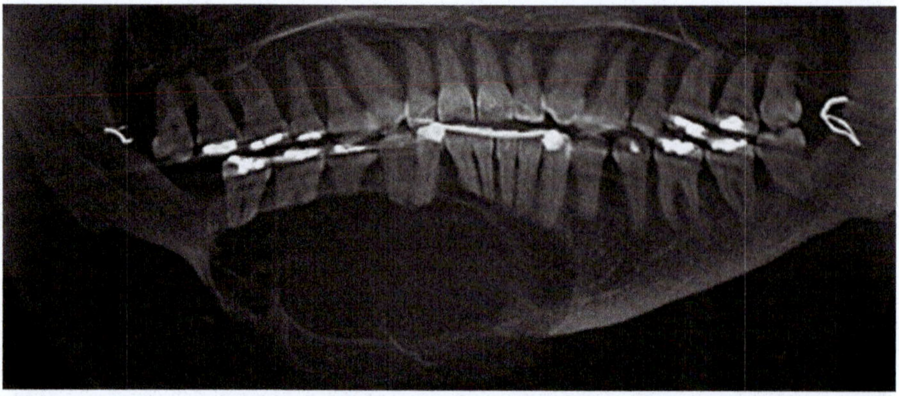

Fig. 2.21 Ossifying fibroma of mandible. Note expansile lesion with evidence of root resorption

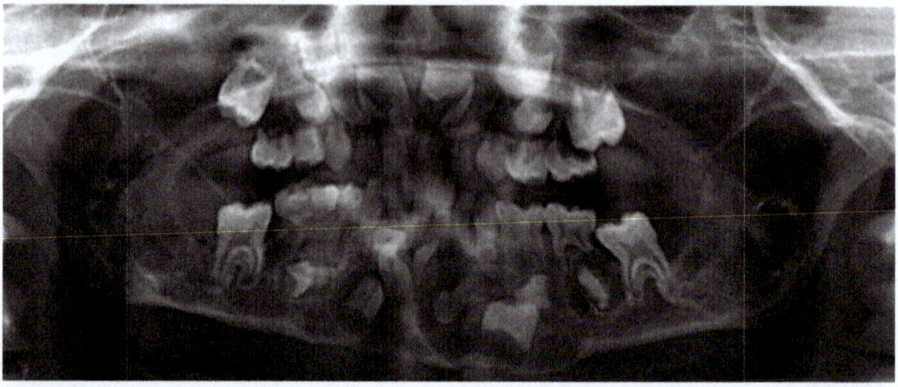

Fig. 2.22 Cherubism involving bilateral maxilla and mandible

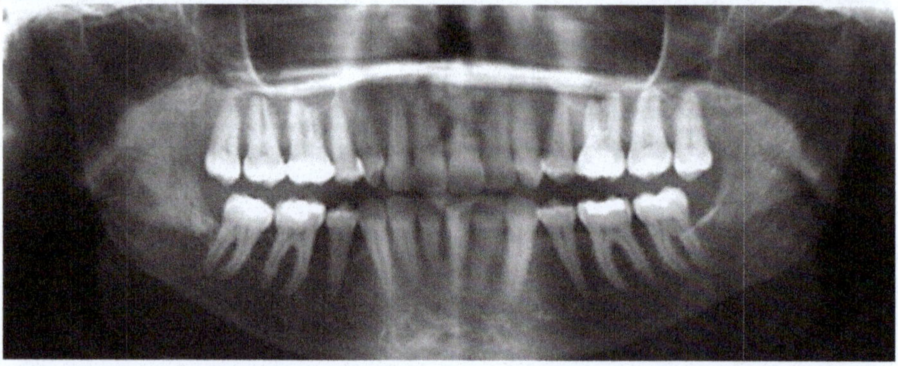

Fig. 2.23 Brown tumor of hyperparathyroidism. Note moderately defined radiolucent lesion in mandibular left premolar region

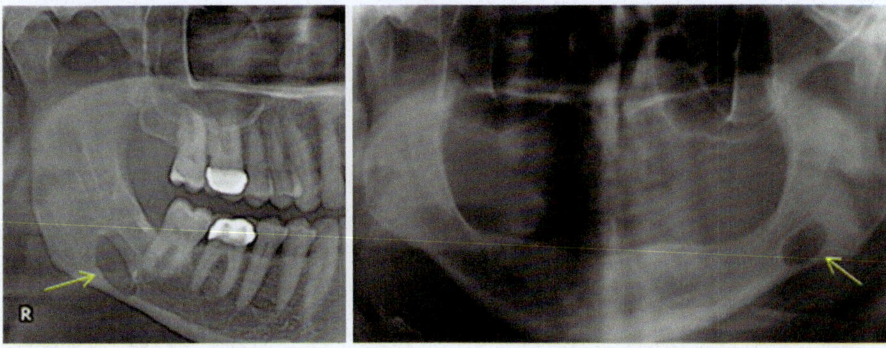

Fig. 2.24 Submandibular salivary gland inclusion defect (Stafne defect)

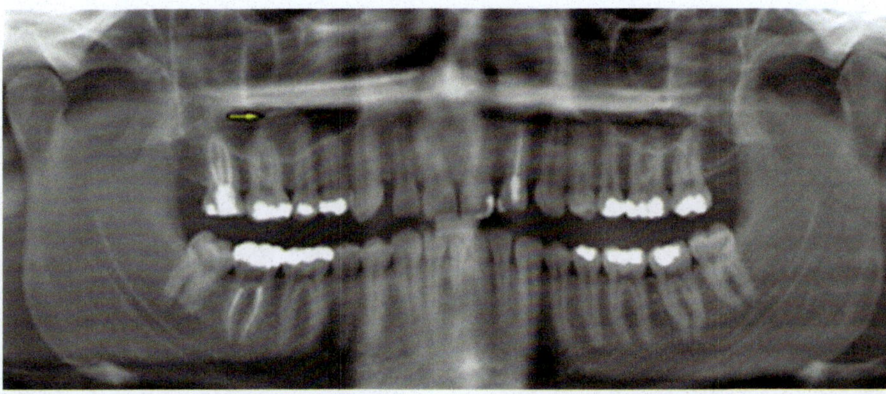

Fig. 2.25 Mucus retention phenomenon in right maxillary sinus

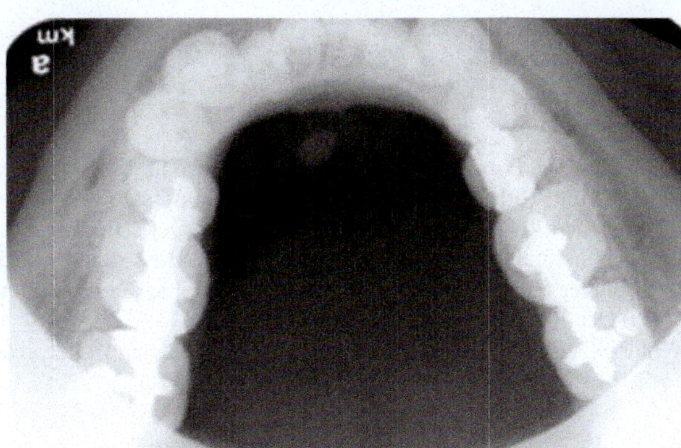

Fig. 2.26 Sublingual sialolith

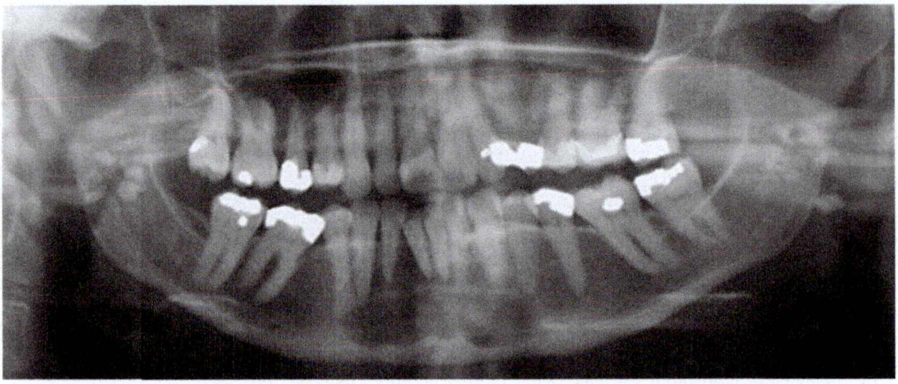

Fig. 2.27 Bilateral tonsilloliths superimposed over mandibular rami. Also note a well-defined corticated lesion in anterior mandible which was diagnosed as glandular odontogenic cyst

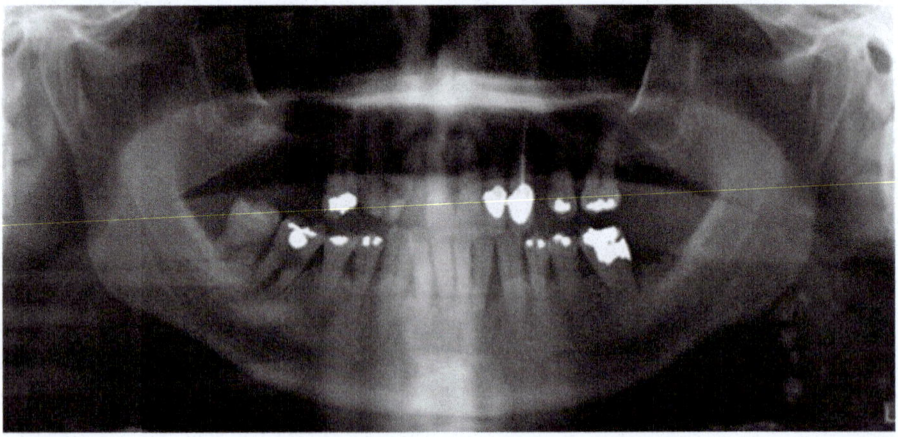

Fig. 2.28 Phleboliths in hemangioma. Note multiple circular radiopaque entities in the soft tissue inferior to the left mandibular angle, representing calcifications in soft tissue hemangioma

References

ISSN FDA US Food and Drug Administration. The ISSN register. http://www.fda.gov/Radiation-EmittingProducts/RadiationEmittingProductsandProcedures/MedicalImaging/MedicalX-Rays/ucm116503.htm (2015). Accessed 30 Oct 2015.

ISSN American Dental Association. The ISSN register. http://www.ada.org/~/media/ADA/Member%20Center/FIles/Dental_Radiographic_Examinations_2012.ashx (2012). Accessed 30 Oct 2015.

White SC, Pharoah M. Oral radiology: principles and interpretation. 7th ed. Mosby: St. Louis; 2014.

Caries Risk Assessment, Remineralizing, and Desensitizing Strategies in Preventive-Restorative Dentistry

3

Saulo Geraldeli and Alex J. Delgado

Contents

Abstract

In the spirit of primum non nocere, latin for first do no harm, it is our responsibility as dentists to correctly evaluate our patients and counsel them regarding their disease prior to treating them surgically. We must also critically evaluate dental materials for treating or arresting dental caries as these become available and efficacious in the years to come.

S. Geraldeli, DDS (✉) • A.J. Delgado, DMD, MS
Department of Restorative Dental Sciences, University of Florida, College of Dentistry, Gainesville, FL, USA
e-mail: sgeraldeli@dental.ufl.edu

G.M. Weinstein, M.T. Zientz (eds.), *The Dental Reference Manual*,
DOI 10.1007/978-3-319-39730-6_3

3.1 Caries Risk Assessment

Dental caries is defined as a localized dynamic disease with multifactorial etiology. In order for this disease to develop, four factors must occur:

1. Host: The patient's diet must consist of frequent ingestion of refined carbohydrates.
2. Bacteria: *Streptococcus mutans*. This specific bacteria must be present in the plaque.
3. Tooth: Resistance to the disease decreases and susceptibility to caries increases.
4. Time: Over a period of time.

Dental caries is caused by specific bacteria which produce acids that destroy the tooth enamel and dentin. There are many types of bacteria that live in the mouth. *Streptococcus mutans* plays an important role in the early stages of the caries process, whereas the bacteria *Lactobacillus* contributes to the progression of the disease. When refined carbohydrates are introduced into the oral cavity, lactic acid production occurs as an end product of *S. mutans* metabolic activity. This causes the saliva pH to drop from a neutral pH of approximately 7 to an acidic pH of 4.5–5.0. *S. mutans* lactic acid production begins to demineralize the enamel.

Caries lesions must be diagnosed in conjunction with tactile and radiographic assessment, but also as clinicians we have to determine the caries risk assessment (CRA), which by definition is to predict future caries activity or development before the clinical onset of the disease. Risk factors are the lifestyle and biochemical status that contribute to the development and progression of the disease.

An evidence-based approach to prevention and treatment of dental caries has been termed as caries management by risk assessment (CAMBRA) (Young and Featherstone 2013; Kutsch 2014). This system requires the understanding that dental caries is an infectious bacterial biofilm disease with a shift of the balance of the microflora due to a change in local environmental conditions. CAMBRA is the assessment of each patient for his/her unique individual disease indicators, risk factors, and protective factors to determine current risk. Identifying the risks allows for individualized, focused treatment strategy (Kutsch 2014). The American Dental Association created two forms that determine low, moderate, or high risk: one for patients 0–6 years old (Fig. 3.1a) and one for patients older than 6 years old (Fig. 3.1b). The CAMBRA philosophy identifies nine risk factors that are outcome measures of the risk for current or future caries disease, and each of these is supported with research. Dental clinicians are advised to use them regularly since insurance companies may request the caries risk assessment as part of the treatment plan. This is critical as the presence of recurrent/secondary caries is the major cause of replacement of existing restorations. Failure to control the disease process prior to surgical intervention and placement of dental restorative biomaterials can lead to recurrent disease (Mount 2005).

Clinical treatment recommendations after patients have been classified through use of CAMBRA forms have been developed and are as follows. These recommendations were adapted from those published by a number of authors (Jenson et al. 2007; Ramos-Gomez et al. 2010; American Academy of Pediatrics 2014). A comprehensive article that is available online can be found at http://www.rdhmag.com/

a **Caries Risk Assessment Form (Ages 0-6)**

Patient Name: **Score:**
Birth Date: **Date:**
Age: **Initials:**

		Low Risk (0)	Moderate Risk (1)	High Risk (10)	Patient Risk
	Contributing Conditions				
I.	**Fluoride Exposure** (through drinking water, supplements, professional applications, toothpaste)	Yes	No		
II.	**Sugary or Starchy Foods or Drinks** (including juice, carbonated or non-carbonated soft drinks, energy drinks, medicinal syrups)	Primarily at mealtimes	Frequent or prolonged between meal exposures/day	Bottle or sippy cup with anything other than water at bed time	
III.	**Eligible for Government Programs** (WIC, Head Start, Medicaid or SCHIP)	No		Yes	
IV.	**Caries Experience of Mother, Caregiver** and/or Other **Siblings**	No carious lesions in last 24 months	Carious lesions in last 7-23 months	Carious lesions in last 6 months	
V.	**Dental Home:** established patient of record in a dental office	Yes	No		
	General Health Conditions				
I.	**Special Health Care Needs***	No		Yes	
	Clinical Conditions				
I.	Visual or Radiographically Eviednt **Restorations/Cavitated Carious Lesions**	No carious lesions or restorations in last 24 months		Carious lesions or restorations in last 24 months	
II.	**Non-cavitated (incipient) Carious Lesions**	No new lesions in last 24 months		New lesions in last 24 months	
III.	**Teeth Missing Due to Caries**	No		Yes	
IV.	**Visible Plaque**	No	Yes		
V.	**Dental /Orthodontic Appliances** Present (fixed or removable)	No	Yes		
VI.	**Salivary Flow**	Visually adequate		Visually inadequate	
				TOTAL:	

Instructions for Caregiver:

*Patients with developmental, physical, medical or mental disabilities that prevent or limit performance of adequate oral health care by themeselves or caregivers.

ADA American Dental Association®

Fig. 3.1 (**a**) Table from the American Dental Association, this form and detailed instructions can be found athttp://www.ada.org/en/~/media/ADA/Member%20Center/FIles/topics_caries_instructions (Accessed on March 5, 2016) ("Copyright © 2009, 2011, American Dental Association. All rights reserved. Reprinted with permission") (**b**) Fig. 3.1a Table from the American Dental Association, this form and detailed instructions can be found at: http://www.ada.org/en/~/media/ADA/Member%20Center/FIles/topics_caries_instructions (Accessed on March 5, 2016) ("Copyright © 2009, 2011, American Dental Association. All rights reserved. Reprinted with permission")

b **Caries Risk Assessment Form (Ages >6)**

Patient Name: **Score:**
Birth Date: **Date:**
Age: **Initials:**

		Low Risk (0)	Moderate Risk (1)	High Risk (10)	Patient Risk
	Contributing Conditions				
I.	**Fluoride Exposure** (through drinking water, supplements, professional applications, toothpaste)	Yes	No		
II.	**Sugary or Starchy Foods or Drinks** (including juice, carbonated or non-carbonated soft drinks, energy drinks, medicinal syrups)	Primarily at mealtimes		Frequent or prolonged between meal exposures/day	
III.	**Caries Experience of Mother, Caregiver** and/or Other **Siblings** (for patients ages 6-14)	No carious lesions in last 24 months	Carious lesions in last 7-23 months	Carious lesions in last 6 months	
IV.	**Dental Home:** established patient of record, receving regular dental care in a dental office	Yes	No		
	General Health Conditions				
I.	**Special Health Care Needs***	No	Yes (over age 14)	Yes (ages6-14)	
II.	**Chemo/Radiation Therapy**	No		Yes	
III.	**Eating Disorders**	No	Yes		
IV.	**Smokeless Tobacco Use**	No	Yes		
V.	**Medications that Reduce Salivary Flow**	No	Yes		
VI.	**Drug/Alcohol Abuse**	No	Yes		
	Clinical Conditions				
I.	**Cavitated or Non-cavitated** (incipient) **Carious Lesions or Restorations** (visually or radiographically evident)	No new carious lesions or restorations in last 36 months	1 or 2 new carious lesions or restorations in last 36 months	3 or more carious lesions or restorations in last 36 months	
II.	**Teeth Missing Due to Caries in past 36 months**	No		Yes	
III.	**Visible Plaque**	No	Yes		
IV.	**Unusual Tooth Morphology** that compromises oral hygiene	No	Yes		
V.	**Interproximal Restorations - 1or more**	No	Yes		
VI.	**Exposed Root Surfaces** Present	No	Yes		
VII.	**Restorations with Overhangs** and/or **Open Margins: Open Contacts** with Food Impaction	No	Yes		
VIII.	**Dental/Orthodontic appliances** (fixed or removable)	No	Yes		
IX.	**Severe Dry Mouth (Xerostomia)**	No		Yes	
				TOTAL:	

Patient Instructions:

*Patients with developmental, physical, medical or mental disabilities that prevent or limit performance of adequate oral health care by themeselves or caregivers.

ADA American Dental Association®

Fig. 3.1 (continued)

etc/medialib/new-lib/rdh/site-images/volume-31/issue-10/1110RDH095-109.pdf (Accessed on March 6, 2016) (Table 3.1A, 3.1B, and 3.1C).

In the United States, there are a number of insurance companies that provide coverage for CAMBRA-related dental procedure codes (Table 3.2). This is not a complete list of possible procedures, but it is a start in encouraging patients in the importance of caries risk assessment and prevention.

Table 3.1A Clinical recommendations for low-risk patients

Low risk	Recall exam	Radiographs	Saliva testing	Fluoride	Xylitol	Antimi-crobials	Calcium phosphate
Age: under 6 years	Annual exam	Bitewings every 12–24 months	Optional	3–5 year old smear of toothpaste; twice daily[a]	No	No	
Age: 6+ years	Every 6–12 months	Bitewings every 24–36 months	Optional	Twice daily brush with fluoridated toothpaste	Optional	If required	Adults for root sensitivity

[a]Smear of toothpaste on the toothbrush was a recent recommendation of American Academy of Pediatric Dentistry (AAPD) (American Academy of Pediatrics 2014)

3.2 Current Therapeutics Available on the Market to Remineralize Active White Spot Lesions

What Are White Spot Lesions?
As an outcome of an ecological imbalance in the physiological equilibrium between tooth minerals and oral microbial biofilms (Fejerskov 2004; Scheie and Petersen 2004; Pitts-Fejerskov 2004; Scheie and Peterson 2004), *white spot lesions* (WSL) may be found when active caries develops on smooth surfaces of the tooth (Fig. 3.2). These lesions typically are the first manifestation of caries lesions. They are characterized as small areas of subsurface demineralization beneath the dental plaque, and present themselves as "milk white opacity" on smooth surfaces (Selwitz et al. 2007; Hilton et al. 2013). Whether dental caries progresses, stops, or reverses is dependent on the undergoing balance between demineralization and remineralization in the oral environment. Management to repair these demineralized enamel lesions can be done with several preventive approaches such as reduction of dietary sugar intake, oral hygiene education, and delivery of remineralizing/repair products.

Can Fluoride Remineralize Active White Spot Lesions (WSL)?
According to Kutsch (2014), prescriptive strategies can be organized into three categories: reparative nonsurgical strategies, therapeutic materials, and behavioral changes. Reparative nonsurgical strategies are well developed by the dental profession and include remineralization and restoration.

Patients at high risk for caries such as those undergoing orthodontic treatment have poor oral hygiene, and non-advised diet are in great risk of developing enamel white spot lesions. If not well cleaned, fixed orthodontic appliances facilitate increase in volume and therefore have reduction in biofilm ph. Development of WSL during fixed appliance therapy can occur rapidly and becomes clinically visible in 4 weeks or even less (Oreilly and Featherstone 1987; Ogaard et al. 1988). Recent studies indicate a prevalence of almost 70 % of WSL in those patients (Benkaddour et al. 2014; Julien et al. 2013; Hadler-Olsen et al. 2012). Fluoride varnish, resin infiltrants, and silver diamine fluoride are a few ways that have promise in remineralizing teeth.

Table 3.1B Clinical recommendations for moderate-risk patients

Moderate risk	Recall exam	Radiographs	Saliva testing	Fluoride	Xylitol	Antimicrobials	Calcium phosphate
[a]Age: under 6 years	Every 3–6 months	BW every 6–12 months	Recommended at baseline and recall	Brushing twice daily with F toothpaste Supervised daily use of over-the-counter fluoride rinse In office fluoride varnish at initial visit and recall	Xylitol wipes can be used especially when unable to brush	None	AAPD states: consider fluoride levels in the drinking water prior to prescribing
Age: 6+ years	Every 4–6 months	BW every 18–24 months	Recommended at baseline and recall	Brushing twice daily with F toothpaste and fluoride rinse In office F varnish application 1–3 times initially then at recall appts.	6–10 g/day = 2 sticks of xylitol gum	Chlorhexidine if required	Adults for root sensitivity

[a]For children who are at moderate through extreme risk for caries, there are recommendations for their caregivers as well. This is to prevent transmission of bacteria from caregiver to child. For the caregiver, it is recommended to use over-the-counter fluoride rinse daily, xylitol gum (2 sticks = 6–10 g xylitol), and possibly chlorhexidine if the child is under the age of 6 (Jenson et al. 2007). In addition, diet counseling to reduce cariogenic food is a highly recommended intervention that the dentist can do while the caregiver and child are in the office. The comprehensive review of recommendations for pediatric patients can be found on http://www.aapd.org/media/policies_guidelines/g_cariesriskassessment.pdf (Accessed on March 6, 2016)

Table 3.1C Clinical recommendations for high- and extreme-risk patients

High risk and extreme risk	Recall exam	Radiographs	Saliva testing	Fluoride	Xylitol	Antimicrobials	Calcium phosphate
Age: under 6 years	Every 1–3 months	Every 6–12 months	At baseline and recall exams	Brushing twice daily with F toothpaste Supervised daily use of over-the-counter fluoride rinse In office fluoride varnish at initial visit and recall	Xylitol wipes can be used especially when unable to brush	Recommended use of chlorhexidine for the *caregiver* to prevent transmission of bacteria	*AAPD states*: consider fluoride levels in the drinking water prior to prescribing
Age: 6+ years	Every 3–4 months	Every 6–12 months	At baseline and recall exams	Brushing twice daily with F toothpaste and fluoride rinse In office F varnish application 1–3 times initially then at recall appts	6–10 g/day = 2 sticks of xylitol gum	0.12% chlorhexidine gluconate 10 ml rinse for 1 min/day for one week each month	If required

Table 3.2 An example of ADA codes that are covered by insurance companies when performing caries risk assessment of a patient

ADA code number	Description
D0425	Caries susceptibility testing (CariScreen)
D1206	Therapeutic applications of fluoride varnish for moderate- or high-caries-risk patients
D1310	Nutritional counseling for the control of dental disease
D9630	Other drugs, medicaments, or fluoride dispensed by the office for at-home use

For more information visit (http://carifree.com/dentist/learn/resource-guide/dental-insurance.html) (Accessed on March 5, 2016)

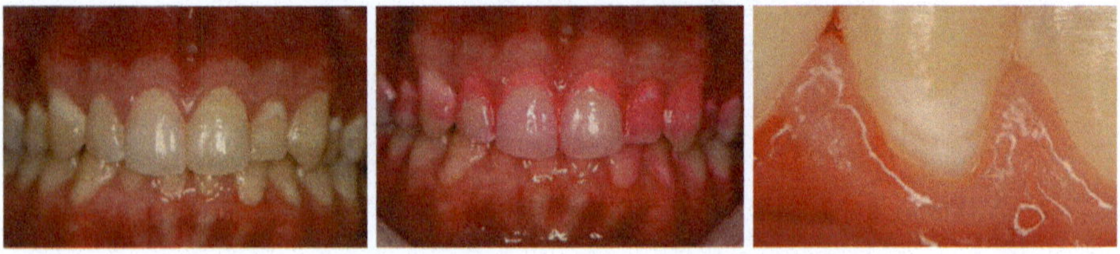

Fig. 3.2 Digital images of a patient undergoing a unbalanced diet and poor tooth brushing technique. Upon application of the disclosing agent, the dental biofilm became evident. The patient was given oral hygiene instruction followed by biofilm removal with mid-grit prophylaxis paste, the white spot became visible then facilitating its diagnosis

3.2.1 Fluoride Varnish

Although clinical studies on WSL have been performed mostly on children, current scientific evidence points for effective remineralization/repair when fluoride is used, and the best form is fluoride varnish (Lenzi et al. 2016; Gibson et al. 2011). In high-caries-risk patients, recommendation is an application of fluoride varnish every 3–4 months (Newbrun 2001; Garcia et al. 2015). Below is a sequence that might be considered for clinical application of fluoride varnish. A number of fluoride varnish materials available in the market are UltraThin (WaterPik), Duraphat (Colgate), Vanish™ 5 % Sodium Fluoride White Varnish with Tri-Calcium Phosphate (3 M-ESPE), Duraflor Fluoride Varnish Tube (Medicom), PreviDent® 5 % Sodium Fluoride Varnish (Colgate).

Procedure for Application of Fluoride Varnish:

1. Use gauze or light air to remove excess moisture from a quadrant at a time.
2. Dispense fluoride varnish in a well or pad.
3. Use a Benda Brush or microbrush applicator to apply the material to all surfaces of the tooth (Fig. 3.3).
4. Give clear, if possible written, instructions to the patient:
   (a) Avoid hard and hot foods or alcohol-containing items such as mouthwashes for 4 h.
   (b) Do not brush or use other oral hygiene devices, if possible, for the remainder of *the day*.

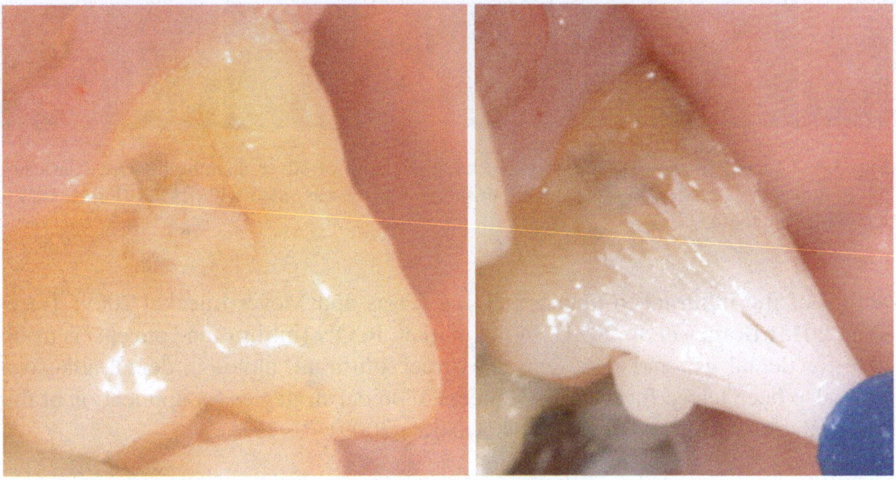

Fig. 3.3 Application of fluoride varnish over white spot lesion

3.2.2 NovaMin

NovaMin is a particulate bioactive glass used for dental application developed in the 1960s. When in contact with saliva, it releases ions such as sodium that reduces pH and favors precipitation of a layer of calcium phosphate ions. These chemical reactions along with continuous depositions eventually crystallize into hydroxycarbonate apatite. Based on this rationale, it was thought then that it will be helpful if incorporated into toothpaste for preventive purposes (Du et al. 2008; Zhu et al. 2015). A recent prospective randomized clinical trial evaluated a prescription-strength dentifrice containing NovaMin (ReNew™), and an over-the-counter commercial fluoride in treating WSL. The findings were that there were no differences in the outcome for change in the WSL appearance in orthodontic-treated patients (Hoffman et al. 2015).

3.2.3 Resin Infiltrants

Resin infiltrants are optimized low-viscosity light-curing resins developed to quickly infiltrate the microporosities present in the lesion's body of demineralized enamel or WSL. Overall this approach poses advantages such as mechanical stabilization of the demineralized enamel, permanent occlusion of superficial micropores and cavities, minimizes risk of secondary caries, no risk of postoperative sensitivity and pulpal inflammation, etc. (Kielbassa et al. 2009). In addition, its potential for changing the aesthetic appearance of white spot lesion is appealing. A few in vitro and in vivo studies had been performed using such approach (Meyer-Lueckel and Paris 2010; Kantovitz et al. 2010; Paris and Meyer-Lueckel 2009). The overall observation is that this approach seems to help change the aesthetic appearance of WSL, but more studies are required, especially regarding the long-term

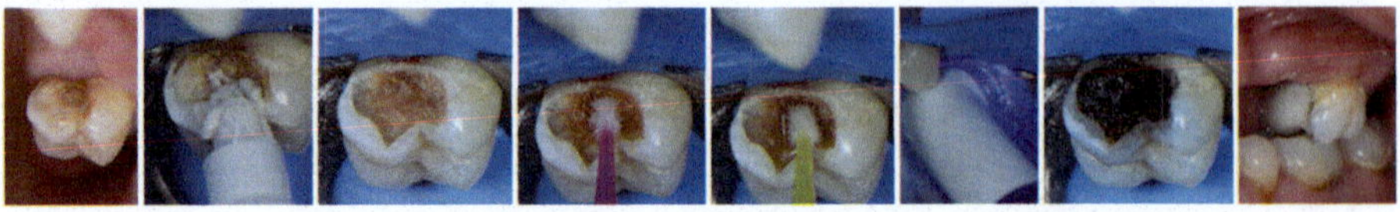

Fig. 3.4 Clinical sequence demonstrating the application of silver diamine fluoride (Cariestop 12 %) in active caries lesion of a vital upper molar. Cavity was filled with RMGI (Fuji II LC) to temporize the tooth

ability of the infiltrant to uptake staining (Paris and Meyer-Lueckel 2009; Torres et al. 2011; Borges et al. 2014). In the market, ICON (infiltration concept) is available for dental use and represents the "true" infiltrant, although dental adhesives have also been tested for the same concept. Clinical strategies for application of this material are as follows (ISSN DMG-America 2009):

Procedure for Application of ICON:

1. Clean the affected and adjacent tooth from biofilm with rubber cup and pumice.
2. Isolate tooth/teeth with rubber dam not made with thermoplastic rubber dam. Make sure the rubber dam is tightly adapted to the cervical area of the tooth. This prevents diffusion of the hydrochloric gel to the gingiva.
3. Apply an ample amount of the etchant (15 % hydrochloric acid) over the lesion site and let it sit for 2 min.
   (a) Unless white spot lesions are being treated shortly (1–2 months) after bracket removal, it is recommended that the etchant be applied twice.
   (b) If a white spot is still visible after rinsing/drying the hydrochloric acid, another etching is recommended.
   (c) For isolated white spot lesions, etching should extend up to 2 mm beyond the lesion.
   (d) For extensive white spot lesions, and at the discretion of the practitioner, the entire smooth surface should be etched.
4. Rinse the etchant for at least 30 s and then dry with oil-free and water-free air.
5. Etched surface should be "dehydrated" by application of 99 % ethanol for 30 s then evaporated through application of dry oil-free and water-free air.
   (a) When wetted with ethanol, the whitish opaque appearance of the etched enamel should diminish. If that is not the case, reapply the etchant for 2 min and rinse and dry, followed by application of the ethanol solution as in step 5.
6. Deliver an ample amount of the resin infiltrant on the etched surface and let it sit for 3 min. Excess of the material can be removed with microbrushes.
   (a) Since the infiltrant is set under light exposition, turn off the operating light.
7. Placing the tip of the light-curing unit as close as possible to the infiltrant, light cure the material for 40 s using a light-curing unit of at least 800 mW/cm (Kutsch 2014).
8. Remove rubber dam.
9. Use polishing cups for removal of material excess and final polishing.

3.2.4 Silver Diamine Fluoride

Silver diamine fluoride (SDF) has also great potential for remineralizing white spot lesions; however, it remains to be validated clinically. Currently there have been no randomized clinical trials testing its effectiveness in such lesions (Gao et al. 2016). Below is a sequence that might be useful for clinical application of SDF (Horst et al. 2016) that has been adapted to arrest caries. Biannual application of SDF along with fluoride varnish has been shown to be effective in arresting early childhood caries when conventional treatment is not available (Chu et al. 2015). Although not all types of carious lesions have been arrested by application of SDF, further studies are required (Featherstone and Horst 2015). Clinically, it could be a useful way to arrest caries that is approaching the pulp in order to prevent pulpal exposure and ultimately endodontic treatment. Patients who are to receive SDF must be aware of the staining risks; consent must be obtained prior to application.

The use of potassium iodide (SSKI) immediately after application of SDF is believed to reduce staining. However, studies are still ongoing as to the efficacy of this. SSKI is off-label in the United States at this time, and its use is contraindicated in pregnant women (Horst et al. 2016).

3.2.4.1 Procedure for Application of Silver Diamine Fluoride (Fig. 3.4):

1. Plastic-lined cover for counter, plastic-lined bib for patient.
2. Standard personal protective equipment (PPE) for provider and patient.
3. One drop of SDF into the deep end of a plastic dappen dish (also obtain one drop of SSKI in a separate dappen dish if selected).
4. Remove saliva with saliva ejector.
5. Isolate tongue and cheek from affected teeth with 2-inch by 2-inch gauze or cotton rolls.
6. If near the gingiva, consider applying petroleum jelly with a cotton applicator for safety.
7. Dry affected tooth surfaces with triple syringe or if not feasible dry with cotton.
8. Bend microsponge, immerse into SDF, and remove excess on side of dappen dish.
9. Apply directly onto the affected tooth surface(s) with microsponge.
10. Allow SDF to absorb for up to 1 min if reasonable then remove excess with gauze or cotton roll. (If using potassium iodide (SSKI), apply with a different microsponge. Repeat one to three times until no further white precipitates are observed. Wait 5–10 s between applications. Remove excess with cotton.)
11. Rinse with water.
12. Follow up with patient in a few weeks.

3.3 Desensitizing Agents

Dentin hypersensitivity may be defined as brief, sharp pain arising from exposed dentin. It occurs typically in response to chemical, thermal, evaporative, or osmotic stimuli and cannot be explained as arising from other dental defects or pathology. The hydrodynamic theory has been accepted as the theory as an explanation of the symptoms. The primary culprit is the loss of enamel, dentin exposed with subsequent loss of cement, or gum recession.

Dentin contains many dentinal tubular structures that radiate outward from the pulp. These tubules are typically between 0.5 and 2 microns in diameter and contain plasma-like biological fluid that is connected to the pulp. Each tubule contains a cytoplasmic cell process called Tomes fiber and an odontoblast that communicates with the pulp. Within the dentinal tubules, there are two types of nerve fibers, myelinated (A-fibers) and unmyelinated (C-fibers). The A-fibers are responsible for dentin hypersensitivity, perceived as pain in response to all stimuli.

3.3.1 Management of Dentin Hypersensitivity with Desensitizers

- Ask patient to describe pain (look for sharp pain, intensity, duration).
- Ask patient to identify the pain trigger (look for thermal, tactile, chemical, osmotic).
- Ask patient for diet habits (acids).
- Ask patient for oral hygiene habits (brushing technique, type of toothbrush, type of toothpaste, type of mouth rinse).
- Examine patient and eliminate these possible sources of sensitivity:
  - Dentin exposure
  - Fractured tooth
  - Fractured/defective restoration
  - Gingival inflammation
  - Gingival recession
  - Pulp vitality
  - Caries
  - Trauma
- Confirm dentin hypersensitivity.
- Educate patient to remove risk factors (OHI, diet).
- Initiate noninvasive treatment:
  - Desensitizing toothpaste
  - Topical fluoride or varnishes
  - Topical desensitizing agents

Noninvasive contemporary treatments are:

- Cavity varnishes: Duraphat
- Fluoride compounds: Sodium fluoride (NaF), phosphate fluoride (APF), stannous fluoride
- Calcium compounds: Calcium phosphate ($Ca(OH)_2$), casein phosphopeptide-amorphous calcium phosphate (CPP-ACP)
- Potassium nitrate
- Oxalates
- Dentin resins: Bonding agents
- Gluma or G5 (glutaraldehyde)
- Silver diamine fluoride
- Teethmate (kuraray)

References

American Academy of Pediatrics. Guideline on Caries-risk Assessment and Management for Infants, Children and Adolescents. The ISSN register. 2014. http://www.aapd.org/media/policies_guidelines/g_cariesriskassessment.pdf. Accessed 6 Mar 2016.

Benkaddour A, Bahije L, Bahoum A, Zaoui F. Orthodontics and enamel demineralization: clinical study of risk factors. Int Orthod. 2014;12(4):458–66.

Borges AB, Caneppele TMF, Luz M, Pucci CR, Torres CRG. Color stability of resin used for caries infiltration after exposure to different staining solutions. Oper Dent. 2014;39(4):433–40.

Chu CH, GaoSS, Li SK. The effectiveness of the biannual application of silver nitrate solution followed by sodium fluoride varnish in arresting early childhood caries in preschool children: study protocol for a randomized controlled trial. The ISSN register. 2015. http://www.ncbi.nlm.nih.gov/pubmed/26407698. Accessed 6 Mar 2016.

Du MQ, Bian Z, Jiang H, et al. Clinical evaluation of a dentifrice containing calcium sodium phosphosilicate (NovaMin) for the treatment of dentin hypersensitivity. Am J Dent. 2008;21(4):210–4.

Featherstone J, Horst J. Alternative approach to managing caries. J Multidiscip Care Decisions Dent. 2015;1(1):39–44.

Fejerskov O. Changing paradigms in concepts on dental caries: consequences for oral health care. Caries Res. 2004;38(3):182–91.

Gao SS, Zhang SN, Mei ML, Lo ECM, Chu CH. Caries remineralisation and arresting effect in children by professionally applied fluoride treatment – a systematic review. BMC Oral Health. 2016;16(12):1–9.

Garcia R, Borrelli B, Dhar V, et al. Progress in early childhood caries and opportunities in research, policy, and clinical management. Pediatr Dent. 2015;37(3):294–9.

Gibson G, Jurasic MM, Wehler CJ, Jones JA. Supplemental fluoride use for moderate and high caries risk adults: a systematic review. J Public Health Dent. 2011;71(3):171–84.

Hadler-Olsen S, Sandvik K, El-Agroudi MA, Ogaard B. The incidence of caries and white spot lesions in orthodontically treated adolescents with a comprehensive caries prophylactic regimen–a prospective study. Eur J Orthod. 2012;34(5):633–9.

Hilton TJ, Ferracane JL, Broome JC. Caries management: diagnosis and treatment strategies. In: Grisham B, editor. Fundamentals of operative dentistry: a contemporary approach. 4th ed. Hanover Park: Quintessence Publishing; 2013. p. 2–4.

Hoffman DA, Clark AE, Rody WJ, McGorray SP, Wheeler TT. A prospective randomized clinical trial into the capacity of a toothpaste containing NovaMin to prevent white spot lesions and gingivitis during orthodontic treatment. Prog Orthod. 2015;16(25):1–6.

Horst JA, Ellenikiotis H, Milgrom PL. UCSF protocol for caries arrest using silver diamine fluoride: rationale, indications and consent. J Calif Dent Assoc. 2016;44(1):16–28. Review.
ISSN DMG-America: The ISSN register. 2009. http://www.dmg-america.com/files/product/literature/[nid]/New_Icon_8pg_Brochure.pdf. Accessed 5 Mar 2016.
Jenson L, Budenz AW, Featherstone JDB, Ramos-Gomez FJ, Spolsky VW. Clinical protocols for caries management by risk assessment. J Calif Dental Assoc. 2007;35(10):714–23.
Julien KC, Buschang PH, Campbell PM. Prevalence of white spot lesion formation during orthodontic treatment. Angle Orthod. 2013;83(4):641–7.
Kantovitz KR, Pascon FM, Nobre-dos-Santos M, Puppin-Rontani RM. Review of the effects of infiltrants and sealers on Non-cavitated enamel lesions. Oral Health Prev Dent. 2010;8(3):295–305.
Kielbassa AM, Muller J, Gernhardt CR. Closing the gap between oral hygiene and minimally invasive dentistry: a review on the resin infiltration technique of incipient (proximal) enamel lesions. Quintessence Int. 2009;40(8):663–81.
Kutsch VK. Dental caries: an updated medical model of risk assessment. J Prosthet Dent. 2014;111(4):280–5.
Lenzi TL, Montagner AF, Soares FZ, de Oliveira Rocha R. Are topical fluorides effective for treating incipient carious lesions?: a systematic review and meta-analysis. J Am Dent Assoc. 2016;147(2):84–91.
Meyer-Lueckel H, Paris S. Infiltration of natural caries lesions with experimental resins differing in penetration coefficients and ethanol addition. Caries Res. 2010;44(4):408–14.
Mount GJ. Defining, classifying, and placing incipient caries lesions in perspective. Dent Clin North Am. 2005;49(4):701–23. v.
Newbrun E. Topical fluorides in caries prevention and management: a North American perspective. J Dent Educ. 2001;65(10):1078–83.
Ogaard B, Rolla G, Arends J. Orthodontic appliances and enamel demineralization. 1. Lesion development. Am J Orthod Dentofacial Orthop. 1988;94(1):68–73.
Oreilly MM, Featherstone JDB. Demineralization and remineralization around orthodontic appliances – an invivo study. Am J Orthod Dentofacial Orthop. 1987;92(1):33–40.
Paris S, Meyer-Lueckel H. Masking of labial enamel white spot lesions by resin infiltration-A clinical report. Quintessence Int. 2009;40(9):713–8.
Pitts-Fejerskov O. Changing paradigms in concepts on dental caries: consequences for oral health care. Caries Res. 2004;38:182–91.
Ramos-Gomez F, Crystal YO, Ng MW, Crall JJ, Featherstone JDB. Pediatric dental care: Prevention and Management Protocols based on Caries risk assessment. J Calif Dent Assoc. 2010;38(10):746–51.
Scheie AA, Petersen FC. The biofilm concept: consequences for future prophylaxis of oral diseases? Crit Oral Biol Med. 2004;15(1):4–12.
Scheie A, Peterson F. The biofilm concept: consequences for future prophylaxis of oral diseases? Crit Rev Oral Biol Med. 2004;15:4–12.
Selwitz RH, Ismail AI, Pitts NB. Dental caries. Lancet. 2007;369(9555):51–9.
Torres CRG, Borges AB, Torres LMS, Gomes IS, de Oliveira RS. Effect of caries infiltration technique and fluoride therapy on the colour masking of white spot lesions. J Dent. 2011;39(3):202–7.
Young DA, Featherstone JD. Caries management by risk assessment. Community Dent Oral Epidemiol. 2013;41(1):e53–63.
Zhu MJ, Li JL, Chen B, et al. The effect of calcium sodium phosphosilicate on dentin hypersensitivity: a systematic review and meta-analysis. Plos One. 2015;10(11):6.

Local Anesthesia Challenges

4

Sidni Paige Manne and Rosalia Rey

Contents

Abstract

In the span of a dental career, there will be patients one encounters that have difficulty achieving anesthesia. There are physiologic explanations for this and clinical techniques to manage the situation. The chapter illustrates the latest on evidence-based dentistry in providing patients with adequate anesthesia to allow dental procedures to occur.

4.1 Difficult Anesthesia

A. Why it occurs?
- The trigeminal pain system is a complex multilevel system that begins with the *detection* of tissue-damaging stimuli in the periphery, the PROCESSING

S.P. Manne, DMD, MS
Private Practice, Ormond Beach, FL, USA

Department of Endodontics, University of Florida College of Dentistry, Gainesville, FL, USA

R. Rey, DDS (✉)
University of Florida College of Dentistry, Gainesville, FL, USA
e-mail: rrey@dental.ufl.edu

G.M. Weinstein, M.T. Zientz (eds.), *The Dental Reference Manual*,
DOI 10.1007/978-3-319-39730-6_4

of that input at the level of the medullary spinal cord, and the final PERCEPTION of what is felt as pain in the cerebral cortex.

- Noxious stimuli → A-delta/C-fibers (primary afferent fibers with cell bodies located in the trigeminal ganglion) → synapse in the medullary dorsal horn (oralis, interpolaris, caudalis) → second-order projection neurons cross midline to the thalamus via the trigeminothalamic tract → third-order neurons → cerebral cortex via the thalamocortical tract (pain perception).

B. Reasons for failure of anesthetic (Fig. 4.1).
- Hyperalgesia due to inflamed nerves and lowered thresholds (Byers et al. 1990).
- Low pH of infected/inflamed tissues reduces the amount of uncharged basic form to penetrate nerve bundle.
- Operator error: missing the block.
- Tetrodotoxin-resistant (TTX-R) sodium channels which are resistant to local anesthetics (LA) (increased expression in symptomatic irreversible pulpitis (SIP) cases).
- Apprehensive patients have decreased pain thresholds.
- Acute tachyphylaxis: depletion of available neurotransmitters or receptors (Hargreaves 2003).
- Accessory innervation:
  - Mylohyoid nerve may supply accessory innervation (Frommer et al. 1972) (Fig. 4.2).
  - Cross innervation of mandibular incisors (Pogrel et al. 1997).

C. Management of local anesthetic failures:
- Provide supplemental local anesthesia:
  - Increase the dosage to expose a greater length of the inferior alveolar nerve (IAN) and increase the likelihood of a conduction blockade (Franz and Perry 1974) (Fig. 4.1).
  - Block the population of tetrodotoxin-resistant (TTX-R) sodium channels that may be elevated in the inflamed state (Novakovic et al. 1998).
- Aim higher on the 2nd IAN block: Gow–Gates or Vazirani–Akinosi (*closed mouth mandibular block*) (Fig. 4.3a, b).
- Mental nerve block: The mental foramen can also be located via palpation, periapical radiographs, and panoramic radiographs (Aminoshariae et al. 2014). Additionally, the average location of the mental foramen is 60 % of the distance from the tip of the buccal cusp of the mandibular 2nd premolar to the inferior border of the mandible (Phillips et al. 1990).

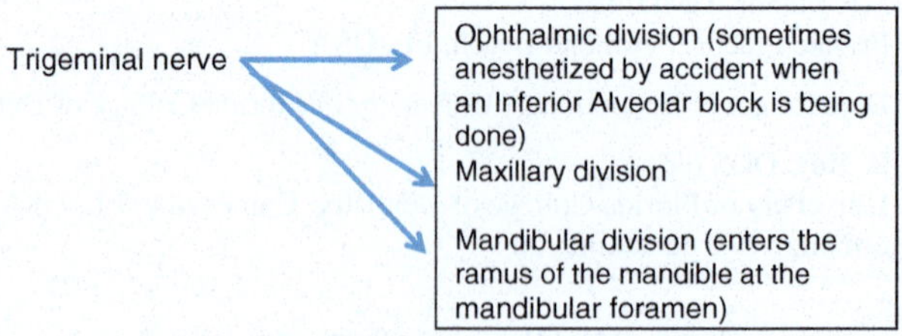

Fig. 4.1 The trigeminal nerve distribution

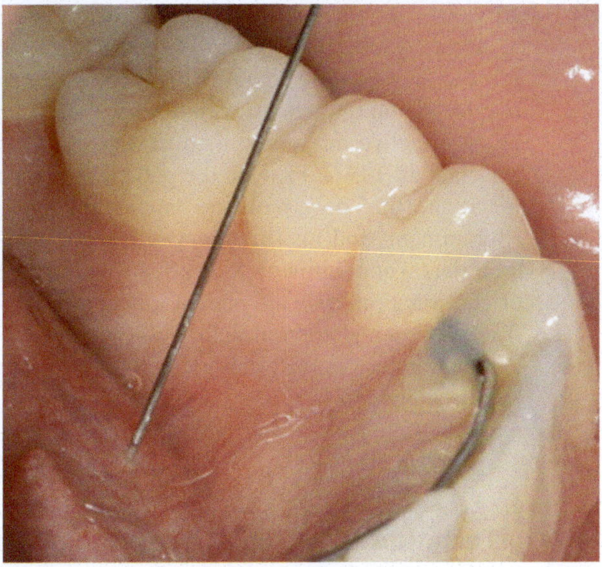

Fig. 4.2 Needle placement for mylohyoid needle

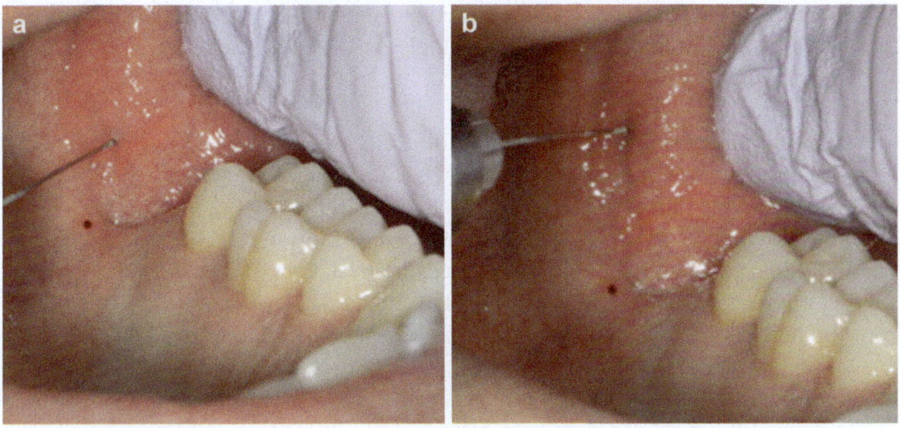

Fig. 4.3 (**a**) Inferior alveolar block and (**b**) aiming higher on the 2nd inferior alveolar block

- Use an anesthetic with a lower pKa 3% mepivacaine since it decreases the potential for ion trapping, increases the concentration of local anesthetic molecules in their base form, and increases diffusion of the LA across nerve terminals, thus increasing onset of anesthesia.
- Adjunctive injections: intraligamentary, intraosseous (IO), intrapulpal (see descriptions below in Section 2).
- Adjunctive drugs: fast-acting nonsteroidal anti-inflammatory drugs (NSAIDs). Ibuprofen in a liquid gel form reduces levels of inflammatory mediator prostaglandin E_2 (PGE_2); this is a hypothesis and has not been evaluated in endodontic patients.

- Anxious patients may benefit from nitrous oxide prior to giving any type of injection. Additionally, anxiolytic therapy my also be provided for the patient prior to their dental appointment. These medications are both safe and effective for dental outpatients. Studies have shown that triazolam (0.25 mg) can be an effective anxiolytic than diazepam (5.0 mg) for endodontic patients (Erich et al. 1997). Provide the patient with a prescription for two tablets of triazolam (0.25 mg), have the patient take one, one hour before their dental appointment, and instruct them to bring the remaining tablet with them to their dental appointment. Side effects include dizziness, drowsiness, and loss of coordination, thus the patient must have a driver accompany them to and from their dental appointment.
- Distraction techniques such as jiggling the patient's lip or quickly pulling the soft tissue over a stationary needle tip may aide in anesthetizing the anxious patient.

4.2 Techniques for Delivery of Anesthesia

A. *Mandibular block:*
   - If the initial block does not anesthetize a patient after 10 min, a second block should be attempted at a higher angle as the mandibular foramen may be positioned higher.

B. *Infiltration:*
   - Supplemental buccal and lingual infiltrations of 4 % articaine or 2 % lidocaine increase the success rate of IAN block in patients with symptomatic irreversible pulpitis (SIP) (Aggarwal et al. 2009).

C. *Intraosseous (IO):* Delivers a local anesthetic solution directly into the cancellous bone adjacent to the tooth to be anesthetized. Given once signs of lip numbness have developed (Hargreaves 2010) (Fig. 4.4).
   - The two IO systems that have been researched include the Stabident system (Fairfax Dental Inc, Miami, FL) and X-tip (Dentsply, Tulsa, OK). Both IO, systems demonstrated similar success onset, duration, and perceived heart rate increases (Gallatin et al. 2003) (Fig. 4.5).
   - Research has demonstrated that 67 % of patients had an increase in heart rate with an IO injection. No contraindications with healthy patients, but consider using an anesthetic without epinephrine, such as 3 % mepivacaine.
   - Stabident with 2 % lidocaine was shown to be 88 % effective for patients experiencing SIP.
   - Stabident with 3 % mepivacaine for SIP was 80 % successful with one injection and 98 % with two injections (Nusstein et al. 1998).

D. *Intrapulpal injection:*
   - Produces profound anesthesia if given under back pressure. The onset of anesthesia is immediate. Strong back pressure is a major factor in achieving

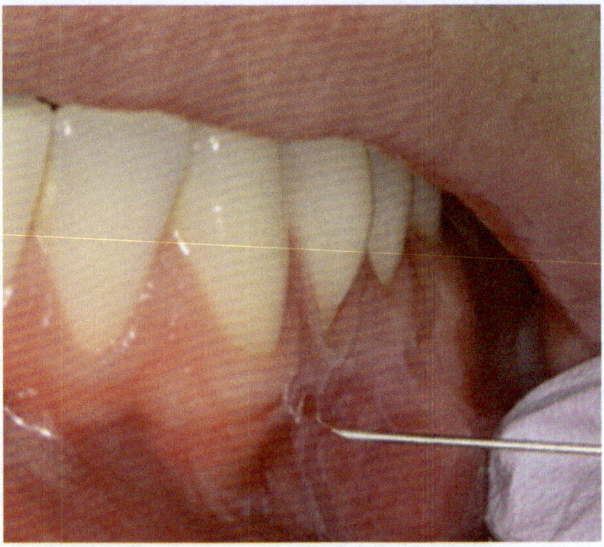

Fig. 4.4 Intraosseous anesthesia needle position

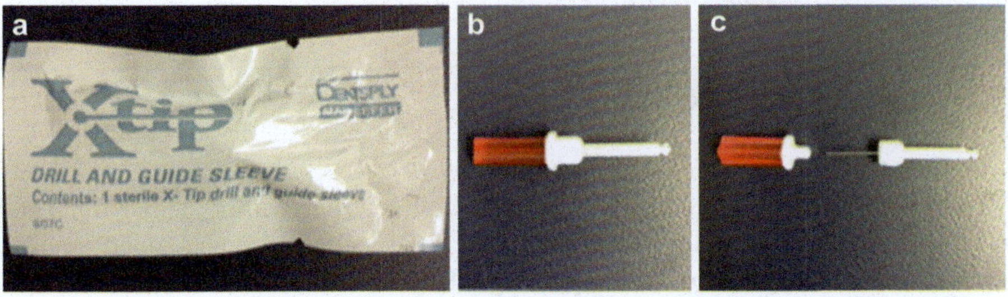

Fig. 4.5 Intraosseous anesthesia: X-tip. (**a**) package; (**b**) guide sleeve (inside *red* cap); (**c**) drill

successful intrapulpal anesthesia. Depositing the anesthetic passively into the chamber will not produce profound anesthesia because the solution will not diffuse throughout the pulp (Birchfield and Rosenberg 1975; VanGheluwe and Walton 1997).

E. *Intraligamentary injection or periodontal ligament injection* (PDL):
   - Experimental studies in volunteers without dental pathology have shown that the addition of a PDL injection with 2 % lidocaine with 1:100,000 epinephrine (delivered with a high-pressure syringe) to a mandibular block significantly increased the success of pulpal anesthesia for 23 min (Childers et al. 1996).

F. *Palatal injections:*
   - These include the greater palatine nerve block, the nasopalatine nerve block, and palatal infiltrations. To reduce discomfort to the patients, apply topical

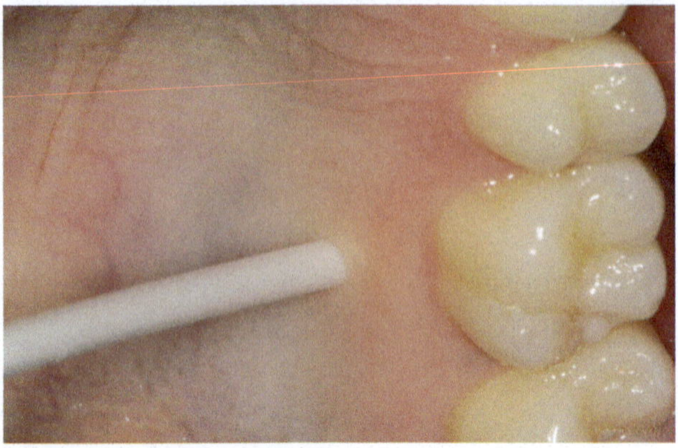

Fig. 4.6 Cotton applicator placement: note the blanched appearance of the tissue

anesthetic for approximately 2 min prior to giving the injection. Next, press cotton applicator, rather than the handle of a mouth mirror until the tissue become ischemic (blanched) in appearance (Fig. 4.6). Maintain this pressure while inserting the needle tip into the soft tissue, and deposit the anesthetic slowly (Malamed 2004).

4.3 Pearls for Success

A. *Antibiotics: when and when not to prescribe*?
   - Do prescribe antibiotics for progressive infections with systemic signs and symptoms such as fever (100 ° F), malaise, cellulitis, unexplained trismus, and swelling that are not improving (Hargreaves 2010).
   - Do not prescribe antibiotics for pain. There is no evidence to support that antibiotics should be prescribed for SIP cases (Keenan et al. 2006). Penicillin is ineffective for pain relief and should not be prescribed for untreated SIP (Nagle et al. 2000).

B. *NSAIDs:*
   - Prophylactic administration of an NSAID, such as 400 mg of ibuprofen 30–60 min before the procedure, has been shown to reduce or prevent post-treatment dental pain (Jackson et al. 1989).

C. *Managing endodontic emergencies* (Torabinejad and Walton 1991):
   - With pretreatment emergency cases of SIP, symptomatic apical periodontitis (SAP), acute apical abscess (AAA), and necrosis, a complete pulpectomy is preferred, and if time permits cleaning and shaping.
   - Post-obturation emergencies are less frequent and might be caused by trauma and/or extension of filling material to PA tissues; however, inform the patient of the possible discomfort for the first few days, and administer minor analgesics.
   - Persistent pain and/or swelling after completion of RCT might require re-treatment or surgery depending on the factors.

D. *Flare-ups of endodontically treated teeth:*
- Occlusal adjustment works for SIP preoperative pain (percussion sensitivity) (Rosenberg et al. 1998).
- Re-enter for complete debridement.
- For swelling, establish incision and drainage.
- Evaluate for analgesics. Research has shown that a combination of ibuprofen and acetaminophen is more effective at reducing pain than ibuprofen alone (76 %), ibuprofen/acetaminophen (96 %). Recommended regimen for moderate pain is 600 mg ibuprofen + 325 mg acetaminophen taken every 6 h (Menhinick et al. 2004).
- Evaluate for antibiotics if patient is experiencing systemic involvement or is immunocompromised (see chapter on prescriptions).
- Evaluate for steroids, oral Medrol Dose Pack (48 mg methylprednisolone).

References

Aggarwal V, Jain A, Kabi D. Anesthetic efficacy of supplemental buccal and lingual infiltrations of articaine and lidocaine after an inferior alveolar nerve block in patients with irreversible pulpitis. J Endod. 2009;35(7):925–9.

Aminoshariae A, Su A, Kulild JC. Determination of the location of the mental foramen: a critical review. J Endod. 2014;40(4):471–5.

Birchfield J, Rosenberg PA. Role of the anesthetic solution in intrapulpal anesthesia. J Endod. 1975;1(1):26–7.

Byers MR, Taylor PE, Khayat BG, Kimberly CL. Effects of injury and inflammation on pulpal and periapical nerves. J Endod. 1990;16(2):78–84.

Childers M, Reader A, Nist R, Beck M, Meyers WJ. Anesthetic efficacy of the periodontal ligament injection after an inferior alveolar nerve block. J Endod. 1996;22(6):317–20.

Erich D, Lundgren JP, Dionne RA, Nicoll BK, Hunter JW. Comparison of triazolam, diazepam, and placebo as outpatient oral premedication for endodontic patients. J Endod. 1997;23(3):181–4.

Franz D, Perry R. Mechanisms for differential block among single myelinated and non-myelinated axons by procaine. J Physiol. 1974;236:193–210.

Frommer J, Mele FA, Monroe CW. The possible role of the mylohyoid nerve in mandibular posterior tooth sensation. J Am Dent Assoc. 1972;85(1):113–7.

Gallatin J, Reader A, Nusstein J, Beck M, Weaver J. A comparison of two intraosseous anesthetic techniques in mandibular posterior teeth. J Am Dent Assoc. 2003;134(11):1476–84.

Hargreaves KCS. Cohen's pathways of the pulp. St. Louis: Mosby Elsevier; 2010.

Hargreaves KMKK. Local anesthetic failure in endodontics: mechanisms and management. Endod Top. 2003;1:26.

Jackson DJ, Moore P, Hargreaves KM. Preoperative non- steroidal anti-inflammatory medication for the prevention of postoperative dental pain. J Am Dent Assoc. 1989;119:641–7.

Keenan JV, Farman A, Fedorowicz Z Z, Newton JT. A Cochrane systematic review finds no evidence to support the use of antibiotics for pain relief in irreversible pulpitis. J Endod. 2006;90(5):636–40.

Malamed S. Handbook of local anesthesia. St. Louis: Elsevier Mosby; 2004.

Menhinick KA, Gutmann J, Regan JD, Taylor SE, Buschang PH. The efficacy of pain control following nonsurgical root canal treatment using ibuprofen or a combination of ibuprofen and acetaminophen in a randomized, double-blind, placebo-controlled study. Int Endod J. 2004;37(8):531–41.

Nagle D, Reader A, Beck M, Weaver J. Effect of systemic penicillin on pain in untreated irreversible pulpitis. Oral Surg Oral Med Oral Pathol Oral Radiol Endod. 2000;90(5):636–40.

Novakovic STE, McGiven J, Haragauchi M, San-gameswaran L, Gogas K, Eglen R, Hunter J. Distribution of the tetrodotoxin-resistant sodium channel PN3 in rat sensory nerves in normal and neuropathic conditions. J Neurosci. 1998;18:2174–87.

Nusstein J, Reader A, Nist R, Beck M, Meyers WJ. Anesthetic efficacy of the supplemental intraosseous injection of 2% lidocaine with 1:100,000 epinephrine in irreversible pulpitis. J Endod. 1998;24(7):487–91.

Phillips JL, Weller RN, Kulild JC. The mental foramen: 1. Size, orientation, and positional relationship to the mandibular second premolar. J Endod. 1990;16(5):221–3.

Pogrel MA, Smith R, Ahani R. Innervation of the mandibular incisors by the mental nerve. J Oral Maxillofac Surg. 1997;55(9):961–3.

Rosenberg PA, Babick PJ, Schertzer L, Leung A. The effect of occlusal reduction on pain after endodontic instrumentation. J Endod. 1998;24(7):492–6.

Torabinejad M, Walton RE. Managing endodontic emergencies. J Am Dent Assoc. 1991;122(5):99, 101, 103.

Van Gheluwe J, Walton R. Intrapulpal injection: factors related to effectiveness. Oral Surg Oral Med Oral Pathol Oral Radiol Endod. 1997;83(1):38–40.

Modern Day Treatment Planning Dilemmas; Natural Tooth Versus Implants

5

Sharon C. Siegel, John R. Antonelli, and Mauricio Hervas

Contents

Abstract

Decision-making about a treatment plan whether to preserve a compromised tooth with endodontic therapy and a protective, functional restoration or to extract and replace it with an implant requires evidence-based diagnosis and recommendations based on patient factors, tooth and periodontium-based factors, and treatment-based factors. The first consideration should be the preservation of the natural dentition as long as possible, since the extraction and implant placement can be done at anytime and the implant treatment is not without risk. This component of the chapter outlines the evidence to recommend and plan the most appropriate treatment when faced with restoring the compromised tooth.

S.C. Siegel, DDS, MS, MBA (✉) • J.R. Antonelli, DDS, MS • M. Hervas, DDS, MS, FACP
Department of Prosthodontics, Nova Southeastern University College of Dental Medicine, Fort Lauderdale, FL, USA
e-mail: scsiegel@nova.edu

G.M. Weinstein, M.T. Zientz (eds.), *The Dental Reference Manual*,
DOI 10.1007/978-3-319-39730-6_5

5.1 Restorative Choices Between an Endodontically Treated Tooth (RCT) Versus Single Tooth Implant (ISC) or Fixed Partial Dental Prosthesis (FPDP)

5.1.1 Introduction

Contemporary dental practice requires decision-making about either preserving a compromised tooth with root canal treatment (RCT) or by extracting the tooth and placing an implant and a single crown (ISC). Preserving the natural dentition is a principal objective in dentistry and one that many patients desire (Devan 1952). The treatment decision to save a compromised tooth with RCT or to extract the tooth and place an implant is difficult when considering multiple factors and multiple risks since each additional factor and risk jeopardizes the survival and success of the treatment (Wolcott and Meyers 2006). The treatment-planning decision should be based on factors related to the local, site-specific factors to include the tooth specifically and the periodontium, general patient-related factors, and ethics of patient treatment. Each of these criteria is discussed and related to the prognosis for making this decision.

5.1.2 Treatment Outcomes for the Compromised Tooth

The first and foremost treatment plan for the compromised tooth that should be considered with the utmost of diligence is to preserve the natural tooth with root canal treatment and to complete the definitive restoration to coronally seal and restore to function as soon as possible (Doyle 2015). The justification and evidence for the first consideration of preserving the compromised tooth with a root canal without apical periodontitis and an adequate, functional restoration is a successful outcome and is based on three overarching rationales. One is that the literature has shown that the long-term survival of both treatments is similar (Levin and Halperin-Sternfeld 2013; Torabinejad et al. 2007; Tomasi et al. 2008; Holm-Pedersen et al. 2007), but there are associated risks with both treatment alternatives. Second, the patient's quality of life with both treatments is similar, but many patients prefer to save their teeth (Azarpazhooh et al. 2013; Gatten et al. 2011). Finally, a tooth can always be extracted and the implant placed as the last resort (Doyle 2015). The extraction is final, and all associated adjunctive treatments and risks will need to be addressed for the remainder of the patient's life.

The alternative treatment of extraction and implant placement should be considered as a complementary treatment for the appropriate patient situation rather than a competing alternative treatment to root canal therapy and an esthetic functional restoration that is the best in all situations (Doyle 2015; Pradeep et al. 2013). The treatment option of replacing missing teeth with cylindrical endosseous implants has significantly affected treatment planning in prosthodontics and periodontics. Patient factors must be considered carefully before defaulting automatically to an "implant only treatment plan" without considering also the endodontic therapy first (Torabinejad and Goodacre 2006; Schroeder et al. 1996; Curtis et al. 2002) (Fig. 5.1). As more specialists (prosthodontists, endodontists) and more general dentists are

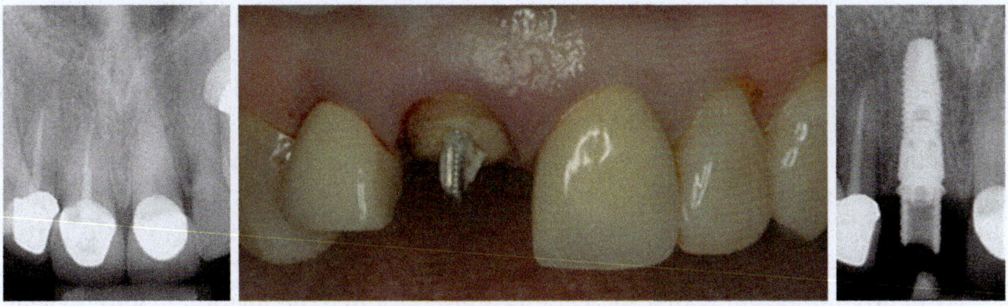

Fig. 5.1 Mobile crown, recurrent caries, nonrestorable tooth #8 resulting in extraction and implant placement

placing implants and restoring them, instead of only restoring them, and risks are being mitigated, treatment-planning bias has had a tendency away from the consideration of saving the tooth through endodontic therapy (Barth 2015; AAE Position Statement 2013) to extraction and placing the implant. Even though more dentists are being required to become competent at implant placement, the first consideration should be maintaining the tooth through RCT and a definitive restoration.

Some experts are reconsidering osseointegration, which has been traditionally defined as the anchorage of an implant by direct bony contact (Brånemark et al. 1977; Albrektsson et al. 1981; Zarb and Albrektsson 1991; Albrektsson and Johansson 2001). Reevaluation of the osteointegrative process by several experts may help to explain marginal bone loss and implant failures. They are considering that osseointegration is a foreign body reaction and foreign body equilibrium response whose clinical function depends on the tissue equilibrium in the patient (Albrektsson et al. 2013; Chrcanovic et al. 2014). This equilibrium could easily change depending on the patient's medical and clinical situation in the future. Conservative treatment planning and preserving the tooth should be the first consideration, not knowing when in the patient's future health or life a change could tip the balance of this equilibrium away from implant survival or success. Implant success and long-term survival are not 100 % guaranteed.

Compromised teeth that will require root canal treatment may also require adjunctive therapy to include periodontal therapy, orthodontic extrusion, post and core, and a final crown (Doyle 2015). When extensive treatment is required, the patient must consider the cost and time commitment of preserving the tooth and returning it to normal form and function as compared to the cost and time commitment of the implant placement and restoration (Goodacre 2016).

Differentiating the cutoff in deciding when a tooth with multiple risk factors should be deemed to have a hopeless prognosis, with extraction as the best possible treatment, is difficult to determine. But the dental practitioner must carefully determine the limit that preserving the tooth will result in short-term failure. One publication differentiates a "compromised" tooth from an "end-stage" failing tooth. The compromised tooth is a "complex, clinical situation" where the tooth is in a structural or pathologic condition that impairs its ability to function without some type of restoration (Iqbal and Kim 2008, p. 520). Tooth pathology requires the removal of enamel and dentin, possibly the surgical removal of the pulp, and/or periodontal treatment. The end-stage failing tooth is one that "is in a pathological or structural deficient state that cannot be successfully repaired with reconstructive therapies, including root canal treatment and/or retreatment and continues to exhibit progressive pathologic changes and clinical dysfunction of the tooth" (Iqbal and Kim 2008, p. 521). The strategies for definitive treatment of "end-stage" tooth failure include extraction and restoring form and function with an implant or a fixed or removable partial denture (Fig. 5.2). Studies have recommended that both RCT teeth and ISC have higher survival rates as compared to fixed partial dental prosthesis (Torabinejad et al. 2007; Scurria et al. 1995, 1998).

Critically important is that for a compromised tooth to be restorable with reasonably predictable long-term success with little or no risk of failure, enough tooth structure (enamel and/or dentin) must be available for a minimal, uniform, 2 mm ferrule, 360° around the tooth (Jotkowitz and Samet 2010; Zhi-Yue and Yu-Zing 2003; Tan et al. 2005) (Fig. 5.3). A caries risk assessment should be completed for the patient as part of the decision making process (Featherstone 2007). Jotkowitz and Samet show the anticipated risk for a tooth with varying amounts of tooth structure is available to retain the final restoration following endodontic treatment and the loads under which those teeth are placed. Taking into account this defined risk assists the dentist in determining the reasonable restorability of the tooth. Determining the reasonable restorability of the tooth should be the first consideration the dentist has in making a treatment decision for the compromised tooth.

Treating a diseased tooth can be influenced by the dental practitioner's background and training. Bader and Shugars (1993) examined the treatment of approximately 1200 teeth in 43 patients and found 62 % of the practitioners agreed on the

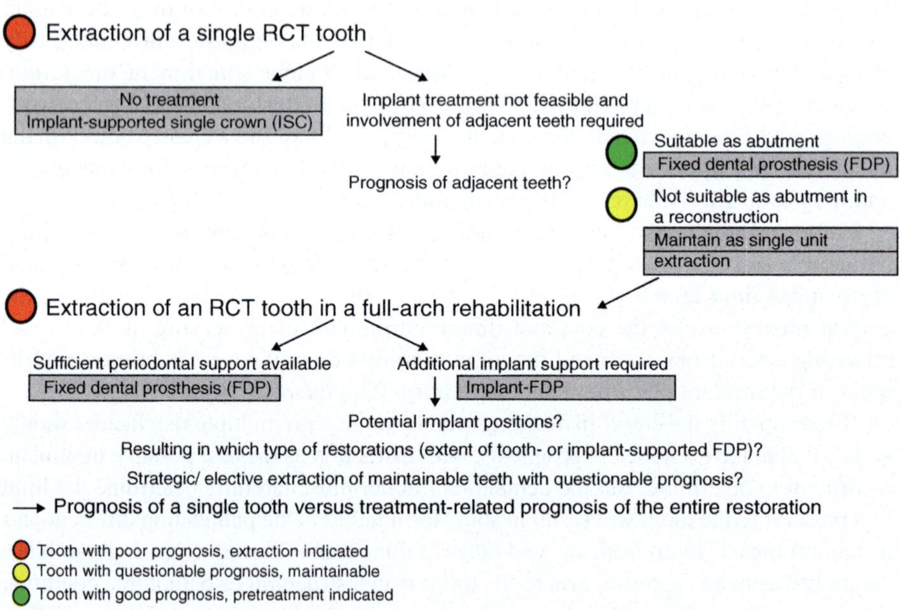

Fig. 5.2 Reconstructive aspects in treatment planning (Zitzmann et al. 2009)

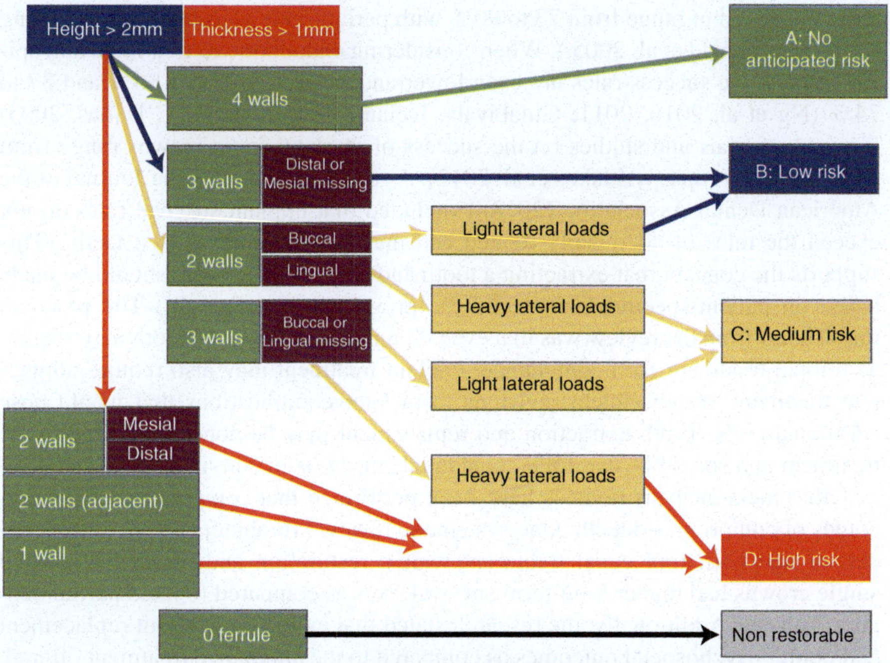

Fig. 5.3 Risk assessment analysis (Reprinted by permission from Macmillan Publishers Ltd. [*British Dental Journal*] (Jotkowitz and Samet 2010) copyright (2010))

treatment plan for individual teeth that were to be treated for the first time but much less agreement for previously restored teeth (Bader and Shugars 1993). The recommendation in this paper was to develop objective criteria for treating teeth with previous restorations. Iqbal and Kim (2008) have also suggested the development of evidence-based guidelines so that patients have sufficient information to select the optimal treatment plan for their situation and not one based on the experience, skills, and interests of the dentist since other members of the dental team can provide specialized care. The best treatment plan for the patient uses the best evidence and specific case factors as well as the patient's desires and needs. This chapter continues with evaluating the best evidence.

5.2 Survival Versus Success

Dentists should know current evidence-based success rates of the treatment they are recommending for the patient to respond to patients' questions. There have been a number of meta-analyses and systematic reviews in the literature comparing long-term endodontically treated tooth and implant survival rates that can assist the dental practitioner in making decisions (Levin and Halperin-Sternfeld 2013; Torabinejad et al. 2007; Tomasi et al. 2008; Holm-Pedersen et al. 2007; Jung et al. 2012). Endodontic success rates on teeth without periapical pathology have been reported to be 92–98 % but range from 73 to 90 % with periapical lesions that heal following RCT (Torabinejad et al. 2005). When considering endodontic re-treatment and apical surgery, the success rates are even lower and range from 74 to 86 % and 37 to 74 % (Ng et al. 2010, 2011; Gulabivala, Iceland, Freedman, AAC Dallas, 2005) Reviews of trials and studies on the success of implant single crowns range from 57.5 to 100 % (Papaspyridakos et al. 2012). A recent review from the Journal of the American Dental Association (2013) concluded that implant survival rates do not exceed the rates of adequately treated and maintained compromised teeth. (This supports the concept that extracting a tooth and placing an implant should be made based on patient-specific factors and the prognosis of the tooth.) The practical implication from the review was that even though a compromised tooth may require additional treatment for maintenance, implant treatment may also require adjunctive treatment or subsequent revisions from later complications that would pose additional risks. Tooth extraction and replacement may be done at anytime in the treatment and should be carefully considered since it is irreversible.

Other meta-analysis reviews have been performed that compare treatment outcomes of compromised teeth. One systematic review (Torabinejad et al. 2007) concluded that both root canal treatment with a restoration and implant-supported single crowns had higher long-term survival rates as compared to fixed partial dental prosthesis. Additionally, the research stated that extraction without replacement had poorer psychosocial outcomes as compared to the alternative treatment offered. Another systematic review found difficulty in making comparisons between RCT and implant treatment due to the heterogeneity in the findings (Tomasi et al. 2008). A systematic review comparing natural untreated teeth, compromised treated natural teeth, and implant treatment concluded that "oral implants when evaluated after 10 years of service do not surpass the longevity of even compromised but successful root canaltreated natural teeth" (Holm-Pedersen et al. 2007).

It is important when reviewing evidence for treatment recommendations that the reader ensures that the authors of the reviews make similar comparisons. Much of the implant literature considers survival rates in reporting outcomes, and the endodontic literature reports statistics in terms of success and survival (Norton 2001; Gotfredsen 2004; Gibbard and Zarb 2002; Morris et al. 2001). Only recently have reviews been conducted to evaluate criteria for implant success (Papaspyridakos et al. 2012) to include evaluating the "long-term primary outcome of the implant prosthetic complex as a whole" (p 247 Papaspyridakos). Survival rates will typically be higher than success rates. So when these meta-analyses are compared, the studies that are used need to be comparable, and survival levels are used since very few implant studies report success rates.

Root canal therapy and implant placement are "complementary treatment options for the appropriate patient situation" (Doyle, p. 2, 2015). There can be many complicating factors depending on the patient that need to be considered in each case. But simply stated, root canal treatment should be the primary consideration in general for restorable, periodontally healthy teeth that have irreversible pulpitis and/or periapical periodontitis (Doyle 2015; Iqbal and Kim 2008; Zitzmann et al. 2009). Implant placement should be considered in general for nonrestorable teeth and/or teeth with severe periodontal unhealthy conditions. To preserve the endodontically treated tooth successfully, there must be enough sound tooth structure to place a core or a post and core and to have an adequate ferrule for the crown margin of 2 mm surrounding the natural sound tooth structure (Sorensen and Engelman 1990; Libman and Nicholls 1995; Isidor et al. 1999). This situation would make the tooth clinically restorable. The presence of multiple risk factors though can jeopardize the compromised tooth and may weigh the decision toward extraction and implant placement or maintain the decision for RCT and final restoration. These other risk factors that must be considered include outcomes assessment, systemic conditions, tooth and periodontium factors, and patient-specific considerations (Torabinejad and Goodacre 2006; Salinas and Eckert 2007; Torabinejad et al. 2014).

5.3 Outcomes Assessment and Prognosis

Studies analyzing outcomes of RCT and ISC can be conflicting (Stockhausen et al. 2011), yet patients want to know whether a procedure that is recommended will be successful. It has been recommended that guidelines be in place so that these decisions can be made by the dentist to appropriately inform the patient. While both RCT and ISC have been found to be successful, studies predicting long-term outcomes concerning RCT have traditionally used "success and failure" as outcomes measures, while implant studies have used survival as outcome measures, making direct comparisons challenging. Long-term survival levels are comparable for both treatments. However, other factors must be taken into consideration.

5.3.1 Systemic Factors

Systemic factors are important to consider when recommending RCT or extraction and an implant for a patient. Table 5.1 outlines contraindications to implant placement from the National Institutes of Health Consensus Conference (NIHC 1988) that include both systemic factors and patient factors. In these situations, the recommended treatment option would weigh more in favor of RCT.

Table 5.1 Contraindications to implant placement

Contraindications to implant placement (National Institutes of Health Consensus Conference)
1. Acute illness
2. Terminal illness
3. Pregnancy
4. Uncontrolled metabolic disease
5. Tumoricidal irradiation of the implant site
6. Unrealistic patient expectation
7. Improper patient motivation
8. Lack of operator experience
9. Inability to restore with a prosthesis

Adapted from Rosenstiel et al. (2016); Yilmaz and McGlumphy (2016), VitalBook file, p. 321

The risk factors for periimplantitis and implant failure include systemic disease, genetic traits, chronic drug or alcohol consumption, smoking, periodontal disease, diabetes, osteoporosis, and poor oral hygiene (Doyle 2015; Dawson and Jasper 2015). Systemic risk factors that are associated with lower survival of endodontically treated teeth include smoking, diabetes, systemic steroid therapy, and hypertension (Doyle 2015; Bowles et al. 2010; Ng et al. 2010, 2011; Wang et al. 2011). The use of antiangiogenic or antiresorptive medications affect treatment planning for root canal treatment and implant placement due to the risk of medication-related osteonecrosis of the jaw. Additionally it is recommended for the completion of skeletal and dental growth before implant placement is considered (Mankani et al. 2014). Thus for adolescents or young adults that are continuing to grow, the first consideration for the compromised tooth should be RCT and the definitive restoration. It has been shown that growth continues throughout a lifetime such that vertical steps can occur after anterior implant restorations of implant placement similar to that of adolescents that are actively growing (Bernard et al. 2004) and thus are considered esthetic risk factors for implant placement (Table 5.2).

5.3.2 Site-Specific Factors

In the endodontic literature, the factors that must be considered are preexisting factors that include severe periodontal disease or post-endodontic factors such as recurrent caries, inadequate restoration, and reinfection or fracture (Iqbal and Kim 2007; Aquilino and Caplan 2002). Since these are factors that are listed as ones that contribute to endodontic failures, treatment planning for extraction and implant placement and a single crown should be the treatment plan of choice (Table 5.3).

In the implant literature, there are four factors that are listed as being taken into account when measuring implant success. These are implant level criteria, periimplant soft tissue, prosthesis, and the patient's subjective evaluations. There are various types of abutments for single implants and the definitive crown restorations (Fig. 5.4). The implant level criteria that are considered include lack of mobility, lack of pain, lack of radiolucency, and minimal periimplant bone loss (<1.5 mm at first year and <0.2/year after) (Papaspyridakos et al. 2012). The authors of this study suggest when including success criteria in evaluating implants, the reported success rate consistently decreased when the number of parameters included for success increased (Papaspyridakos et al. 2012, p 247). Since these are factors that must be considered for implant success, when there is poor quality of the bone (type IV), a thin biotype, anterior teeth that are to be considered, and high esthetics, the tooth should be maintained at all possible costs and RCT and a definitive restoration.

5.3.3 Local Factors

Local factors must be addressed for each particular tooth involved. First and foremost an accurate diagnosis must be made along with an assessment of the restorability of the tooth. This assessment should include the amount of tooth structure remaining to

Table 5.2 Contraindications and increased risk for failure for implant failures

	Disease	Assessment
Medical contraindications	Acute infectious diseases	Absolute, but temporarily; wait for recovery
	Cancer chemotherapy	Absolute, but temporarily; reduced immune status
	Systemic bisphosphonate medication (>2 years)	Risk of bisphosphonate induced osteonecrosis (BON)
	Renal osteodystrophia	Increased risk for infection, reduced bone density
	Severe psychosis	Absolute; risk of regarding the implant as foreign body and requesting removal despite of successful osseointegration
	Depression	Relative
	Pregnancy	Absolute, but temporarily; to avoid additional stress and radiation exposure
	Unfinished cranial growth with incomplete tooth eruption	Relative, but temporarily; to avoid any harm to the growth plates, to avoid in adequate implant position in relation so the residual dentition; utilize hand wrist radiograph to evaluate end of skeletal growth; single tooth implants in the anterior region not before a 25th year of age
Intraoral contraindications	Pathologic findings at the oral soft- and/or hard tissues	Temporarily; increased risk for infection, wait unit healing is completed
Increased risk for implant failure or complications	History of (aggressive) periodontitis	Relative, requires supportive periodontal care; increased risk to develop peri-implantitis
	Heavy smoking ≥10 pack-years (particularly in combination with HRT/oestrogen), alcohol and drug abuse	Relative or absolute, indicates cessation protocol; would healing problems, locally reduced vascularisation, impaired immunity, reduced bone turn over
	Insufficient oral hygiene	Absolute; wound healing problems, infection
	Uncontrolled parafunctions	Relative; increased risk for technical complications
	Post head and neck radiation therapy	Absolute, but temporarily; reduced bone remodelling, risk of osteoradionecrosis, implant placement 6–8 weeks before or ≥1 year after radiotheraphy
	Osteoporosis	Relative; reduced bone-to-implant contact; consider calcium substitution, prolong healing period and avoid high torque levels for abutment screw fication
	Uncontrolled diabetes	Relative, requires medical treatment; wound healing problems (impaired immunity, microvascular diseases)
	Status post chemotherapy, immune-suppressants or steroid long-term medication, uncontrolled HIV infection	Absolute, but temporarily; wound healing problems, medical advice required (consider corticosteroid cover)

With permission Zitzmann et al. (2009)

Table 5.3 Factors influencing endodontic and treatment-planning outcome

	Initial RCT	Endodontic retreatment	Apical surgery	Implant treatment
Preoperative	+Vital pulp tissue – Periapical lesion	+ Root canal filling >2 mm short of the apex +No periapical lesion – Large periapical lesion – Altered root-canal morphology or perforation – Adequate existing root canal filling	+Orthograde retreatment feasible +Significant overfill or root canal filling >2 mm short of the apex – Lesion ≥5 mm – Persisting lesion despite satisfactory root canal filling – Combined endo-perio lesion – Previous surgical treatment	– Insufficient bone volume – Specific anatomic findings – History of periodontitis – Previous implant failure – Insufficient oral hygiene and smoking (see also Table 5.3)
Intraoperative	+ Root canal filling with no voids extending to 2 mm within apex (radiographically) + Sufficient coronal restoration – Missed canals and inadequate cleaning – Errors such as ledging, instrument fracture, root perforations – Inadequate obturation – Root canal filling >2 mm short of the apex or overfill	+ Addressing previous technical shortcomings + Adequate root canal filling feasible	+ Root-end filling – Poor accessibility	+/– Type of implant and surface +/– Type of bone – Fenestration, bone defects – Specific anatomic findings – Bone augmentation – Immediate implant placement
Postoperative	– Restoration failure (coronal leakage)	– Restoration failure (coronal leakage, no cuspal coverage)	+/– No obvious influence by antibiotics	– Wound healing problems – Iatrogenic factors (e.g., excess cement) – Insufficient oral hygiene and smoking – Peri-implantitis

With permission Zitzmann et al.(2009)
+ positively influencing factors, – negatively influencing factors

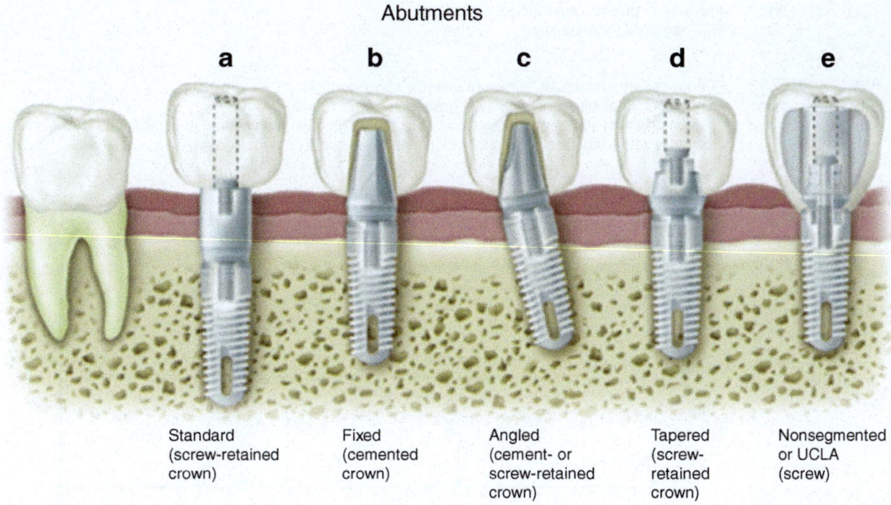

Fig. 5.4 Implant abutment types for single implants and the definitive crown. *A* Standard, length can be selected for the margin to be subgingival or supragingival. *B* Fixed, abutment is similar to a post and core restoration, but it is screwed into the implant and has a prepared finished line to receive a cemented crown. *C* Angled (fixed), used to correct implant orientation for biomechanical or esthetic reasons. *D* Tapered, used to improve emergence profile transition from smaller implant to larger restoration. *E* Nonsegmented or direct, used in limited interocclusal space situations where esthetics are important. This UCLA abutment has the crown and abutment in one piece (With permission from Rosenstiel et al. (2016, p. 338) Modified from Hupp, Ellis (2006))

allow restorability with a 2 mm, uniform ferrule, if there is a periapical pathosis associated with the root, whether this is the first time treating the tooth with a root canal; the periodontal condition of the area, whether multiple areas of the mouth are involved with compromised teeth; the caries risk assessment of the patient; the patient's periodontal biotype; and the area of the mouth that the tooth is located. Figure 5.5 is a decision tree that lists a starting point of a compromised tooth with irreversible pulpitis with or without periapical pathosis. It continues with factors that positively or negatively affect the treatment decision.

Additionally, in the presence of cracks, root fractures, or root resorption, the extent must be taken into account, and the treatment recommendation should lean toward extraction and implant placement (Figs. 5.6a, b and 5.7). The use of CBCT or microCT is being utilized more frequently to assist in the diagnosis and appropriate treatment of compromised teeth (Fig. 5.8).

5.3.4 Ethical Factors

Ethical standards for dental practitioners prescribe that patients be informed of all reasonable treatment options that include an explanation of the risks and benefits of these options and an informed consent to sign before treatment starts. This should

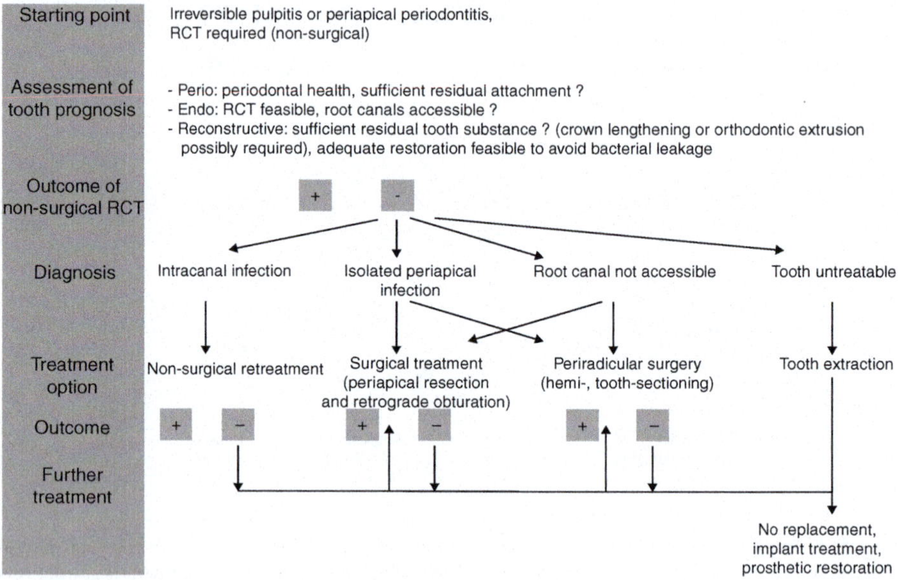

Fig. 5.5 Treatment considerations for root canal-treated teeth or implant placement (With permission from Zitzmann et al. (2009))

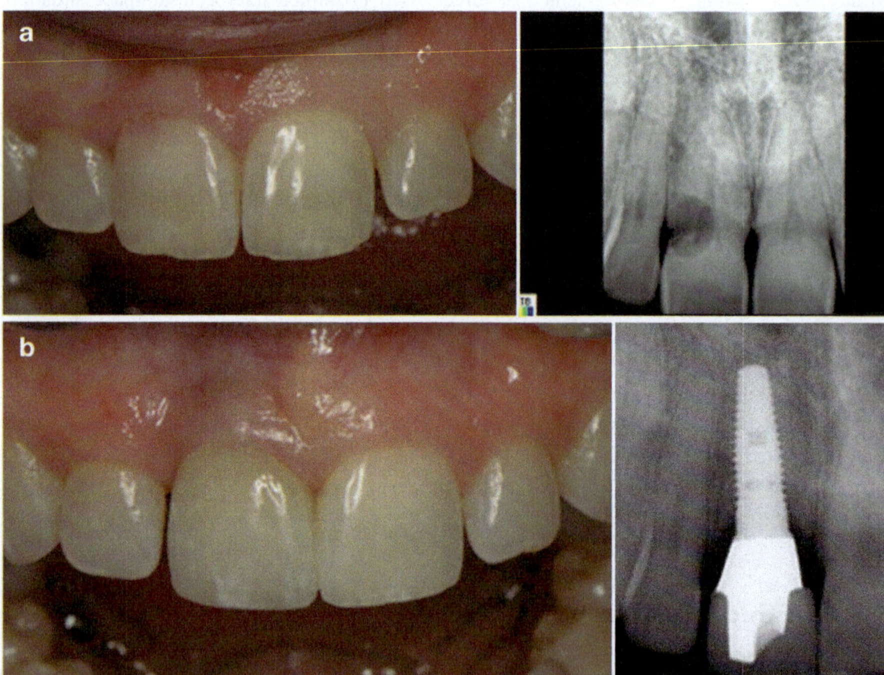

Fig. 5.6 (**a**) Before extraction photo of a nonrestorable tooth due to internal root resorption #8. (**b**) After the replacement photo of tooth #8 with an implant

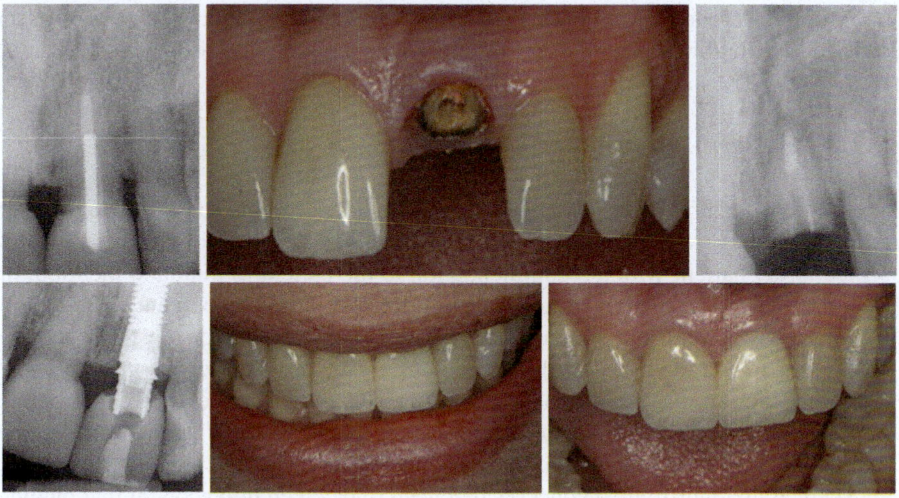

Fig. 5.7 Nonrestorable tooth following crown fracture that was also periodontally compromised. An implant was placed to replace it

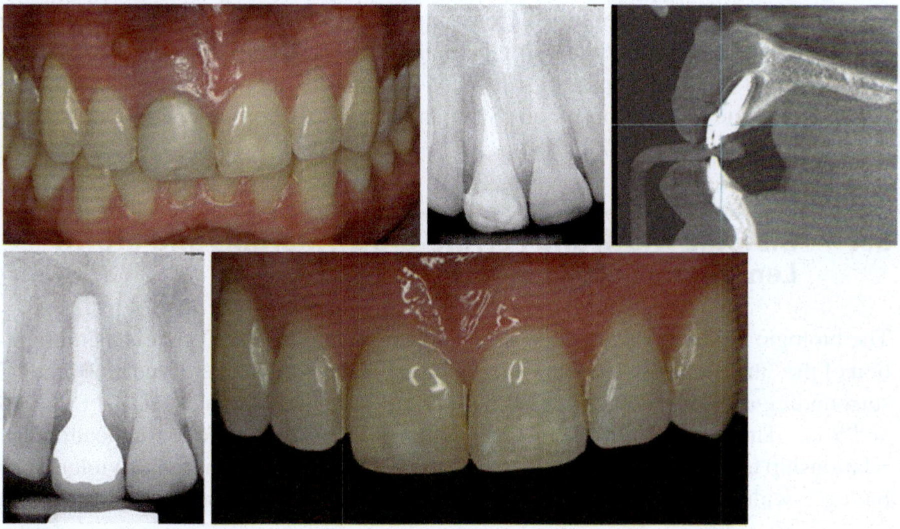

Fig. 5.8 CBCT or microCT assists in diagnosis and appropriate treatment

be done in an impartial manner (Doyle 2015). Treatment of the patient should always be done in the patient's best interests using the most current evidence-based information whether RCT is performed or if tooth extraction and implant placement and restoration are done.

It may be necessary to refer some or all components of the treatment so that the patient receives the highest quality and most appropriate care that will result in the best possible outcome. Specialists should be considered as partners in the delivery of complicated care for patients. Questionable teeth may need the expertise of an endodontist and/or prosthodontist to preserve the natural dentition.

5.3.5 Patient-Related Factors

Various treatment alternatives must be given as valid options for the patient rather than competing treatments. The evidence should be taken into account and presented to the patient with a recommendation to the patient to maintain the tooth or to extract the tooth (with or without implant, RCT, or FPDP placement). The definitive choice rests with the patient regarding whether to accept or reject the recommendation to preserve the tooth with a root canal, post and core, and crown or accept extraction and an implant restoration. When either the root canal or the implant procedure is more demanding, it is most appropriate to refer to a specialist (endodontist or prosthodontist/implant specialist).

There are patient-related concerns that need to be taken into account that include cost, length of treatment, and the potential for adverse outcomes. Figure 5.9 shows implant esthetic failures. A patient's decision can be influenced by finances to include whether the patient has dental insurance that may cover all or some of the treatment. RCT and the definitive crown may require less time to restore the tooth to final form and function than a single implant crown. Potential postoperative treatment can also influence a patient's decision for treatment. One study showed a longer average time to function for an ISC than for a similarly restored endodontically treated tooth (Doyle et al. 2006).

5.4 Biologic Width and Ferrule-Crown Margins and Crown Lengthening Considerations

The biologic width can be defined as an "essential dental space" that is a combination of the "junctional epithelium and the supracrestal connective tissue attachment" surrounding all teeth (Kina, p.1913; Schmidt, p.493; Ingber et al. 1977) (Figs. 5.10 and 5.11). The biologic width must be maintained to ensure periodontal health in its relationship to any dental prosthetic restoration (Kina). When there is a violation of biologic width during crown preparation to ensure an adequate uniform 2 mm

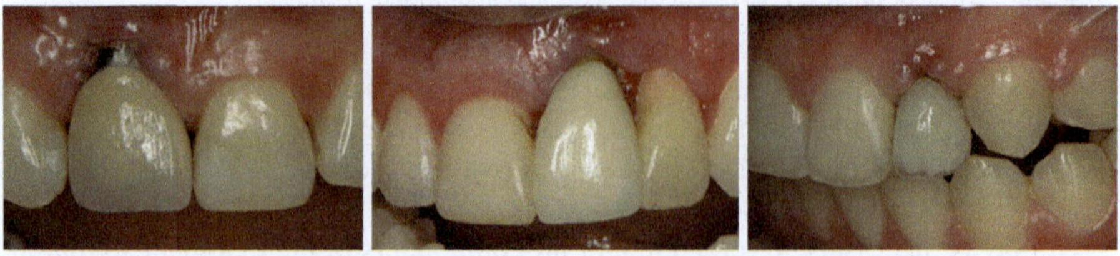

Fig. 5.9 Implant esthetic failures

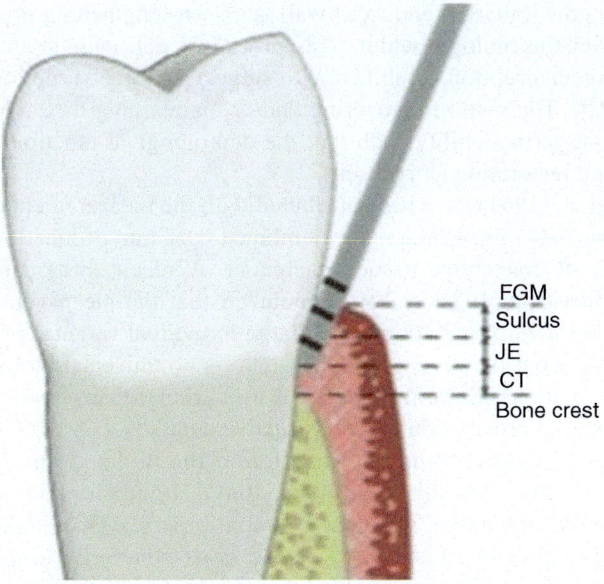

Fig. 5.10 "A probe placed into the sulcus of a tooth goes through the sulcus and the epithelial attachment. It is stopped by the connective tissue attachment. The biologic width of a natural tooth has a connective tissue (CT) zone that inserts into the cementum of the tooth. A periodontal probe can penetrate the sulcus and the junctional epithelium (JE). FGM (free gingival margin)" (Image with permission Misch (2015)

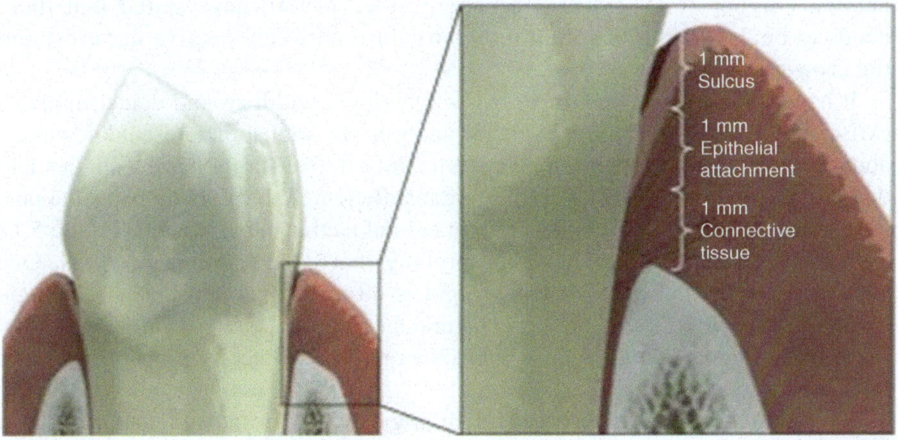

Fig. 5.11 The biologic width for a natural tooth is approximately 1 mm of connective tissue above the bone and 1 mm of epithelial attachment between the sulcus and the connective tissue (Image with permission from Misch (2015)

ferrule of the crown margin and axial wall, a crown-lengthening procedure can be done to recover the biologic width. This procedure can include an apically positioned flap, forced eruption combined with surgery or forced eruption with fiberotomy (Oh 2010). The goal of recovering and/or maintaining the biologic width for all teeth is long-term stability such that the dentogingival junction is in harmony with any dental restoration (Jorgensen).

Gargiulo et al. (1961) have been attributed with the measurement of the biologic width as being 2.04 mm, which is the combined 0.97 mm of junctional epithelium and 1.07 mm of connective tissue attachment. A recent systematic review that included studies from 1924 to 2012 concluded that the mean values of biologic width varied from 2.15 to 2.30 mm, and large individual variances were observed. The conclusion from the review was that there is no universal biologic width that appears to exist (Schmidt et al. 2013), but it is crucial that periodontal health be established prior to prosthodontic reconstructive dentistry.

Experts have suggested that the function of the biologic width is of a "protective barrier" for the subjacent periodontal ligament and alveolar bone (Bosshardt and Lang 2005). A recent systematic review (Kosyfaki 2010) found that supragingival crown margins were the most beneficial to the periodontal health of the patient. Comparatively, this study found that equigingival and subgingival margins resulted in increased plaque. This increased plaque accumulation could lead to gingival inflammation, increased pocket depths, loss of attachment, and thus gingival recession (Reitemeier et al. 2002). It has been proposed that a minimal dimension of 3 mm from the crown margin to the coronal crest must be maintained to have a stable periodontium and proper healing (Ingber et al. 1977). Rosenberg et al. (1980) have stated that there needs to be 3.5–4 mm of sound tooth structure between the alveolar crest and the crown margin.

It has been proposed that there exists a biologic width around dental implants (Misch et al. 2008, 2015). But evidence analysis shows that the present knowledge about biologic width around implants is mainly derived from animal studies and that clinical controlled human studies are insufficient. Table 5.4 compares the proposed measurements of biologic width in natural teeth and in implants. Figure 5.12 presents a schematic diagram of the probing that occurs around implants. One author has stated that the gingival margin is more coronal and that the biologic width (BW) is closer in dimension to natural teeth around one-piece nonsubmerged implants as compared to two-piece nonsubmerged or two-piece submerged implants (Hermann).

In conclusion, the dimensions for biologic width are not universal and can vary between 2.04 and 2.3 mm, but this essential dental space must be maintained around the tooth and dental restorations for a stable periodontium. Recommendations vary for the best distance to maintain between the crestal bone and a crown margin, but the literature supports that supragingival margins of crowns support a healthier periodontium than either equigingival margins or subgingival margins.

Table 5.4 Comparison of tooth and implant support structures

	Tooth	Implant
Connection	Cementum, bone, periodontal ligament	Osseointegration, bone functional ankylosis
Junctional epithelium (JE)	Hemidesmosomes and basal lamina (lamina lucida and lamina densa zones)	Hemidesmosomes and basal lamina (lamina lucida, lamina densa, and sublamina lucida zones)
Connective tissue (CT)	Thirteen groups: perpendicular to tooth surfaces	Only two groups: parallel and circular fibers No attachments to the implant surface and bone
Biological width (BW)	JE: 0.97–1.1.4 mm CT: 0.77–1.07 mm BW: 2.04–2.91 mm	JE:1.88 mm CT:1.05 mm BW:3.08 mm
Vascularity	More	Less
Probing depth	3 mm in health	2.5–5.0 mm (depending on soft tissue depth)
Bleeding on probing	More reliable	Less reliable

Image with permission Misch (2015)

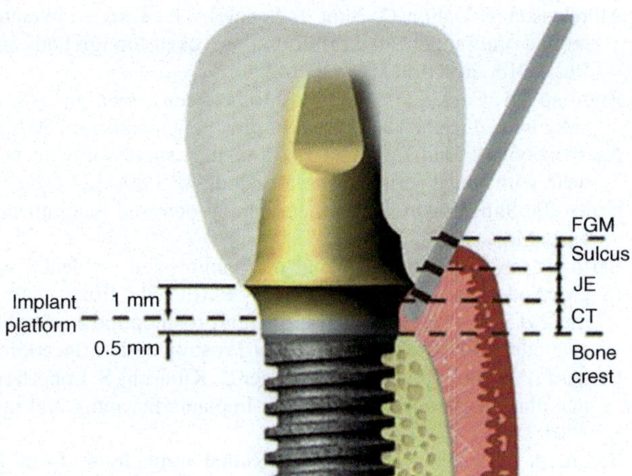

Fig. 5.12 An implant has no connective fibers in the connective tissue zone that insert into the implant. The periimplant probe penetrates the sulcus, junctional epithelium (JE) attachment, and most of the connective tissue zone. *FGM* free gingival margin, *JE* junctional epithelium, *CT* connective tissue (Image with permission Misch (2015)

5.5 Concluding Remarks

Preserving the natural dentition for a lifetime is a primary tenet of dentistry and a desire for most patients. Since patients are living longer, treatment planning to preserve the natural teeth through RCT and a definitive restoration should be the first treatment option presented to patients when teeth are compromised rather than defaulting to extraction and a single implant-retained crown. Studies support this philosophy of preservation of the restored endodontically treated tooth as a "long-term approach to retaining nature's implant—a tooth with an intact periodontal ligament" (Doyle 2015, p.7), which have similar survival rates to single implant-retained crowns. The dental practitioner needs to consider contributing factors that will influence treatment-planning decision for the compromised tooth toward the RCT or toward extraction and implant placement with a single crown. These factors are systemic, site specific, local, and patient related.

Clinical photographs are all courtesy of Dr. Mauricio Hervas, D.D.S., M.S., F.A.C.P.

References

AAE Position Statement. Scope of endodontics: dental implants. 2013. Retrieved from http://www.aae.org/uploadedfiles/publications_and_research/guidelines_and_position_statements/scopeofendo_implants.pdf.

Albrektsson T, Johansson C. Osteoinduction, osteoconduction and osseointegration. Eur Spine J. 2001;10(2):S96–101.

Albrektsson T, Brånemark PI, Hansson HA, Lindström J. Osseointegrated titanium implants. Requirements for ensuring a long-lasting, direct bone anchorage in man. Acta Orthop Scand. 1981;52:155–70.

Albrektsson T, Dahlin C, Jemt T, Sennerby L, Turri A, Wennerberg A. Is marginal bone loss around oral implants the result of a provoked foreign body reaction? Clin Implant Dent Relat Res. 2013. doi:10.1111/cid.12142.

Aquilino SA, Caplan DJ. Relationship between crown placement and the survival of endodontically treated teeth. The Journal of prosthetic dentistry. 2002;87(3):256–63.

Azarpazhooh A, Dao T, Figueiredo R, et al. A survey of patients' preferences for the treatment of teeth with apical periodontitis. J Endod. 2013;39:1534–41.

Bader JD, Shugars DA. Agreement among dentists' recommendations for restorative treatment. J Dent Res. 1993;72:891–6.

Barth C. Prosthodontists applaud the commission on dental accreditation's new standards for prosthodontic education. 2015. Retrieved from https://globenewswire.com/news-release/2015/08/11/759829/10145651/en/Prosthodontists-Applaud-the-Commission-on-Dental-Accreditation-s-New-Standards-for-Prosthodontic-Education.html.

Bernard JP, Schatz JP, Christou P, Belser U, Kiliaridis S. Long-term vertical changes of the anterior maxillary teeth adjacent to single implants in young and mature adults. J Clin Periodontol. 2004;31(11):1024–8.

Bosshardt DD, Lang NP. The junctional epithelium: from health to disease. J Dent Res. 2005;84(1):9–20.

Bowles WR, Drum M, Eleazer PD. Endodontic and implant algorithms. Dent Clin N Am. 2010;54(2):401–13.

Brånemark PI, Hansson BO, Adell R, Breine U, Lindström J, Hallén O, Öhman A. Osseointegrated titanium implants in the treatment of the edentulous jaw. Scand J Plast Reconstr Surg. 1977;11 Suppl 16:1–175.

Chrcanovic BR, Albrektsson T, Wennerberg A. Reasons for failures of oral implants. J Oral Rehabilit. 2014;41(6):443–76. doi:10.1111/joor.12157.

Curtis DA, Lacy A, Chu R, et al. Treatment planning in the 21st century: what's new? J Calif Dent Assoc. 2002;30:503–10.

Dawson DR, Jasper S. Key systemic and environmental risk factors for implant failure. Dent Clin N Am. 2015;59(1):25–39.

DeVan MM. The nature of the partial denture foundation: suggestions for its preservation. J Prosthet Dent. 1952;2:210.

Doyle SL. Treatment planning: retention of the natural dentition and replacement of missing teeth. Colleagues for Excellence Newsletter from the Am Assoc Endodont. 2015:1–7.
Doyle SL, Hodges JS, Pesun IJ. Retrospective cross-sectional comparison of initial nonsurgical endodontic treatment and single tooth implants. J Endodont. 2006;32:822–7.
Featherstone JD, Domejean-Orliaguet SOPHIE, Jenson L, Wolff M, Young DA. Caries risk assessment in practice for age 6 through adult. J Calif Dent Assoc. 2007;35(10):703.
Gargiulo AW, Wentz FM, Orban B. Dimensions and relations of the dentogingival junction in humans. J Periodontol. 1961;32(3):261–7.
Gargiulo A, Krajewski J, Gargiulo M. Defining biologic width in crown lengthening. CDS review. 1995;88(5):20–3.
Gatten DL, Riedy CA, Hong SK, et al. Quality of life of endodontically treated versus implant treated patients: a university-based qualitative research study. J Endod. 2011;37:903–9.
Gibbard LL, Zarb G. A 5-year prospective study of implant-supported single-tooth replacements. J Can Dent Assoc. 2002;68(2):110–7.
Goodacre C. Tooth retention through root canal treatment or tooth replacement using implants or fixed partial dentures: which treatment is best? American Academy of Fixed Prosthodontics 2016 Conference; 2016.
Gotfredsen K. A 5-year prospective study of single-tooth replacements supported by the Astra Tech® implant: a pilot study. Clin Implant Dent Relat Res. 2004;6(1):1–8.
Hermann JS, Buser D, Schenk RK, Higginbottom FL, Cochran DL. Biologic width around titanium implants. A physiologically formed and stable dimension over time. Clin Oral Implants Res. 2000;11(1):1–11.
Holm-Pedersen P, Lang NP, Müller F. What are longevities of teeth and oral implants? J Clin Oral Implant Res. 2007;18 Suppl 3:15–9.
Ingber JS, Rose LF, Coslet JG. The "biologic width" – a concept in periodontics and restorative dentistry. Alpha Omegan. 1977;70(3):62–5.
Iqbal MK, Kim S. For teeth requiring endodontic treatment, what are the differences in outcomes of restored endodontically treated teeth compared to implant-supported restorations? Int J Oral Maxillofac Implants. 2007;22(Suppl):96–116.
Iqbal MK, Kim S. A review of factors influencing treatment planning decisions of single-tooth implants versus preserving natural teeth with nonsurgical endodontic therapy. J Endod. 2008;34:519–29.
Isidor, F, Brøndum K, and Ravnholt G. The influence of post length and crown ferrule length on the resistance to cyclic loading of bovine teeth with prefabricated titanium posts. Int J Prothodont. 1999;12(1):78–82.
Jorgensen MG, Nowzari H. Aesthetic crown lengthening. Periodontol 2000. 2001;27(1):45–58.
Jotkowitz A, Samet N. Rethinking ferrule–a new approach to an old dilemma. Br Dent J. 2010;209(1):25–33.
Jung R, Zembic A, Pjetursson BE, Zwahlen M, S Thoma D. Systematic review of the survival rate and the incidence of biological, technical, and aesthetic complications of single crowns on implants reported in longitudinal studies with a mean follow-up of 5 years. Clinical Oral Implants Research. 2012;23(s6):p2–21.
Kina JR, dos Santos PH, Kina EFU, Suzuki TYU, dos Santos PL. Periodontal and prosthetic biologic considerations to restore biological width in posterior teeth. J Craniofacial Surg. 2011;22(5):1913–6.
Levin L, Halperin-Sternfeld M. Tooth preservation or implant placement: a systematic review of long-term tooth and implant survival rates. J Am Dent Assoc. 2013;144:1119–33.
Libman WJ, Nicholls JI. Load failure of teeth restored with cast posts and cores and complete crowns. Int J Prothodont. 1995;8:155–60.
Linkevicius T, Apse P. Biologic width around implants. An evidence-based. Stomatologija. 2008;10(1):27–35.
Mankani N, Chowdhary R, Patil BA, Nagaraj E, Madalli P. Osseointegrated dental implants in growing children: a literature review. J Oral Implantol. 2014;40(5):627–31.
Misch CE. Dental implant prosthetics. 2nd edn. Elsevier Publishing, Inc.; 2015, p. 52.

Misch CE, Perel ML, Wang HL, Sammartino G, Galindo-Moreno P, Trisi P, Steigmann M, Rebaudi A, Palti A, Pikos MA, Schwartz-Arad D. Implant success, survival, and failure: the International Congress of Oral Implantologists (ICOI) pisa consensus conference. Implant Dent. 2008;17(1):5–15.

Morris HF, Winkler S, Ochi S. A 48-month multicentric clinical investigation: implant design and survival. J Oral Implantol. 2001;27(4):180–6.

National Institutes of Health Consensus Development Conference statement on dental implants (June 13–15, 1988). J Dent Educ. 1988;52:824.

Ng YL, Mann V, Gulabivala K. Tooth survival following non-surgical root canal treatment: a systematic review of the literature. Int Endod J. 2010;43(3):171–89.

Ng YL, Mann V, Gulabivala K. A prospective study of the factors affecting outcomes of nonsurgical root canal treatment: part 1: periapical health. Int Endod J. 2011;44(7):583–609.

Norton MR. Biologic and mechanical stability of single-tooth implants: 4-to 7-year follow-up. Clin Implant Dent Relat Res. 2001;3(4):214–20.

Oh SL. Biologic width and crown lengthening: case reports and review. Gen Dent. 2010;58(5):e200–5.

Padbury A, Eber R, Wang HL. Interactions between the gingiva and the margin of restorations. J Clin Periodontol. 2003;30(5):379–85.

Papaspyridakos P, Chen CJ, Singh M, Weber HP, Gallucci GO. Success criteria in implant dentistry a systematic review. J Dent Res. 2012;91(3):242–8.

Pradeep K, Rajesh H, Rao PK, et al. Implant or root canal treatment: clinical guidelines and decision making. J Dent Implant. 2013;3:67–72.

Reitemeier B, Hänsel K, Walter MH, Kastner C, Toutenburg H. Effect of posterior crown margin placement on gingival health. J Prosthet Dent. 2002;87(2):167–72.

Rosenberg ES, Garber DA, Evian CI. Tooth lengthening procedures. Compend Contin Educ Gen Dent. 1979;1(3):161–72.

Rosenstiel SF, Land MF, Fujimoto J. Contemporary fixed prosthodontics.5th end. Elsevier Health Sciences. St Louis, Missouri; 2015.

Salinas TJ, Eckert SE. In patients requiring single tooth replacement, what are the outcomes of implants as compared to tooth-supported restorations? Part I of a descriptive analysis. Int J Oral Maxillofac Imp. 2007;22(Suppl):71–95.

Sanavi F, Weisgold AS, Rose LF. Biologic width and its relation to periodontal biotypes. J Esthet Restor Dent. 1998;10(3):157–63.

Schmidt JC, Sahrmann P, Weiger R, Schmidlin PR, Walter C. Biologic width dimensions–a systematic review. J Clin Periodontol. 2013;40(5):493–504.

Schroeder A, Sutter F, Buser D, Krekeler G, editors. Oral implantology. 2nd ed. New York: Thieme Medical Publishers; 1996.

Scurria MS, Shugars DA, Hayden WJ, Felton DA. General dentists'patterns of restoring: endodontically treated teeth. J Am Dent Assoc. 1995;126(6):775–9.

Scurria MS, Bader JD, Shugars DA. Meta-analysis of fixed partial denture survival: prosthesis and abutments. J Prosthet Dent. 1998;79(4):459–64.

Sorensen JA, Engelman MJ. Ferrule design and fracture resistance of endodontically treated teeth. J Prosthet Dent. 1990;63:529–36.

Stockhausen R, Aseltine Jr R, Matthews JG, et al. The perceived prognosis of endodontic treatment and implant therapy among dental practitioners. Oral Surg Oral Med Oral Pathol Oral Radiol Endod. 2011;111:42–7.

Tan PL, Aquilino SA, Gratton DG, Stanford CM, Tan SC, Johnson WT, Dawson D. In vitro fracture resistance of endodontically treated central incisors with varying ferrule heights and configurations. J Prosthet Dent. 2005;93(4):331–6.

Tomasi C, Wennström JL, Berglundh T. Longevity of teeth and implants – a systematic review. J Oral Rehabil. 2008;35 Suppl 1:23–32.

Torabinejad M, Goodacre CJ. Endodontic or dental implant therapy: the factors affecting treatment planning. J Am Dent Assoc. 2006;137(7):973–7.

Torabinejad M, Kutsenko D, Machnick TK, Ismail A, Newton CW. Levels of evidence for the outcome of nonsurgical endodontic treatment. J Endod. 2005;31(9):637–46.

Torabinejad M, Anderson P, Bader J, Brown JB, Chen LH, Goodacre CJ, Kattadiyil MT, Kutsenko D, Lozada J, Patel R, Petersen F, Puterman I, White SN. Outcomes of root canal treatment and restoration, implant-supported single crowns, fixed partial dentures, and extraction without replacement: a systematic review. J Prosthet Dent. 2007;98:285–311.

Torabinejad M, Salha W, Lozada JL, et al. Degree of patient pain, complications, and satisfaction after root canal treatment or a single implant: a preliminary prospective investigation. J Endod. 2014;40:1940–5.

Wang CH, Chueh LH, Chen SC, Feng YC, Hsiao CK, Chiang CP. Impact of diabetes mellitus, hypertension, and coronary artery disease on tooth extraction after nonsurgical endodontic treatment. J Endod. 2011;37(1):1–5.

Wolcott J, Meyers J. Endodontic re-treatment or implants: a contemporary conundrum. Compend Contin Educ Dent (Jamesburg, NJ: 1995). 2006;27(2):104–10.

Yilmaz B, McGlumphy E. Implant-supported fixed prosthesis. In: Rosensteil S, Land M, Fujimoto J (editors) Contemporary fixed prosthodontics. 5th edn. Elsevier; 2016, p. 318–66.

Zarb G, Albrektsson T. Osseointegration – a requiem for the periodontal ligament? – An editorial. Int J Periodont Rest Dentistry. 1991;11:88.

Zhi-Yue L, Yu-Xing Z. Effects of post-core design and ferrule on fracture resistance of endodontically treated maxillary central incisors. J Prosthet Dent. 2003;89(4):368–73.

Zitzmann NU, Krastl G, Hecker H, Weiger R. Endodontics or implants? A review of decisive criteria and guidelines for single tooth restorations and full arch reconstructions. Int Endod J. 2009;42(9):757–74.

Restorative Considerations for Endodontically Treated Teeth

6

John R. Antonelli

Contents

Abstract

Most nonvital teeth suffer from a loss of structural integrity. The amount of remaining tooth structure dictates the type of restoration that can be used to restore pulpless teeth. There remains some controversy about the quantity of lost coronal tooth structure that justifies the need to use a post as well as how to restore an endodontically treated tooth to protect all remaining tooth structure. The variety of post and core buildup systems available contributes to the level of uncertainty.

J.R. Antonelli, DDS, MS
Professor Director of fixed Prosthodontics Courses, Department of Prosthodontics, Nova Southeastern University College of Dental Medicine, Fort Lauderdale, FL, USA

Adjunct Professor, Department of Prosthodontics, The University of Tennessee Health Science Center College of Dentistry, Memphis, TN, USA
e-mail: antonell@nova.edu

G.M. Weinstein, M.T. Zientz (eds.), *The Dental Reference Manual*,
DOI 10.1007/978-3-319-39730-6_6

Preparation design parameters of nonvital teeth are a critical consideration in the restoration of endodontically treated teeth. The ferrule effect or the encircling band of cast metal around circumferential axial dentin coronal to the preparation finish line improves the integrity of an endodontically treated tooth. The benefits of a ferrule or circumferential area of axial dentin superior to the preparation finish line has been shown in the literature to minimize tooth fracture by counteracting functional forces. This chapter seeks to help the dental student and practitioner make evidence-based decisions to complete a thorough diagnosis and develop the most appropriate treatment plan for the restoration of endodontically treated teeth.

6.1 Endodontically Treated Teeth: To Post or Not to Post?

When planning to restore an endodontically treated tooth, clinicians often must decide whether or not to use a post. On this issue, there continues to be much confusion among students, and there is a diversity of "opinion" among dentists about the need for posts in different clinical situations. The indication for placing a post depends on the amount of tooth structure remaining in a tooth being considered for root canal therapy. Evidence-based decisions should be made by:

1. Quantifying tooth loss and relating it to the decision whether or not to place a post
2. Examining evidence that might influence treatment decisions and strategies regarding post placement
3. Providing some tooth preparation design parameters to guide clinicians and students in restoring endodontically treated teeth with posts and cores

Along with an assessment of the quantity of remaining tooth structure, an accurate evaluation of root canal treatment must be completed before considering whether to place a post-core or a definitive restoration. An accurate evaluation of root canal treatment should be based on a diagnosis of clinical symptoms and observation of follow-up radiographs. The tooth's dentinal structure must be solid—without craze lines or fissures, which might be the origin of later fractures. Clinical evaluation of any endodontically treated tooth must not reveal (1) sensitivity to percussion, (2) exudate, (3) fistula, and (4) apical sensitivity to palpation.

There is a common belief that endodontically treated teeth are weaker or more brittle than teeth that have not been treated endodontically. This has not been demonstrated experimentally. An in vitro study (Sedgley and Messer 1992) of endodontically treated teeth that compared them to their contralateral vital pairs showed that there was no significant biomechanical (strength) change to indicate that the endodontically treated teeth had become more brittle. These findings were supported by another study of matched tooth pairs, conducted 2 years later, which found that vital dentin and dentin from endodontically treated teeth had moisture contents of 12.35 % and 12.10 %, respectively (Papa et al. 1994). Both studies showed no significant difference in the moisture content between endodontically treated teeth and vital teeth.

Table 6.1 Reduction in cuspal stiffness for tooth preparations (3)

Type of tooth preparation	% reduction in stiffness
Conservative endodontic access	5
Occlusal cavity preparation	20
MO or DO preparation involving at least one marginal ridge	46
MOD preparation involving both marginal ridges	63

The quantity of tooth structure remaining—not moisture content or brittleness—has the greatest influence on tooth stability (strength). The evidence that follows should help to clarify the relationship between tooth loss and tooth stability.

6.1.1 The Need for Cuspal Protection

When the effects of conservative endodontic and restorative procedures on tooth strength were compared, it was found that a conservative endodontic access preparation resulted in only a 5 % reduction in cuspal stiffness (Reeh et al. 1989a) (Table 6.1). Strand et al. (1995) found that the distance of the tooth preparation from the marginal ridge is more important to tooth strength than its bucco-palatal width. Preservation of the marginal ridge seems to be important to the overall structural stability of teeth. Cuspal deflection during function increases with increasing cavity size and is greatest following endodontic access preparation (Panitvisai and Messer 1995; Faria et al. 2011). Increased cuspal deflection raises the likelihood of cusp fracture and microleakage at the margins of restorations. The loss of structural integrity resulting from access preparation—not changes in the dentin—will lead to a higher incidence of tooth fracture in endodontically treated teeth compared with vital teeth (Reeh et al. 1989a). Axial reduction for full-coverage crown preparation (peripheral destruction) combined with tooth reduction from endodontic access preparation (central destruction) often results in insufficient remaining dental tissue to withstand occlusal loads without cuspal coverage (Shillingburg et al. 2012). As we shall see, this is especially true of premolars.

The prognosis of an endodontically treated tooth depends on the quality of endodontic treatment and minimizing the chances for leakage of oral fluids and microbes into the canal space by prompt placement of a coronal restoration. In fact, it has been shown that only after 3-day exposure to artificial saliva, there was extensive coronal leakage through apparently sound endodontic gutta-percha fillings (Saunders and Saunders 1994). In a retrospective study of 1273 endodontically treated posterior teeth without coronal coverage (i.e., lacking a restoration that at least covers cusps), the failure rate was between 39 and 50 % (Sorensen and Martinoff 1984a). In another study, endodontically treated teeth that were not crowned after obturation failed at a rate six times greater than teeth crowned after obturation (Aquilino and Caplan 2002). When 220 endodontically treated permanent molars without coronal coverage were evaluated, overall survival (i.e., lack of tooth fractures) at 1, 2, and 5 years were 96 %, 88 %, and 36 %, respectively (Nagasiri and Chitmongkolsuk 2005). The 5-year survival rate of molars with Class I access cavity preparations and at least 2.0 mm of axial wall thickness was 78 % (i.e., 22 % had failed). More than 50 years ago, Rosen (1961) described the hugging action (encirclement) of vertical axial tooth structure provided by a crown, and he referred to it as the extracoronal brace. Encirclement of a circumferential area of axial dentin superior to the preparation finish line is known today as the ferrule effect, which protects a tooth from fracture. This concept will be described further.

The advantages of adhesive restorations (dentin bonding) have misled some clinicians into believing that the creation of a monoblock dentin-post-core complex would enable more uniform distribution of forces along the root, maximize a tooth's ability to absorb stresses, and minimize the possibility of root fracture. This belief has caused some clinicians to minimize the benefits of coronal coverage and the ferrule effect (Morgano 2015). Costa's in vitro study (Costa and Pegoraro 1997) evaluated the fracture resistance (strength) of endodontically treated teeth with MOD preparations restored with (1) amalgam restorations, (2) bonded cast inlays, and (3) onlays cemented with zinc phosphate. Fracture resistance proved to be the greatest for group 3 and least for group 1. The need for cuspal coverage of endodontically treated posterior teeth is revealed further in a clinical study in which bonded Empress inlays were evaluated (Stoll et al. 2007). Results of this long-term study revealed a survival rate of 53 % (or 47 % failure rate) after only 23 months, and failures began to surface early in the study. Restoration of endodontically treated teeth with inlays was not recommended. The amount of remaining coronal tooth structure appears to have the most influence on survival rates of endodontically treated teeth. According to Rosenstiel (2016), posterior teeth are subjected to greater occlusal loads than anterior teeth because they are closer to the fulcrum of the jaw (the temporomandibular joint) in what is a Class III lever system. The longest lever arm in a Class III lever has the weakest force, which is why much less force can be applied to an object placed between the central incisors than between molars. Consequently, this fact and the morphology that characterizes posterior teeth (a divided occlusal surface with cusps that can be wedged apart) make them susceptible to fracture, especially during excursive movements when working and/or balancing interferences are present. Endodontically treated posterior teeth should be restored with cuspal coverage to prevent bite forces from causing tooth fracture. Although they are in a minority, endodontically treated premolars or molars with sufficient remaining sound tooth structure should be restored with a cast or bonded all-ceramic restoration with occlusal coverage, such as an MOD onlay. Perhaps the only exceptions are when mandibular premolars and first molars have conservative access preparations and substantial remaining marginal ridge widths of at least 2.0 and 1.6 mm, respectively, and are protected by canine guided occlusion. Endodontically treated maxillary premolars especially are at higher risk for failure, and complete coverage restorations are recommended to protect against fracture.

6.1.2 Rationale for Using Posts to Restore Anterior Teeth

The decision to use a post to restore and endodontically treated tooth should be based on the quantity of remaining coronal tooth structure after removal of all caries and remaining restorative materials and the type of tooth. Traditionally, an

Table 6.2 Efficacy of post placement in anterior teeth

Studies on anterior teeth endodontically treated	No post	Post placed	Years of survival of tooth after treatment
Ross (1980)	61 %	Nonapplicable	5 years or more
Sorensen and Martinoff (1984a, b)	84.7 %	89.4 %	1–25 years

endodontically treated tooth received a post to reinforce it and a full- or partial-coverage crown to protect it from occlusal load forces. Retrospective clinical studies have prompted a reevaluation of this strategy (Table 6.2). Similar success rates were uncovered for endodontically treated anterior teeth with and without crowns—87.5 % and 85.4 %, respectively. Lovdahl and Nicholls (1977) found that the mean failure load of endodontically treated maxillary central incisors with intact crowns was approximately 3.6 times greater than those restored with cast gold post-cores. Two in vitro studies revealed that inserting posts in relatively intact endodontically treated anterior teeth does not increase their fracture resistance (Guzy and Nicholls 1979; McDonald et al. 1990). Clearly, endodontically treated anterior teeth do not always require complete coverage with a crown. A crown might be indicated when composite restorations will have a limited prognosis, as in the case of large proximal restorations and unsupported tooth structure. Previous research has demonstrated that endodontic access only in an otherwise intact tooth has only a minimal effect on the strength of the tooth (Steele and Johnson 1999; Reeh et al. 1989b). If the crown structure is largely intact and occlusal loading is favorable, as it often is on an anterior tooth far from the fulcrum (temporomandibular joint), then an endodontically treated anterior tooth with a conservative access preparation may be restored with composite placed in the access cavity. In cases where the crown is nearly intact, the tooth is better served with a conservative, bonded restoration (Fig. 6.1). If tooth devitalization results in discoloration of the crown, and shade change is needed, then bleaching is a better option than crown placement when the tooth is relatively intact (Goerig and Mueninghoff 1983a). When a restoration is necessary, the facial surface of a tooth could be restored less destructively with a porcelain laminate veneer.

6.1.3 Quantifying Tooth Loss

The primary purpose of a post is to retain core material that substitutes for missing extensive crown structure resulting from caries, previous restorations, trauma, and/or endodontic access. Often, in these teeth, insufficient axial tooth structure remains after tooth preparation for a full- or partial-coverage definitive restoration. The indication for post placement depends on the degree of coronal tooth destruction in a tooth that is being evaluated for endodontic treatment. Unfortunately, the amount of tooth destruction necessary to justify placing a post has not been defined clearly. An attempt to quantify the extent of destruction was detailed by Peroz et al. (2005). They used a classification that described five categories of crown destruction, based on the number of remaining axial walls. In the Class I category (the most conservative), the endodontic access cavity is surrounded by all four axial walls. Class II

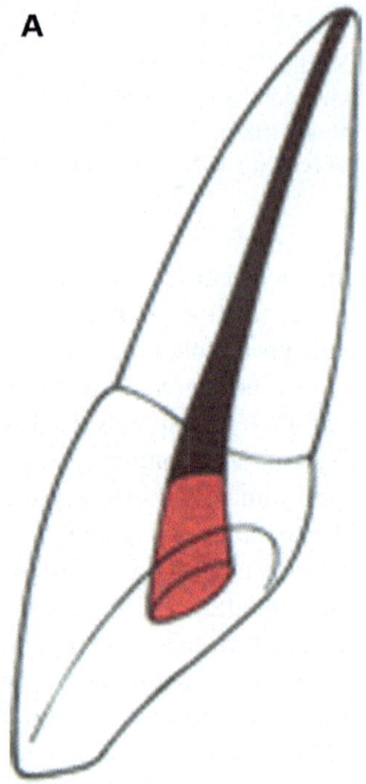

Fig. 6.1 Anterior teeth with intact crowns can be restored with composite restorations in the endodontic access cavity (Reproduced from Rosenstiel et al. (2016))

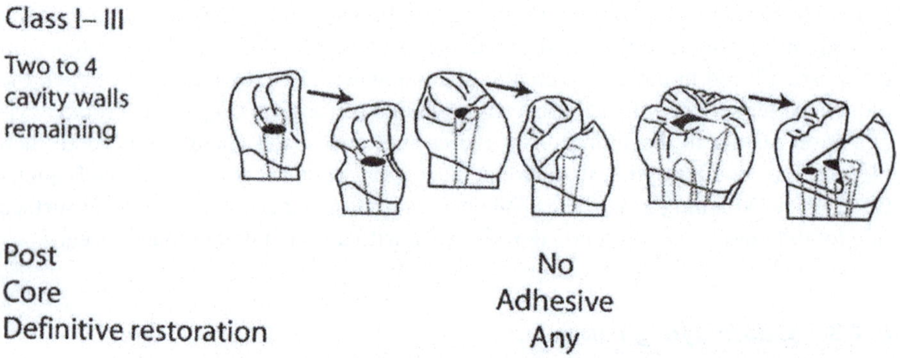

Fig. 6.2 A post is not required when at least two axial walls remain. If axial wall thickness after tooth preparation is >1 mm, a post is not required. When axial wall thickness prior to preparation is <2 mm, it must be considered as missing (Reproduced from Peroz et al. (2005))

describes the typical mesio-occlusal (MO) or disto-occlusal (DO) cavity in which one cavity wall is missing. Class III represents the MOD cavity with two remaining axial walls. In the Class IV category, a single axial wall—either buccal or lingual—remains. Class V depicts the crownless tooth with no remaining axial walls (Figs. 6.2, 6.3, and 6.4). A cavity wall thickness greater than 1.0 mm after tooth preparation should retain core material for a crown and is considered the absolute

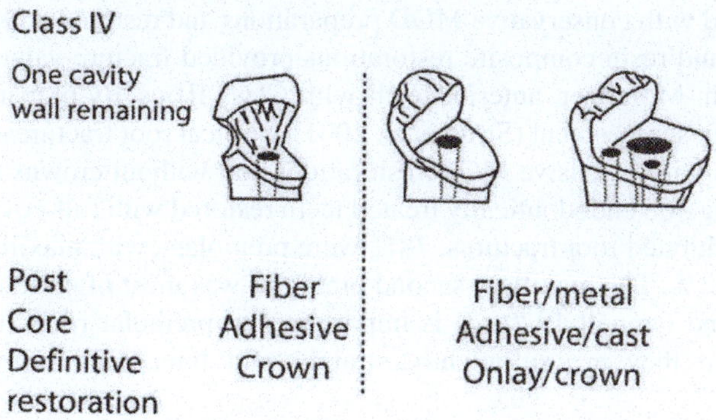

Fig. 6.3 A post is indicated when one cavity wall remains. Fiber posts are used in anterior teeth (metal is used with porcelain-metal crowns); fiber or metal posts are used in posterior teeth. A bonded composite core or cast post-core may be used. Full-coverage crowns should be made for anterior teeth; crowns or onlays are indicated for posterior teeth (Reproduced from Peroz et al. (2005))

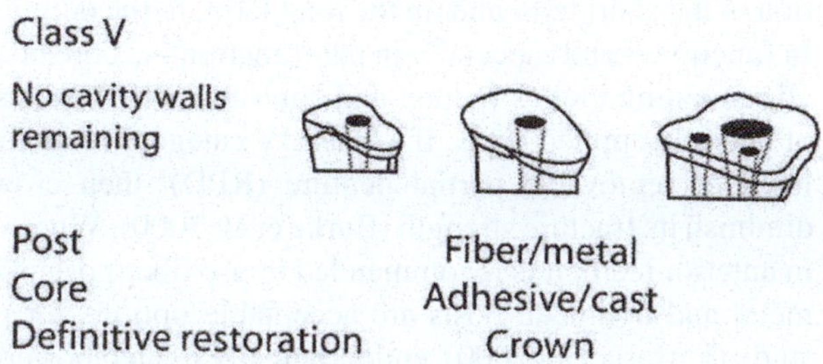

Fig. 6.4 A post (fiber or metal) must be used when no axial walls remain. A ferrule of at least 2 mm is needed to minimize root fracture (Reproduced from Peroz et al. (2005))

minimum to resist functional loads (Peroz et al. 2005; Pilo and Tamse 2000). When cusp thickness is less than 1.0 mm, teeth prepared for crowns will lose all remaining axial tooth structure (ferrule) for strength and stability. The ferrule may be defined as a circumferential area of axial dentin superior to the preparation finish line. The design of the ferrule will be discussed further.

According to Peroz et al. (2005), if Class I, II, and III cavity walls have thicknesses greater than 1.0 mm and axial heights of at least 2.0 mm, then a post is not recommended. Most types of definitive restorations may be considered in these situations because remaining coronal tissues provide sufficient surface area for building cores with adhesive systems. Research by Steele and Johnson (1999) compared the fracture resistance (strength) of endodontically treated premolars with conservative MOD cavity preparations and endodontic access preparations. The teeth received either amalgam or composite resin restorations. Their study revealed that the addition of both restorations increased the resistance to fracture, although never approaching the strength of unaltered (control) teeth or teeth with standard endodontic access preparations only. They noted that teeth with access preparations only were more resistant to fracture than MOD preparations. A study by Ausiello et al. (1997), using maxillary premolars, disclosed that the fracture resistance of teeth prepared with conservative MOD preparations and restored with dentin bonding systems and resin composite restorations provided fracture values comparable to intact teeth. Moreover, anterior teeth with Class III cavity preparations do not benefit from post placement (Strub et al. 2001). Vertical root fractures were noted in 28 % of teeth with extensive MOD restorations and without crowns (Testore et al. 1993). Among 468 endodontically treated teeth restored with full-coverage crowns, and which exhibited root fractures, 78 % were premolars, with maxillary premolars comprising 62 %. The maxillary second premolar was most often found to be fractured (Rud and Omnell 1970). It is important that premolar roots have sufficient bulk and that they are sufficiently straight and long prior to restoring with post-cores.

When only one cavity wall remains (as in the Class IV category), the fracture resistance of endodontically treated mandibular molars is not enhanced by core buildups with different materials (Foley et al. 1997). A core buildup restoration must be capable of withstanding the rigors of crown preparation and impression procedures. It must contribute to the retention and support of a provisional restoration in the short term and, in the long term, to the definitive extracoronal restoration. In function—and especially in parafunction—a core buildup transmits axial loads to all remaining tooth structure and contributes to the resistance form and distribution of laterally applied loads. If a Class IV category tooth must serve as an abutment for fixed or removable partial denture (RPD), then crown preparation will further diminish its fracture strength (Burke et al. 2000). When only one cavity wall remains in anterior teeth, it is recommended to use fiber posts with all-ceramic crowns; both metal and nonmetal posts are acceptable options for posterior teeth. In a clinical study (Ferrari et al. 2000), endodontically treated posterior teeth with one remaining coronal wall and a post experienced a restorability success rate of 95 % after 2 years. When posts were omitted, the success rate declined to 30 % over the same period.

6.1.4 Ferrule

When there are no remaining cavity walls (as in the Class V category), a post is needed to secure the core to the root. Also, the post must transfer bite forces to surrounding root structure. The post is most effective when it distributes those forces over the entire wall of the post space to minimize concentration of stresses to any particular area. In extensively damaged crowns, the post provides the definitive crown restoration with retention that would have otherwise been obtained from coronal tooth structure. In the Class V category, the ferrule makes a major contribution toward preserving the fracture resistance of a tooth because it provides the major anchorage for the core. When a crown encircles 1.5–2.0 mm of vertical axial tooth structure (with a minimum horizontal thickness of 1.0 mm) above the finish line, it will help minimize the risk of a root splitting open under stresses generated by the post (Shillingburg et al. 2012).

Endodontically treated posterior teeth with no remaining cavity walls and ferrules less than 2.0 mm showed a success rate of 80 % when posts were inserted.

When posts were omitted, the success rate fell to 40 % (Ferrari et al. 2000). In an in vitro study, maxillary central incisors restored with cast post-cores and full-coverage crowns were subjected to cyclical fatigue loads within the range of physiological masticatory loads (Libman and Nicholls 1995). Teeth prepared with 1.0-mm ferrules survived 10 times more cyclical loads before their cement seals fractured at the crown margins than those with 0.5-mm ferrules. Crowns on teeth with 1.5-mm ferrules survived 63 times as many cyclical loads as those with 1.0-mm ferrules. Although most studies concur that ferrules improve fracture resistance and help protect the integrity of the cement seal of the artificial crown, sufficient coronal tooth structure is absent in many instances. A study of endodontically treated incisors by Rendez da Silva et al. (2010) showed that teeth lacking a ferrule that were restored with ceramic crowns exhibited higher fracture resistance than those restored with metal crowns. In fact, the use of ceramic crowns in this study seemed to nearly overcome the problem of lack of ferrule; however, the fracture patterns seen in teeth without ferrules, and restored with ceramic crowns, were more serious compared to teeth restored with metal crowns. In a review of available clinical studies, Dietschi et al. (2008) stated that fatigue studies support conservation of tooth structure and the presence of a circumferential ferrule to optimize tooth biomechanical properties. The studies clearly indicate that resistance to failure of core buildups and natural crown structure increases with the amount of tooth structure remaining. Every attempt should be made to incorporate a ferrule bracing of at least 1.5 mm (optimally 2.0 mm) because with sufficient ferrule, post length and post design features (i.e., parallel sided or tapered) take on a subordinate role (Weine et al. 1991; Assif et al. 1993; Sorensen and Engelman 1990).

Goodacre et al. (2003) reviewed 12 clinical studies, which evaluated almost 3000 posts and cores. A mean complication incidence of 10 % was reported over a time span ranging from 1 to 25 years. Among the most common complications relating to post and cores, post dislodgement accounted for 5 % and root fracture 3 %. The ferrule helps minimize root fracture by encircling tooth structure.

A Ferrule Performs Three Additional Functions

1. Protects the post against fracture
2. Minimizes post dislodgement
3. Protects the cement seal at the margin of the crown

A search of the literature on fracture threshold revealed that if the intaglio surface of the crown apposes 1.5–2.0 mm of ferrule, then the force needed to fracture the tooth is increased. Among the 788 posts studied by Torbjőrner et al. (1995), 5.7 % dislodged from the canal space and 2.7 % failed because of root fracture. All 6 (0.8 %) post fractures were attributed to a lack of ferrule. These findings are in agreement with those of Goodacre et al. (2003). The results of both studies show that if the margin of a crown and the core-tooth interface are at the same cervical level, then all forces of occlusion will be placed on the post that exits the post space; eventually, the post could fatigue and fracture. When a crown rests entirely on core material, occlusal stresses are concentrated on root structure, close to the crown

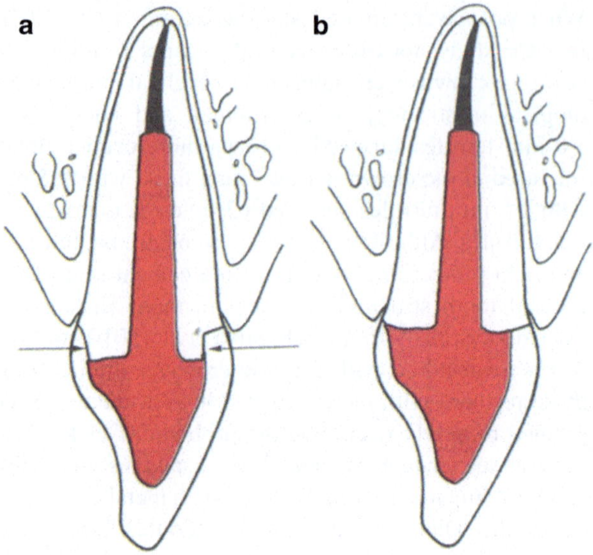

Fig. 6.5 Preparation of a ferrule (*arrows* in **a**) minimizes fracture of an endodontically treated tooth during function. (**b**) Preparation of tooth without a ferrule (Reproduced from Rosenstiel et al. (2016))

margin. In this scenario, vertical root fracture is more likely. The complete coverage crown with a 2-mm ferrule on sound tooth structure will change the distribution of forces to the root and the post-core complex. A circumferential ferrule helps minimize the chances for damage to the tooth and the post-core complex when they are subjected to occlusal loads (Ree and Schwartz 2010; Morgano et al. 2004). The most important design feature of the tooth preparation to protect it from fracture is likely to be a 360° ferrule, with a minimal vertical height of 1.5–2.0 mm above the finish line (Eissmann and Radke 1976; Schwartz and Robbins 2004) (Fig. 6.5).

A classical study by Kaufman et al. (1961) showed that most retention in full-coverage crown preparation designs is derived from the cervical areas of the preparations; therefore, inclusion of a circumferential ferrule provides sound tooth structure in a critical area. When a core is added to increase the axial height of a tooth preparation, it enhances resistance, or the ability of the preparation to prevent dislodgment of the restoration by forces directed in an apical, oblique, or horizontal direction.

6.1.5 Biologic Width and Crown Lengthening

One microleakage study found that with dynamic loading, as the height of the ferrule increases, the potential for leakage into the crown decreases (Libman and Nicholls 1995). Microleakage was observed to progress between the crown margin and finish line, up the ferrule, and then into the tooth-core interface. Leakage patterns that invade the tooth-core junction eventually progress into the post space. Often, if a crown is placed on a tooth that lacks an adequate ferrule, then fracture of the underlying preparation is likely, most probably in the region of the crown margin where stress is greatest and the tooth is thinnest. Perhaps a modification in treatment planning should be considered when a tooth lacks a circumferential ferrule of at least 1.5 mm, especially when the final restoration will be subjected to increased occlusal loads, as a fixed partial denture (FPD) abutment, or an abutment for a distal extension RPD. Increasing ferrule height might be accomplished by preparing the finish line farther apically without invading the biologic width (i.e., the combination of connective tissue attachment and epithelial adhesion to root. Two millimeters is the average minimum space of the biologic width). In general, to avoid biologic width impingement, the minimum distance required from the osseous crest to the final restoration margin is approximately 2.5 mm. Subgingival margin placement should not exceed half the depth of the gingival sulcus (Rosenstiel et al. 2016). If this is not possible for those teeth with severe coronal destruction, then it might be necessary to perform periodontal crown lengthening or orthodontic extrusion to increase ferrule height. The choice between each option should be based on the effect each procedure will have on the esthetic outcome of the case (e.g., gingival margin location and symmetry), the possibility of creating an unfavorable crown-to-root ratio, or uncovering furcations in the tooth and in neighboring teeth as well. When little crown structure remains and the furcation is high, crown lengthening is usually not indicated because the long-term prognosis of the tooth is poor. Extraction is a better alternative than placing a well-executed restoration on a questionable tooth (Faria et al. 2011).

Kovarik et al. (1992) have shown that the type of core material one uses also impacts on the integrity of the cement seal. When teeth were prepared with less than 1.0-mm ferrules (where occlusal forces were shouldered by the post-core materials), and restored with prefabricated posts and flexible composite cores, 83 % of the cores eventually failed. Fifty percent of the failures occurred as a result of failure of the zinc phosphate cement at the crown-core interface, the post-root interface, or both. Forty percent of the failures were the result of fractured posts. Failures were attributed to the flexure of composite cores under dynamic loading, which placed increased shearing stresses at the cement interface, and just below the junction of the post with the core material. In these situations, leakage of a crown is often impossible to detect clinically because the crown will remain on the tooth as long as the post and core are cemented. Although everything appears to be intact, microleakage can occur along the cement crack, and this can result in a radiographically undetectable carious lesion in the structure of the tooth beneath the crown. The core material that held up best in this study was amalgam, although the failure rate was still unacceptably high at 33 %. All core buildups with glass ionomer failed.

Conclusions by Kovarik et al. (1992) Regarding Cores

1. Almost any core material might be acceptable with 2 mm of circumferential vertical dentin that extends coronally from the finish line of the preparation (i.e., the ferrule).
2. When remaining tooth structure is scarce, the choice of core materials is critical.
3. The use of composite resin or reinforced glass ionomer core buildup materials should be avoided when very little axial tooth structure remains.

6.1.6 Restorative Problems Associated with Premolars

Thin roots and radicular fluting (a mesio-proximal invagination of the tooth, near the cemento-enamel junction [CEJ]), characteristic of many maxillary first premolars, can pose a particularly great restorative challenge. When there is little remaining crown structure, crown lengthening or orthodontic eruption might be needed to obtain adequate ferrule. Either procedure could result in uncovering the fluted area or furcation, which could create prosthodontic or periodontal maintenance problems. Another potential problem associated with restoring premolars involves the location and number of posts to be placed. The problem was uncovered in a study that was designed to investigate the point at which cyclic loads, directed at maxillary first premolars, would cause crack propagation in the cement seals of full-coverage crowns cemented over cores maintained with prefabricated and cast posts (Fan et al. 1995). Each tooth in the study was prepared with a 1.0-mm ferrule and received an occlusal load, within a functional range, that was directed to the palatal incline of the buccal cusp. Posts and crowns were cemented with zinc phosphate. When posts—cast and prefabricated stainless steel (with amalgam cores)—were cemented into palatal canals, all specimens exceeded the upper limits of 250,000 cyclic loads without evidence of crack propagation in the cement layer of the crowns. Similar results were observed when two stainless-steel prefabricated posts (with amalgam cores) were cemented. However, when posts were placed in buccal canals only, failure occurred after an average of 164 cyclic loads. The authors recommended placing two posts when restoring endodontically treated and structurally compromised premolars to ensure protection from occlusal forces from either the buccal or palatal/lingual directions. Cracks in the cement seal are impossible to detect clinically; therefore, the choice of post location could have a profound effect on the survival of a restoration. When teeth with full-coverage crowns experience preliminary failure (i.e., cracks in the luting cement caused by cyclic loading), leakage of microbes could progress to the coronal level of the gutta-percha and compromise the root canal seals (Freeman et al. 1998). Gutta-percha does not present an effective barrier to leakage down the canal space. The evidence presented highlights the importance of adequate ferrule height for teeth being considered for full-coverage restorations and the need for crown lengthening or orthodontic eruption when there is minimal coronal tooth structure available to design a ferrule.

While some groups of teeth will not require a post in many clinical situations, Sadan (2002) recommended placing post-cores in the majority of premolars that must be restored with full-coverage crowns. His concerns were based on their relatively narrow diameter at the CEJ and their relatively wide buccolingual dimension at the height of contour—i.e., many premolars have "narrow waists" and "broad shoulders." Current design parameters for finish lines for full-coverage crowns advocate deep chamfer or shoulder widths in the range of 0.9–1.2 mm for maximum esthetics in porcelain (Rosenstiel et al. 2016). With this in mind, when an endodontically treated premolar is prepared for a full-coverage crown and a deep finish line is prepared, a significant quantity of crown structure will be eliminated at the height of contour before the chamfer or shoulder can be fashioned, even when the prepared tooth is tapered minimally (6–10°), which is not likely on many posterior teeth. Often, what remains is a tooth preparation with very thin axial wall structure. The crown of the tooth is further compromised structurally as additional dentin is removed from inside the crown to create an access preparation for endodontic treatment. The resultant tooth preparation often contains paper thin axial walls or areas that lack axial dentin. It must be remembered that in function, complete coverage crowns distribute stresses over axial dentin, transfer loads to the post-core, and provide the ferrule effect to minimize root fracture. When a crack propagates within the luting cement, any resisting force provided by the cement is increasingly transferred to the post. Eventually, the post could become the last remaining structure to resist applied loads, which could result ultimately in catastrophic failure of the restoration.

Older retrospective studies often failed to specify whether a ferrule was present in the teeth that were tested. Conversely, the concept of a ferrule and its importance to the survival of restorations is addressed in some newer prospective studies. For example, a study by Ellner et al. (2003) examined fifty single-rooted teeth in need of single full-coverage crowns. Especially meaningful was the fact that the study evaluated four different post-core systems over a period of up to 10 years. All teeth had a ferrule at least 2.0 mm in height. The following post-core systems were evaluated: system 1, conventional tapered post-cores cast in gold alloy; system 2, prefabricated gold ParaPosts and cast gold cores; system 3, the ParaPost system (using burnout patterns) with cast gold post-cores; and system 4, Radix Anchor-threaded titanium posts with resin cores. Teeth receiving Radix Anchor posts were excluded from the randomization process as the shape of the core sections was too large and could not be used to restore teeth. The overall failure rate for all four groups was 6 %. When the Radix Anchor posts were excluded, the failure rate diminished to 3 % over the 10-year period, which represented a very good success rate. In the literature, threaded posts are associated with greater failure rates (Mentink et al. 1993). A meta-analysis of ten in vitro and six in vivo studies revealed no significant difference in the performances of direct and cast post-cores (Heydecke and Peters 2002). Also, no statistically significant differences were found between prefabricated (direct) and cast post-core systems that would justify recommending one over the other (Reagan et al. 1999).

In a prospective study by Creugers et al. (2005), in which the follow-up rate was 5 years, 319 teeth were studied to determine whether (1) the survival rate of cast post-core restorations was greater than the survival of direct metal post and resin core restorations and post-free (all-composite) restorations; and (2) the survival rate of the buildup restoration was influenced by the length of the ferrule in teeth restored with full-coverage crowns. Two hundred one prepared teeth contained a collar of dentin sufficient in height for a classical ferrule; 118 teeth contained a minimal collar of dentin—not sufficient for a classical ferrule. Restorations made on teeth with sufficient ferrule had a 98 % survival rate; restorations made on teeth with a minimal collar of dentin had a survival rate of 93 %. Post-core restorations fabricated for teeth with a sufficient ferrule performed significantly better than those placed on teeth that lacked sufficient ferrule. The evidence is compelling that ferrule height is more important to the survival of the restoration than the design of the core buildup.

A prospective study from the endodontic literature compared the survival rates of endodontically treated teeth restored by different post-core systems and compared them to endodontically treated teeth without post-core restorations (Salvi et al. 2007). Restored teeth served as abutments for single metal-ceramic crowns, composite crowns, or FPDs. Post-cores were omitted only in teeth in which approximately two-thirds of the remaining clinical crown structure was still available. A dentin ferrule was incorporated in all tooth preparations. Although it was not specifically stated by the authors, it is assumed that a substantial ferrule (1.5–2.0 mm) characterized all preparations. After 5 years, success rates for teeth restored with prefabricated titanium posts, cast post-cores, and teeth without posts amounted to 93 %, 97 %, and 94 %, respectively. The high rates of success attest to the importance of the dentin ferrule in increasing tooth fracture resistance. When uniform and nonuniform ferrule heights were incorporated into the designs of full-coverage crown preparations of maxillary central incisors that were restored with cast post-cores and crowns, Tan et al. (2005) found that teeth with nonuniform ferrules (0.5–2.0 mm vertical height) withstood 27 % fewer static loads than those with uniform (2.0 mm) ferrules. Teeth that lacked ferrules withstood 55 % fewer static loads than teeth with uniform ferrules. Based on the magnitude of forces at which the teeth fractured, it was concluded that teeth without a ferrule are at risk of fracture when subjected to maximal clenching forces, whereas teeth with nonuniform ferrules could resist forces from maximal clenching.

6.1.7 Fiber-Reinforced Posts

Various post systems have been used to restore endodontically treated teeth in many different clinical situations (Sorensen and Martinoff 1984a; Fraiman 2010). The first composite reinforced fiber post systems were made with carbon fibers arranged longitudinally in an epoxy resin. The potential disadvantage of carbon fiber posts is their black color, which could transmit through all-ceramic crowns, especially those made for anterior teeth. Black fibers were replaced subsequently by more esthetic white or translucent glass and quartz fibers, which have become standard components of fiber posts; they are the better choice for cases with greater esthetic demands. The manufacturers of these posts claim that as they will flex with dentin under occlusal loading, they will distribute forces and guard against tooth fracture. As mentioned previously, this has caused some clinicians to believe that the classic concept of a ferrule is not applicable when fiber posts are used. In fact, the use of posts has been associated with fractures of teeth; this occurs in many more teeth with posts than without. With this in mind, it should be remembered that the purpose of the post is to retain the core while minimizing the risk for tooth fracture. A 3-year prospective clinical study by Mancebo et al. (2010) that evaluated the survival of fiber posts where more than one-quarter of the teeth are restored with fiber posts, but without ferrules, failed after 3 years (Table 6.3). When Soares et al. (2008a) subjected endodontically treated teeth with major loss of crown structure (i.e., MOD cavity preparation + $\frac{2}{3}$ loss of occluso-cervical (O-C) cusp

Table 6.3 Clinical results of study done by Mancebo et al. (2010) on survival rate of fiber-reinforced posts

3-year study of teeth with fiber posts cemented with Rely-X	45 teeth with ferrule of at least 2 mm	42 teeth without ferrule
1. Teeth restored with metal-ceramic crowns or ceramic crowns 2. Not used as a part of an FPD or RPD	6.7 % failure	26.2 % failure

height + composite resin restoration and MOD cavity preparation + $\frac{2}{3}$ loss of O-C cusp height + glass fiber post + composite resin restoration) to compression loads at 30°, their fracture resistance decreased. Adding a glass fiber post to these teeth did not restore the fracture resistance significantly. However, inserting a fiber post in teeth exhibiting minor structural loss significantly reduced their fracture resistance. Although posts did not reinforce endodontically treated teeth, they were found to reduce catastrophic root fractures in teeth with major loss of crown structure. Endodontically treated teeth with MOD cavity preparations, two-thirds loss of O-C cusp height and composite resin restorations suffered 80 % catastrophic root fractures, whereas inserting a fiber post reduced catastrophic fractures to 40 %. Obviously, the use of fiber posts in this situation promoted more favorable fracture patterns that were considered retreatable. Their results seem to reinforce the main function of posts in endodontically treated teeth with major crown structure loss—retention of restorative core material and not reinforcement of the dental unit. Despite the loss of fracture resistance in teeth with major loss of crown structure, studies show that the combination of a fiber (glass or quartz) post with an adhesive restoration created a higher incidence of rerestorable failure types (Soares et al. 2008a; Akkayan and Gülmez 2002; McLaren et al. 2009; Zhi-Yue and Yu-Xing 2003). It appears that when a post is needed to retain a foundation restoration (core), the best option is a fiber-reinforced post with physical properties that resemble natural dentin, bonded to tooth structure (Dietschi et al. 2008).

6.1.8 Ceramic Posts

Ceramic posts are made of zirconium oxide. They are weaker than metal posts; therefore, a thicker post is necessary, which might require removal of additional root dentin. Theoretically, an intact root should permit retreatment of a tooth. However, removal of zirconia posts cemented in canal spaces with adhesive cements—normally a tedious and risky process—is not always successful. Retrieval of cemented zirconia posts often results in tooth fractures or removal of considerable remaining dentin, which might result in a nonrestorable outcome. A metallic post could produce a gray discoloration in translucent, all-ceramic crowns and in the adjacent gingiva of a patient with a thin periodontal biotype. Ceramic posts were designed originally to be used with composite resin cores for all-ceramic crowns, primarily for esthetic purposes. Research by Butz et al. (2001) on survival rate and fracture strength of endodontically treated teeth restored with four different post-core materials revealed that zirconia posts with composite cores had the lowest survival rates (63 %). When natural central incisors were restored with zirconia posts (with cores made of either composite or heat-pressed ceramic) and full-coverage cast metal crowns, and the crowns were subjected to 30 N forces (well within the normal clinical range), all zirconia posts fractured. However, tooth fractures in both groups rarely extended below the crown margin. Restoration of endodontically treated teeth with zirconia post-cores resulted in fewer vertical root fractures than prefabricated metal posts with composite cores or cast metal post-cores.

An in vitro study by Oblak et al. (2004) examined the strength (load to fracture values) of 1.3-mm- and 1.5-mm-diameter zirconium oxide posts that were (1) ground with a coarse diamond bur, (2) air particle abraded, and (3) left untreated. Posts were then luted into artificial (stainless-steel) canal spaces and subjected to a universal testing machine to evaluate the effect of the different surface treatments on fracture resistance. It was found that strength depended primarily on post diameter—thicker posts were significantly stronger. For both diameter posts, surface grinding weakened posts. Airborne-particle-abraded posts exhibited significantly higher resistance to fracture than posts in the other two groups. All posts fractured in the cervical region. Based on the results of the study, it is recommended to avoid grinding zirconium posts because microcracks might be introduced that could likely propagate through the body of the material and result in catastrophic failure. However, as these posts are prefabricated, grinding with diamond burs is often necessary to achieve a satisfactory fit in the canal space. Although airborne-particle abrasion increased the strength of posts, it appears to be at the expense of creating thousands of microcracks on the surface. It is conceivable that if any one of the microcracks propagated, then the post could fracture in the short or long term. Zirconium posts are very hard and difficult to remove from the canal space; therefore, their clinical application might be limited. Studies of survival rates of zirconium and fiber posts showed a significantly lower survival value for zirconium posts because of cracks within the post (Mannocci et al. 1999; Martinez-Gonzalez et al. 2001). Fiber posts exhibited an additional advantage when compared to zirconium oxide, gold, and titanium posts—they were readily retrievable subsequent to failure. The other post systems proved to be nonretrievable (Cormier et al. 2001). A retrospective in vivo study by Ferrari et al. (2000) found that failure rates after a 4-year recall were 2 % for fiber posts (mostly because of endodontic failure) and 14 % for cast post-cores (root fracture was the most frequent type). Perhaps black carbon posts are easier to remove after catastrophic failure because of enhanced visibility resulting from the color contrast. Black posts should be avoided for buildups of endodontically treated anterior teeth without crown coverage (Mannocci et al. 1999).

Some have suggested that a post system should have the same modulus of elasticity as canal space dentin to distribute forces along the length of the post (Ferrari et al. 2000; Mannocci et al. 1999). Carbon fiber posts seem to fulfill this requirement. The modulus of elasticity of carbon fiber posts is approximately 21 GPa, well within the range of dentin at 18 GPa. However, Morgano (2015) warned that the modulus of elasticity of dentin will vary among different teeth. Also, Kovarik et al.

(1992) claimed that when ferrule tooth structure is inadequate, the majority of forces are borne by the core material itself. The extra flexure exhibited by composite resin core materials places greater shearing stresses on the posts and tooth-cement interface, thus endangering the cement seal of the crown. When the resin core and the post have similar inherent flexibilities, then the potential for failure of the cement seal of a crown might be relatively high (Morgano 2015). In an in vitro leakage study, Chang et al. (2012) loaded extracted natural incisors with ferrules of 1.5 mm (considered the absolute minimum for restoration of a tooth). They determined that there was a significantly higher incidence of leakage when teeth were restored with fiber posts compared with teeth restored with stiffer metal posts. There was evidence of leakage through dentinal tubules, penetrating ferrule dentin and, ultimately, reaching the post space. Apparently, fiber posts allowed movement of the crown during function, which lead to percolation at the margin and subsequent leakage. The higher modulus of elasticity of the stainless-steel posts might have deterred the buildup of cervical stresses and micromovement at the crown margins. One study, with a very large data base comprising 12 clinical studies of clinical complications among almost 3000 post-cores, reported that 5 % dislodged from the canal space, 3 % were involved with fractured roots, and 2 % failed because of caries (Goodacre et al. 2003). The authors revealed that four studies evaluated 1047 post-cores and reported a 9 % mean incidence of caries. It is safe to assume that marginal leakage played a major role in the appearance of caries; consequently, we may infer further from these investigations that the rigidity of the post determines the marginal seal of the post-core and the crown. All information to date appears to cast some doubt on the purported advantages of flexible post-core systems.

What is the best post-core system for all-ceramic crowns on anterior teeth? If we examine the study by Carossa et al. (2001), extracted anterior teeth were mounted in a denture model with simulated gingiva. Four types of post-cores and three types of all-ceramic crowns were fabricated for each tooth. Of the four post-core types, two were cast in gold alloy (one polished and one matte finished), one was made of pressed lithium disilicate glass ceramic, and one was cast in palladium alloy, with porcelain on the facial surface to mask the color of metal. Two types of all-ceramic crowns were made: one was glass ceramic (Empress2) and the other was made of aluminous ceramic (In-Ceram). A spectrophotometer was used to analyze the different post-cores on light transmission through the all-ceramic crowns. When ten prosthodontists were asked to evaluate the chromatic appearance of each all-ceramic crown restored with each post-core type, they could not detect clinical differences among the different post-core types. The best optical effect was produced when all-ceramic posts were used; polished gold produced the second best effect. When the translucency of CAD-CAM crowns made with three different all-ceramic materials (alumina crowns, CAD-CAM Procera; zirconia, CAD-CAM Lava; and lithium disilicate, pressable IPS e.max Press) were evaluated, pressable lithium disilicate crowns, IPS e.max Press, showed the greatest translucency (Sravanthi et al. 2015). Translucency of material will dictate to the clinician the choice of post-core materials to be used in the different zones and which material is best for restorations in the esthetic zone to mimic the patient's natural dentition. A prospective study by

Malament and Socransky (2001) examined the effect of natural dentin and cast gold cores on the survivability of 1444 single-unit, all-ceramic restorations. Over a 16-year period, acid-etched restorations luted to a gold core exhibited 91 % survivability; when luted to natural dentin, survivability was 75 % over the same period. The higher rigidity of cast gold was responsible for the dramatic difference in survival probability. Nonacid-etched restorations luted to dentin had a significantly lower probability of survival (43 %) after 16 years. Consequently, it is recommended to use polished, yellow cast gold alloy cores with anterior all-ceramic crowns, providing that an adequate ferrule is present.

6.2 Factors Affecting Post Retention

There are four factors that affect post retention: length, taper, diameter, and surface configuration (i.e., smooth, threaded, serrated). If we consider the issue of post length, then arguably the best information can be found in a study by Sorensen and Martinoff (1984b), in which 1273 endodontically treated teeth were evaluated retrospectively. When the success and failure rate associated with post length was assessed, they found that the longer the post, the greater its chances for success. Inadequate post length is probably the most common reason for failure of crowns on endodontically treated teeth. It was found that when the length of the post equaled the length of the crown, the failure rate was 2.5 %. At one-quarter the length of the crown, the failure rate was 25 %—ten times the restorative failure rate (and, one out of four crowns failed). When post length exceeded crown length, the success rate was 100 %. In a controlled study by Fuss et al. (2001), endodontically treated teeth with vertical root fractures were examined after extraction. They discovered that 69.5 % of the fractures occurred in teeth with posts in the coronal third of the root; only 30.5 % occurred in teeth where posts reached the middle third of the root. Cohen et al. (2003) also evaluated endodontically treated teeth with vertical root fractures and attributed the failures to posts that were either too long, too wide, or both. Post length influences the stress load along the root. Shorter posts are associated with a higher incidence of root fracture because of the law of leverage. When the length of the lever arm that receives the applied force (the length of the clinical crown) is three times the length of the resisting arm (the section of post embedded in the pulp canal), the stress applied to the root is magnified by a factor of three. When the post is as long as the crown, then the forces transmitted to the root are one to one. These results support observations that longer posts are preferable to shorter ones. Perhaps a good rule to follow is that the length of the post should be approximately two-thirds the length of the root. It is recommended that at least 4.0–5.0 mm of apical gutta-percha should remain to avoid dislodging the endodontic seal and subsequent leakage. Furthermore, when considering post length, it should be remembered that length is less critical to fracture resistance than the ferrule effect (Isidor et al. 1999). Also, post length that exceeds two-thirds of the root length does not decrease stress in the cervical region; rather, it increases the possibility of inadvertently losing the apical gutta-percha seal and perforating the root by increasing stress at the apex (Hunter et al. 1989).

In their study of extracted maxillary and mandibular molars, Abou-Rass and colleagues (1982) exposed some of the difficulties that are encountered when preparing canal spaces for molars. They used numbers 2, 3, and 4 Peeso reamers to enlarge canal spaces to a depth of 8 mm from the canal orifices. Roots were then sectioned at the 7- and 4-mm levels. Based on their findings, the authors made the following recommendations: (1) when preparing canal spaces for posts, it is best to avoid the mesial roots of mandibular molars as their distal walls are usually thin and concave, and perforations or stripping are more likely to occur here. Root concavities (termed "danger zones") are not always obvious on radiographs; (2) canal spaces should be made in the distal canals of mandibular molars, using only a number 2 Peeso reamer to a depth of 7–8 mm from the canal orifice to avoid perforating the canal walls; (3) avoid the buccal roots of maxillary molars because Peeso reamers cannot negotiate their natural curvatures; and (4) canal spaces for posts should be made in the palatal roots of maxillary molars, and number 2 or 3 Peeso reamers should be used to a depth of 7 mm. Studies confirm that at least 4–5 mm of gutta-percha should remain at the apex after post preparation to minimize the degree of apical leakage in teeth (Mattison et al. 1984; Raiden and Gendelman 1994).

Removal of dentin to prepare a post space weakens an endodontically treated tooth and can lead to root fracture. Preservation of tooth structure is the most critical factor in the long-term success of an endodontically treated tooth. There is relatively little data to recommend an optimal post space diameter. Lloyd and Palik (1993) offered two philosophies: the first, starting post space preparation at approximately 5 mm from the anatomic apex and developing a post space that is one-third the diameter of the root at its narrowest dimension. The second philosophy also recommended maintaining 5 mm of gutta-percha and preserving 1.75 mm of tooth structure in any direction from the margin of the prepared post. A good general rule to follow is to avoid enlarging the post space one or two endodontic file sizes beyond the largest size required for endodontic treatment (Eakle 1985). Post diameter can affect post retention—the greater the diameter, the greater the retention. That explains why cylindrical posts are more retentive than conical posts. However, cylindrical posts often require excessive preparation of the canal space, which could weaken the dentin and increase the risk of root fracture. This does not apply as much to conical posts that resemble the shape of the canal space; their fabrication often requires much less removal of dentin, especially in apical areas (Weine et al. 1991; Nergiz et al. 1997). The retention of posts might be overrated in the literature because the major force to which posts are subjected is usually directed perpendicular to their long axes. Some believe that resistance (the ability of the post to resist dislodgment along an axis other than the path of placement), rather than retention (the ability of the post to resist forces of dislodgement along the path of placement), is the major contributor to a post's stability (Lloyd and Palik 1993).

Some controversy exists about how to remove gutta-percha from the canal to create space for a post. It has been shown that a hot endodontic condenser could be used at the fill appointment without compromising the apical seal (Goerig and Mueninghoff 1983b). At the fill appointment, a rotary instrument such as a Peeso reamer should not be used to remove gutta-percha to create a post space as dislodgement of the filling material and loss of apical seal is likely to occur. Also, significantly greater leakage along apical root fillings with gutta-percha was found after a 1-week delay in post space preparation than with immediate preparation (Fan et al. 1999; Safavi et al. 1987). The authors stressed maintaining proper rubber dam isolation, especially during delayed post space preparation and subsequent post cementation, and immediate construction of a post-core. In view of the increasing likelihood of recurrent caries around deteriorating provisional restorations, the vulnerability of coronal tooth structure to fracture, and the enhanced probability of marginal leakage and leakage of the endodontic seal, it is best to direct efforts at appropriate and prompt permanent restoration of teeth subsequent to endodontic therapy (Abramovitz et al. 2000).

The surface texture of passive posts (those which adapt to the dentinal walls of the post space when cemented into place) presents in a variety of configurations. When Standlee and Caputo (1993) compared the retentive capacity of four post designs (serrated, cross-hatched, threaded, and longitudinally spiraled) that were cemented with resin cement, they found that the most retentive were the serrated and cross-hatched designs. Threaded and longitudinally spiraled post surface designs were the least retentive by a significant factor. The least retentive post design—those with longitudinal spirals that were nearly parallel with the long axis of the post—failed to resist dislodgement because they offered less resistance to withdrawal compared with serrated and cross-hatched designs. In fact, this design dislodged with most of the luting cement remaining within the endodontic post space, which is indicative of failure of the adhesive at the post-cement interface. Enhancing a post's surface texture positively influences its retentive properties. Nergiz et al. (1997) altered the surface texture of tapered titanium posts and measured their retentive strengths after cementation with zinc phosphate. Post spaces were shaped with the use of post drills corresponding to the size of the post. Various surface textures were tested; they included smooth, smooth with grooves, sandblasted, and sandblasted with grooves. Smooth posts were the least retentive. Sandblasting the surface more than doubled the retentive strength (218 N vs. 491 N), and adding grooves to sandblasted surfaces increased retentive strength significantly (694 N). Also demonstrated clearly was that the retentive strength of posts can be increased significantly when a prepared post space is roughened with a diamond that conforms to the shape of the space. When the walls of post spaces were roughened in this manner, retention of sandblasted posts and sandblasted-and-grooved posts increased almost four and five times, respectively, compared with smooth posts cemented in unaltered post spaces. The retention of resin luting agents to roughened post space dentin, or to dentin in which undercuts were placed, enhanced the mechanical bond significantly by a keying effect (Tjan et al. 1997). In this study, placement of 100-μm-deep grooves in canal dentin increased the retention (i.e., tensile force applied to the post-core) of prefabricated steel post-cores cemented with resin cement by a factor of almost four. These studies highlight the large role that surface configuration plays in the overall retention of posts. Increasing the length of a post increases retention by engaging greater surface area in the canal walls. Longer posts also distribute stress over a larger area of bone-supported root.

Increasing post diameter has been shown to have little effect on retention and can increase cervical stress (Sorensen and Martinoff 1984b; Stockton 1999). As the predominant canal shape is ovoid, and the walls of prefabricated posts are commonly parallel or cylindrical, the majority of prefabricated posts will not adapt well along the entire interface with canal walls. Consequently, luting agent might not completely fill the post-dentin interface, with negative implications for post retention and resistance.

Post design also influences the success of the restoration. A prospective study of 788 tapered and parallel-sided posts by Torbjorner et al. (1995) showed that the cumulative failure rate for tapered posts (15 %) was nearly twice that for parallel-sided posts (8 %). Failure resulting from loss of retention—the most frequent mode of failure for both types of posts—was 6.7 % for tapered and 4.2 % for parallel-sided posts; failure resulting from root fracture was 3.5 % for tapered posts and 1.5 % for parallel-sided posts. Parallel-sided fiber posts are more retentive than tapered posts (Sahafi et al. 2004; Teixeira et al. 2006). The highest tooth fracture rates occurred among tapered posts that were intimately adapted to the canal space and those that engaged only minimal dentin at the apical end of the canal space. Photoelastic studies reveal that with vertical loading, parallel-sided posts generate the highest apical stresses, whereas tapered posts produced equal stress concentrations at the apex and CEJ areas. In the area of the CEJ, tapered posts exerted slightly more force than parallel-sided posts (Assif et al. 1989; Burns et al. 1990; Standlee et al. 1972; Cooney et al. 1986). During cementation, tapered posts tend to be self-venting (i.e., there is little buildup of hydraulic pressure when the post is cemented into the canal space). However, cementation of parallel-sided posts generates significant hydraulic pressure in teeth, especially when the cement is viscous. To minimize pressure, it is recommended to vent parallel-sided posts by creating a longitudinal channel along which cement can escape (Trabert and Cooney 1984). Without a channel, excessive hydraulic back pressure can cause a root to fracture or incomplete seating of the post. If fracture resistance is to be maximized, then post design must be considered along with other design features of the prepared, endodontically treated tooth. The ferrule effect might be a more important variable than post design in optimizing fracture resistance (Assif et al. 1993). When preparing a tooth for a full-coverage crown, if the design parameters for a circumferential ferrule cannot be satisfied, then another restorative modality or extraction should be considered.

Peroz et al. (2005) suggested that metal post-cores should be fabricated with materials that closely match the metals used to construct the definitive restorations. The authors recommended gold alloy, cobalt-based alloy, or titanium. Use of screw posts has been associated with higher incidences of root fractures. In one study (Creugers et al. 2005), the root fracture rate after 6 years was 19 %. In a second study that examined 178 teeth, the fracture rate was 25 % at the first examination and 19.9 % after a second examination of 218 teeth 5–7 years later (Eckerbom et al. 1991). When glass fiber composite, carbon/quartz fiber epoxy composite, carbon fiber epoxy composite, zirconium oxide, palladium gold alloy, and titanium posts were bonded and luted in endodontically treated teeth, and then fracture resistance-tested, fracture resistance for glass fiber composite posts and cores was the weakest

(Cormier et al. 2001). In the presence of catastrophic forces of occlusion, fiber-reinforced posts differed from all other posts tested in that they had demonstrated the ability to fracture at the coronal portion of the tooth restoration—at the core-root interface—without root fracture. Posts that fracture at this location are considered to have a higher retrievability rate; consequently, the teeth have a higher probability of being restored. Teeth restored with titanium and zirconia posts tended to display catastrophic fractures when subjected to 130° angle, in vitro load tests (Akkayan and Gülmez 2002). Teeth restored with titanium posts tended to display oblique root fractures at more apical locations. The more catastrophic fractures were found in this group. No serious damage to the root was detected in teeth restored with quartz fiber and glass fiber posts, although failure was observed at the interface between core and root. When interpreting the results of these studies, it should be kept in mind that the magnitude and angle of the forces to which the specimens were subjected often mimicked the worst case scenario of force application to a restoration. These forces often simulated a traumatic blow to a tooth as one might encounter in an accident. Teeth restored with adequate ferrules and full-coverage crowns, and loaded axially, might require greater forces to cause failure; therefore, the various post systems tested, especially the fiber posts, might perform well clinically (i.e., have sufficient fracture thresholds to warrant their use). Keep in mind that angulation of loading is a factor determining the failure load of an endodontically treated tooth. As teeth are subjected to increasing loads, failure rates appear to increase concomitantly. When the crowns of post-restored maxillary central incisors were subjected to loads at angles of 110-, 130-, and 150° (closer to the long axes of the teeth), the mean load required to fracture teeth was 372 N, 598 N, and 1274 N, respectively (Loney et al. 1995). When determining the prognosis of a tooth to be restored, it is recommended to consider the quantity and strength of remaining tooth structure and the load to which it will be subjected.

In an in vitro study, the canal spaces of 40 maxillary central incisors were deliberately instrumented to compromise wall thicknesses to be in the range of 0.50–0.75 mm at the CEJ to simulate extensive clinical structural damage (Saupe et al. 1996). One group of 20 teeth was restored with cast post-cores (ten teeth with and ten without ferrules) that adapted intimately to the canal space walls. The canal walls of the second group of 20 teeth were reinforced with visible light-cured composite and then restored with a fiber post-core system (ten teeth with and ten without ferrules). All restorations were cemented with a self-curing resin system. Teeth were subjected to static loads of 3 kg (well within physiologic loads to which central incisors are usually subjected). All teeth restored with the fiber posts system exhibited significantly increased resistance to load failure (up to 50 %) when compared to teeth restored with conventional cast post-cores, irrespective of whether a ferrule was provided. It appears that reinforcing structurally compromised roots with resin, and a fiber post can significantly increase their fracture resistance, with or without the presence of a ferrule. In general, fiber posts should be cemented with adhesive cements. Penetration with a curing light is limited in the post space; therefore, dual-cured bonding agent or self-cure resin adhesives must be used. Dual-cure resins will polymerize quickly where light penetrates effectively and much more slowly in areas where light is not available. Dual-cure resin produces a resin-dentin penetration zone higher than that seen with light-cured bonding agent or a one-step bonding system (Ferrari et al. 2001).

6.3 Role of the Tooth in Survivability of the Restoration

What role does the tooth play in the survival of restorations? Three retrospective studies help to provide answers to the question. The first study examined the survivability of more than 1300 single crowns—a large data set—with or without custom-cast post-cores, made at a dental school over a period of 18 years (De Backer et al. 2006a). Survival rates of full-coverage crowns, with and without post-cores, were 79.4 % and 74.9 %, respectively. Differences in survival rates between post-core crowns and full-coverage crowns made for vital teeth were not statistically significant. The investigators then examined 134 three-unit FPDs grouped into vital and nonvital groups (i.e., one abutment tooth was endodontically treated). Survival of restorations in the vital and nonvital groups after 20 years was 83.2 % and 60.5 %, respectively. The differences in survivability became greater only as they approached the 20-year period. They then examined 322 FPDs with 1–6 pontics and 2–4 abutments, made over a period of 20 years (De Backer et al. 2006b). When they focused on the FPD itself as the variable to be considered, the survival rate of FPDs with vital abutments was 77.4 %; FPDs with post-cores in at least one abutment had a survival rate of 56.7 %. The difference between both groups was statistically significant. In their third study, De Backer et al. (2007) looked only at the abutment itself—with and without a post—and found survival rates of 69.4 % and 81.1 %, respectively. Again, the differences were statistically significant. When the findings of these studies are considered, it appears that when a single crown is made for a vital tooth and for an endodontically treated tooth restored with a post-core, survival rates should be the same. When abutments are part of a FPD, then vitality and loss of vitality makes a significant difference in survivability. The prognosis of FPDs with spans longer than three units is not as good. Their study also evaluated cantilever FPDs (C-FPDs) over the same period. As expected, survival of C-FPDs in the vital group after 16 years was 73.5 %. Survival of those in the endodontically treated group was 52.3 % over the same period. The difference was statistically significant. Cantilever FPDs constructed on teeth with post-cores can be expected to have more problems and fail sooner.

The prognosis of an endodontically treated tooth is best if it is part of a complete dental arch. In this situation, mesial and distal proximal contacts are the stabilizing factors (Sorensen and Martinoff 1985). When an endodontically treated tooth must serve as an abutment for a RPD, the insertion of a post increases treatment success significantly (Hatzikyriakos et al. 1992). Endodontically treated teeth serving as abutments for RPDs have a higher risk for failure than those serving as abutments for FPDs and single crowns. The success rate for all endodontically treated RPD abutments was 77.4 % compared with FPDs (89.2 %) and single crowns (94.8 %). There is an increase in the stresses to which teeth are subjected as we proceed from single crowns to FPDs and to RPDs. Fixed partial dentures exhibited three times the number of restorable and nonrestorable tooth fractures than single crowns; RPDs had up to eight times the number (Sorensen and Martinoff 1985). As part of the informed consent requirement, patients should be told about the higher risk for failure when endodontically treated teeth must serve as abutments for cantilever FPDs or as terminal abutments for RPDs (Peroz et al. 2005). In the latter case, endodontically treated teeth have been shown to fail at rates greater than four times when compared with endodontically treated teeth not serving as abutments (Sorensen and Martinoff 1985). It is best to avoid recommending endodontically treated teeth to serve as abutments in either case.

6.4 Post Cementation

Some cements that are available for use with post-cores include zinc phosphate, polycarboxylate, glass ionomer, resin (filled and unfilled), resin-modified glass ionomer, and compomer (although not used commonly for cementing post-cores). All have been used with success. Reeh et al. (1989b) found that the use of enamel and dentin etching increased the relative stiffness (strength) of a tooth to a level close to that of an unprepared tooth. Acid etching and placing composite resin in the root canal space strengthens the tooth; adding a post does not strengthen endodontically treated teeth; however, cementing a post with bonded resin cement strengthens weakened coronal dentin that surrounds the post (Eakle 1985). A post should be used only to retain the core and restoration. Mendoza et al. (1997) showed that teeth were approximately 56 % more resistant to fracture when adhesive cements were used to cement posts than when zinc phosphate cement was used. There was a 44 % increase in retention (tensile strength) of posts that were cemented with resin cement compared with zinc phosphate cement (Utter et al. 1997). However, resin cements are not compatible with eugenol, which is contained in some sealers used by dentists. When Tjan and Nemetz (1992) luted posts with resin cement into canal spaces contaminated with eugenol, they found that post retention was diminished by approximately 64 %; when zinc phosphate cement was used with posts in eugenol-contaminated canal spaces, retention decreased by almost 19 %. Clearly, the presence of eugenol in canal dentin has a major effect on the behavior of resin cements and, to a lesser extent, on zinc phosphate cement. Whenever possible, it is best to use a resin endodontic sealer when performing endodontic therapy. Also, one should consider that the ability of resin to bond to canal dentin is less reliable than adhesion to coronal dentin. Bond strength values to canal dentin vary among studies—from 5 to 28 MPa (Bouillaguet et al. 2003; Mallmann et al. 2007; Soares et al. 2008b). On the other hand, bond strengths to pulpal floor dentin are in the range of 15.58 ± 4.24 MPa to 22.48 ± 7.08 MPa (Kijsamanmith et al. 2002). Bonding to dentin is more difficult than bonding to enamel because dentin is a wet substrate (20 % fluid by volume) and resins are hydrophobic. Also, the relative lack of mineralized surface also makes adhesion to dentin a challenge. If metal posts are used, then it is recommended to use glass ionomer, resin composite, or self-adhesive composite

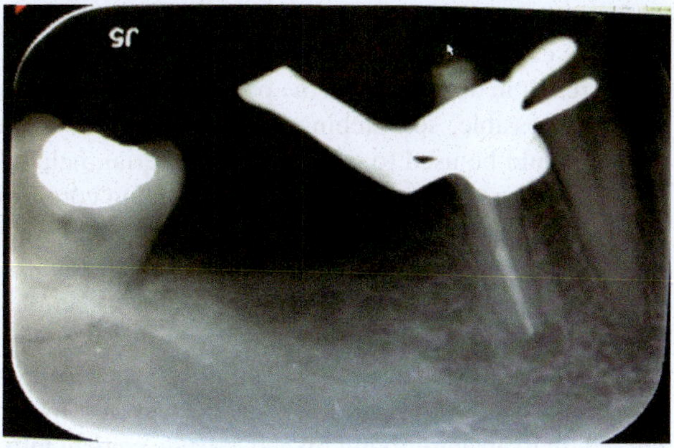

Fig. 6.6 The fiber post used to restore the premolar is sufficiently radiopaque in this radiograph. The apical end of the post should contact gutta-percha

cement. After the tooth is isolated with rubber dam, rinse the canal space thoroughly with 0.2 % chlorhexidine. Then dry the post space thoroughly with paper points. Mix the cement and extrude it into the canal with a Jiffy tube. To maximize contact between cement and dentin, use a Lentulo spiral to carry the cement to the canal walls. Avoid overfilling. Place cement on the metal post and seat the post in the canal. After the cement is set partially, break off any excess that is displaced from the canal space. Allow all intraradicular cement to polymerize fully, undisturbed.

If a fiber-reinforced post is used, then isolate the tooth with rubber dam and rinse the canal space with 0.2 % chlorhexidine. Rinse and dry the canal space. Insert the post in the canal space to ensure that it fits passively. If the post binds inside the canal space, choose a narrower diameter post or make any necessary adjustments to ensure passivity of fit. If the post extends occlusal to the cavosurface margin of the tooth preparation, adjust the length by cutting according to manufacturer's directions (generally, while using a diamond bur and copious water). Ensure that the post head is cut back a few millimeters below the cavosurface margin. Avoid sandblasting a fiber post as it will incorporate aluminum oxide crystals on the surface of the post, which will diminish bond strength between luting agent and post. In general, it is probably best to avoid sandblasting fiber posts unless manufacturer's directions specify otherwise. Confirm with a radiograph that the apical end of the post contacts gutta-percha. Notwithstanding the fact that most fiber posts are relatively radiolucent, they are detectable on radiographs (Fig. 6.6).

It is essential to use eye protection for all etching and bonding procedures. Separate etching and rinsing are recommended. Next, etch canal dentin with 35 % phosphoric acid gel for approximately 15 s; use a long syringe needle to extrude etchant. Place etchant gel on coronal dentin and peripheral enamel. All remaining peripheral enamel must be etched for 30 s. After etching is completed, rinse the canal space and all remaining enamel and dentin with water for approximately 15 s. Blot the canal walls dry with paper points as far apically as possible. Reirrigate the canal space with water to remove residual etchant gel. If a dry paper point is reintroduced into the canal space and appears to be stained with etchant gel, reirrigate until a new paper point inserted into the canal appears free of etchant. Although the etch and rinse system still remains the “gold standard,” failing to remove all etchant from the canal might diminish the bond strength of the luting agent and eventually might result in debonding of the post. For clinicians who wish to eliminate as many steps as possible, self-etching dentin adhesive systems might be used. A matrix system could be used to confine core material, help adapt composite to remaining crown structure and post, and prevent bonding core material to adjacent teeth.

Next, use a small microbrush to coat the canal walls with bonding agent. Work the bonding material into the canal space and on all etched surfaces of the tooth cavity for approximately 30 s or according to manufacturer’s directions. Use a dry paper point to remove bonding agent that might pool inside the canal space, working quickly to avoid premature polymerization of bonding materials. Gently air-blow all tooth surfaces until they appear evenly moist. Attach a narrow-diameter, curved tip to an automixing tip and extrude cement into the canal space. Disperse all intraradicular cement with a Lentulo spiral. Coat the post with cement and seat it into the canal space without exerting too much apical pressure. (Consider placing two posts in premolars with two canals.) Maintain constant apical pressure on the post for approximately 20 s to counteract hydraulic pressure that could unseat the post. Once seated, some excess cement will emerge from the canal orifice. Light cure the excess cement to stabilize the post while cement inside the canal space polymerizes fully.

Finally, the same self-cure or dual-cure composite resins applied to the post space are added to create a core buildup. This procedure can be started immediately because cement at the canal orifice was light polymerized to stabilize the post. To hasten polymerization, a light-cured composite could be used for the core buildup. It is generally best to light-cure composite in small increments to minimize polymerization shrinkage. Remove the matrix and adjust the contours and occlusion of the core. A final radiograph could be taken to confirm whether the marginal seal of the core is satisfactory. The crown preparation could be completed at the same session. All finish lines must be located on natural tooth structure, ideally 1.5–2.0 mm apical to the core.

The technique employed when using zinc phosphate cement might play a role in the overall retention of a post. Jacobi and Shillingburg used two techniques to cement posts into plexiglass tooth analogs, using zinc phosphate cement (Jacobi and Shillingburg 1993). The walls of one canal space were coated with zinc phosphate, using a Lentulo spiral to distribute the cement prior to post placement. The other posts were coated first with cement and then placed in the canal spaces. Large voids were noted between the cement and the plexiglass walls when the latter technique was employed. When Panavia composite resin cement was used to lute posts in canal spaces, it appeared to trap air as the posts exhibited large air voids in the cement to the extent that only a small fraction of the cement surface was involved in actual contact with dentin (Tjan and Nemetz 1992). Since the polymerization of Panavia is diminished by the presence of oxygen, Oxygard gel is placed around the restoration to cover any exposed cement. However, if air is already trapped in the cement, then the effectiveness of Oxygard gel is questionable.

Cementation technique does indeed play a major role in the retention of posts when zinc phosphate is used. In one study (Fakiha et al. 2001), when zinc phosphate was inserted into the canal space with a pipette and then applied to the post, retention was nearly doubled compared to a post on which cement was applied with a plastic instrument (the control) prior to placement in the canal. When cement was extruded into the canal with a pipette, and a Lentulo spiral was used to further distribute the cement into the canal space, followed by application of cement over the post prior to its placement in the canal, retention more than doubled when compared to the control. In another study, when a Lentulo was employed to distribute zinc phosphate cement in the canal, followed by coating the post with cement, retention was increased more than 64% (Goldman et al. 1984). With both techniques, air entrapment in the cement is minimized, resulting in significant increases in post retention. The use of adhesive resin for cementation of any kind of post is recommended. Based on the information presented, it appears that the cement that one chooses may not be as important as the cementation technique.

The research cited and the guidelines discussed in this chapter should help the student and clinician make evidence-based decisions for the restoration of endodontically treated teeth. An integration of these parameters into clinical decision-making will enable a treatment plan to be created for the patient that incorporates treatment modalities that should increase the chances for long-term success for the restoration of an endodontically treated tooth.

References

Abou-Rass M, Jann JM, Jobe D, et al. Preparation of space for posting: effect on thickness of canal walls and incidence of perforation in molars. J Am Dent Assoc. 1982;104:834–7.

Abramovitz I, Tagger M, Tamse A, et al. The effect of immediate vs. delayed post space preparation on the apical seal of a root canal filling: a study in an increased-sensitivity pressure-driven system. J Endod. 2000;26(8):435–9.

Akkayan B, Gülmez T. Resistance to fracture of endodontically treated teeth restored with different post systems. J Prosthet Dent. 2002;87:431–7.

Aquilino SA, Caplan DJ. Relationship between crown placement and the survival of endodontically treated teeth. J Prosthet Dent. 2002;87:256–63.

Assif D, Oren E, Marshak BL, et al. Photoelastic analysis of stress transfer by endodontically treated teeth to the supporting structure using different restorative techniques. J Prosthet Dent. 1989;61:535–43.

Assif D, Bitenski A, Pilo R, et al. Effect of post design on resistance to fracture of endodontically treated teeth with complete crowns. J Prosthet Dent. 1993;69:36–40.

Ausiello P, De Gee AJ, Rengo S, et al. Fracture resistance of endodontically-treated premolars adhesively restored. Am J Dent. 1997;10:237–41.

Bouillaguet S, Troesch S, Wataha JC, et al. Microtensile bond strength between adhesive cements and root canal dentin. Dent Mater. 2003;19:199–205.

Burke FJ, Shaglouf AG, Combe EC, et al. Fracture resistance of five pin-retained core build-up materials on teeth with and without extracoronal preparation. Oper Dent. 2000;25:388–94.

Burns DA, Krause WR, Douglas HB, et al. Stress distribution surrounding endodontic posts. J Prosthet Dent. 1990;64:412–8.

Butz F, Lennon AM, Heydecke G, et al. Survival rate and fracture strength of endodontically treated maxillary incisors with moderate defects restored with different post-and-core systems: an in vitro study. Int J Prosthodont. 2001;14:58–64.

Carossa S, Lombardo S, Pera P, et al. Influence of posts and cores on light transmission through different all-ceramic crowns: spectrophotometric and clinical evaluation. Int J Prosthodont. 2001;14:9–14.

Chang JW, Soo I, Cheung SP. Evaluation of fiber post-supported restorations under simulated occlusal loading. J Prosthet Dent. 2012;108:158–64.

Cohen S, Blanco L, Berman L. Vertical root fractures: clinical and radiographic diagnosis. J Am Dent Assoc. 2003;134:434–41.

Cooney JP, Caputo AA, Trabert KC. Retention and stress distribution of tapered-end endodontic posts. J Prosthet Dent. 1986;55:540–6.

Cormier CJ, Burns DR, Moon P. In vitro comparison of the fracture resistance and failure mode of fiber, ceramic, and conventional post systems at various stages of restoration. J Prosthodont. 2001;10:26–36.

Costa LC, Pegoraro LF. Influence of different metal restorations bonded with resin on fracture resistance of endodontically treated maxillary premolars. J Prosthet Dent. 1997;77:365–9.

Creugers N, Mentink AG, Fokkinga WA, et al. 5-year follow-up of a prospective clinical study on various types of core restorations. Int J Prosthodont. 2005;18(1):34–9.

De Backer H, Van Maele G, De Moor N, et al. An 18-year retrospective survival study of full crowns with or without posts. Int J Prosthodont. 2006a;19:136–42.

De Backer H, Van Maele G, De Moor N, et al. A 20-year retrospective survival study of fixed partial dentures. Int J Prosthodont. 2006b;19:143–53.

De Backer H, Van Maele G, Decock V, et al. Long-term survival of complete crowns, fixed dental prostheses, and cantilever fixed dental prostheses with posts and cores on root canal-treated teeth. Int J Prosthodont. 2007;20:229–34.

Dietschi D, Duc O, Krejci I, et al. Biomechanical considerations for the restoration of endodontically treated teeth: a systematic review of the literature, part II [Evaluation of fatigue behavior, interfaces, and in vivo studies]. Quintessence Int. 2008;39:117–29.

Eakle WS. Increasing the resistance of teeth to fracture: bonded composite resin versus glass ionomer cement. Dent Mater. 1985;1:228–30.

Eckerbom M, Magnusson T, Martinsson T. Prevalence of apical periodontitis, crowned teeth and teeth with posts in a Swedish population. Endod Dent Traumatol. 1991;7:214–20.

Eissmann HF, Radke Jr RA. Postendodontic restoration. In: Cohen S, Burns RC, editors. Pathways of the pulp. Saint Louis: C.V. Mosby Co; 1976.

Ellner S, Bergendal T, Bergman B. Four post-and-core combinations as abutments for fixed single crowns: a prospective up to 10-year study. Int J Prosthodont. 2003;16(3):249–54.

Fakiha Z, Al-Aujan A, Al-Shamrani S. Retention of cast posts cemented with zinc phosphate cement using different cementing techniques. J Prosthodont. 2001;10:37–41.

Fan P, Nicholls JI, Kois JC. Load fatigue of five restoration modalities in structurally compromised premolars. Int J Prosthodont. 1995;8(3):213–20.

Fan B, Wu M-K, Wesselink PR. Coronal leakage along apical root fillings after immediate and delayed post space preparation. Endod Dent Traumatol. 1999;15:124–6.

Faria AC, Rodriguez RC, Antunes RP, et al. Endodontically treated teeth: characteristics and considerations to restore them. J Prosthodont Res. 2011;55:69–74.

Ferrari M, Vichi A, Garcia-Godoy F. Clinical evaluation of fiber-reinforced epoxy resin posts and cast post and cores. Am J Dent. 2000;13:15B–8.

Ferrari M, Vichi A, Grandini S, et al. Efficacy of a self-curing adhesive-resin cement system on luting glass-fiber posts into root canals: an SEM investigation. Int J Prosthodont. 2001;14:543–9.

Foley J, Saunders E, Saunders WP. Strength of core build-up materials in endodontically-treated teeth. Am J Dent. 1997;10:166–72.

Fraiman HP. Post and core: clinical factors. Compend Contin Educ Dent. 2010;31(1):80–1.

Freeman MA, Nicholls JI, Kydd WL, et al. Leakage associated with load fatigue-induced preliminary failure of full crowns placed over three different post and core systems. J Endod. 1998;24(1):26–32.

Fuss Z, Lustig J, Katz A, et al. An evaluation of endodontically treated vertical root fractured teeth: impact of operative procedures. J Endod. 2001;27(1):46–8.

Goerig AC, Mueninghoff LA. Management of the endodontically treated tooth. Part I: concept for restorative designs. J Prosthet Dent. 1983a;49:340–5.

Goerig AC, Mueninghoff LA. Management of the endodontically treated tooth. Part II: technique. J Prosthet Dent. 1983b;49:491–7.

Goldman M, DeVitre R, Tenca J. Cement distribution and bond strength in cemented posts. J Dent Res. 1984;63(12):1392–5.

Goodacre CJ, Bernal G, Rungcharassaeng K, et al. Clinical complications in fixed prosthodontics. J Prosthet Dent. 2003;90:31–41.

Guzy GE, Nicholls JI. In vitro comparison of intact endodontically treated teeth with and without endo-post reinforcement. J Prosthet Dent. 1979;42:39–44.

Hatzikyriakos AH, Reisis GI, Tsingos N. A 3-year postoperative clinical evaluation of posts and cores beneath existing crowns. J Prosthet Dent. 1992;67:454–8.

Heydecke G, Peters MC. The restoration of endodontically treated, single-rooted teeth with cast or direct posts and cores: a systematic review. J Prosthet Dent. 2002;87:380–6.

Hunter AJ, Feiglin B, Williams JF. Effects of post placement on endodontically treated teeth. J Prosthet Dent. 1989;62:166–72.

Isidor F, Brøndum K, Ravnholt G. The influence of post length and crown ferrule length on the resistance to cyclic loading of bovine teeth with prefabricated titanium posts. Int J Prosthodont. 1999;12:78–82.

Jacobi R, Shillingburg Jr HT. Pins, dowels, and other retentive devices in posterior teeth. Dent Clin N Am. 1993;37(3):367–90.

Kaufman EG, Coelho DH, Colin L. Factors influencing the retention of cemented gold castings. J Prosthet Dent. 1961;11:487–502.

Kijsamanmith K, Timpawat S, Harnirattisai C, et al. Micro-tensile bond strengths of bonding agents to pulpal floor dentine. Int Endod J. 2002;35:833–9.

Kovarik RE, Breeding LC, Caughman WF. Fatigue life of three core materials under simulated chewing conditions. J Prosthet Dent. 1992;68:584–90.

Libman WJ, Nicholls JI. Load fatigue of teeth restored with cast posts and cores and complete crowns. Int J Prosthodont. 1995;8:155–61.

Lloyd PM, Palik JF. The philosophies of dowel diameter preparation: a literature review. J Prosthet Dent. 1993;69:32–6.

Loney RW, Moulding MB, Ritsco RG. The effect of load angulation on fracture resistance of teeth restored with cast post and cores and crowns. Int J Prosthodont. 1995;8:247–51.

Lovdahl PE, Nicholls JI. Pin-retained amalgam cores vs. cast-gold dowel-cores. J Prosthet Dent. 1977;38:507–14.

Malament KA, Socransky SS. Survival of Dicor glass-ceramic dental restorations over 16 years. Part III: effect of luting agent and tooth or tooth-substitute core structure. J Prosthet Dent. 2001;86:511–9.

Mallmann A, Jacques LB, Valandro LF, et al. Microtensile bond strength of photoactivated and autopolymerized adhesive systems to root dentin using translucent and opaque fiber-reinforced composite posts. J Prosthet Dent. 2007;97:165–72.

Mancebo JC, Jiménez-Castellanos E, Cañadas D. Effect of tooth type and ferrule on the survival of pulpless teeth restored with fiber posts: a 3-year clinical study. Am J Dent. 2010;23:351–6.

Mannocci F, Ferrari M, Watson TF. Intermittent loading of teeth restored using quartz fiber, carbon-quartz fiber, and zirconium dioxide ceramic root canal posts. J Adhes Dent. 1999;1(2):153–8.

Martinez-Gonzalez A, Amigó-Borrás V, Fons-Font A, et al. Response of three types of cast posts and cores to static loading. Quintessence Int. 2001;32(7):552–60.

Mattison GD, Delivanis PD, Thacker RW, et al. Effect of post preparation on the apical seal. J Prosthet Dent. 1984;51:785–9.

McDonald AV, King PA, Setchell DJ. An in vitro study to compare impact fracture resistance of intact root-treated teeth. Int Endod J. 1990;23:304–12.

McLaren JD, McLaren CI, Yaman P, et al. The effect of post type and length on the fracture resistance of endodontically treated teeth. J Prosthet Dent. 2009;101:174–82.

Mendoza DB, Eakle WS, Kahl EA, et al. Root reinforcement with a resin-bonded preformed post. J Prosthet Dent. 1997;78:10–4.

Mentink AG, Creugers NH, Meeuwissen R, et al. Clinical performance of different post and core systems—results of a pilot study. J Oral Rehabil. 1993;20:577–84.

Morgano S. Restoring pulpless teeth-do traditional principles still apply? Chicago: Scientific Session/American Academy of Crown & Bridge Prosthodontics; 2015. 27–28 Feb 2015.

Morgano SM, Rodrigues AH, Sabrosa CE. Restoration of endodontically treated teeth. Dent Clin N Am. 2004;48:397–416.

Nagasiri R, Chitmongkolsuk S. Long-term survival of endodontically treated molars without crown coverage: a retrospective cohort study. J Prosthet Dent. 2005;93:164–70.

Nergiz I, Schmage P, Platzer U, et al. Effect of different surface textures on retentive strength of tapered posts. J Prosthet Dent. 1997;78:451–7.

Oblak C, Jevnikar P, Kosmac T, et al. Fracture resistance and reliability of new zirconia posts. J Prosthet Dent. 2004;91:342–8.

Panitvisai P, Messer HH. Cuspal deflection in molars in relation to endodontic and restorative procedures. J Endod. 1995;21(2):57–61.

Papa J, Cain C, Messer HH. Moisture content of vital vs endodontically treated teeth. Endod Dent Traumatol. 1994;10:91–3.

Peroz I, Blankenstein F, Lange K-P, et al. Restoring endodontically treated teeth with posts and cores—a review. Quintessence Int. 2005;36(9):737–46.

Pilo R, Tamse A. Residual dentin thickness in mandibular premolars prepared with Gates Glidden and ParaPost drills. J Prosthet Dent. 2000;83:617–23.

Raiden GC, Gendelman H. Effect of dowel space preparation on the apical seal of root canal fillings. Endod Dent Traumatol. 1994;10:109–12.

Reagan SF, Fruits TJ, Van Brunt C, et al. Effects of cyclic loading on selected post-and-core systems. Quintessence Int. 1999;30:61–7.

Ree M, Schwartz RS. The endo-restorative interface: current concepts. Dent Clin N Am. 2010;54:345–74.

Reeh ES, Messer HH, Douglas WH. Reduction in tooth stiffness as a result of endodontic and restorative procedures. J Endod. 1989a;15(11):512–6.

Reeh ES, Douglas WH, Messer HH. Stiffness of endodontically-treated teeth related to restoration technique. J Dent Res. 1989b;68(11):1540–4.

Rezende da Silva N, Raposo LH, Versluis A, et al. The effect of post, core, crown type, and ferrule presence on the biomechanical behavior of endodontically treated bovine anterior teeth. J Prosthet Dent. 2010;104:306–17.

Rosen H. Operative procedures on mutilated endodontically treated teeth. J Prosthet Dent. 1961;11:973–86.

Rosenstiel SF, Land MF, Fujimoto J. Contemporary fixed prosthodontics. 5th ed. St Louis: Elsevier; 2016.

Ross IF. Fracture susceptibility of endodontically treated teeth. J Endod. 1980;6(5):560–5.

Rud J, Omnell K-A. Root fractures due to corrosion. Scand J Dent Res. 1970;78:397–403.

Sadan A. Post placement and cementation: part 1. Pract Proced Aesthet Dent. 2002;14(9):716.

Safavi KE, Dowden WE, Langeland K. Influence of delayed coronal permanent restoration on endodontic prognosis. Endod Dent Traumatol. 1987;3:187–91.

Sahafi A, Peutzfeldt A, Asmussen E, et al. Retention and failure morphology of prefabricated posts. Int J Prosthodont. 2004;17:307–12.

Salvi GE, Guldener S, Amstad T, et al. Clinical evaluation of root filled teeth restored with or without post-and-core systems in a specialist practice setting. Int J Prosthodont. 2007;40:209–15.

Saunders WP, Saunders EM. Coronal leakage as a cause of failure in root-canal therapy: a review. Endod Dent Traumatol. 1994;10:105–8.

Saupe WA, Gluskin AH, Radke RA. A comparative study of fracture resistance between morphologic dowel and cores and a resin-reinforced dowel system in the intraradicular restoration of structurally compromised roots. Quintessence Int. 1996;27:483–91.

Schwartz RS, Robbins JW. Post placement and restoration of endodontically treated teeth: a literature review. J Endod. 2004;30(5):289–301.
Sedgley CM, Messer HH. Are endodontically treated teeth more brittle? J Endod. 1992;18(7):332–5.
Shillingburg Jr HT, et al. Fundamentals of fixed prosthodontics. 4th ed. Hanover Park: Quintessence Publishing Co.; 2012.
Soares CJ, Soares PV, Santos-Filho PC, et al. The influence of cavity design and glass fiber posts on biomechanical behavior of endodontically treated premolars. J Endod. 2008a;34(8):1015–9.
Soares CJ, Santana FR, Pereira JC, et al. Influence of airborne-particle abrasion on mechanical properties and bond strength of carbon/epoxy and glass/Bis-GMA fiber-reinforced resin posts. J Prosthet Dent. 2008b;99:444–54.
Sorensen JA, Engelman MJ. Ferrule design and fracture resistance of endodontically treated teeth. J Prosthet Dent. 1990;63:529–36.
Sorensen JA, Martinoff JT. Intracoronal reinforcement and coronal coverage: a study of endodontically treated teeth. J Prosthet Dent. 1984a;51(6):780–4.
Sorensen JA, Martinoff JT. Clinically significant factors in dowel design. J Prosthet Dent. 1984b;52:28–35.
Sorensen JA, Martinoff JT. Endodontically treated teeth as abutments. J Prosthet Dent. 1985;53:631–6.
Sravanthi Y, Ramani YV, Asha M, et al. The comparative evaluation of the translucency of crowns fabricated with three different all-ceramic materials: an in vitro study. J Clin Diagn Res. 2015;9(2):30–4.
Standlee JP, Caputo AA. Effect of surface design on retention of dowels cemented with a resin. J Prosthet Dent. 1993;70:403–5.
Standlee JP, Caputo AA, Collard EW, et al. Analysis of stress distribution by endodontic posts. Oral Surg Oral Med Oral Pathol. 1972;33(6):952–60.
Steele A, Johnson BR. In vitro fracture strength of endodontically treated premolars. J Endod. 1999;25(1):6–8.
Stockton LW. Factors affecting retention of post systems: a literature review. J Prosthet Dent. 1999;81:380–5.
Stoll R, Cappel I, Jablonski-Momeni A, et al. Survival of inlays and partial crowns made of IPS empress after a 10-year observation period and in relation to various treatment parameters. Oper Dent. 2007;32(6):556–63.
Strand GV, Tveit AB, Gjerdet NR, et al. Marginal ridge strength of teeth with tunnel preparations. Int Dent J. 1995;45:117–23.
Strub JR, Pontius O, Koutayas S. Survival rate and fracture strength of incisors restored with different post and core systems after exposure in the artificial mouth. J Oral Rehabil. 2001;28:120–4.
Tan P, Aquilino SA, Gratton DG, et al. In vitro fracture resistance of endodontically treated central incisors with varying ferrule heights and configurations. J Prosthet Dent. 2005;93:331–6.
Teixeira E, Teixeira F, Piasick J, et al. An in vitro assessment of prefabricated fiber post systems. J Am Dent Assoc. 2006;137:1006–12.
Testore T, Badino M, Castagnola M. Vertical root fractures in endodontically treated teeth: a clinical survey of 36 cases. J Endod. 1993;19(2):87–90.
Tjan AH, Nemetz H. Effect of eugenol-containing endodontic sealer on retention of prefabricated posts luted with an adhesive composite resin cement. Quintessence Int. 1992;23(12):839–44.
Tjan AH, Tjan AH, Sun JC. Retention of luminex post system. Oral Health. 1997;87(8):31–5.
Torbjörner A, Karlsson S, Ödman PA. Survival rate and failure characteristics for two post designs. J Prosthet Dent. 1995;73:439–44.
Trabert KC, Cooney JP. The endodontically treated tooth. Dent Clin N Am. 1984;28(4):923–51.
Utter JD, Wong BH, Miller BH. The effect of cementing procedures on retention of prefabricated metal posts. J Am Dent Assoc. 1997;128:1123–7.
Weine FS, Wax AH, Wenckus CS. Retrospective study of tapered, smooth post systems in place for 10 years or more. J Endod. 1991;17(6):293–7.
Zhi-Yue L, Yu-Xing Z. Effects of post-core design and ferrule on fracture resistance of endodontically treated maxillary central incisors. J Prosthet Dent. 2003;89:368–73.

Fixed Restorative Materials

7

Mauricio Castellanos and Alex Delgado

Contents

Abstract

The clinical basis for selection of any restorative material should be based on scientific evidence and clinical experience. It is necessary to evaluate the information gathered from randomized clinical studies, where experimental materials are compared with a control group or a systematic review that answers a specific

M. Castellanos, DDS, MS (✉)
Division of Prosthodontics, Department of Restorative Dental Sciences, University of Florida, College of Dentistry, Gainesville, FL, USA
e-mail: ECastellanos@dental.ufl.edu

A. Delgado, DMD, MS
Department of Restorative Dental Sciences, University of Florida, College of Dentistry, Gainesville, FL, USA

G.M. Weinstein, M.T. Zientz (eds.), *The Dental Reference Manual*,
DOI 10.1007/978-3-319-39730-6_7

question relating to the material. It is important that the clinician takes into consideration factors that will affect the longevity of the restoration.

7.1 Clinical Basis for Selection of Restorative Material (All Ceramic, Zirconia, PFM, All Gold)

1. *The restorative material* – Clinicians have to be aware of the success and survival rate of the material as each material has a mode of fatigue and/or failure. The clinician should recognize and think critically about the choice of materials. Another important issue is the skills necessary in handling each material. In general, success of adhesive procedures for all ceramic crowns can be dependent on the skill of the practitioner and the ability to isolate the tooth.
2. *The patient* – Since all patients are not the same, it is imperative that we assess the caries risk, oral hygiene, occlusion (parafunctional habits, bruxism), diet, medications, and any habits (smoking, alcohol, drugs) of patients. In doing a general assessment, we can determine the best material of choice for the patient. Patients who are susceptible to staining in their teeth would not be good candidates for ceramic restorations unless the source of the stain is determined and the patient is counseled appropriately.
3. *The tooth* – It is very important to determine the restorability of the tooth and the periodontal condition in order to select a specific material. In fixed prosthodontics, it is critical to determine the ferrule (1.5–2 mm) or as Shillingburg's text describes is the amount of tooth structure remaining in the coronal area. Other considerations would be if the tooth is endodontically treated, its position in the arch and the occlusal load (See Chap. 6 Restorative Considerations).
4. *The operator* – Clinical experience plays an important role; it is essential that the clinician has the ability to communicate with the patient and inform him/her about the different options. The ability to pay attention to details and the relevant evidence-based knowledge will lead to a better decision.
5. *The laboratory* – There are many laboratories with different degrees of expertise, equipment, training, and technology. It is vital to communicate with your laboratory to achieve the expected outcome (See Chap. 20 Communicating with the Dental Laboratory).

7.2 Types of Materials Available for Fabrication of Fixed Restorations

7.2.1 Noble Alloys

In a laboratory prescription, it is crucial that you request the type of alloy that you selected for the patient. Gold is the standard metal alloy in dentistry. This alloy is composed mainly of gold that provides tarnish resistance. Because gold is not particularly strong enough to withstand the forces of mastication, it must be mixed with

Table 7.1 Types of gold

Type	AU %	Hardness	Indication
I	98	Soft	Class V, gold foils
II	77	Soft enough to make great margins	Inlays or small onlays with finishable margins on tooth surfaces
III	72	Hard	Crowns, nonfinishable margins
IV	69	Harder	Removable partial dentures

other metals. The other alloys that are added are silver (Ag) and copper (Cu) to give strength to the gold (Table 7.1).

Noble metals are the most popular when fabricating a fixed prosthodontic restoration. These include gold (Au), platinum (Pt), and palladium (Pd). Below is an illustration of the composition of noble metal alloys:

A. High gold: 80–85 % Au, 7–10 % Pt
B. High noble: 53 % Au, 38 % Pd, 0–12 % Ag
C. Pd-Ag alloy: 60 % Pd, 30 % Ag (shading problems, must use a low-sodium ceramic)

Base metal alloys are sometimes utilized due to the reduced cost. An example of this composition is nickel-chrome-beryllium: 65 % Ni, 20 % Cr, and 2 % Be. The problem with base metal alloys is the oxide. Oxide affects the porcelain bond, making that bond unreliable. Margin integrity is an issue as base metal alloys shrink significantly more than noble alloys. The margin distortion is a function of the geometry of the margin and the composition of the alloy. Due to the lower melting temperature, the casting has a greater probability of distorting.

7.2.2 All-Ceramics Restorations

A. *Feldspathic porcelain*: Is derived from the natural feldspar; it is predominantly a glass material with amorphous (noncrystalline) structure. It is a glass ceramic that is mainly composed of silicon dioxide (silica quartz) and some amount of alumina. It provides excellent esthetics, and its major concern is strength. Feldspathic porcelain has traditionally been used to veneer porcelain-fused-to-metal (PFM) restorations.
   Indications: *porcelain veneers*
B. *Leucite-reinforced pressed glass ceramic*: There is significant literature to support its use. This is a glass ceramic which has incorporated fillers to increase its strength. Pressed leucite-reinforced ceramic has been found to have better marginal adaptation than more traditional porcelain-fused-to-metal restorations (Goldin et al. 2005).
   Indications: Esthetic inlays, onlays, porcelain veneers, and anterior crowns
   Brand names: IPS Empress, Ivoclar Vivadent; 3G All-Ceramic System, Pentron; Finesse All-Ceramic, Dentsply; Authentic, Jensen Industries
C. *Lithium disilicate glass ceramic*: These are traditionally milled with computer-aided design/computer-aided milling (CAD/CAM) in the laboratory and pressed

with layers of porcelain for improved esthetics. The milled full contour form (monolithic) has been found to have very good survival rate in a 3-year study (Fasbinder et al. 2010). In three unit bridges, Kern et al. in 2012 have found that following manufacturer's directions, the survival of IPS e.max over 5–10 years is similar to the more traditional porcelain-fused-to-metal bridges. In addition, the cement type used for final cementation did not affect the longevity of the survival of the bridge. The restoration has to be characterized to obtain acceptable esthetics. It is the strongest glass ceramic in the market. Dental laboratories in the United States fabricate IPS e.max through a digital pathway and ultimately utilizing milling machines (see Fig. 7.1). In any milled ceramic, careful tooth preparation considerations should be observed to have successful outcomes (See Chap. 10 Indirect Restorations Utilizing CAD/CAM).

The long-term success of lithium disilicate crown is dependent on the bonding of the cement to the restoration and the tooth. Careful preparation of the restoration after the try in process removes contaminants like saliva and blood. Current recommendation is to "clean" the restoration using 5 % hydrofluoric etch for 20 s, rinse and dry, followed by silane application (Kern 2014). It is thus not necessary to have the laboratory etch the restoration prior to try in. Air abrasion of lithium disilicate is contraindicated as it may alter the marginal integrity. Following manufacturer's directions on the use of your chosen cement is also essential for success.

Indications: Anterior and posterior single crowns and three unit bridges, inlays and onlays, and veneers (Cortelli 2012; Sulaiman et al. 2015)

Brand name: IPS e.max, Ivoclar Vivadent

7.2.3 Other Metal

Zirconia: Is a shiny gray-white metal, which may look blue-black when in powder form. It is an oxide which has high tensile strength, high hardness, and high

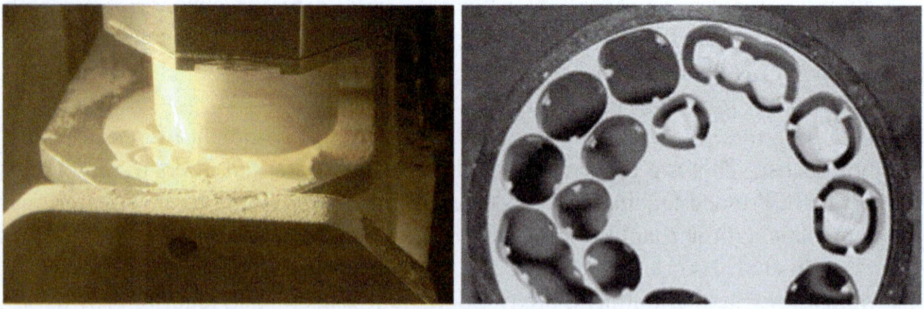

Fig. 7.1 Commercial milling units and a lithium disilicate puck which can accommodate 25–30 restorations and are milled in a few hours (Photo Courtesy of Mr. Kevin Hudi, DSG Americus Laboratories, Saint Petersberg, Florida)

corrosion resistance. It is a strong core that can be fabricated as a monolithic restoration or can be layered with porcelain over the core. The esthetic result is not comparable with the glass ceramics. Zirconia is milled and sintered in high-heat ovens to attain the correct fit on the tooth. An interesting video of this process can be found on https://www.youtube.com/watch?v=HDedHm5SWR4 (Accessed on March 22, 2016). A chairside zirconia CAD/CAM workflow was introduced by Dentsply Sirona and Glidewell laboratories in 2016.

There has not been a consensus on the best way to achieve adhesion of zirconia to the tooth. It is especially an issue when mechanical retention is not present. A recent review of the literature by Ozcan and Bernasconi revealed that adhesion of zirconia to the tooth is increased when two things are done (Ozcan and Barnasconi 2015):

1. Conditioning of the zirconia prior to bonding (use of silane or primers).
2. The use of an MDP monomer-based resin cement had slightly higher results.

In a literature review by Agustin-Panadero et al., their findings report high fracture rates of porcelain-veneered zirconia, 6–15 % over a 3–5-year period. This is compared to PFM which is 6–10 % over 10 years. Minimizing the thickness of the veneered surface decreases the risk of fracture (Grob and Sisera 2014). The monolithic zirconia on the other hand is heralded for its resistance to fracture even in limited occlusal clearance areas and feather edge (or shoulder-free preparations) (Nakamura et al. 2015).

Preparation of a zirconia crown prior to cementation should include air abrasion with alumina particles after try in to remove saliva or blood contaminants (Kern 2014):

Indications: (Monolithic) core for anterior and posterior crowns, nonesthetic zones, bridges, abutments for implants

Some brand names: BruxZir® Solid Zirconia and Prismatik™ Clinical Zirconia restorations

7.3 Design Guidelines for the Restoration

7.3.1 Laboratory Techniques (Our Special Acknowledgment to Mr. Lee Culp for Assisting Us in Writing This Section)

Beginning with the end in mind is a great way to understand what we as dentists need to provide our laboratory technicians in order for them to have the ability to fabricate functional and esthetic restorations. The techniques below are examples of how dental laboratories can improve the esthetics of all ceramic crowns. The basic foundation is keeping the majority of the tooth as a monolithic piece (milled as a solid structure Vazquez 2012) to preserve the strength of the zirconia or lithium disilicate restoration. If the restoration is to be fabricated from zirconia, the restoration will be designed in dental CAD/CAM software and then milled out to achieve

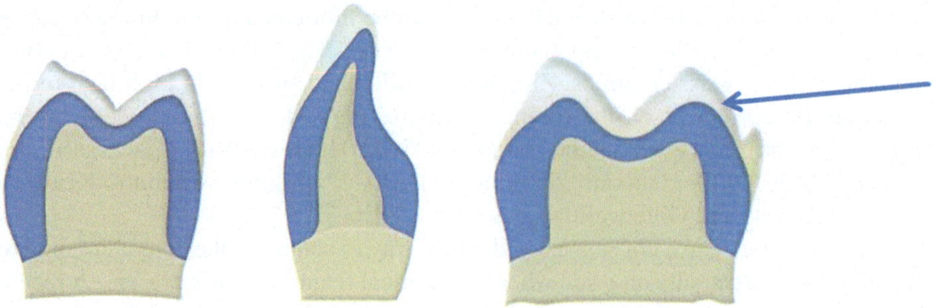

Fig. 7.2 Cutback. The full contour is utilized in essence to determine where the cutbacks are needed to maximize esthetics

the final tooth form. If the restoration is to be fabricated from lithium disilicate, the restoration can be "waxed up" by hand, similar to the creation of a gold crown, or it can be designed and milled in a dental CAD/CAM system.

For final esthetic enhancement, the porcelain is then layered in different shades and translucencies to achieve the correct esthetics for the different parts of the tooth. Strength and esthetics become possible when these techniques are adapted. For best results on esthetic cases, communication with the laboratory is an essential element even at the planning stage (See Chap. 20 Communicating with Dental Laboratories):

A. *Cutback technique*: Design is done as a full contour crown (blue and white layers together) utilizing design software, CAD. The design is then modified and a coping (blue layer) is milled through CAM. Porcelain layers (white) are pressed onto the coping to achieve the desired esthetics. The cutback technique was developed by Mr. Lee Culp in 2002. Ivoclar's Empress Esthetic system was based on this technique (Fig. 7.2 Images reprinted with permission from Ivoclar Vivadent).
B. *Full layering technique*: After the coping frame is milled, the entire anatomical shape of the tooth is layered by hand using the brush technique and fired over the CAD/CAM coping design in order to achieve better esthetics.
C. *Staining technique*: The entire crown is milled through a CAD/CAM pathway. The porcelain is then stained to characterize the crown.

7.3.2 Tooth Preparation Guidelines

7.3.2.1 Veneer Preparations (Table 7.2)

These illustrations are step-by-step guidelines in preparing a veneer. The same basic principles apply when preparing full coverage posterior or anterior teeth:

Table 7.2 Prior to large esthetic cases in the anterior, a wax up of the desired final result should be done. This would also be useful in fabricating provisional restorations and ultimately for the laboratory to fabricate the final restorations

Porcelain veneers	Cervical reduction	Mid-facial reduction	Incisal reduction	Comments
Porcelain veneers feldspathic	0.3 mm	0.5–0.7 mm	1–1.5 mm	Communicate with your lab technician regarding best ways to shade match. Photographs are often helpful Minimal preparation on tooth, bonded to enamel for better results 85 % of porcelain veneers are additive
Porcelain veneers pressed (e.max)	0.6 mm	0.6 mm	1–1.5 mm	Cervical reduction might end in dentin
Porcelain veneers to mask discolored dentin (mildly)	0.6–0.8 mm	0.8–1 mm	1–1.5 mm	Veneer preparation is on dentin. Increase in mm per shade change

Step 1 Depth guides are established and marked.

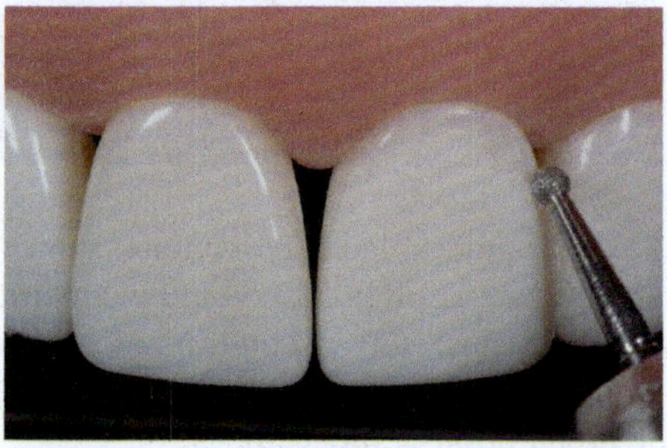

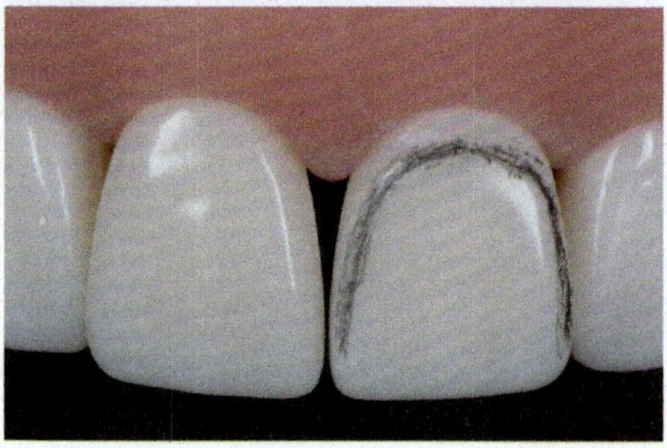

Step 2 Incisal reduction guides, followed by actual incisal reduction is critical in preventing over-reduction of the facial surface of the tooth.

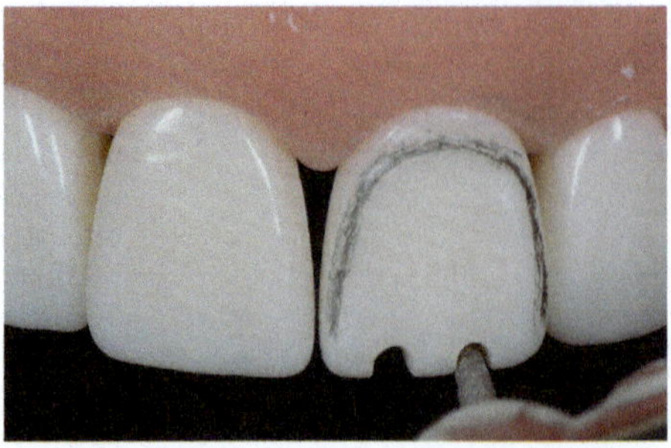

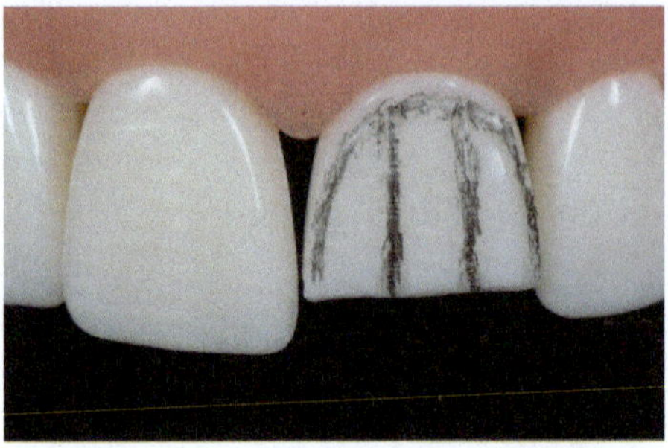

Step 3 In following the depth guides, facial reduction is done (Rosentiel 1995). The decision to break the contact is often based on the condition of the tooth. If old interproximal restorations exist, these should be incorporated into the preparation. Once again, a diagnostic wax up would help determine the amount of clearance needed for the preparation of the teeth.

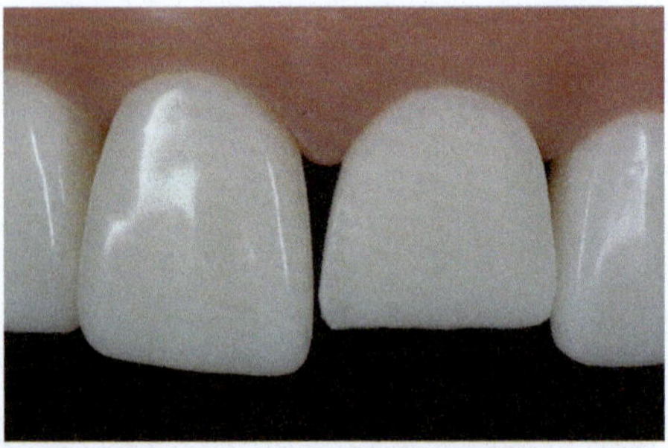

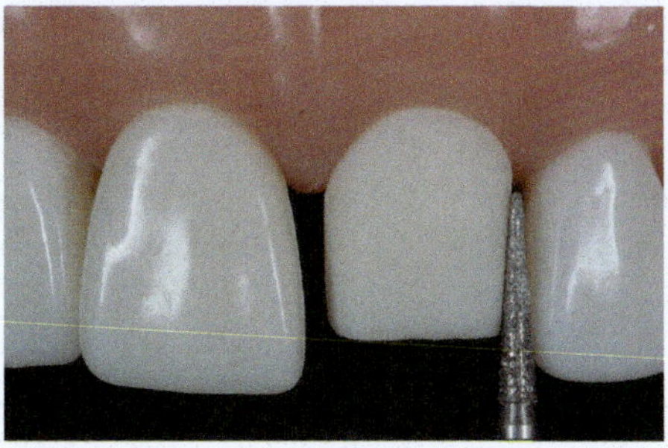

Step 4 The preparations should be very smooth with no sharp angles or corners (Shillimburg 2012). Be mindful of the final material selected to fabricate these veneers as they all have minimum thickness that must be met (Kent 1998; Smith 1999).

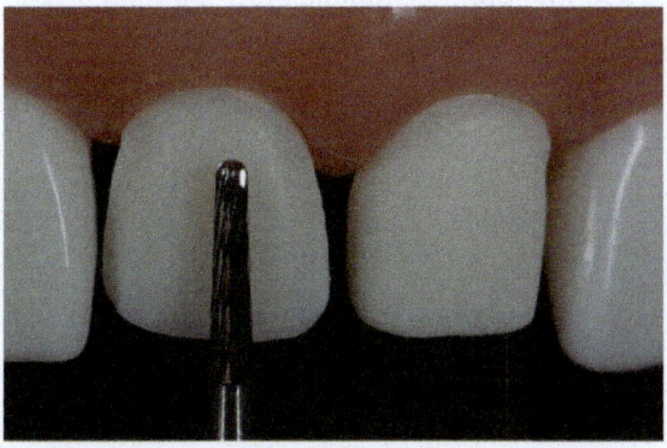

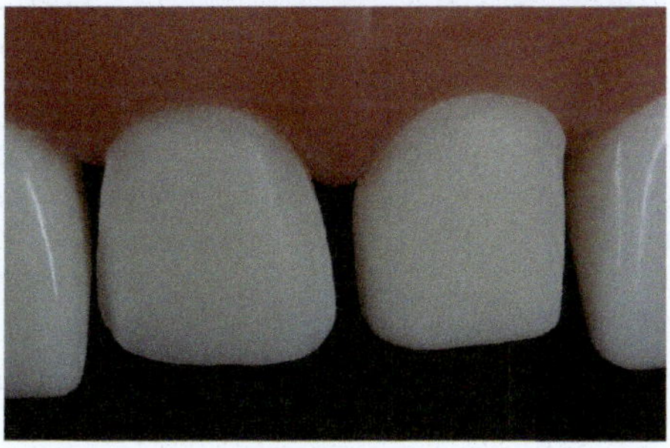

Table 7.3 These guidelines are for the feldspathic or leucite-reinforced ceramics

All ceramic crowns (ACC)	Axial reduction	Incisal/occlusal reduction	Margin	Comments
ACC posterior crowns	1.2–1.4 mm	1.5–2 mm	Shoulder 1–1.5 mm	This applies for zirconia with porcelain layers
ACC anterior crowns	0.6–0.8 mm	2–2.5 mm	Shoulder 1.5 mm	This may vary depending on the esthetics

Annesrtedt (1996)

Table 7.4 Guidelines for more traditional restorations that have served dentistry for many decades

Porcelain fused to metal (PFM)	Axial reduction	Incisal/ occlusal reduction	Margin	Comments
Nobel metals	1.5–1.7 mm	1.5–2 mm	Chamfer/modified Chamfer/shoulder 1–1.5 mm	Increase reduction of functional cusps to compensate for thickness of porcelain + metal Margin design depends on esthetics and function
Base metals	1.0–1.5 mm	1.5–2 mm	Chamfer or modified chamfer 1.5 mm	Less reduction than nobles Not recommended because of metal oxides

Goodacre (2001); Wilson and Chen (1994)

Table 7.5 Full cast gold and monolithic zirconia allow minimal preparation of the tooth

Full cast gold/ monolithic zirconia	Axial reduction	Incisal/occlusal reduction	Margin	Comments
Gold	0.5–1 mm	1–1.5 mm (functional cusps) 0.5–1 mm (nonfunctional cusps)	Chamfer 0.5–1 mm	Fees for high noble metal are significantly more than monolithic zirconia
Monolithic zirconia	0.5–1 mm	1–1.5 mm (functional cusps) 0.5–1 mm (nonfunctional cusps)	Chamfer 1–1.5 mm	Consider mechanical retention when preparing for zirconia

Table 7.6 CAD/CAM-milled restorations are quite common from today's laboratories. These are done in either lithium disilicate or zirconia. Specific guidelines in preparing the tooth for these restorations should be noted to insure a well-adapted restoration

CAD/CAM restorations	Axial reduction	Incisal/occlusal reduction	Margin	Comments
CAD/CAM	1–2 mm	1.5	Shoulder 1 mm	See Chap. 10 indirect restorations

Guidelines for other restorations: (*Tables* 7.3, 7.4, 7.5, *and* 7.6)

7.4 Cements

The selection of the luting agent is dependent on the specific clinical situation, the type of restoration utilized, and the physical, biologic, and handling properties of the luting agent (Donovan 2006). The primary purpose of the luting procedure is to achieve a durable bond and to have good marginal adaptation of the luting material to the restoration and tooth. For cement selections the authors have provided a table to use as a guideline to demonstrate physical properties, indications, and components of current cements available in the market (Table 7.7).

Table 7.7 Dental cements and their properties (Jivraj et al. 2006; Kim et al. 2006)

Cement	Composition	Adhesion to tooth	Adhesion to restoration	Strength	Solubility	Fl-release	Film thick	Biocompatibility	Ease	Indications	Dowel	Technique sensitivity
ZnPO4	ZnO MgO/H3PO4	No	No	15 k psi (CS) 8k psi (DT)	Not good	No	25 μm	Ok	Diff no problem	Metal/Zr	None	None
Polycarboxide	ZnO MgO/PAA	Yes	No	Low 10 k psi (CS/DT)	Not good	No	25 μm No problem	Ok	No problem	Provisional implants	None	None
GI	SiA/PAA	Yes	No	Good	More less	No	25 μm No problem	Ok	Negative	None	None	Yes
RMGI	GI+resin	Yes	No	Good	Good	No	No problem	Ok	More less	Metal/Zr	None	None
	Resin+glass+initiator		Yes				80–200 μm	Shrinkage		Veneers, cream res		
Resin	BisGMA+fillers+silane	Yes	Ceramic/ metal	Very good	Very good	No	400 μm	C factor	Hard		Good	Yes
ZOE	ZnO/Eug	No	No	Very low	Very good	No	No problem	Ok	No problem	Provisionals	None	None

7.4.1 Temporary Cements

1. Intermediate restorative material (IRM) or zinc oxide with eugenol- It is really meant for use as a temporary restoration but can also be used to cement provisional crowns. It contains eugenol which is helpful to reduce sensitivity in vital teeth.
2. Temp bond NE- A zinc oxide with *NO* eugenol (thus the NE). Safe for use in all provisional restorations.
3. Polycarboxylate (Duralon)- This has good film thickness, ideal for provisionals that need to stay in the mouth for an extended period of time.

It is interesting to note that some studies claim that the type of temporary cement and its composition have no effect on the retention of the final ceramic restorations to the tooth (Abo-Hamar et al. 2005). Other publications claim that the presence of eugenol in temporary cements will contaminate the preparation and reduce the bond strength of adhesive systems to the tooth (Ribeiro et al. 2011). Zortuk et al. tested temporary cement removal utilizing an explorer, ER:YAG laser, and a brush with pumice prior to final cementation; each protocol resulted in similar bond strengths (Zortuk et al. 2012).

7.4.2 **Permanent Cements** (Deghan 2014)

1. Glass ionomer- Renown as the cement that releases fluoride in vivo thus having a bacteriostatic effect for the first 24 h (Freedman, 2003). More studies show greater promise for the use of glass ionomer cement to release chlorhexidine over a period of time (Bellis et al. 2016). The bond strength for glass ionomer is significantly less than the resin-modified glass ionomers or resin cements (Tomar et al. 2015), although it is noted to chemically bond to the tooth structure.
2. Resin-modified glass ionomer- In a comparative study utilizing different cements on metal crowns, resin-modified glass ionomer was shown to have the highest bond strength to metal. It was also noted that preparation of the metal crown surface prior to cementation with sandblasting with alumina and ultrasonic cleaning improved the bond strength significantly (Tomar et al. 2015). Ease of use and clean up after cementation has made this a widely used cement.
3. Resin cement- It is the cement with more technique-sensitive in today's market. It is the cement of choice for all ceramic restorations as it prevents fracture of the porcelain. These cements are manufactured as light-cured, dual-cure, or auto-cure resins. Following specific manufacturer's instructions is the key to successful bonding.
4. Zinc phosphate- A good cement that is still in use with long-term clinical success. There have been concerns for its low pH causing pulpal irritation. This is often manifested by post-cementation sensitivity by the patient. It is recommended that in tooth preparations that are near the pulp of the tooth, other cements should be considered. In patients that have sensitivity, resolution often takes 3 weeks to resolve, basically the pulp reacting and placing reparative dentin and distancing itself from the cement (Pameijer 2012).

References

Abo-Hamar S, Federlin M, Hiller KA, Friedl KH, Schmalz G. Effect of temporary cements on the bond strength of ceramic luted to dentin. Dent Mater. 2005;21(9):794–803.

Annerstedt AL, Engström U, Hansson A, Jansson T, Karlsson S, Liljihagen H, et al. Axial wall convergence of full veneer crown preparations. Documented for dental students and general practitioners. Acta Odontol Scand. 1996;54:109–12.

Bellis C, Nobbs A, O'Sullivan D, Holder J, Barbour M. Glass ionomer cements functionalised with a concentrated paste of chlorhexidine hexametaphosphate provides dose-dependent chlorhexidine release over at least 14 months. J Dent. 2016;45:53–8.

Cortellini D, Canale A. Bonding lithium Disilicate ceramic to feather-edge tooth preparations: a minimally invasive treatment concept. J Adhes Dent. 2012;14:7–10.

Dehghan M, Braxton A, Simon J. An overview of permanent cements. Inside Dentistry. 2012;8(11). The ISNN: https://www.dentalaegis.com/id/2012/11/an-overview-of-permanent-cements. Accessed 25 Mar 2016.

Donovan TE. The selection of contemporary restorative materials: anecdote vs. evidence-based? J Calif Dent Assoc. 2006;34(2):129–34.

Fasbinder D, Denninson JB, Heys D, Neiva G. A clinical evaluation of chairside lithium Disilicate CAD/CAM crowns: a two-year report. J Am Dent Assoc. 2010;141:10S–14S.

Freedman R, Diefenderfer KE. Effects of daily fluoride exposures on fluoride release by glass ionomer-based restoratives. Oper Dent. 2003;28(2):178–85.

Goldin E, Boyd N, Goldstein G, Hittelman E, Thompson V. Marginal fit of leucite-glass pressable ceramic restorations and ceramic pressed-to-metal restorations. J Prosthet Dent. 2005;93(2):143–7.

Goodacre CJ, Campagni WV, Aquilino SA. Tooth preparations for complete crowns: an art form based on scientific principles. J Prosthet Dent. 2001;85(4):363–76.

Grob E, Sisera M. Monolithic zirconia complete arch reconstructions. In: Ferencz J, editor. High strength ceramics interdisciplinary perspectives. 1st ed. Chicago: Quintessence; 2014. p. 188–203.

Jivraj SA, Kim TH, Donovan TE. Selection of luting agents, part 1. J Calif Dent Assoc. 2006;34(2):149–60.

Kent WA, Shillingburg Jr HT, Duncanson Jr MG. Taper of clinical preparations for cast restorations. Quintessence Int. 1988;19:339–45.

Kern M. Cementation procedures for ceramics. In: Ferencz J, editor. High strength ceramics interdisciplinary perspectives. 1st ed. Chicago: Quintessence; 2014. p. 173–85.

Kern M, et al. Ten-year results of three-unit bridges made of monolithic lithium Disilicate ceramic. J Dent Assoc. 2012;143(3):234–40.

Kim TH, Jivraj SA, Donovan TE. Selection of luting agents, part 2. J Calif Dent Assoc. 2006;34(2):161–6.

McLaren EA, Whiteman YY. Ceramics: rationale for material selection. Compend Contin Educ Dent. 2010;31(9):666–8.

Nakamura K, Harada A, Inagaki R, Kanno T, Niwano Y, Milleding P, Örtengren U. Fracture resistance of monolithic zirconia molar crowns with reduced thickness. Acta Odontol Scand. 2015;73(8):602–8.

Ozcan M, Bernasconi M. Adhesion of zirconia used for dental restorations: a systematic review and meta-analysis. J Adhes Dent. 2015;17(1):7–26.

Pameijer C. A review of luting agents. Int J Dent. 2012. ISSN: http://www.ncbi.nlm.nih.gov/pmc/articles/PMC3296365/. Accessed 1 Apr 2016.

Ribeiro JCV, Coelho PG, Janal MN, Silva NRFA, Monteiro AJ, Fernandes CAO. The influence of temporary cements on dental adhesive systems for luting cementation. J Dent. 2011;39(3):255–62.

Rosenstiel SF, Land MF, Fujimoto J. Contemporary fixed prosthodontics. 2nd ed. St. Louis: Mosby–Year Book; 1995. p. 137–8, 170–3, 184–5, 229.

Shillingburg H, et al. Fundamentals of fixed prosthodontics. 4th ed. Illinois: Quintessence; 2012.
Smith CT, Gary JJ, Conkin JE, Franks HL. Effective taper criterion for the full veneer crown preparation in preclinical prosthodontics. J Prosthodont. 1999;8:196–200.
Sulaiman T, Delgado A, Donovan TE. Survival rate of lithium Disilicate restorations at 4 years: a retrospective study. J Prosthet Dent. 2015;114(3):364–6.
Tomar SS, Bhattacharyya J, Ghosh S, Goel P, Das S, Chakarvarty K. Comparative evaluation of bond strength of all-metal crowns with different luting agents after undergoing various modes of surface treatments: an in-vitro study. J Indian Prosthodont Soc. 2015;15(4):318–25.
Vasquez J. The canvas cutback technique for IPS e-maxPress and emax CAD. Inside Dental Technology. 2012;3(6). The ISSN: https://www.dentalaegis.com/idt/2012/06/the-canvas-cutback-technique-for-ips-emax-press-and-emax-cad. Accessed 29 Mar 2016.
Wilson A, Chan DC. The relationship between preparation convergence and retention of extracoronal retainers. J Prosthodont. 1994;3:74–8.
Zortuk M, Gumus HO, Kilinc H, Tuncdemir AR. Effect of different provisional cement remnant cleaning procedures including Er:YAG laser on shear bond strength of ceramics. J Adv Prosthodont. 2012;4(4):192–6.

Removable Partial Dentures (RPD) Treatment: A Clinical Guide

8

Mauricio Castellanos and Luisa F. Echeto

Contents

M. Castellanos, DDS, MS
Division of Prosthodontics, Department of Restorative Dental Sciences, University of Florida, College of Dentistry, Gainesville, FL, USA

L.F. Echeto, DDS, MS (✉)
Division of Prosthodontics and Predoctoral Prosthodontics Program, Department of Restorative Dental Sciences, University of Florida, College of Dentistry, Gainesville, FL, USA
e-mail: LECHETO@dental.ufl.edu

G.M. Weinstein, M.T. Zientz (eds.), *The Dental Reference Manual*,
DOI 10.1007/978-3-319-39730-6_8

Abstract

Removable partial denture is an integral component of treatment plan development. Its primary goal is the preservation of the integrity of remaining teeth and adjacent structures. Other objectives include the elimination of disease and the replacement of missing teeth and structures as well as the restoration of function in an esthetically pleasing manner. These objectives cannot be achieved without a thorough clinical and radiographic evaluation, complete diagnosis, and adequate treatment plan arranged in a logical sequence.

Designing a removable partial denture is challenging since there is rarely one correct design. There may be differences in what dentists may consider appropriate for a particular situation. We will endeavor to guide you with foundation knowledge in removable partial denture design based on the fundamental, biological, and mechanical concepts.

This clinical guide includes all of the aspects to be considered in the treatment of the partially edentulous patients with removable partial dentures (RPD). Step-by-step procedures will be described including the objectives of each visit, the materials and instruments needed, and the techniques involved for a successful treatment with predictable results.

8.1 Classification of Removable Partial Dentures (RPD)

Partially edentulous patients are classified using the *Kennedy classification* system. This classification is a universally accepted classification that has been created by Dr. Edward Kennedy in 1925 for easy communication among dentists and laboratory technicians.

The Kennedy classification is composed of four major categories based on their clinical occurrence. It allows visualization of the type of partially edentulous arch, permits differentiation between tooth-supported and tooth-tissue supported partial dentures, and serves as a guide to the type of design to be used. Each Kennedy classification, except class I, refers to a single edentulous area. If another edentulous area is present, those are called *modification spaces.*

8.1.1 Class I (Fig. 8.1)

1. Bilateral edentulous areas posterior to the remaining teeth
2. Bilateral distal extension

8.1.2 Class II (Fig. 8.2)

1. Unilateral edentulous area posterior to the remaining teeth
2. Unilateral distal extension

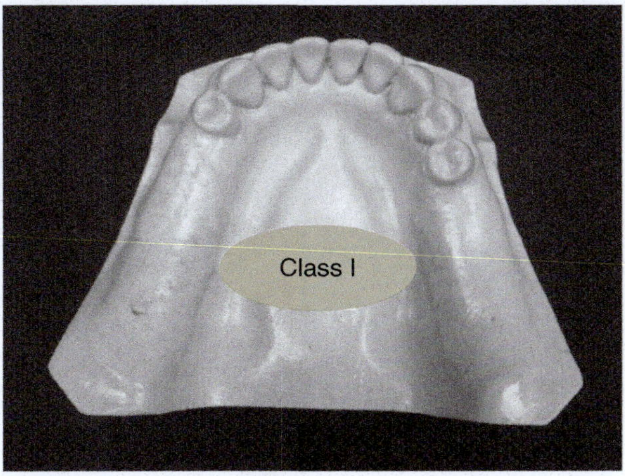

Fig. 8.1 Kennedy class I – mandibular case

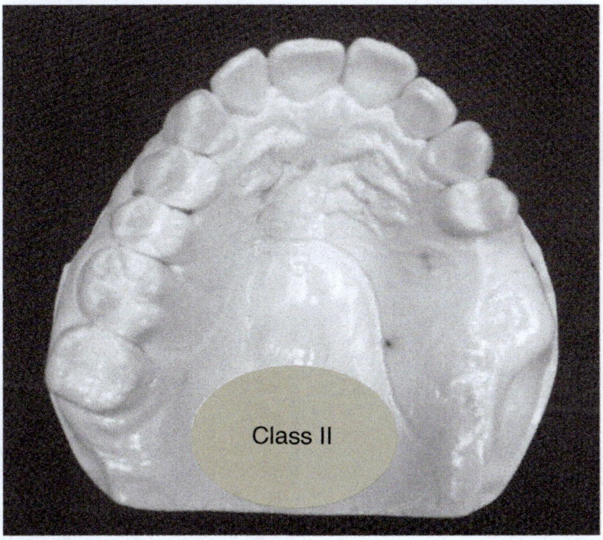

Fig. 8.2 Kennedy class II – maxillary case

8.1.3 **Class III** (Fig. 8.3)

1. Unilateral edentulous area with natural teeth both anterior and posterior to it.

8.1.4 **Class IV** (Fig. 8.4)

1. Single bilateral edentulous area located anterior to the remaining natural teeth.
2. It *MUST* cross the dental midline.
3. *Does NOT allow modification or additional spaces.*

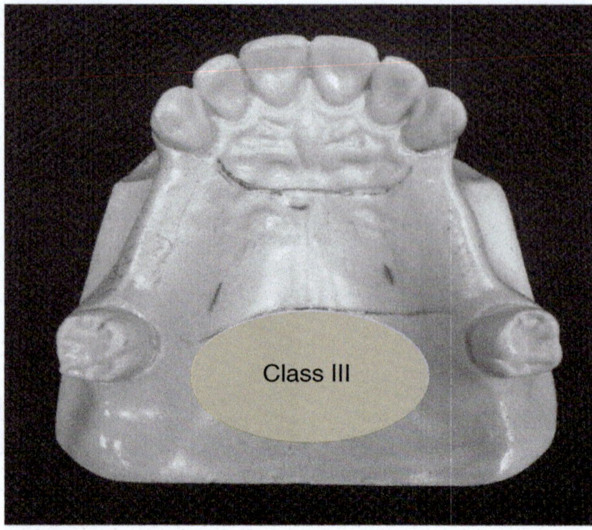

Fig. 8.3 Kennedy class III – maxillary case

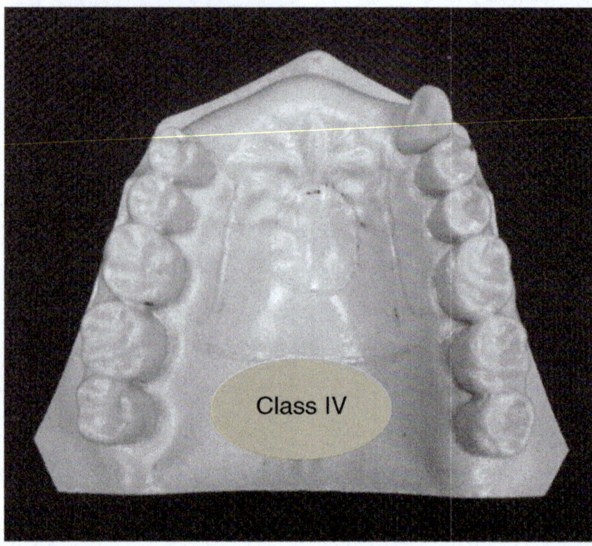

Fig. 8.4 Kennedy class IV – maxillary case

8.1.5 Applegate Rules

1. Each additional edentulous area (*NOT* each additional missing tooth).
2. The most posterior edentulous area *ALWAYS* determines the classification.
3. Edentulous areas other than those determining the classification are referred to as modification spaces and are designated by their number (i.e., mod 1, 2, or 3).
4. The extent of the modification or number of teeth missing is not considered, *only the number of additional edentulous areas.*
5. If the second molar is missing and it will *NOT* be replaced, it is not considered in the classification.

6. Classification should follow extractions that might alter the classification.
7. If the third molar is missing and it will *NOT* be replaced, it is not considered in the classification.
8. If the third molar is present and it will be used as abutment, it is considered in the classification.

8.2 Fundamentals of RPD Design Considerations

Significant *displacement differences* should be considered when designing a removable partial denture that is supported by teeth and soft tissues, i.e., Kennedy class I RPD situations – Distal extension cases:

1. Healthy teeth – displaced ~ 0.2 mm
2. Soft tissue – displaced ~ 1.0 mm or more

To prevent displacement of RPD away from oral tissues and rotational movements, *retention* is obtained by *direct* and *indirect* retainers. Optimum *support* of distal extension denture base is necessary as well as the use of flexible direct retention to prevent the torquing forces transmitted to the abutment teeth. Additionally, the equitable distribution of occlusal forces preserves the remaining teeth and residual ridges.

Kennedy class I RPD is a significantly challenging denture since it has a rotational fulcrum:

1. Two flexible direct retention retainers are needed with the use of stress relief clasps that prevent torquing forces to the abutment.
2. Provision of indirect retention retainers prevents the rotation of the denture.

Kennedy class III RPD is supported *by abutments only* (teeth or implants) anterior and posterior to the edentulous space. This class does not tend to move or rotate in function. It is considered the most stable RPD:

1. Denture bases do not rotate or lift away if there are enough remaining teeth to place four retainers in a quadrilateral configuration.
2. Compensation of rotational forces is *NOT* needed.
3. Residual ridges used for support in long-span cases only.
4. Direct retention is needed to prevent dislodgment of the denture when functioning.
5. Any clasp could be designed – There are no restrictions.

Kennedy class II RPD has features of both, class I for the tooth-tissue supported side and class III for the tooth-supported side:

1. Well-adapted denture base is necessary.
2. Properly designed direct retention is needed. Three clasps (two must be stress relieve clasps) positioned in a tripodal configuration.
3. Appropriately positioned *indirect* retention is also needed.

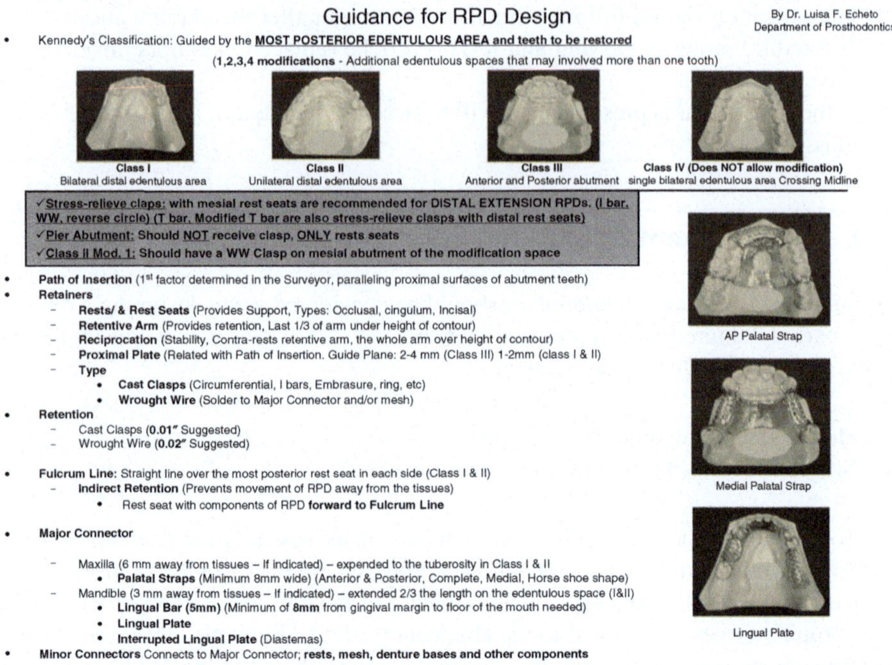

Fig. 8.5 Guidance for RPD design created by Dr. Luisa F. Echeto

Kennedy class IV RPD does not allow for modifications as any additional posterior space will change the classification:

1. Long span acts as a reserved class I RPD. In these cases appropriately positioned indirect retention is needed.
2. Well-adapted denture base is necessary.
3. Properly designed direct retention is needed. Four clasps placed on posterior teeth is the most common design (i.e., bilateral embrasure clasps – if occlusion allows) (Figs. 8.5, 8.6, and 8.7).

8.3 RPD Fabrication Steps

The removable partial dentures fabrication consists of six visits.

Visit 1: Preliminary impressions, diagnostic casts, and RPD design
Visit 2: Mouth preparations and final impressions
Visit 3: Framework try-in and records
Visit 4: Teeth try-in
Visit 5: Delivery
Visit 6: 24-h check

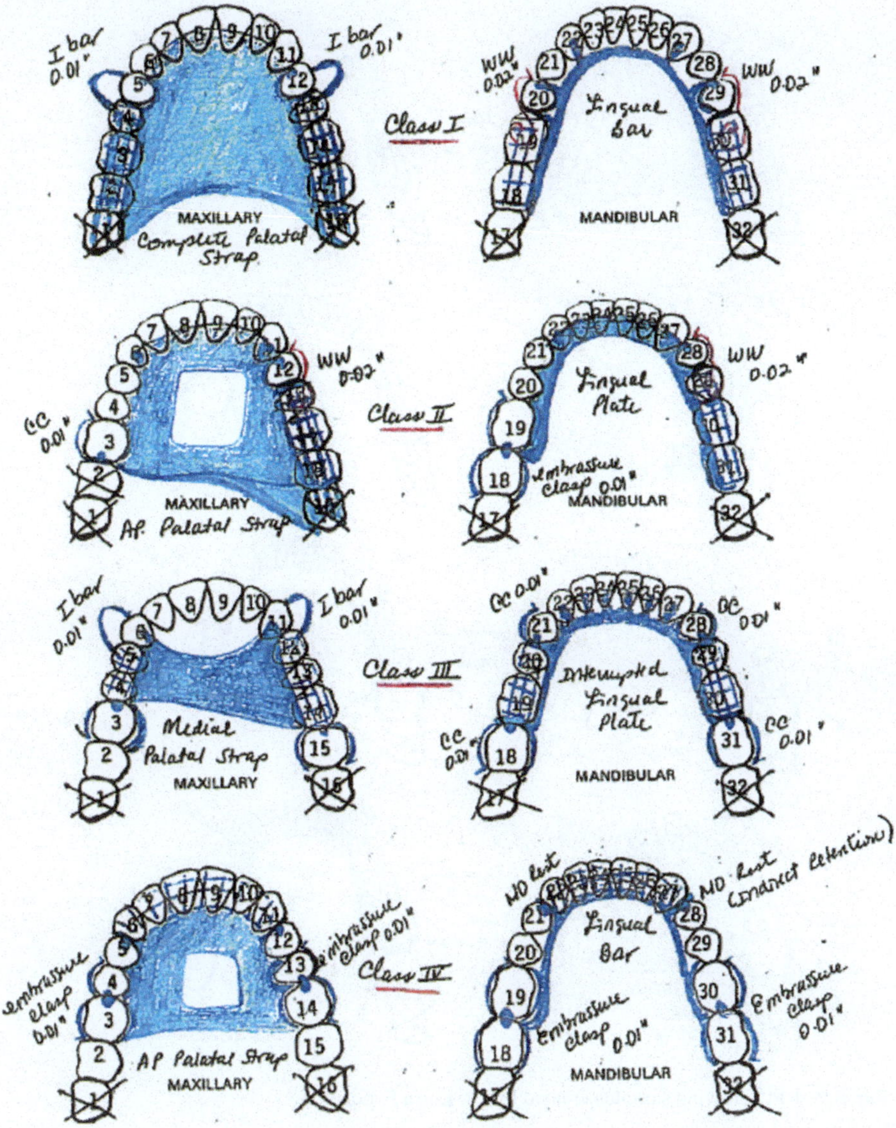

Fig. 8.6 RPD drawing samples created by Dr. Luisa F. Echeto

8.3.1 Visit 1: Preliminary Impressions, Diagnostic Casts, and RPD Design

Objectives:

1. Fabrication of diagnostic casts and articulation using facebow and MMR record
   (a) Class III and IV cases will be mounted in maximum intercuspation.
   (b) Class I and II cases will be mounted in centric relation using record bases and wax rims.

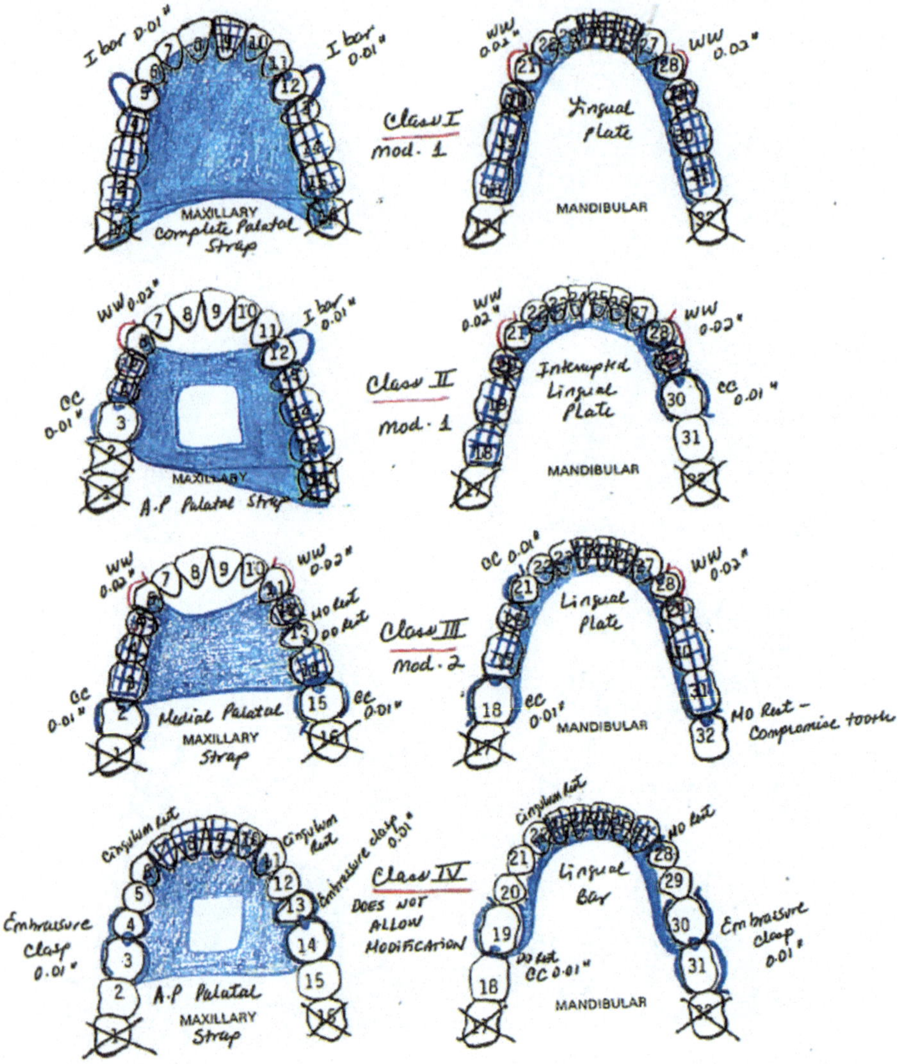

Fig. 8.7 RPD drawing samples created by Dr. Luisa F. Echeto

2. Clinical and radiographic examination along with diagnostic casts evaluation
3. Establishment of the RPD design

See Chap. 9 Occlusion.

At the Treatment Plan Visit We Should Consider:

1. Disease control on RPD patients.
2. High caries/periodontal risk.
3. Previous RPDs and failures.
4. The distance (8 mm) of the tongue frenulum insertion with a periodontal probe in order to determine the use of the lingual bar or lingual plate as major connector.
   (a) Clinical evaluation is necessary by asking the patient to raise the tongue.

5. Deep bites/interference/no clearance for the maxillary major connector.
6. Evaluate for loss of vertical dimension of occlusion.
7. Evaluate the periodontal prognosis of abutments for RPDs.
   (a) Plan for RPD repairs – by the use of lingual plates.
   (b) Do not use compromised tooth for a distal extension partial when the tooth adjacent may be a better abutment.
8. Determine if the tooth requires a survey crown as opposed to clasping a tooth with multiple restorations. Can the patient afford the treatment?
   (a) Survey crowns – RPD design done prior to crown fabrication
9. Risk assessment of endodontically treated teeth with posts for distal extension partials.
   (a) Most of the time they will fail within 5 years.
   (b) Extraction.
   (c) Should receive rest seat only.

See Chap. 6 Restorative Considerations of Endodontically Treated Teeth.

10. Number of teeth present and the location/distribution of remaining teeth can be critical for the success of the RPD.
    (a) Canines are crucial for maxillary RPD success when no posterior teeth are present.
11. Full Valplast (recommended only for interim RPD).
    (a) Combination with metal major connectors must be planned.
    (b) It should not be an option for distal extension RPDs.

Materials

Alginate, adhesive, rope wax, boxing wax, stone – microstone, Blu-Mousse, record base triad, base plate wax, lead pencil, red/blue pencil, RPD worksheet

Instruments

Mirror, explorer, probe, cotton pliers, stock plastic tray (S,M,L), facebow, articulator, surveyor, removable burs, waxing instruments, curing unit

Technique

1. Complete clinical and radiographic examination is performed.
2. The case is classified using the four Kennedy classification for partially dentate dental arches.
3. A plastic stock tray is selected (S,M,L).
4. Corresponding adhesive is applied to the tray.
5. Maxillary and mandibular preliminary impressions are made with irreversible colloid (alginate).
6. Facebow transfer is made using Blu-Mousse in the articulator fork to index.
7. MI record is made with Blu-Mousse if hand articulation is not achievable for class III and IV cases.
8. Maxillary and mandibular impression are poured with microstone to fabricate diagnostic casts.
9. Diagnostic casts are then indexed in the bottom with a tripod round channels.

10. Record bases and wax rims are fabricated in Kennedy class I and II cases for proper MMR record.
    (a) Patient is reappointed for CR record using the record bases and wax rims.
11. Diagnostic casts are then mounted on the articulator using the facebow record and MI or CR record using the record bases and wax rims.
12. Begin the RPD design process using the mounted diagnostic casts and the surveyor following the RPD principles.
13. Using accumulated diagnostic information, formulate a sequential treatment plan for a partially edentulous patient.
14. Given a partially edentulous patient, discuss the factors influencing the prognosis of the patient's treatment.

8.3.2 Visit 2: Mouth Preparations and Final Impression

Objective

Properly prepare enamel, restoration, or crown surfaces according to the RPD treatment plan design to receive a metal removable partial denture.

At the Teeth Preparation Appointment We Should Consider:

1. Space for the minor connector to avoid occlusal interference.
2. Use the occlusal paper to determine where the opposing tooth contacts before make the preparation to avoid interference of the metal structure on the occlusion.
3. Adding composite to the tooth to gain retention.
   (a) Dimples are created when you are going to use a cast clasps as a retainer.
4. Rest seats should go on restoration and enamel.
5. Evaluate the inter-occlusal space using mounted models.
6. Evaluate restoration where rest seats will be placed and make sure that the remaining restoration is strong enough to hold the RPD without fracture.
7. Inform the patient about the risks of making mouth preparations in existing crowns.

Materials

Chamfer bur, #2 round bur, #330 inverted cone bur

Instruments

Removable denture tray to include but not limited to, mouth mirror, explorer, probe, Bard Parker holder, wax spatula #7, #32 impression spatula, cleoid-discoid wax carver, and high-speed handpiece

8.3.3 Visit 2A: Mouth Preparations

1. Evaluate the previously approved treatment plan RPD design with the patient.

2. The following procedures detail how to prepare the appropriate rest seats and other mouth preparation components:
   (a) Occlusal rest seat – Depending on whether the tooth is a molar or a premolar, take a #2 round bur mounted on a high-speed handpiece and cut the tooth or the crown to a depth of 1.5 mm and a buccolingual and mesio-distal width of 2–3 mm in the position of the rest seat.
   (b) Cingulum rest seat – Use a #330 inverted cone bur or a chamfer bur and follow the outline of the cingulum on the maxillary canines. Create a positive shelf as shown in the shape of the cingulum.
   (c) Ball rests – These types of rests are indicated for mandibular canines since they do not have a large cingulum OR for maxillary canines where placement of a cingulum rest is not feasible.
      (i) Using a chamfer bur, angle the bur directly parallel to the long axis of the tooth and make a notch where the center of the cingulum is. This establishes the location of your ball rest. Use articulating paper to identify the location of the rest seat away from the occlusal contact at all possible.
      (ii). Using a #330 bur, drill a triangular-shaped hole with the base on the gingival side of the cingulum, to the depth of an amalgam preparation (1.5 mm).
      (iii) Fill the preparation with amalgam and using a ball burnisher to create a positive rest seat on the gingival portion of the preparation.
      (iv) Test the support of your rest seat by placing a probe on the rest and pushing gingivally. If the probe slips, then the rest is ineffective for support and needs to be modified.
   (d) Guide planes – Using a chamfer bur, angle the handpiece parallel to the long axis of the tooth on the proximal surface adjacent to the edentulous area. Make a 0.25 mm vertical slice on the tooth and the other proximal surfaces. Make vertical slices parallel to each other.
   (e) Tooth modifications – If modification is for reducing the height of the contour, use a chamfer and remove tooth structure similar to making guide planes. If the tooth needs an undercut, use an oval-shaped bur to create an undercut where needed.
3. It is recommended to make a quick alginate impression and pour with slurry water to evaluate preparations in the surveyor prior to final impression.
4. Once preparations are completed and polished, fluoride application should be done unless final impression will be done in the same session. In this case it should be applied after the final impression.

8.3.4 Visit 2B: Final Impression

Objective

Accurately capture the different components of the RPD for fabrication of metal framework with the appropriate impression material and custom tray. Altered cast technique might be considered.

Materials

A custom tray made out of triad light-cured material (for class I and II), stock metal/plastic tray (class III and IV), modeling compound, Bunsen burner, alcohol torch

Alcohol torch, polysulfide or vinylpolysiloxane light and medium body or regular set alginate, 2x2 gauze, aluwax, or VPS bite registration material

Instruments

Removable denture tray to include but not limited to, mouth mirror, explorer, probe, Bard Parker holder, wax spatula #7, #32 impression spatula, cleoid-discoid wax carver, and high-speed handpiece

Technique

1. For class I and class II RPDs, a custom tray needs to be fabricated to capture the edentulous areas and prior to this visit. Class III and IV RPDs will need a properly fitting stock metal tray. Make sure to use the proper size tray.
2. Prior to making the impression for class I and II, border mold the edentulous areas only.
3. Dry the patient's teeth with 2x2 gauze prior to making the impression.
4. Mix the impression material according to manufacturer's instructions.
5. Wait for the proper setting time for the impression material and remove from patient's mouth.
6. Check if the patient is doing alright and then rinse the impression with water. Inspect the impression to see if all the rest seats and teeth included in the RPD were properly captured. Inspect for the presence of bubbles or blebs in the impression.
7. Make sure that when you are making the mandibular final impression, the patient is in a relaxed position to avoid flexure of the mandible that may distort the master cast and consequently the RPD framework may not fit.

8.3.5 Visit 3: Framework Try-In and Records

Objective

Cast RPD framework fits properly intraorally (passively).

(a) Rest seats fully seated.
(b) Major connector fully seated (seated against the soft tissue and tooth structures as designed).
(c) Retentive clasps and reciprocating clasps properly positioned.
(d) Minor connectors properly positioned.
(e) Framework is stable across the arch (seats fully on both sides simultaneously) and does not rock.
(f) Ensure that RPD framework does not interfere with normal dentate occlusion (does not prevent normal tooth-to-tooth contacts).

Materials
Occlude indicator spray, pink baseplate wax, Blu-Mousse occlusal registration, articulating paper

Instruments
High-speed and low-speed handpieces, mirror, explorer, perio-probe, articulating paper holder, bur block for pros, two prong pliers, #8 wax spatula, Bunsen burner, alcohol torch

Technique

1. Check fit of RPD framework on master cast, compare to design cast, and work authorization.
2. Seat gently in patients' mouth (IF SIGNIFICANT RESISTANCE IS FELT IN PLACEMENT, DO NOT FORCE).
3. Assess possible interference to path of insertion: Consider guide planes, retentive clasps, and areas which are plated. Some adjustment may be needed. Make adjustments to cast framework with a high speed and carbide bur. Frameworks get HOT when adjusting with a high speed (be careful).
4. If framework seats but not fully or there is a discrepancy between sides, use the occlude spray to identify interferences. Teeth must be dry and the framework must be dry. Apply a thin spray coat (remember only spray where you are looking for interference).
   (a) Adjust incrementally to achieve full seating of framework.
   (b) Check occlusion. Are the same tooth-to-tooth contacts present with or without the framework seated? Make adjustments as needed. Do not significantly thin and weaken critical design components (rest seats, clasp arms). (If seating both a maxillary and mandibular framework, check them individually at first then with both seated to ensure there are no occlusal interferences.)
5. Once proper occlusion is achieved, add wax rim(s) in the edentulous areas. Kennedy class I or II partials need distal extension record bases for accurate mounting of master models. Class III partials that can be accurately hand articulated and do not need additional occlusal registration.
   (a) A centric relation record or occlusal registration is needed for any case that cannot be accurately hand articulated. The wax rims in the edentulous areas should be properly contoured and adjusted to articulate against an opposing dentition, an opposing RPD, or an opposing complete denture. Wax rims should be notched with V-shaped grooves to index the occlusal registration material.
6. Rehearse the proper closure into the desired occlusion with the patient prior to placing the registration material intraorally (Blu-Mousse).
7. A facebow mounting is needed for the maxillary cast, and it can be taken (again) or properly mounted from an index of the master model articulation prior to framework fabrication.

8. Select denture teeth for trial arrangement: Anterior teeth for esthetics and posterior teeth by cuspal inclination and occlusal scheme. Evaluate the cuspal inclination of opposing or adjacent natural teeth to select 33, 22, 15, or monoplane. An RPD arrangement opposing a complete denture or P/P posterior tooth selection is dictated by occlusal scheme (monoplane, balanced, lingualized).

8.3.6 Visit 4: Teeth Try-In

Objective
Verify an accurate mounting of RPD case, confirm appropriate occlusal scheme, and determine that arrangement of teeth for esthetics is approved by patient.

Materials
Bunsen burner, alcohol torch, articulating paper, wax spatula (#7), acrylic burs, straight low-speed handpiece, occlusal registration material (Blu-Mousse or aluwax)

Instruments
High-speed and low-speed handpieces, mirror, explorer, perio-probe, articulating paper holder, bur block for crown and bridge and operative bur block, two prong pliers, #8 wax spatula, Bunsen burner

Technique

1. Denture teeth should have been set on the articulated master cast(s) and RPD. Selection of denture teeth is done according to esthetic and phonetic criteria for anterior teeth and esthetic and functional requirements for posterior teeth. Posterior denture teeth selection for RPDs is generally determined by evaluating the cuspal inclination of opposing or adjacent teeth (33, 22, 15, or monoplane Blu-Line).
2. The plane of occlusion for posterior teeth may be dictated by existing natural teeth or if opposing a complete denture or *Kennedy Class I* or II RPD an idealized occlusal plane.
3. Denture teeth may have to be modified significantly to fit properly around framework components or adjacent natural teeth.
4. At patient try-in verify the accuracy of your articulator mounting by assessing the RPD intraorally and making a verification bite registration (Blu-Mousse or aluwax). Guide the patient to proper closure for a CR mounting or allow the patient to close to normal natural tooth contact for a MI record. As in the framework try-in, the RPD should not prevent natural teeth from making normal contact.
5. When doing a try-in of opposing RPDs, first try in each setup individually and then together to evaluate proper occlusion.

6. If the bite registration indicates that the mounting is off, it will be necessary to remount the mandibular cast. *DO NOT* reset denture teeth if the mounting is the problem. Slight adjustments of tooth position for esthetics or cusp/fossa occlusion can be made if the mounting is accurate.
7. Assess the esthetics and phonetics of anterior tooth arrangement.
8. Do not forget to select an acrylic shade.
9. Complete work authorization lab form for processing of RPD

8.3.7 Visit 5: Delivery

Objectives

(a) Fit, adjust, and delivery of the removable denture.
(b) Instruct the patient about their dental care and the denture care.

Materials
Pressure-indicating paste, occlude disclosing spray, articulating paper

Instruments
Articulator, casts, jigs, handpieces (high speed, low speed, and straight), burs, mandrels, exam kit, patient's mirror, gauze, and cotton rolls

Technique

1. Before appointment check partials and remove acrylic flash over guide planes, under rest seats, or on the occlusal surfaces of the teeth. Check acrylic flanges for sharp spots and evident undercuts.
2. Seat partial dentures *one at a time* making sure:
   (a) The acrylic for proper seating
   (b) The framework seats fully
   (c) Occlusion to opposing dentition[1]
3. Only after each partial has been checked individually should the partials be evaluated together.
4. If a significant occlusal discrepancy exists, then the case should be remounted on the articulator to be adjusted. If the occlusal discrepancy is determined to be minor, then intraoral adjustment is permitted.
5. Patient instructions should be reviewed with the patient regarding use, limitations, and maintenance.
6. 24-h check should be scheduled.

[1] *There should be no occlusal interferences of the frameworks as this should have been corrected at the previous framework try-in appointment. Interferences of the frameworks should be remounted to determine if the case needs to be redone or if it can be adjusted.*

8.3.8 Visit 6: 24-h Check

Objectives

(a) Address the patient's complains, signs, and symptoms and adjust the RPD accordingly.
(b) Evaluate the fit and function of the RPD.

Materials
Pressure-indicating paste, occlude disclosing spray, articulating paper

Instruments
Articulator, casts, jigs, handpieces (high speed, low speed, and straight), burs, mandrels, exam kit, patient's mirror, gauze, and cotton rolls

Technique

1. Listen carefully to the patient to list any problems or concerns.
2. Inspect the tissues under and around the partials for signs of redness and lacerations.
3. Cheek biting, tongue biting, speech.
4. Adjust the tissue side of the acrylic using PIP.
5. Inspect the occlusion with articulating paper for even, bilateral marks.
6. Review instructions and address all patient concerns.
7. Determine appropriate interval of periodontal maintenance and periodic exam.
8. Remind the patient about the limitations of the RPDs and that it takes time and practice to get use to them.

References

Aviv I, Ben-Ur Z, Cardash HS. An analysis of rotational movement of asymmetrical distal-extension removable partial dentures. J Prosthet Dent. 1989;61:211–4.

Browning JD, Jameson WS, Stewart CD, McGarrah HE, Eick JD. Effect of positional loading of three removable partial denture clasp assemblies on movement of abutment teeth. J Prosthet Dent. 1986;55:347–51.

Cecconi BT, Asgar K, Dootz E. The effect of partial denture clasp design on abutment tooth movement. J Prosthet Dent. 1971;25:44–56.

Christidou L, Osborne J, Chamberlain JB. The effects of partial denture design on the mobility of abutment tooth movement. Br Dent J. 1973;135:9–18.

Devan MM. Preserving natural teeth through the use of clasps. J Prosthet Dent. 1955;5:208–14.

Frechette AR. The influence of partial denture design on distribution of force to abutment teeth. J Prosthet Dent. 1956;6:195–212.

Kratochvil FJ, Caputo AA. Photoelastic analysis of pressure on teeth and bone supporting removable partial dentures. J Prosthet Dent. 1974;32:52–61.

Kratochvil FJ, Davidson PN, Guijt J. Five-year survey of treatment with removable partial dentures part I. J Prosthet Dent. 1982;48:237–44.

Krol AJ. Clasp design for extension-base removable partial dentures. J Prosthet Dent. 1973;29:408.

Phoenix RD, Cagna DR, DeFreest CF, Stewart KL. Stewart's clinical removable partial prosthodontics, 4th ed. Quintessence Pub., 2008.

Shohet H. Relative magnitudes of stress on abutment teeth with different retainers. J Prosthet Dent. 1969;21:267–82.

Tebrock OC, Rohen RM, Fenster RK, Pelleu Jr GB. The effect of various clasping systems on the mobility of abutment teeth for distal-extension removable partial dentures. J Prosthet Dent. 1979;41:511–6.

Thompson WD, Kratochvil FJ, Caputo AA. Evaluation of photoelastic stress patterns produced by various designs of bilateral distal-extension removable partial dentures. J Prosthet Dent. 1977;38:261–73.

Introduction to Occlusion

9

Margarete C. Ribeiro-Dasilva, James Nguyen, Keith Kiskaddon, and Peter E. Dawson

Contents

M.C. Ribeiro-Dasilva (✉)
Department of Restorative Dental Science, University of Florida, Gainesville, FL, USA
e-mail: mdasilva@dental.ufl.edu

J. Nguyen, DMD
Advanced Education in General Dentistry Program,
University of Florida College of Dentistry, Seminole, FL, USA

K. Kiskaddon, DMD
Private Practice St Petersburg, Florida, USA

P.E. Dawson, DMD
The Dawson Academy, St. Petersburg, FL, USA

G.M. Weinstein, M.T. Zientz (eds.), *The Dental Reference Manual*,
DOI 10.1007/978-3-319-39730-6_9

Abstract

Occlusion is one of the most important concepts in dentistry. The success of many dental treatments relies heavily on a stable and harmonious occlusion. All dentists should understand that even when they are making a "simple" occlusal composite or amalgam restoration, they should first diagnose and treat occlusal disharmonies in order to avoid creating iatrogenic occlusal or temporomandibular disorders.

9.1 Introduction

The primary requirement for successful occlusal therapy is the presence of (Shillingburg et al. 2012):

(a) Stable temporomandibular joints: where this complex articulation is capable of comfortably receiving loads.
(b) Anterior teeth are in harmony with the envelope of function; there is perfect disocclusion of molars without any interference during anterior guidance and lateral movements of the mandible (Dawson 2007).

In this chapter, we will review some concepts that all dentists should be familiar with, as well how to avoid iatrogenic occlusion disorders and how to treat simple occlusal imbalances.

9.2 Occlusal Scheme and Clinical Implications

9.2.1 Temporomandibular Joint (TMJ)

The "TMJ" is the most complex joint in the human body. It is capable of rotation and translation; this joint is the basis of occlusion and is also called the posterior determinant of occlusion. There is a neutral point at which the joints are in a position allowing the muscles to rest in equilibrium. This defines the centric relation position. For this harmony to be maintained, the teeth have to occlude (in maximum intercuspation) while the condyles are in the anterior-superior-most position (centric relation).

Clinical Implication Any deviation from this relation will result in a muscular imbalance. This imbalance may result in pain in the masticatory muscles and/or eventual damage to the dentition (e.g., broken teeth, abfraction, splayed tooth) as well as the periodontium and supporting hard tissues (e.g., widening of periodontal ligament space, tooth mobility, bone loss around the tooth) in the body's attempt to adjust to centric relation.

9.2.2 Masticatory Muscles

These are the most important muscles to be familiar with, in order to diagnose temporomandibular disorders (TMD):

1. *Temporalis*: acts as a mandibular elevator and positioner. This muscle is a fan-shaped muscle with its origin connecting to a semilunar infratemporal line covering parietal, temporal, frontal, and sphenoid surfaces of the cranium.
2. *Masseter*: it is one of the principal elevators and closing muscle of the mandible. The rectangular-shaped muscle has its origin at the inferior aspect of the temporal and anterior portion of the zygomatic arch, and it is insertion at the angle of the mandible, extending to the ascending posterior border of the ramus and posterior lower border of the mandible.
3. *Lateral pterygoid muscle* moves the condyle forward, downward, and medially. The larger inferior head originates from the lateral aspect of the lateral pterygoid plate. The smaller superior head originates from the roof of the infratemporal fossa of the greater wing of the sphenoid. The larger inferior head inserts into the anterior aspect of the condylar neck and capsule.
4. *Medial pterygoid* is a strong elevator muscle slightly weaker than the masseter. The medial pterygoid muscle originates from the pterygoid fovea, the medial aspect of the lateral pterygoid plate, and has a tendinous attachment to the pyramidal palatine and maxillary tuberosity. The insertion is at the medial surface of the angle of the mandible. The line of action is superior and oblique, similar to the masseter (Gross 2015).

Clinical Implication Knowing the location of these muscles is very important when the patient presents with orofacial pain. Temporomandibular disorder (TMD) is suspected if the patient has any of these symptoms:

1. Palpation sensitivity to 1 kg pressure
2. Pain in the muscles of mastication
3. Tension-type headaches
4. Clinical evidence of bruxism/clenching (e.g., tongue scalloping, tori/exostosis, cheek ridging, and wear facets)

9.2.3 Centric Relation (CR)

Is the relationship of the mandible to the maxilla when the properly aligned condyle-disk assemblies are in the most superior position against the eminentiae irrespective of the vertical dimension or tooth position. At the most superior position, the condyle-disk assemblies are braced medially, thus centric relation is also the midmost position. A properly aligned condyle-disk assembly in centric relation can resist maximum loading by the elevator muscles with no sign of discomfort (Dawson 2007).

9.2.4 Vertical Dimension at Rest

This is controversial; according to Dawson the rest position is highly variable and should not be used as a reference for restoring occlusion. This should be determined by speech positions in patients with dentures as it is a repeatable position.

9.2.5 Interocclusal Rest Space (IORS)

When the mandible is in the postural rest position, the teeth are separated by the "interocclusal rest space" formerly termed "the freeway space." The mean value ranges from 1 to 3 mm (Gross 2015).

Clinical Implication Vertical dimension is determined by the musculature, and the body will return to the natural physiological VDO if it is changed. Dawson states that: "1. Decreases in tooth height are compensated for by a commensurate increase in alveolar bone height. This is true even in severe abrasive wear by habitual bruxers. 2. Increases in tooth height are compensated for either by regressive remodeling of the alveolar bone to commensurately shortening the dentoalveolar process, or by intrusion into the alveolus of the teeth that had been lengthened" (Dawson 2007).

9.2.6 Protrusion

When the right and left pterygoid muscles contract simultaneously, pulling the condyle and disk forward. This movement is guided anteriorly by the lingual anatomy of the incisors and posteriorly by the condylar guidance and should not be guided by posterior teeth.

Clinical Implication As the condylar guidance and incisal guidance gets steeper, disocclusion occurs faster and results in greater interocclusal space. This increased space allows the dentist to restore cusps with more pronounced anatomy.

Comparatively, with shallower guidance, the interocclusal space is decreased requiring flatter occlusal anatomy to achieve immediate disclusion of posterior teeth during protrusive movements.

9.2.7 Incisal Guidance

Anterior guidance is a functional relationship between the lingual of the maxillary incisors and facial of the mandibular incisor teeth. During protrusive movement, the lower incisors make an angle with the upper incisors, called "incisal guidance angle."

9.2.8 Lateral Movement

In a perfected occlusion, lateral excursive movements will be guided on the upper and lower canine teeth. Posterior cusps should never contact during this jaw movement. Wear facets on posterior teeth are evidence that anterior guidance or canine guidance is not appropriate. Perfected occlusion does not allow wear facets to occur on posterior teeth.

Clinical Implication During this movement it is very important that there isn't any tooth contact on the nonworking side. If dental contacts (interferences) are present in the nonworking side, they can be traumatic to the occlusion as the body will find ways to remove these contacts, i.e., wear facets (Dawson 2007).

Working side: During the lateral movement of the mandible, this is the side that the lower jaw is moving to. For example, if the mandible moves to the right, the right side would be the working side. *Nonworking side:* The opposite side from where the mandible is moving to. In the previous example, the left side would be the nonworking side.

Clinical Implications Verifying lateral or excursive movements is critical in any occlusion. If these movements are not verified and interferences are present, restorations can be fatigued from overloading and may either fracture or fail. For dentures, these interferences may lead to tipping and loss of retention.

9.2.9 Vertical Dimension of Occlusion (VDO)

The vertical relation of the maxilla to the mandible, which is determined by the repetitive contracted length of the elevator muscles, determines the VDO (Dawson 2007) (Fig. 9.1).

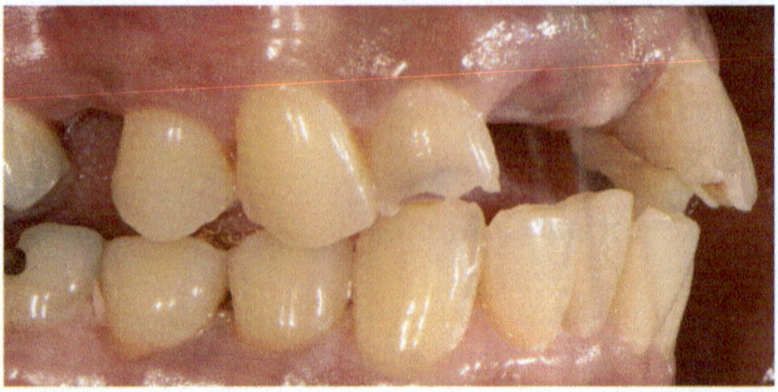

Fig. 9.1 Splayed teeth, broken incisal edge, and wear facets are indicators for a loss of vertical dimension

9.3 Types of Occlusion

Dawson classification (Dawson 2007).

Type I: Maximal intercuspation is in harmony with centric relation

- Centric relation is variable the teeth separated
- Treatment of TMD is not needed
- The jaw can close to maximal intercuspation without premature contacts or deflections
- The patient can close with no sign of discomfort
- Use of occlusal splint is not indicated

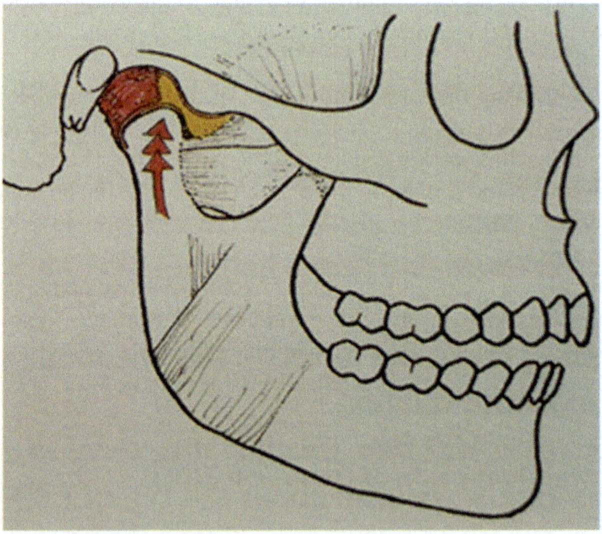

Type IA: Maximal intercuspation occurs in harmony with centric posture

- Intracapsular structures have deformation but have adapted
- TMJs can accept loading with no discomfort
- Treatment for TMD is not needed
- Occlusal correction is not needed because there is no TMJ/occlusion disharmony

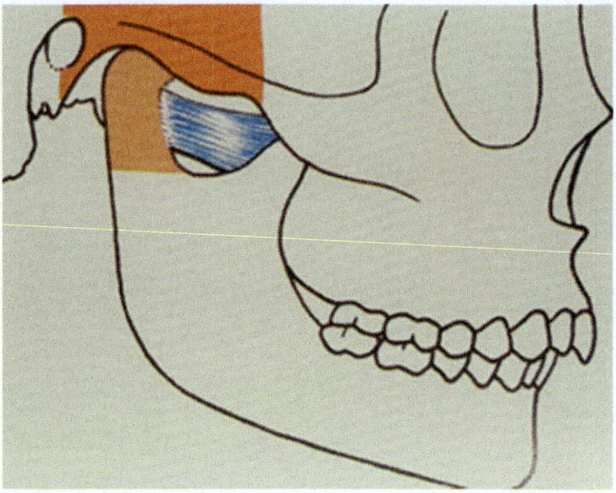

Type II: Type IIA: Condyles must displace from and adapted centric posture for maximum Intercuspation to occur

- Discomfort from an intracapsular disorder has been ruled out.
- The source of pain will be in the muscle or interfering teeth
- Prognosis is excellent when occlusal interferences are eliminated
- Surgical procedure is not indicated

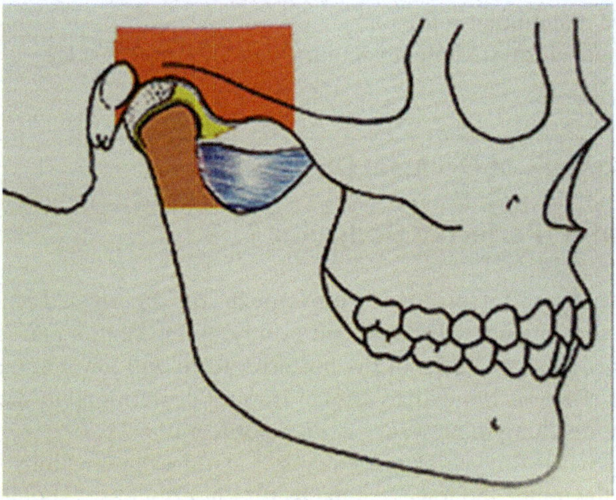

Type III: Centric Relation cannot be verified

- Treatment depends on the type of TMD and varies from a simple permissive occlusal device to relieve muscle spam to surgical procedure to correct certain types of intracapsular disorder.
- The TMJ cannot accept load testing without discomfort.

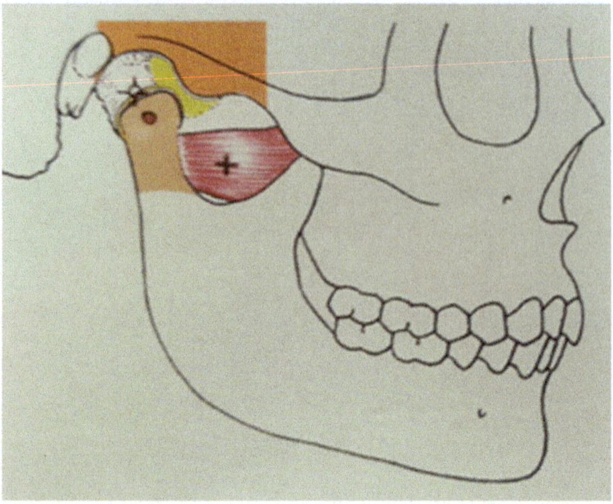

Type IV: The occlusal relationship is in an active stage of progressive disorder because of pathological unstable TMJs.This indicate an actively progressive disorder of the TMJs that makes it impossible to stabilish a stable TMJ/occlusion relationship. Types of signs of Type IV are

- Progressive anterior open bite
- Progressive asymmetry
- Progressive mandibular retrusion
- Irreversible occlusal treatment is contra-indicated at this stage

9.4 Diagnosis of Occlusal Disorder

9.4.1 What Is "Perfected Occlusion"?

1. Anterior guidance for protrusive movements. In a perfected stable occlusion, protrusive movements will be guided evenly on the central and lateral incisors. Most importantly, the cusps of the posterior teeth will never contact during this movement. There is immediate disocclusion of posterior teeth with any anterior movement, resulting in no wear on posterior teeth.
2. Canine guidance for lateral movements. Lateral excursive movements will be guided on the upper and lower canine teeth. Posterior cusps should never contact during this jaw movement. Wear facets on posterior teeth are evidence that anterior guidance or canine guidance is not appropriate along with interferences involving nonworking cups. In a perfected occlusion, the posterior interferences will need to be removed.
3. No CR-MIC shift (stable occlusal centric contacts. A shift indicates interferences of the posterior dentition). There should be no shift from initial centric relation

contact to maximum intercuspation. For example, when watching a mandible close, if the mandible moves to either the right or left side to obtain MIC, then a shift has occurred.

9.4.2 Diagnosis: How to Determine if Occlusal Disorder Exists

1. The initial exam. This is the best time to gain a thorough understanding of the stability of the patient's TMJ. Here are some ideas of how to incorporate this evaluation into a clinical practice.
2. Ask the patient if they currently have headaches or have ever suffered with headaches in the past. Are there any specific muscles that "feel tired" or sore i.e., temporalis, masseter, pterygoids, or neck muscles? Does the patient report any discomfort of their temporomandibular joint? Ask the patient to point to the sources of the pain.

Sequence of the Exam

A. Begin your extra oral exam by palpating the TMJ and have the patient open and close. Document any clicking, popping, crepitus, joint noises, or reported joint discomfort specific to the affected joint (refer to Chap. 1 Comprehensive Head and Neck Exams for how to do this and the form to document your findings) (Dawson 2007).
B. Palpate the masticatory muscles: temporalis, masseter, pterygoids, and neck muscles and concomitant sensitivity to palpation.
C. Next complete your intraoral exam and note the findings as presented in Table 9.1.
D. Regarding the occlusal aspect of the intraoral exam, look for signs of wear, mobility, stress lines on teeth, and abfractions (Figs. 9.2, 9.3, and 9.4).
E. Have the patient go through protrusive and lateral excursive movements. Does the patient have perfected occlusion? Classify the patient according to the Dawson classification system.

Table 9.1 Clinical findings that suggest occlusal disorder

Condition noted	Clinical clues to support these conditions
Fremitus	Mobility of tooth/teeth while in occlusion
Widened periodontal ligament	Teeth that are constantly in a state of unevenly contacting each other with excessive force will compensate by causing the ligaments to thicken
Wear facets (Fig. 9.2)	Worn down incisal or occlusal tooth structure. This suggests a loss of vertical dimension as evidenced by the teeth intercuspating into these wear areas
Muscular pain	Any associated discomfort to palpation or reported discomfort by the patient involving the facial or neck muscles
Fractured teeth or restorations (Fig. 9.2)	Missing cusps, broken restorations, vertical stress lines (craze lines), and abfractions

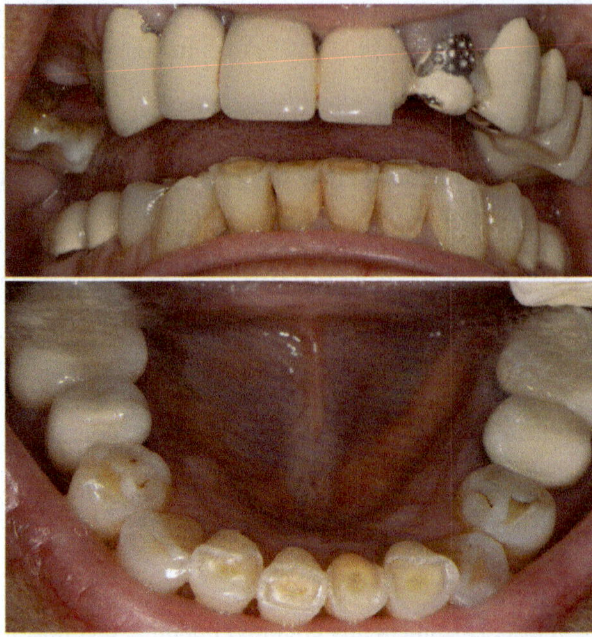

Fig. 9.2 Wear facets on teeth are suggestions of loss in vertical dimension. Wear facets on the lower incisal and broken tooth restoration on the maxillary teeth

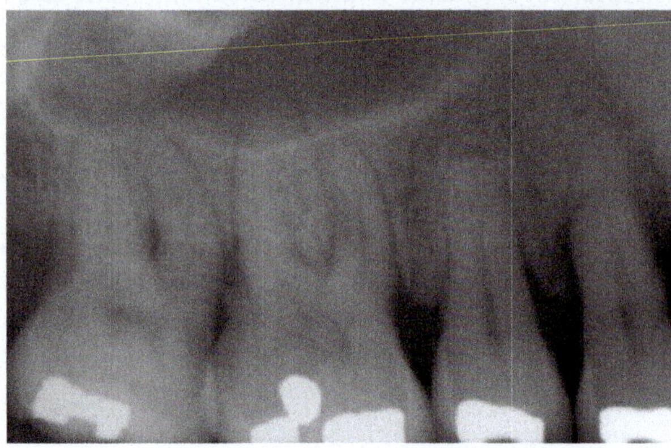

Fig. 9.3 Widened periodontal ligaments as noted on radiographic examination

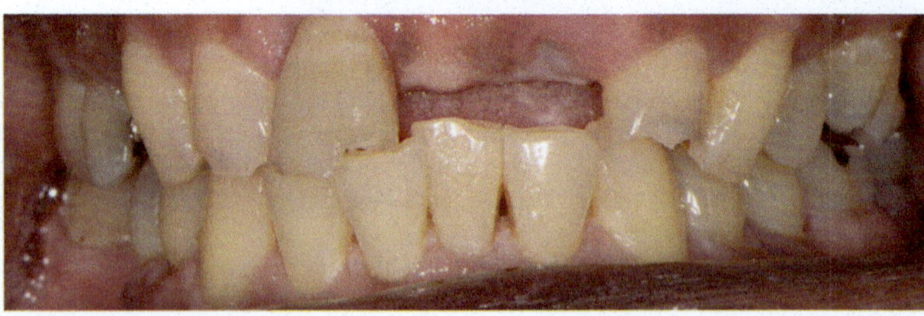

Fig. 9.4 When teeth are not replaced or restored, a patient continues to break down the dentition, causing a loss of vertical dimension

F. After a thorough review of the patient's occlusion, and upon completion of the other intraoral findings, the diagnosis of occlusal disease and proposed plan of action can be considered to help your patient begin the journey of stabilizing their occlusion and temporomandibular joint.

9.5 Treatment of Occlusal Disorder

9.5.1 What Is an Anterior Deprogrammer?

If the patient is in pain, and the origin of pain is determined to be muscular, as evidenced by palpation of muscles of mastication and muscles of the lower neck, the patient will notice immediate relief to muscular pain following the use of an anterior deprogrammer. Pain of the joint origin should be referred to a dentist in one's region who is dedicated to treating TMD disorders. Alterations to occlusion and use of anterior deprogrammers can exacerbate joint issues if the discomfort is associated within the joint capsule. The anterior deprogrammer should not be used for long periods of time as it can create an anterior open bite.

An anterior deprogrammer is any dental device that is placed intraorally to separate the back teeth. Examples of this are cotton rolls placed at the first premolar teeth, with the Lucia Jig placed in the central incisor region or a lab fabricated splint. The anterior deprogrammer will separate the back teeth from contacting, thus stopping any neurologic signals being sent to the muscles of mastication and thus turning off the muscles of mastication. In time, the muscles will relax and the patient will become more comfortable.

9.5.2 Occlusal Guard

An occlusal guard can relieve muscular tension without irreversible alteration of dentition. In cases where an anterior deprogramming device brings relief to the patient's signs and symptoms of masticatory muscle sensitivity, a permanent device can be fabricated for the patient to wear without having to worry about posterior supra eruption of the teeth. In the long run, an occlusal guard can be replaced by completing full mouth equilibration. However, a hard acrylic occlusal guard is a good treatment choice to begin with as it will give the patient comfort while in the process of equilibration. This is a noninvasive way of treating a patient. Occlusal guards are also a good way to prevent damage after placement of new restorations in patients that have a history of bruxism (Fig. 9.5).

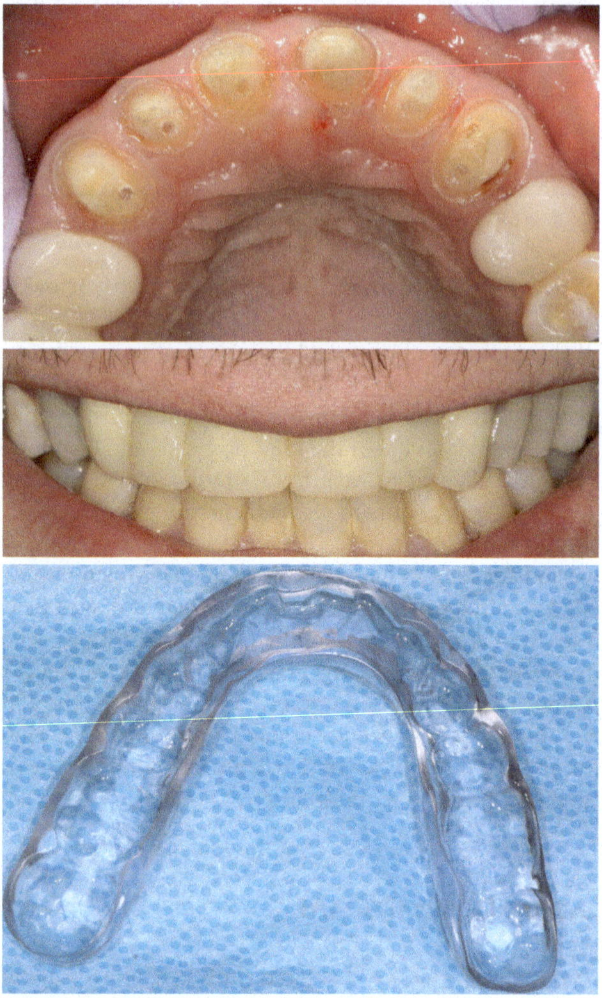

Fig. 9.5 A patient had just received anterior all-ceramic crowns. Part of his treatment plan was delivery of an occlusal guard to protect his teeth from occlusal damage. He is instructed to wear the guard every night

9.6 Preventing Iatrogenic Occlusal Problems

9.6.1 What Are the Results of a High Restoration?

1. Change in occlusal plane – super eruption.
2. Discomfort-hypersensitivity-pain. Usually occurs within 3 days of the restoration being placed.
3. Impaired function (teeth don't come together) – affects chewing.
4. Impaired esthetics – open bite.
5. Fracture of the tooth or the restoration.
6. Occlusal trauma – mobility.

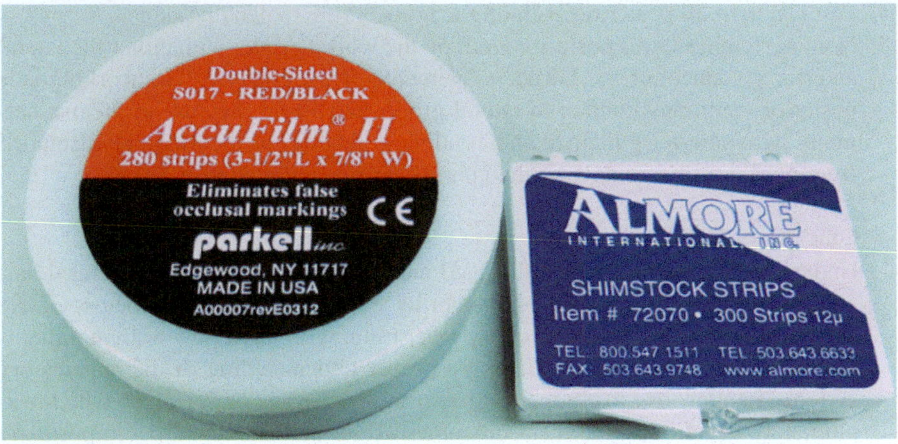

Fig. 9.6 Utilizing articulating paper before and after a restoration is an easy way to visualize correct occlusion

7. TMJ strain – i.e., a high restoration on the right side can cause strain on the left jaw joint since muscles will have to stabilize the unstable joint position.
8. Incomplete dentures: instability of the dentures, "teeth clicking" and impaired speech.

9.6.2 When Restoring Teeth

1. Mark contacts before you start, compare to what you have after the restoration is placed.
2. Use occlusal paper and shim stock (Fig. 9.6).
3. Utilize the red and black colors to your benefit. Before starting a restoration, mark the teeth with the red color of the articulating paper with the patient's bite. After you finish the restoration, use the black color; the contacts should match. Verify that there is an even distribution of centric stops and remove any posterior excursive interferences.
4. Inform the patient of the symptoms associated with a high restoration (tenderness and discomfort to chewing within a few days after the restoration was placed) and encourage them to return immediately for adjustments if symptoms surface.

9.6.3 Five Requirements for Occlusal Stability (Dawson 2007):

1. Stable stops on all teeth when the condyles are in centric relation
2. Anterior guidance in harmony with the border movement of the envelope of function
3. Disclusion of all posterior teeth in protrusive movements

4. Disclusion of all posterior teeth on the nonworking (balancing) side
5. Noninterference of all posterior teeth on the working side, with either the lateral anterior guidance, or the border movements of the condyle. The working-side posterior teeth may contact in lateral group function if they are in precise harmony with anterior guidance and condylar guidance, or they may be discluded from working-side contact by the lateral side anterior guidance.

Conclusion

Understanding the relation of the TMJ and its role in establishing occlusal harmony can help improve the predictability of our dentistry. As doctors of the masticatory system, we can access proper training to learn how to treat patients with occlusal disharmonies. Having a proper understanding of the masticatory system can allow one to come to a greater understanding of occlusion which will ultimately benefit the treatment outcomes of our patients and most importantly improve our patient's quality of life.

References

Dawson P. Functional occlusion from TMJ to smile design. Missouri: Mosby; 2007. p. 525–45.

Gross M. The science and art of occlusion and oral rehabilitation. 4th ed. UK: Quintessence Pub. Co; United Kingdom, 2015:130–4.

Shillingburg Herbert T Jr, Sather David A, Wilson Edwin L Jr, Cain Joseph R, Mitchell Donald L, Blanco Luis J, Kessler James C. Fundamentals of fixed prosthodontics, fourth edition. Illinois: Quintessence Pub. Co; 2012. p. 13–25.

The pictures on this chapter was previously published in Functional Occlusion from TMJ to Smile Design, Book ISBN-13: 978-0323033718 ISBN-10: 0323033717, Vol 17, Peter Dawson, Chapter: Classification of Occlusion, Copyright Elsevier; 2007. p. 107–109.

Indirect Restorations with CAD/CAM Technology

10

Geraldine Weinstein, W. Stephen Howard, and Richard Fox

Contents

Abstract

Computer-aided design/computer-aided milling (CAD/CAM) has grown in popularity over the last decade and is here to stay! The technology as a whole and the materials of choice are continuously evolving, allowing us to fabricate predictable restorations. Perhaps even more importantly, CAD/CAM assists us in becoming better dentists. When proper technique and attention to detail are observed in treatment planning, preparing teeth, and scanning and bonding restorations, we as dentists can predictably fabricate an esthetic and functional

G. Weinstein, DDS
Department of Craniofacial Sciences, DDS University of Connecticut
School of Dental Medicine, Farmington, CT, USA
e-mail: geraldineweinstein@gmail.com

W.S. Howard, DMD (✉)
University of Florida College of Dentistry, Gainesville, FL, USA
e-mail: WSHoward@dental.ufl.edu

R. Fox, DDS
Densply-Sirona Cerec Specialist, CEREC, Detroit, MI, USA

G.M. Weinstein, M.T. Zientz (eds.), *The Dental Reference Manual*,
DOI 10.1007/978-3-319-39730-6_10

restoration for the patient. This chapter is written based on our experiences with Sirona's CEREC and Planmeca's E4D systems. The authors bring to light some basic principles that are applicable to any milled restoration as we expect more systems to emerge in the years to come.

10.1 Material Selection

Computer-aided design/computer-aided milling (CAD/CAM) is an exciting part of modern dentistry which began in the 1980s when CEREC was first introduced (Mormann 2006). Digital dentistry has developed tremendously since and has revolutionized how we do things today. There are many indirect restorations which require weeks in the laboratory for fabrication that are now done in a single visit/day. Some of the basic principles of crown and bridge remain, yet improvements in bonding to enamel have erased many of our previous limitations (Ferencz 2014). There is a significant amount of literature on CAD/CAM to date, evidence-based practice of fabricating restorations in this manner is what we aim to present here.

One must decide on the material to be used for the final restoration prior to preparation of the tooth. Considerations should be made based on occlusal wear, location in the mouth, and full coverage versus partial coverage restorations. It is essential to follow manufacturers' recommendations on the material of choice and prepare the tooth to those specifications. Ivoclar, for instance, has specific guidelines for preparing the tooth for IPS e.max CAD (lithium disilicate) restorations (Fig. 10.1a–d). To date, IPS e.max is the material of choice for full coverage restorations in CAD/CAM (Dennis 2010). A myriad of material choices exist for CAD/CAM; one has to be vigilant in following indications for use when selecting materials.

10.2 Tooth Preparation Guidelines for CAD/CAM Technology

- Prior to tooth preparation and anesthetizing the patient, select a shade. This avoids desiccation of the tooth and improper matching of the shade for the final restoration.
- In preparing the tooth, one must first decide on the design of your preparation. Conservation of the enamel is essential as bond strengths are the greatest in enamel (Heymann 2014). CAD/CAM restorations are a wonderful way to preserve tooth structure (Patel 2013).

10.2.1 Pearls for Tooth Preparation for All-Ceramic Restorations

- Armamentarium selection facilitates preparation of the tooth surface for all ceramic restorations. Several companies have a select set of burs that help accomplish the goals (Fig. 10.2).
- More often than not, occlusal reduction should be the first step in preparing the tooth to avoid excessive removal of tooth structure. Depth cuts on the occlusal with the proper burs ensure that the proper occlusal clearance is obtained for your material of choice (Fig. 10.3).

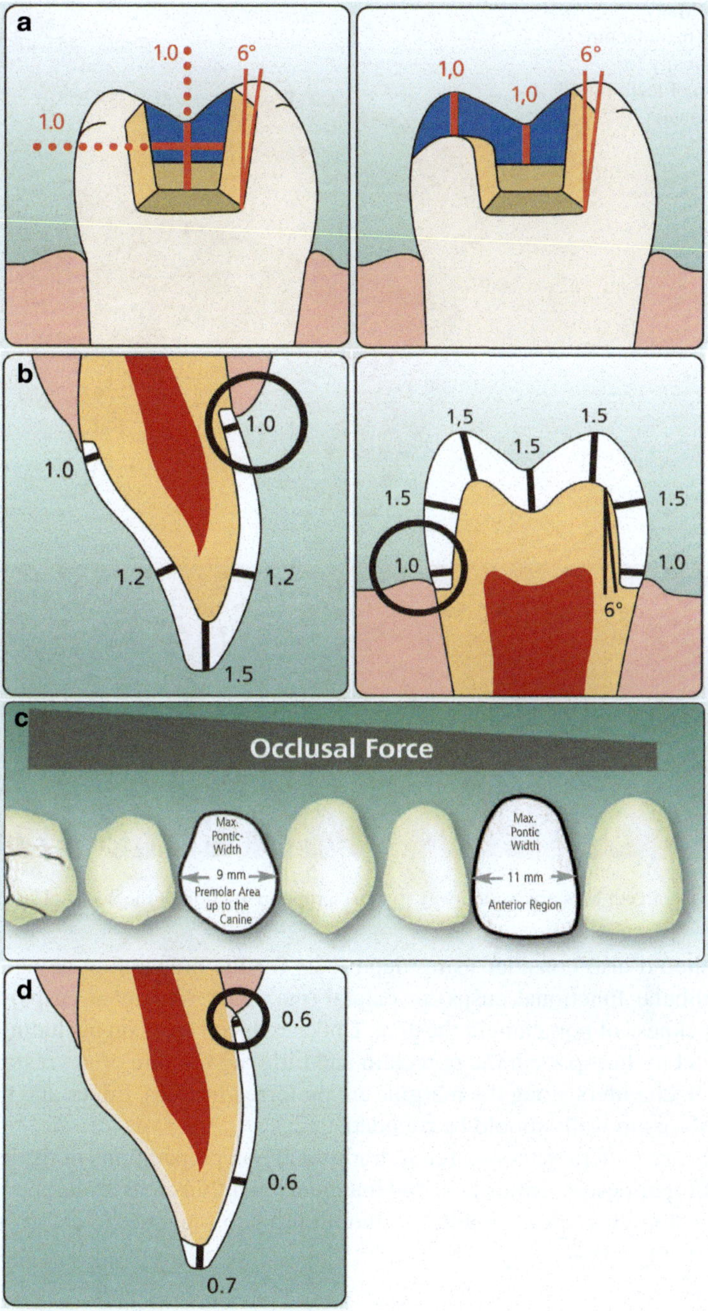

Fig. 10.1 (**a**) Inlay/onlay dimensions for E-max (printed with the permission of Ivoclar Vivadent). (**b**) Anterior and posterior crown dimensions (printed with the permission of Ivoclar Vivadent). (**c**) Bridge span (Printed with the permission of Ivoclar Vivadent). (**d**) Veneer dimensions (Printed with the permission of Ivoclar Vivadent)

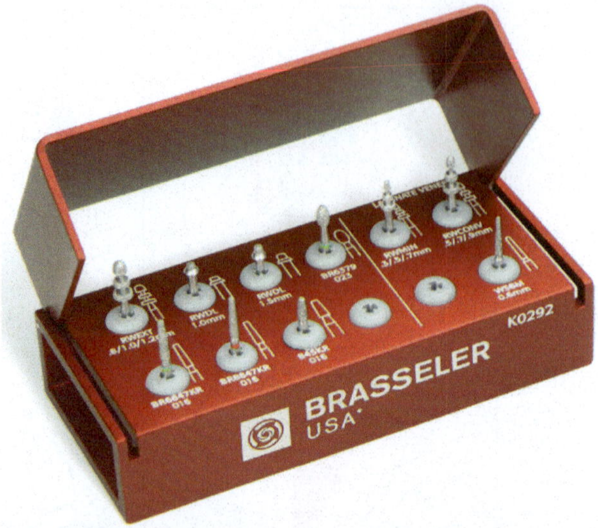

Fig. 10.2 Many companies manufacture burs specifically for preparation of teeth for all ceramic crowns

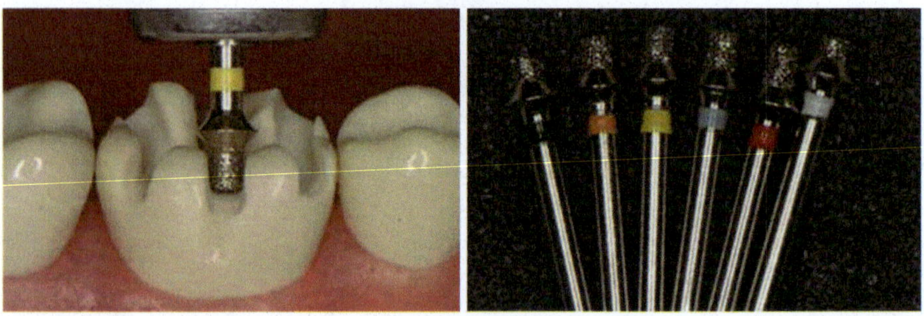

Fig. 10.3 Depth cut burs are a good way to mark proper reduction of the occlusal surface

- One should also consider using depth cuts for the preparation along the facial (mandibular functional cusps) or palatal (maxillary functional cusps) to ensure the thickness of porcelain in the area. Under-reduced areas on occluding surfaces can lead to thin spots in the porcelain and ultimate fracture of the restoration.
- Smooth chamfers along the margins are preferred finishes. Edges and transitions from floors to walls should be rounded.
- Ramps are preferable compared to traditional box preparations in the interproximal. Proper design avoids possible undercuts and thin areas along the margins.
- Adjacent contact areas should be smooth prior to scanning to create a flawless contact (Fig. 10.4).

10.2.2 A Few Pointers on Milled Restorations

- When using all-ceramic restorations from the laboratory or your own milling unit, one must understand the dimensions of the burs that create your restoration. Careful and thoughtful preparation of teeth is essential when using milled restorations (Figs. 10.5 and 10.6).

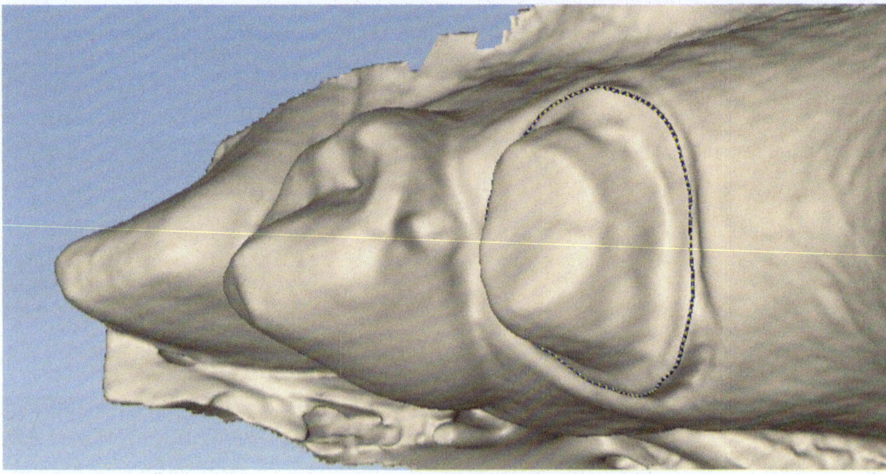

Fig. 10.4 Irregularities in the adjacent tooth will cause problems with cementation and ultimately the contact

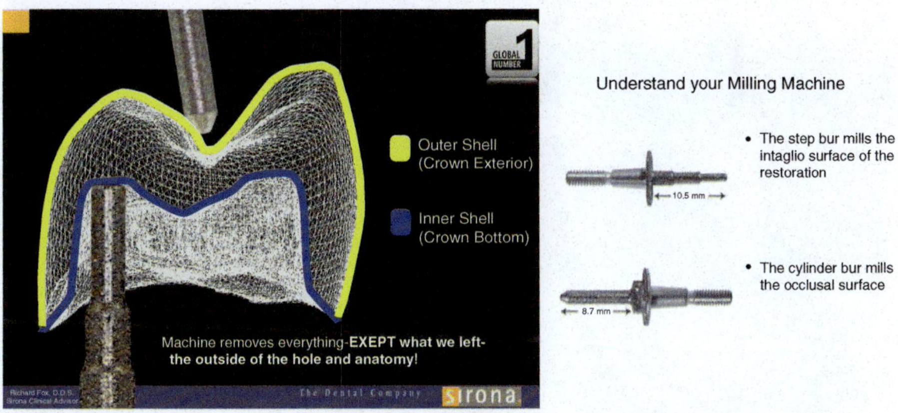

Fig. 10.5 CEREC milling units

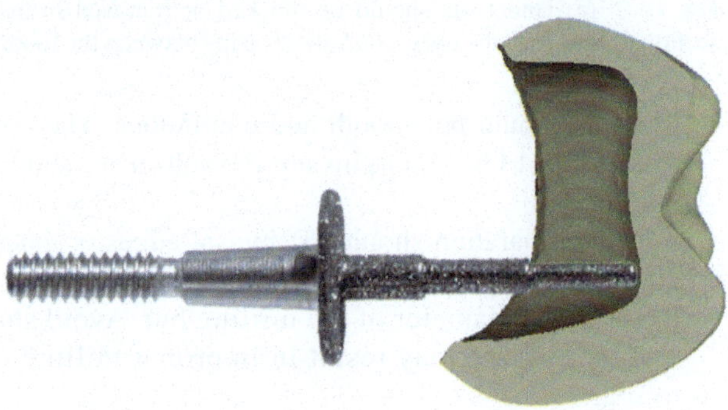

Fig. 10.6 The depth of the preparation should never exceed the length of the bur

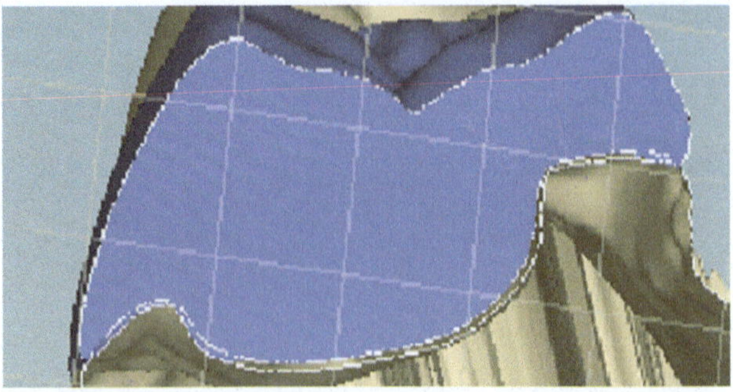

Fig. 10.7 Cross section shows a thin margin. This may lead to the material fracturing during milling. Followed by an open margin in the restoration

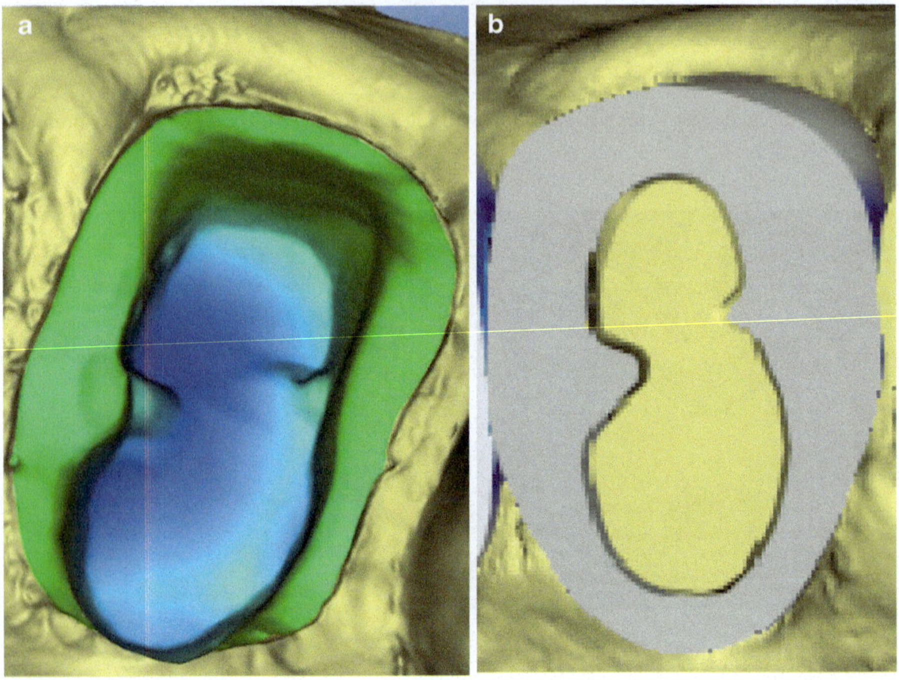

Fig. 10.8 (a) Undercuts should be blocked or removed from the preparation. (**b**) This cross-sectional view with the restoration shows gaps between the tooth and the milled restoration

- Margins should be smooth and continuous. The burs and software cannot mill sharp edges! Open margins are a result of roughness that is ignored around the margins.
- Ensure preparation shoulders; incisal edges or cusp tips are at least 1.3 mm in diameter to allow for proper milling (Fig. 10.7).
- Respect the diameter of the milling bur. Avoid sharp edges along your preparation as these may result in improper milling causing the restoration not to seat.

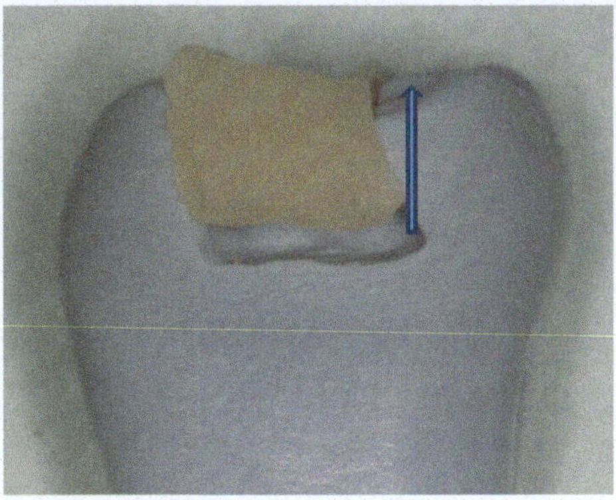

Fig. 10.9 Undercuts in the interproximal boxes prevent a path of draw. Line shows where the preparation should end in order to have a path of draw

- Undercuts in the preparation walls will not be milled by the software. This creates a larger gap between the restoration and the tooth surface that will be filled with cement. Use of your software's mill preview allows you to view these undesirable areas (Fig. 10.8a,b).
- Undercuts in interproximal area should be avoided; the machine will mill these area's causing the restoration not to seat (Fig. 10.9).

10.3 The CAD/CAM Workflow

10.3.1 Scanning

- Prior to scanning, proper isolation of the tooth and visibility of the preparation margins are essential. Occlusal clearance should be checked prior to scanning and can be measured accurately after scanning. Scanning is the final impression and all the old traditional rules apply: use of packing cord, hemostatic agents, or use of a laser/electro surgery to facilitate visualization of the margins.
- The scanned prepared tooth is the perfect opportunity to critique your own work! It is a good time to check if the preparation exhibits a path of draw. Check for undercuts, occlusal clearance, and sharp edges. The contour on adjacent teeth can prevent visualization of the entire tooth from the occlusal view. Corrections must be made, and rescan of the preparation, if necessary, prior to continuing onto the design phase (Fig. 10.10).
- For more information on scanning, see chapter on "Digital Impressions."

10.3.2 Design and Milling

- Learn special features of your chosen CAD/CAM system as this will enhance your abilities to design and mill the best possible restoration (Figs. 10.11; 10.12a,b; 10.13a,b; 10.14a,b; 10.15a,b; and 10.16).

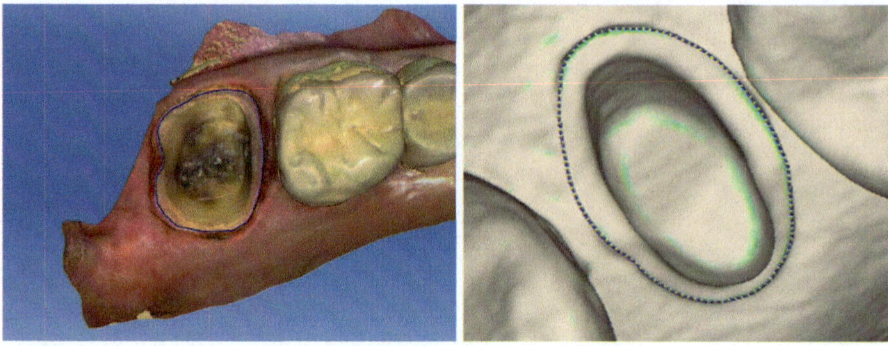

Fig. 10.10 Sirona's CEREC and Planmeca's E4D scan of the preparation

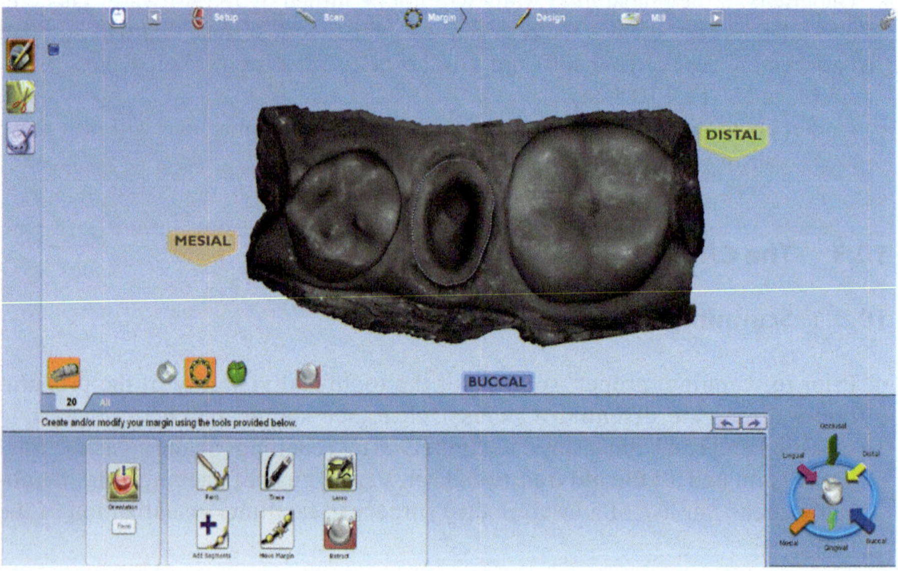

Fig. 10.11 Specific views in the chosen system allow improved visualization of your preparation margin

10.3.3 Glazing the Porcelain and Crystallizing

There are many ways to go about glazing an IPS e.max CAD crown once it has been milled. If you are inclined to do so, characterizing the porcelain prior to firing provides ways to customize the tooth. However, beginners can take the simple step of using glaze spray prior to a combined crystallization and glaze firing cycle (Fig. 10.17). Once again, it is critical to follow the manufacturer's directions on your chosen system.

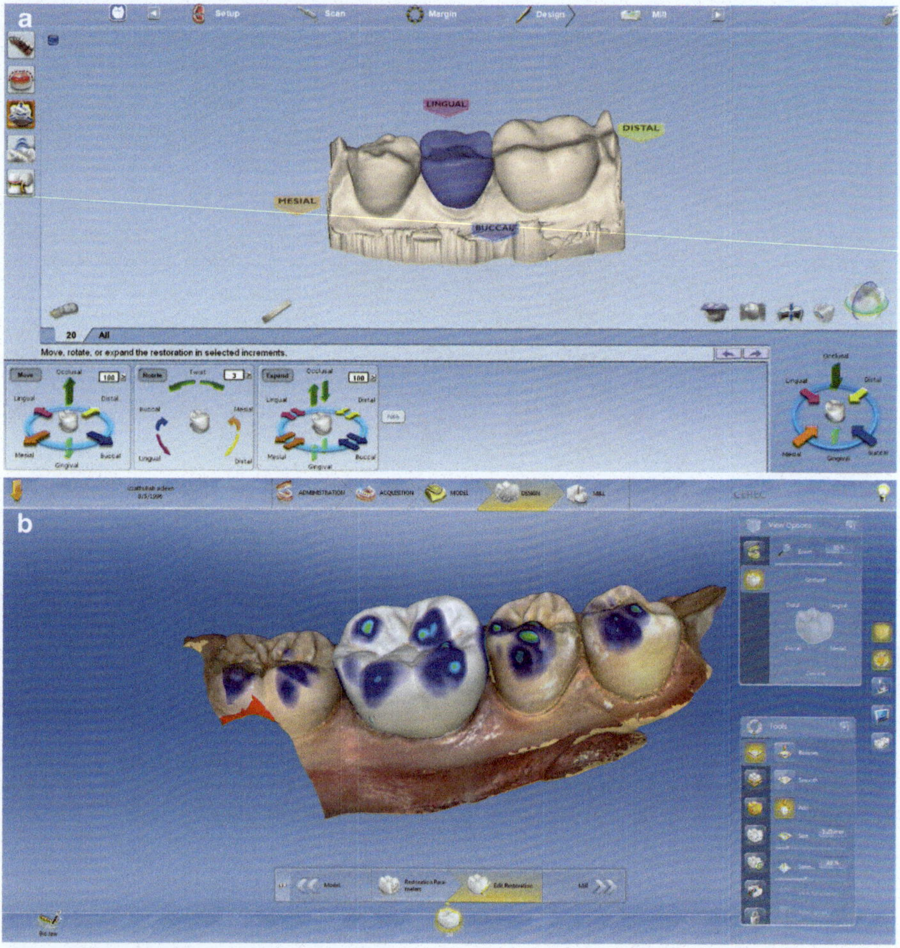

Fig. 10.12 (**a**) The Planmeca-designed crown can be virtually placed to improve esthetics and occlusion. (**b**) Virtual placement of CEREC crown, with tools available for editing of proposed crown and occlusal scheme

10.3.4 Bonding of CAD/CAM Restoration

Success of a bonded restoration lies in following the manufacturer's directions for all of your chosen materials. Flow sheets with specific directions are often found on the manufacturer's websites. In general, you will need to prepare both the crown surface and the tooth surface prior to bonding. It is best to complete preparation of the E-max crown prior to preparing the prepared tooth in order to avoid contamination (Table 10.1).

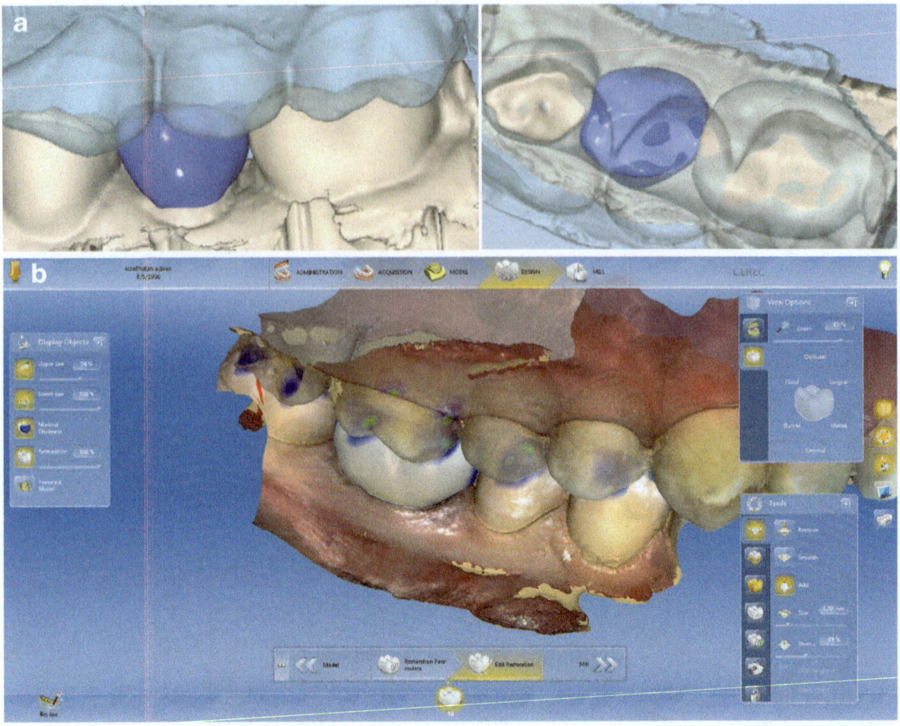

Fig. 10.13 (**a**) Planmeca E4D screen shots show occlusion prior to milling with options to do virtual adjustments. This minimizes the need for adjustments after cementation. (**b**) A screen shot from CEREC showing evaluation of occlusal contacts with available adjusting tools

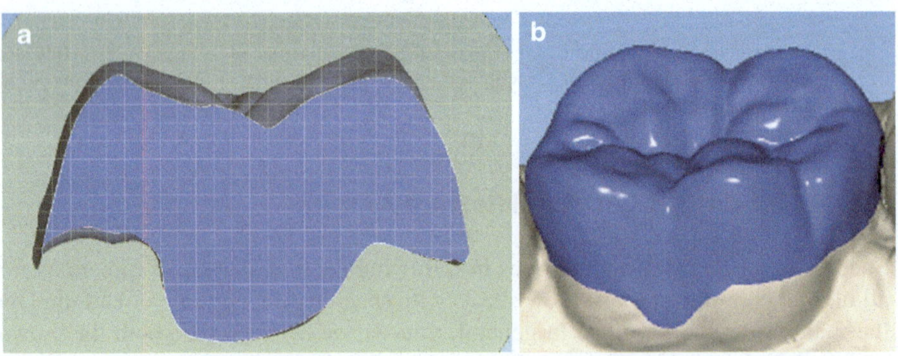

Fig. 10.14 (**a**, **b**) Cross sections of your restorations can reveal proper thickness of the material. In the screen shot from Planmeca, each square represents a square millimeter

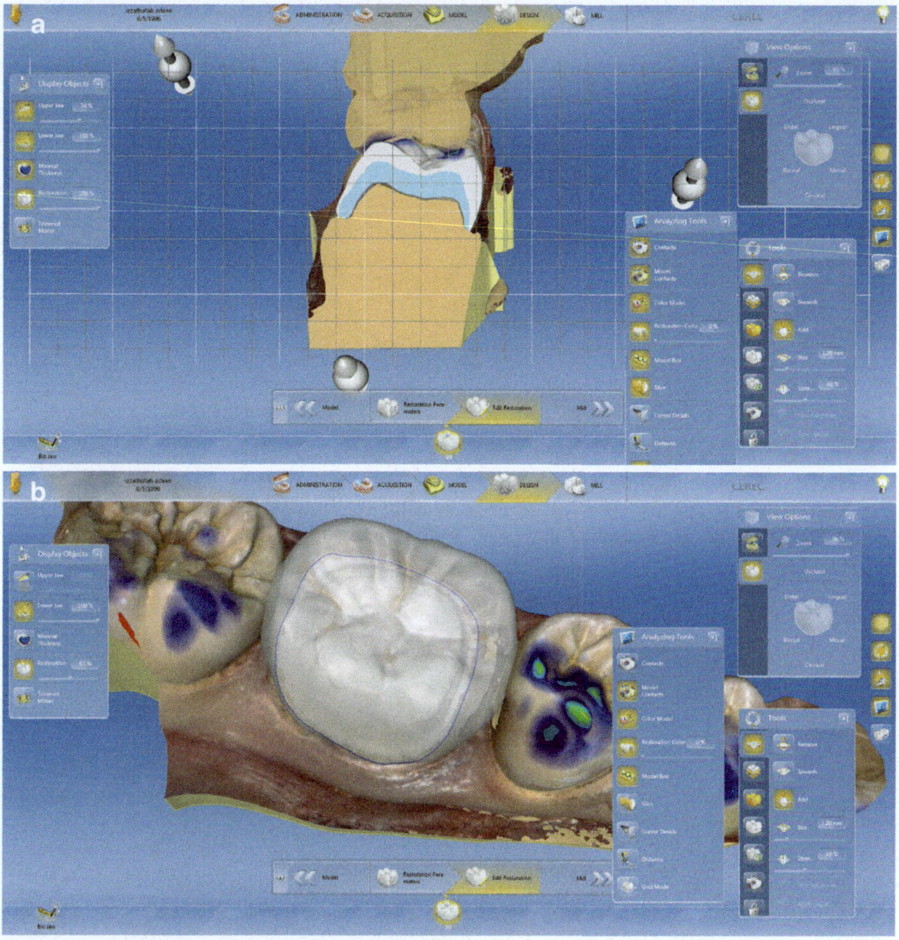

Fig. 10.15 (**a, b**) CEREC with grid lines, in cross section with minimal thickness warning (light blue) activated. Allows the operator to evaluate preparation, minimal thickness, and occlusal contacts at the same time

10.4 Creative Restorations with CAD/CAM

A. *Crownlays*—preserving the enamel is essential for bonding of modern day restorations. For instance, crown margins do not have to be extended to the gingival area. Designs referred to as crownlays are increasing in popularity as the bonding to tooth structure improves and materials such as E-max become readily available. Dr. Walter Renne at the Medical University of South Carolina (MUSC) College of Dental Medicine has videos online illustrating such designs on:

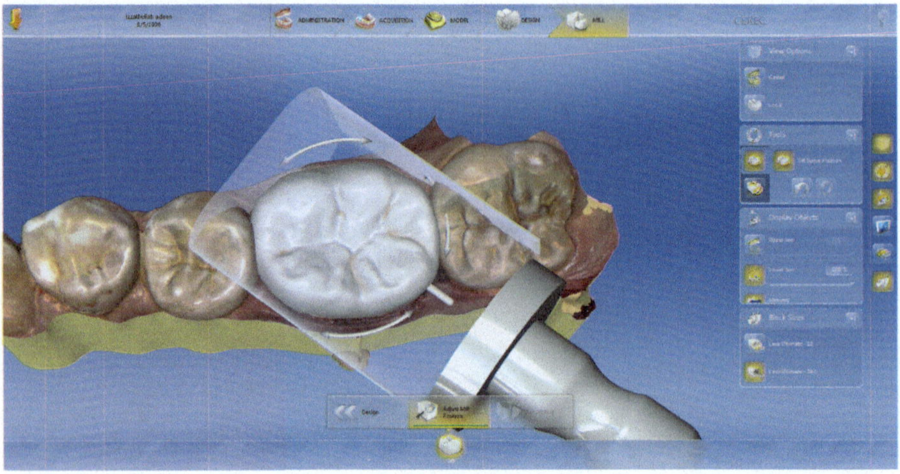

Fig. 10.16 Prior to milling, check the sprue placement, place sprue in an area that can be polished easily. Insure that the restoration is within the confines of the block

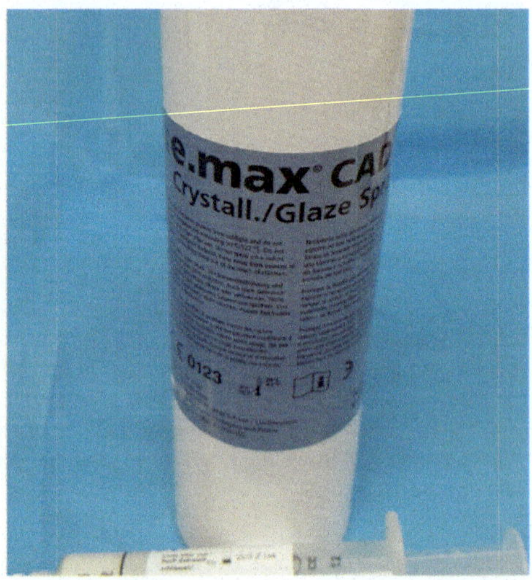

Fig. 10.17 One-step crystallization and glaze spray for E-max

https://learndigitaldentistry.com/video/the-inlay-onlay-and-crownlay-preparation/.

B. *Endocrowns*—In the event of CAD/CAM dentistry, endodontically treated molar teeth can best be treated by a single restoration that incorporates the core and crown as one unit. This not only eliminates the separate traditional steps of a post and core followed by a crown. A bonded single restoration, endocrown utilizes the tooth's chamber for retention and makes the tooth more resistant to fracture (Biacchi and Basting 2012). Studies using lithium disilicate material for endocrowns have shown higher resistance to fracture compared to other materials

Table 10.1 Workflow in preparing e.max CAD restoration and the prepared tooth (Gehrt 2013)

	Prepared tooth surface (Heymann 2014)	Milled E-max crown
Clean	Pumice, rinse with water, and isolate	Clean crown with alcohol, steamer or Ivoclean to remove debris from milling and firing paste
Etch	Phosphoric acid etch (follow manufacturer's directions) Rehydrating the tooth after etching can be done in one of two ways: 1. Apply Consepsis (2% Chlorhexidine) as it improves stability of bonding to dentin and blow off excess 2. Alternatively, in patients with sensitivity, after etching, consider using GLUMA (desensitizer from Heraeus Kulzer) to seal the dentinal tubules	Hydrofluoric acid etch (for E-max, recommendation is 20 s; rinse and dry)
Prime	Wet tooth with one-step primer and bonding agent. Scotchbond Universal (3M) is a popular one which is applied in a thin coat, gently thinned with an air syringe and light-cured	Silanate the crown and blow off excess (follow manufacturer's directions)
Cement	IPS e.max CAD crowns are traditionally bonded to the tooth with resin cement.[a] In addition to following directions of the luting cement, the tooth should be kept isolated from any saliva or blood contaminants. Care should be taken to quickly floss and remove excess cement prior to light curing. A post-cementation radiograph is recommended to insure the crown is seated completely and all excess cement was removed	

[a]Gehtt et al. reported that in 104 single crowns on 41 patients followed over 9 years, there is no difference in success between E-max crowns that were cemented with glass ionomer cement and those that were bonded with resin cement. Kern et al. did a similar experiment using 36 3-unit FPDs on 28 patients. The FPDs were either cemented with glass ionomer or adhesively bonded with resin cement. Success over the 10 years was equal for both groups (Kern et al. 2012).

(Carvahlo 2015). Refer to Chap. 6 "Restorative Considerations for Endodontically Treated Teeth" (Fig. 10.18).

C. *Replacing Missing Laterals*—In the younger adult population when laterals are congenitally missing and the patient is not ready for implant placement, a bonded bridge with one wing has been found to be quite effective (Sailer, 2014). Materials that are available today allow for high bond strengths and resistance to fracture of the porcelain. There are videos available online that demonstrate this concept as well (Renne 2015; Puri 2016) (Fig. 10.19).

D. *Implant Crowns*—Updates in the software for these companies allow the dentist to fabricate same-day crowns for a number of different implant abutments (Fig. 10.20).

E. *Zirconia Restorations*—Dentsply Sirona has just released a CEREC Zirconia and CEREC SpeedFire sintering furnace for same-day in-office sintering of zirconia-milled restorations. Zirconia has its advantages as it can be luted to the

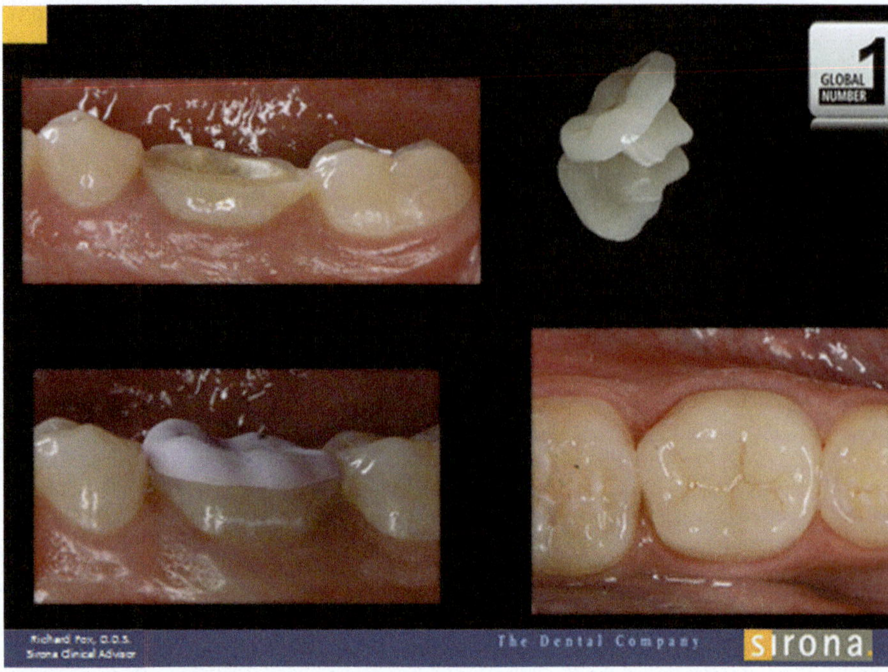

Fig. 10.18 In the endocrown illustrated below, note that the margins of the crown do not go all the way down to the gingiva. This is based on the principle that the bonding to the enamel is stronger and more predictable than any other part of the tooth. If the crown margins are supragingival, the ability to isolate away from crevicular fluids improves bonding abilities and the patient's access to clean and maintain the integrity of the restoration margins

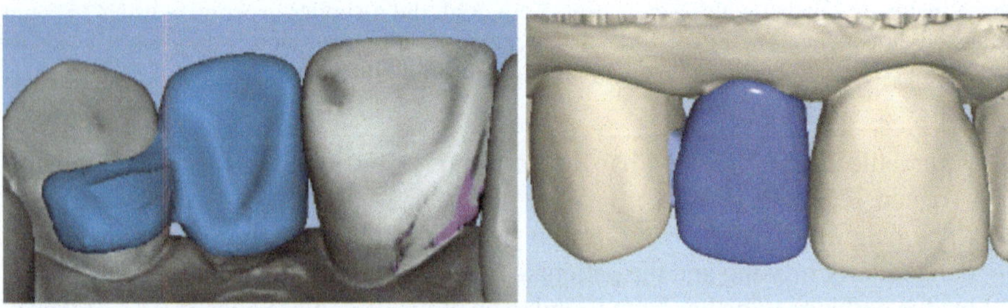

Fig. 10.19 A missing lateral can be replaced by a single wing bridge to satisfy esthetics and maintenance of the space

tooth with traditional cementation as compared to technique-sensitive resin cement (CerecDoctors 2016).

F. *3D Printing in Dentistry*—Additive manufacturing is also termed as "robocasting" wherein the final product is manufactured in layers of material based on the design from the CAD process (Silva et al. 2011). In dentistry this would replace milling units that have dominated the market. Dental laboratories already

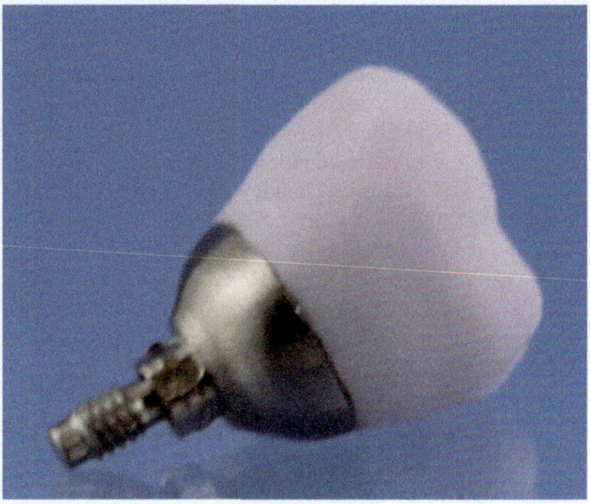

Fig. 10.20 Implant crown seated on an abutment

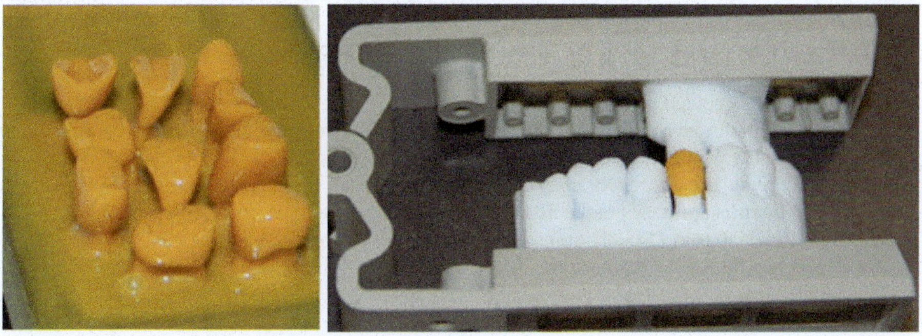

Fig. 10.21 3D-printed copings for a crown that will be cast in gold (Photo courtesy of Mr. Kevin Hudi, DSG Americus Laboratories in St. Petersburg, Fl)

utilized 3D printers (rapid prototyping) for fabricating cores utilizing plastic-like material that can be burned off when casted in either metal or porcelain (Fig. 10.21). In the future, development of "porcelain ink" to fabricate ceramic dental restorations could give better fitting crowns that aren't as technique sensitive as milled restorations and have improved esthetics. An interesting video on how 3D printing has been incorporated into today's dental labs can be found on: ihttps://www.youtube.com/watch?v=LRU0dk0KBJQ (accessed on 3/23/16).

G. See Chap. 11

References

Biacchi GR, Basting RT. Comparison of fracture strength of endocrowns and glass fiber post-retained conventional crowns. Oper Dent. 2012;37(2):130–6.

Carvalho AO, Bruzi G, Anderson RE, Maia HP, Giannini M, Magne P. Influence of adhesive core buildup designs on the resistance of endodontically treated molars restored with lithium.Oper Dent. 2016;41(1):76–82.

Cerecdoctors. Learn how to fabricate chairside Zirconia restorations with Cerec in a single visit. The ISSN register. https://www.cerecdoctors.com/zirconia?utm_campaign=Content+Campaigns&utm_source=hs_email&utm_medium=email&utm_content=26648386&_hsenc=p2ANqtz-_7_-DSbsIQa8Mjkz-Qk8meGpuWIJ6xQzksNEJPyIc7w10K0nGmQNfZNx06MFl7T82BlKGMt_alk5vjLx5FmaDkYo8voA&_hsmi=26648386. 2016. Accessed 29 Feb 2016.

Dennis F. A clinical evaluation of chairside lithium disilicate CAD/CAM crowns: a two-year report. J of American Dental Association. 2010;141(2):10s.

Ferencz J, Silva N, Navarro J, editors. High-strength ceramics: interdisciplinary perspectives. Illinois: Quintessence; 2014.

Gehrt M, Wolfart S, Rafai N, Reich S, Edelhoff D. Clinical results of lithium-disilicate crowns after up to 9 years of service. Clin Oral Investig. 2013;17(1):275–84.

Heymann H, Swift E, Ritter A. Fundamental concepts of enamel and dentin adhesion. In: Sturdevant, Mosby in St. Louis, Missouri (editor). Art and science of operative dentistry, 6th edn. Mosby; 2014.

Kern M, Sasse M, Wolfart S. Ten-year outcome of three-unit fixed dental prostheses made from monolithic lithium disilicate ceramic. J Am Dent Assoc. 2012;143(3):234–40.

Mormann W (editor). State of the art of CAD/CAM restorations. Quintessence in New Malden, Surrey United Kingdom, 2006.

Patel D. Conservative preparation guidelines for CAD/CAM restorations. Compendium. 2013;34(6):472.

Puri S. Digital dentistry: a workflow in the esthetic case. Spear education. 2016. The ISSN register: https://www.speareducation.com/spear-review/2016/02/digital-dentistry-a-workflow-in-the-esthetic-case. Accessed on 11 Feb 2016.

Renne W. E4D planscan adhesive bridge. 2015. The ISSN register: https://www.youtube.com/watch?v=Lq4xyWawPqI. Accessed on 11 Feb 2016.

Sailer I. Fixed dental prostheses for anterior and posterior teeth. In: Ferencz J, editor. High-strength ceramics: interdisciplinary perspectives. 1st ed. Chicago: Quintessence; 2014. p. 188. 146.

Silva NR, Witek L, Coelho PG, Thompson VP, Rekow ED, Smay J. Additive CAD/CAM process for dental prostheses. J Prosthodont. 2011;20(2):93–6.

Digital Impressions

11

Stefanie D. Seitz and Richard L. Zimmermann

Contents

Abstract

Intraoral scanning for digital impressions is a rapidly progressing technology that provides dentists with new capabilities for enhanced patient care. From simple inlays to fusing virtual models with cone beam computed tomography, this technology is changing the way dentistry is accomplished.

11.1 Intraoral Scanners

- Some digital impression systems require powdering of teeth prior to scanning.
- Systems create either a color (Fig. 11.1) or monochromatic (Fig. 11.2) virtual model, or the ability to see both.
- Open and closed systems.
  - Open – digital impression file (usually .stl file) can be imported into other software programs for design and restoration fabrication.

S.D. Seitz, DDS • R.L. Zimmermann, DDS (✉)
Comprehensive Dentistry, University of Texas in San Antonio School of Dentistry, San Antonio, TX, USA
e-mail: zimmermannr@uthscsa.edu

G.M. Weinstein, M.T. Zientz (eds.), *The Dental Reference Manual*,
DOI 10.1007/978-3-319-39730-6_11

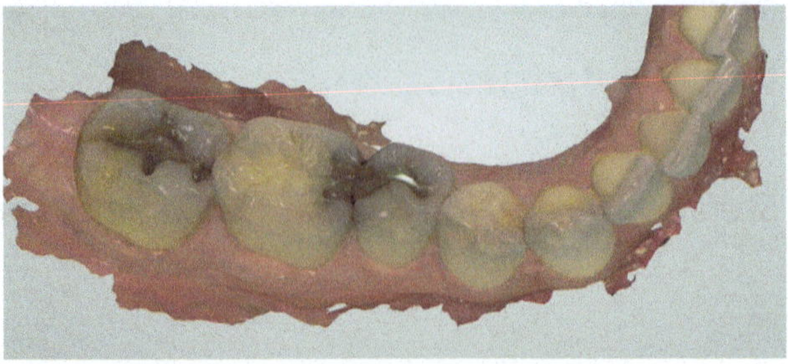

Fig. 11.1 Color virtual model

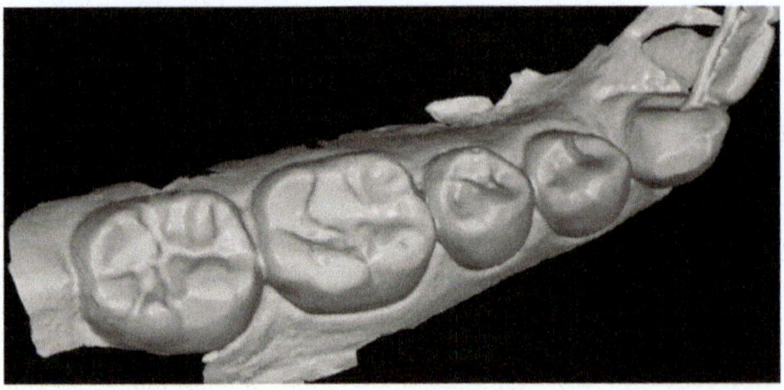

Fig. 11.2 Monochromatic virtual model

- Closed – digital impression file stays within the same software system for design and restoration fabrication.

- Most systems employ continuous image capture or true video during the scanning process.
- Proven accuracy (Ahrberg 2016).
- Secure virtual submission (Digital Dental Exchange 2016).

11.1.1 Capabilities of Intraoral Scanners

- Magnified image and ability to zoom allow better visualization of tooth preparation (Fig. 11.3).
- Occlusal clearance indicated with color-coded ranges so that the dentist can evaluate the need for additional reduction (Fig. 11.4).
- Ability to verify virtual occlusion is identical to intraoral occlusion.
- Preparation undercut detection (Fig. 11.5).
- Ability to edit and modify impressions.
- See chapter on Indirect Restorations with CAD/CAM Technology.

11.1.1.1 Advantages

- Enhanced patient comfort
- Efficient submission to lab virtually
- Improved lab communication – ability to include pictures, mark margins, and annotate on digital impression

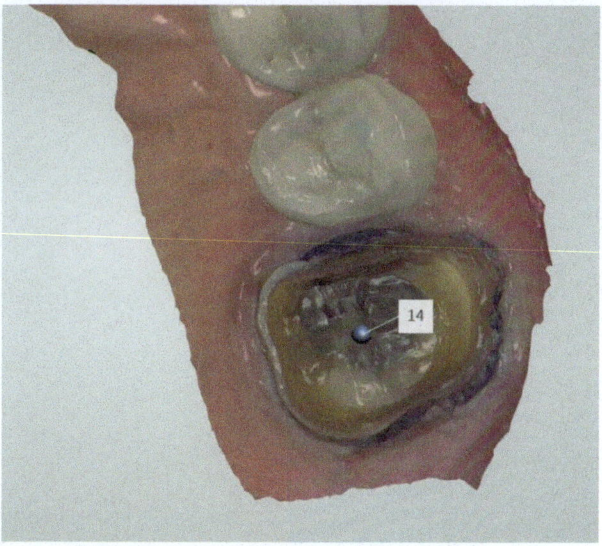

Fig. 11.3 Magnified view of preparation

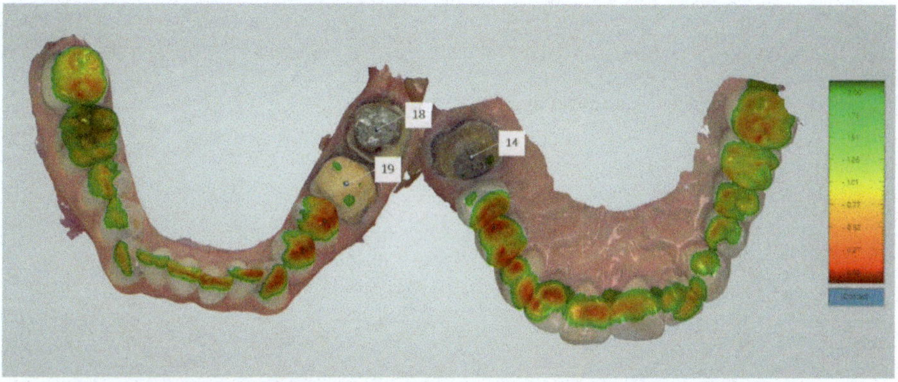

Fig. 11.4 Occlusal clearance on prepared teeth

- Retake impressions at no additional cost
- Reduction of necessary components for implant impressions

11.1.1.2 Disadvantages

- Learning curve associated with initial use
- High initial investment and/or recurring additional fees (i.e., licensing fees/click fees)

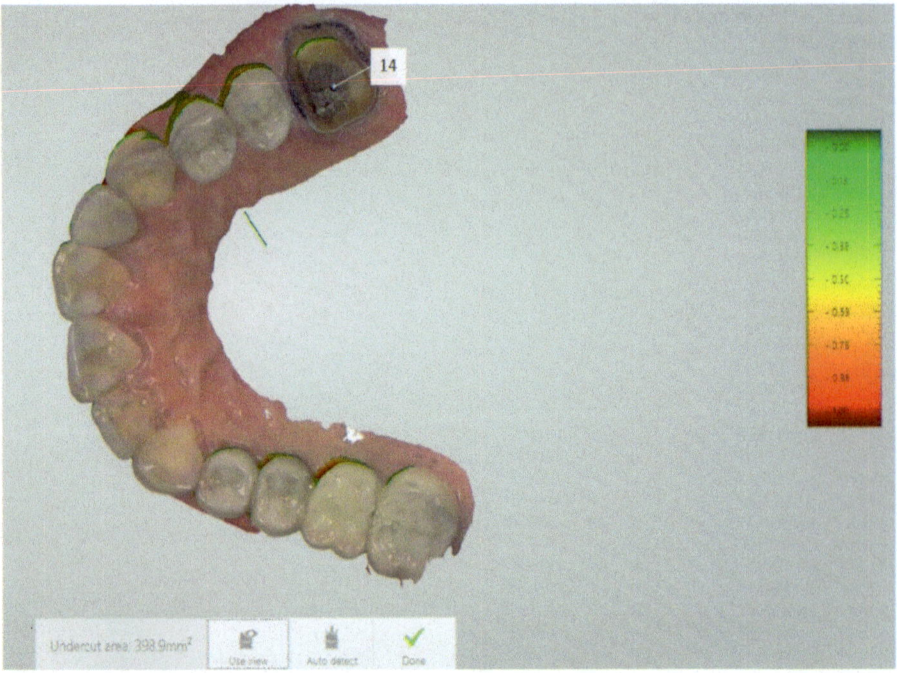

Fig. 11.5 Undercut detection shown in *green*

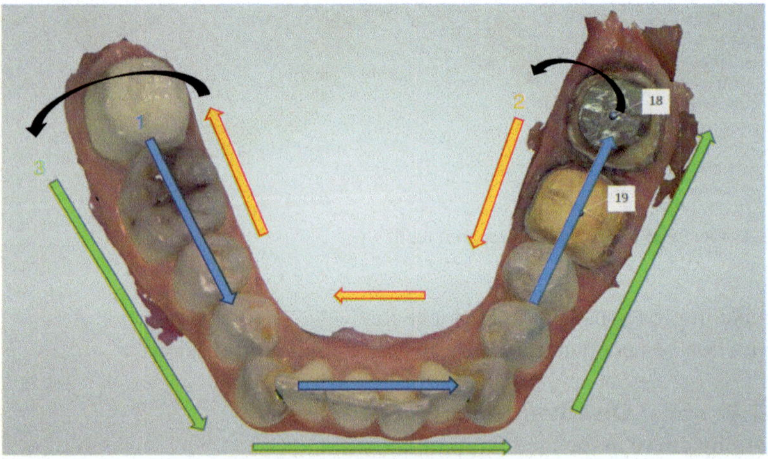

Fig. 11.6 *Suggested scanning path* – start on the occlusal and rotate to scan the lingual and then the buccal

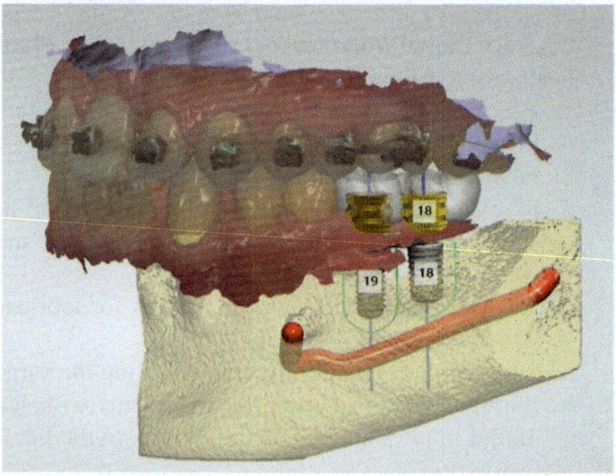

Fig. 11.7 Virtual implant planning with fused surface scan

11.2 Proper Technique for Imaging

(a) Avoid redundancy during scanning – increases accuracy and decreases file size (i.e., begin scanning occlusal surfaces on the most posterior tooth, moving to the anterior; rotate to capture the lingual surfaces and move from anterior to posterior; rotate over tooth to capture buccal surfaces and move anteriorly; end on an occlusal surface) (Fig. 11.6).

(b) Tissue retraction – ensure that the entire margin can be seen utilizing the retraction method of your choice (i.e., cord – this can remain in place or be removed for scanning as long as the entire preparation margin can still be seen).

(c) Ensure that the area to be scanned is free of saliva and blood.

(d) Ensure that the gingival margin is captured in each of the impressions for articulation of the bite.

(e) Always finish scanning on an occlusal surface.

11.3 Applications

(a) Ability to design and mill in-house or virtually submit to a laboratory.
- Single units – inlays, onlays, veneers, and crowns (Nejatidanesh 2015). See *Chap. 10 Indirect Restorations with CAD/CAM.*
- Fixed dental prosthesis.
- Implant restorations (Monaco 2015).
- Removable – doesn't displace tissue.
- Submission for orthodontic appliances.

(b) Fusion of CBCT with surface scan from digital impression (Rinaldi 2016) (Fig. 11.7).

Box 11.1: Digital Workflow for Implant Planning, Placement, and Final Restoration (Baumgarten 2015)

1. Use intraoral scanner of choice to scan teeth with the edentulous area that is to receive an implant.
2. Fusion of CBCT and intraoral scan.
3. Plan and design placement of the implant and final restoration (Fig. 11.7 shows #18/19 as edentulous area). There are many different design software that can be used for this.
4. An STL file of the scans can be sent for fabrication of the surgical guide which can be 3-D printed.
5. Surgical placement of the implant using the surgical guide.
6. Intraoral scan of the implant abutments with scan bodies for an accurate digital impression which will be sent to the lab for fabrication of the final restoration.
7. Delivery of the final restoration.

- Virtual implant planning – the ability to plan implants with the fused surface scan (virtual model) allows a restoratively driven plan utilizing the patient's own teeth as a guide for the restoration (Box 11.1).
- Surgical guides are designed using the surface scan so that the guide fits accurately in the patient's mouth.
- Immediate provisional design for guided implant placement – allows dental laboratory to fabricate a provisional based on virtual implant plan.

References

Ahrberg D, Lauer HC, Ahrberg M, Weigl P. Evaluation of fit and efficiency of CAD/CAM fabricated all-ceramic restorations based on direct and indirect digitalization: a double-blinded, randomized clinical trial. Clin Oral Investig. 2016;20(2):291–300.

Baumgarten HS, Wunsche A. CAD/CAM fabrication of definitive implant prostheses: a digital workflow from planning to implant placement to final restoration. Compend Contin Educ Dent. 2015;36(10):746–55.

Digital Dental Exchange. Discover the advantages of an intelligent online digital exchange. 2016. ISSN: http://www.ddxdental.com/products/dentist/benefits#tabs-2. Accessed 14 Mar 2016.

Monaco C, Evangelisti E, Scotti R, Mignani G, Zucchelli G. A fully digital approach to replicate peri-implant soft tissue contours and emergence profile in the esthetic zone. Clin Oral Implants Res. 2015.

Nejatidanesh F, Amjadi M, Akouchekian M, Savabi O. Clinical performance of CEREC AC Bluecam conservative ceramic restorations after five years–a retrospective study. J Dent. 2015;43(9):1076–82.

Rinaldi M, Ganz S, Mottola A. Computer guided dental implants and reconstructive surgery. Missouri: Elsevier; 2016.

Part II

The Specialties in General Dentistry

Endodontics for the General Practitioner 12

Uma Nair

Contents

12.1 Sequela for *Diagnosis*

- *Chief complaint*: should be noted in patient's own words
- *Medical history:*
  - Conditions/medications that alter dental treatment
  - Conditions that alter the outcomes of endodontic therapy: diabetes mellitus, steroid therapy, and smoking
- *Dental history*: subjective information from patient regarding the chief complaint (Table 12.1)
  - Nature of pain: dull vs. sharp
  - Duration of pain: short vs. prolonged
  - Frequency of pain
  - Spontaneity

U. Nair, DMD, MDS, Dip. ABE
Department of Endodontics, University of Florida College of Dentistry, Gainesville, FL, USA
e-mail: upnayar@gmail.com

G.M. Weinstein, M.T. Zientz (eds.), *The Dental Reference Manual*,
DOI 10.1007/978-3-319-39730-6_12

Table 12.1 When a patient presents with a history of pain from a tooth, answers from a patient can give you a hint on the nature of the diagnosis

Questions to ask	Reversible pulpitis	Irreversible pulpitis or necrotic
Is the pain there all the time?	No	Yes, possibly for hours or days
Is the pain induced by anything? Sweet? Cold? Hot?	Possibly	Pain may start on its own, not induced by anything. This is a clue that the pain is spontaneous
Does the pain go away when the stimulus is removed?	Yes, pain goes away quickly (no more than 10 s or so). Pain should go away when the stimulus is removed	No, the pain lingers for a while, a minute to all day
Is the pain relieved by anything?	Pain goes away on its own upon removal of stimulus	As the infection progresses, pain relief will not always be achieved by over the counter analgesics. Patients will often report taking many tablets of acetaminophen or ibuprofen without getting relief from pain
Can you tell where the pain is coming from?	Often the patient can tell the tooth or quadrant the source of pain is coming from	The patient is not always able to point out the source of pain as referred pain is a distinct possibility
Is the pain sharp or dull?	A sharp ache from biting or chewing can be a sign of a fractured tooth or a loose restoration	Dull throbbing ache on the affected side. A dull ache that keeps a patient from chewing on that side must be differentiated from temporomandibular joint problems by performing endodontic testing on the teeth

 - Stimulus: causes/relieves pain
- *Clinical exam*: intraoral and extraoral exam to evaluate the presence of swelling, symmetry, sinus tracts, soft tissue abnormalities, periodontal status (probing, mobility), caries, and restorations
- *Clinical testing*: clinical tests for objective information about the chief complaint
  - Thermal tests: Determines vitality and inflammation in the pulp (cold, refrigerant spray on a cotton pellet; heat, gutta-percha stick).
  - Electric pulp tester: Determines vitality of pulp.
  - Percussion: Determines presence of apical periodontitis.
  - Palpation: Determines presence of swelling or inflammation in the periodontium.
  - Probing: Determines presence of pockets or sinus tracts; note that probing to the apex of the tooth in a single spot may mean that there is a vertical root fracture.
  - Mobility: Determines presence of periodontal disease.
- *Radiographic analysis*:
  - Bitewing radiographs of the tooth to determine restorability, proximity of caries, and restorations to the pulp (Fig. 12.1a, b)
  - Periapical radiographs: two angles for evaluation of periapical pathology, number of canals, presence of calcifications, resorption, etc.

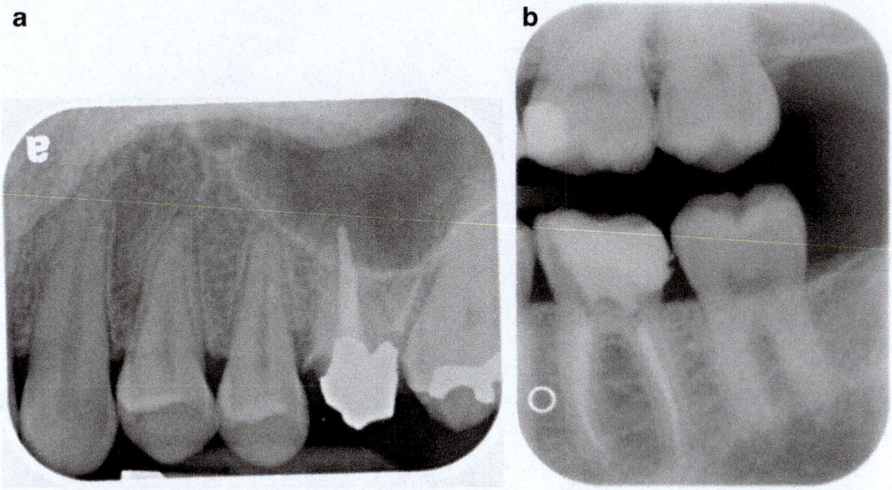

Fig. 12.1 (**a**, **b**). Determine the restorability of the tooth prior to initiating endodontic treatment by evaluating the amount of tooth structure remaining. See Chap. 6 Restorative Considerations of Endodontically Treated Teeth

- *Additional testing*: recommended if diagnosis cannot be reached with the above steps
  - Test cavity: Cavity preparation in the suspected tooth with no anesthesia when vitality is in question. Tooth will be sensitive if vital when dentinoenamel junction is reached.
  - Selective anesthesia: Anesthetizing the maxillary or mandibular quadrant to isolate tooth when referred pain to opposing arch is suspected.

12.2 Arriving at the Diagnosis

Arriving at a diagnosis can be very difficult especially in patients with multiple carious lesions. Careful endodontic testing and clinical exam are essential for proper diagnosis (Fig. 12.2).

The patient's medical/dental history and subjective and objective information should be combined to arrive at a diagnosis which should include a pulpal and periapical diagnosis. The American Association of Endodontics approved terminology should be utilized for diagnosis (Glickman 2009) (Tables 12.2 and 12.3).

12.3 Endodontic Emergencies

Inflammation/infection of the pulp and periapical tissue can cause pain and swelling.

Treatment:

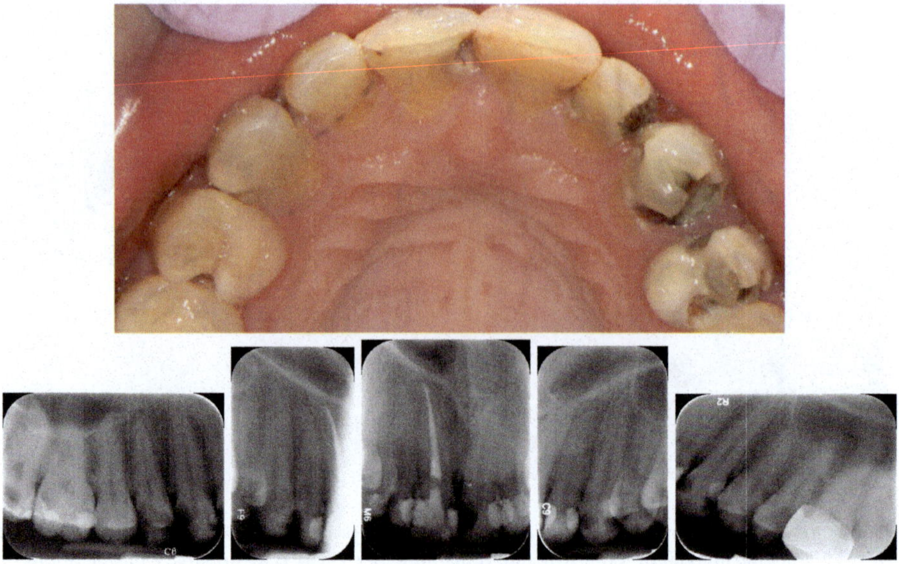

Fig. 12.2 Extensive carious lesions observed clinically and radiographically

(a) Pain caused by irreversible pulpitis can be relieved by complete pulpectomy. In multirooted teeth, removal of pulp from the widest canal provides relief of pain (Pak 2011).
(b) Antibiotics have no effect on pain. Antibiotics are only indicated for swelling in the presence of systemic signs and symptoms such as fever, cellulitis, trismus, malaise, or for progressive increase in the size of the swelling (Aminoshariae 2015).
(c) Incision and drainage are recommended for localized fluctuant or indurated swelling.
(d) Analgesics should be prescribed for control of pain. See Chap. 22 Prescriptions.

12.3.1 Treatment Considerations

(a) Standard of care for endodontic treatment: Use of rubber dam is mandatory.
(b) In cases where there is significant inflammation, anesthesia may be difficult. See Chap. 4 Local Anesthesia Challenges.
(c) Access shapes: Ideal and modifications required under certain conditions. *Access should provide straight line access to the root canal to avoid stresses on the files and to ensure complete removal of pulp tissue* (Fig. 12.3).
(d) Working length determination: Use of an electronic apex locator vs. radiograph. Apex locators are approximately 90 % accurate. Combination of apex locators and radiographs give the most accurate results.
(e) Cleaning and shaping:

Table 12.2 Presumptive clinical diagnosis of pulpal/periapical conditions

Classification	Signs/symptoms	Test results
PULPAL:		
Normal pulp	None	Normal responses to thermal and EPT – responses are definite and well defined and cease on removal of stimulus
Reversible pulpitis	Requires stimulus to evoke a painful response of short (seconds) duration. Pain is mild and with short lingering sensation. Negative for radiographic changes	Hyperresponsive (slightly exaggerated) and/or slightly prolonged (seconds) to cold and/or hot, EPT is within normal limits
Symptomatic irreversible pulpitis	Induced pain – usually more intense and lingers well beyond removal of stimulus (i.e., temperature changes). History of spontaneous pain, usually severe; can be constant or intermittent	Hyperresponsive (grossly exaggerated) and prolonged (>10 s) to cold and/or hot. EPT is within normal limits
Asymptomatic irreversible pulpitis	None	Clinically and radiographically the caries extends to the pulp. EPT is within normal limits. Thermal tests maybe within normal limits
Pulpal necrosis	Usually asymptomatic. May have history of episodic, prolonged, spontaneous, or provoked pain during irreversible pulpitis stage	EPT, no response; thermal tests, no response
Previously treated	Radiographic evidence of root canal filling material in the canal	EPT, no response; thermal tests, no response
Previously initiated	Radiographic evidence of access into the pulp cavity	EPT, may or may not respond; thermal, may or may not respond

- Rotary and hand instrumentation: Rotary instrumentation with nickel – titanium instruments provide a tapered preparation of the canal.
- Irrigants:

NaOCL: Sodium hypochlorite (household bleach) is the most commonly used root canal irrigant. 0.5–8.15 % dilutions are used. Advantages – ability to dissolve organic substances and affordability. Disadvantages – cytotoxicity when injected into periradicular tissues, smell, and staining of clothes.

Chlorhexidine gluconate: Broad spectrum antimicrobial action.

EDTA: Ethylenediaminetetraacetic acid. Chelating agent used to remove the inorganic portion of the smear layer. 17 % EDTA for one minute followed by adjunctive NaOCl final rinse to remove smear layer before final obturation.

Irrigation techniques: Activation of irrigants using sonic or ultrasonic aids, e.g., Endoactivator.

Cleaning and shaping should result in a tapered canal preparation with an adequate apical stop and removal of diseased dentin, microorganisms, and organic material from the canal.

(f) Obturation:

Table 12.3 Periradicular

Classification	Signs/symptoms	Test results
Symptomatic apical periodontitis (with irreversible pulpitis or pulp necrosis)	Intense pain made worse with mastication or percussion. Radiographic changes vary from none, thickened PDL at apex, or periapical radiolucency	EPT and thermal responses range from hyperresponsiveness (irreversible pulpitis) to no response (necrotic pulp). Extreme sensitivity to percussion with or without palpation/sensitivity
Acute apical abscess	Spontaneous moderate to severe pain. Radiating throb. Prolonged duration, but may be episodic. Swelling ranges from barely perceptible to extensive. Later stages will manifest an elevated temperature. Radiographic changes vary from none, thickened apical PDL, or periapical radiolucency	EPT and thermal tests yield no response. Marked sensitivity to percussion and apical palpation; increased mobility
Asymptomatic apical periodontitis (apical granuloma, apical cyst)	Generally asymptomatic. May have had symptoms in the past. Definite radiographic evidence of periapical radiolucency	Nonresponsive to thermal and EPT (except sometimes in multirooted teeth). No response to percussion and palpation. No mobility
Chronic apical abscess	No discomfort, gradual onset, and intermittent discharge of pus through an associated sinus tract. Periapical radiolucency present	Nonresponsive to thermal and EPT. Percussion and palpation negative
Condensing osteitis (focal sclerosing osteomyelitis)	Little or no discomfort. Periapical circumscribed radiopaque lesion. Root outline is visible	May or may not respond to EPT and thermal tests. Percussion and palpation negative

- Lateral condensation: Does not use heat or thermoplasticized gutta-percha
- Warm vertical techniques: Uses heat source, e.g., System B, Calamus, Obtura

(g) Outcomes: Evaluation of endodontic success and failure. Healing of periapical pathology on periapical radiographs may not be evident for up to 6 months. Patient should be free of symptoms and the tooth should not exhibit any signs of pathology such as deep probings or presence of sinus tracts (Fig. 12.4 a, b).

12.4 Endodontic Pearls

(a) The most characteristic radiographic evidence of a vertical root fracture (VRF) is a radiolucent halo surrounding the root. Clinically a narrow, isolated probing may be present. An isolated deep pocket when traced with gutta-percha illustrates the connection between the oral cavity and the apex (Fig. 12.5).
(b) Chloroform is the reagent of choice to soften gutta-percha.
(c) Gutta-percha points may be sterilized by placing in 5.25 % NaOCl for 1 min.

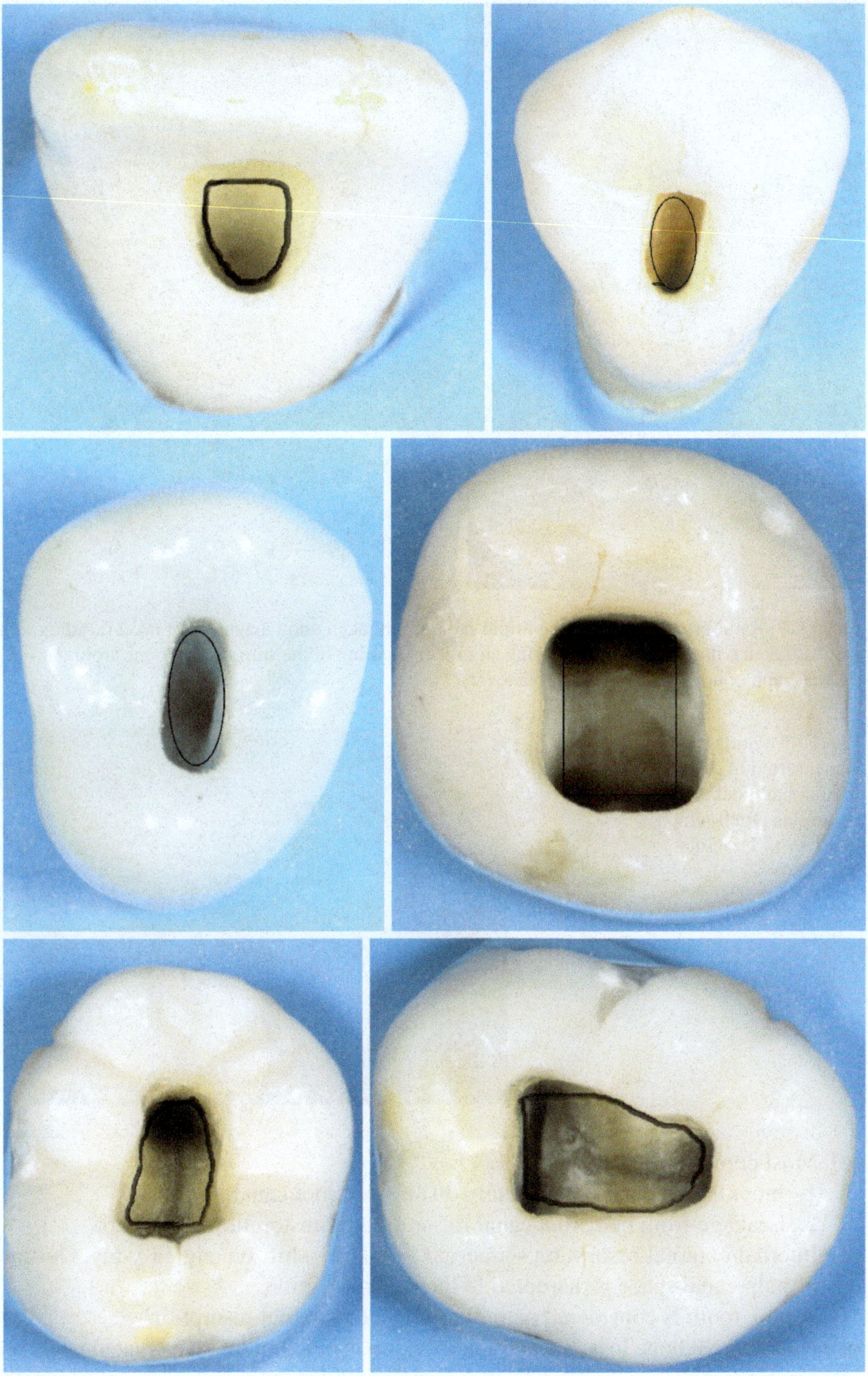

Fig. 12.3 Examples of access shapes that include the canals of a given tooth (Photos courtesy of Dr. Jon Scott)

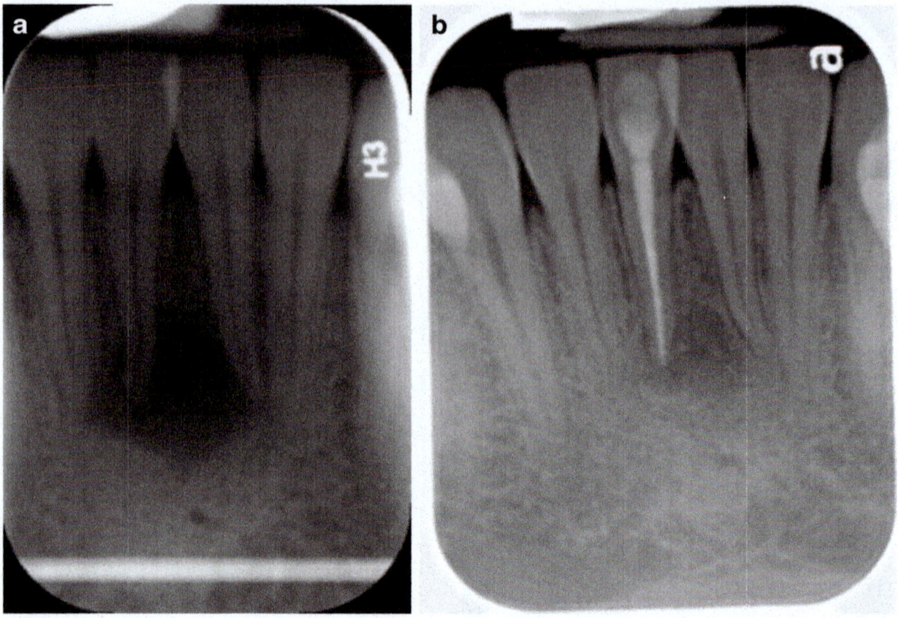

Fig. 12.4 Radiograph (**a**) shows the initial radiograph taken upon diagnosis of no. 24; radiograph (**b**) was taken 6 months after showcasing significant healing of the surrounding bone around no. 25 (Radiograph courtesy of Dr. Joshua Yanover)

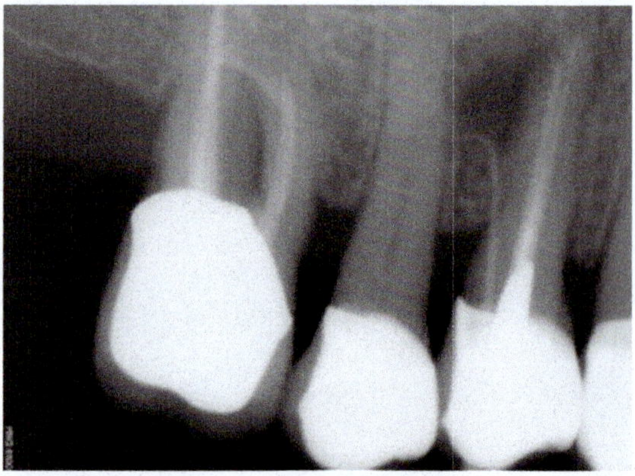

Fig. 12.5 Gutta-percha was inserted in deep periodontal pocket to trace its origins (Radiograph courtesy of Dr. Gina Nicoloso)

(d) Most common causes of failure:
    1. Incompletely and inadequately disinfected root canal
    2. Leakage from poor root canal fill or coronal restoration (Fig. 12.6)
(e) Internal/external resorption – internal will NOT shift on angled x-ray. Outline of pulp canal space is disrupted in internal resorption.
(f) A pink tooth is considered pathognomonic of internal resorption.
(g) Histological bone loss in a periapical lesion is much more than what appears on a radiograph.

(h) The root formation is completed 2–3 years after tooth eruption (*see Pediatric chapter for Sequence of Tooth Eruption*).
(i) The lower incisors have 30–40 % chance of a second canal.

12.5 **When to Refer** (Endodontic Case Difficulty Assessment)

The following factors should be taken into consideration when assessing case difficulty and need for referral to an endodontists:

(a) Unusual length.
(b) Unusual canal shape: open apex, C-shape canals, dens en dente, taurodontism, and roots with bulbous tips (Fig. 12.7).
(c) Extreme root curvatures (Fig. 12.8).

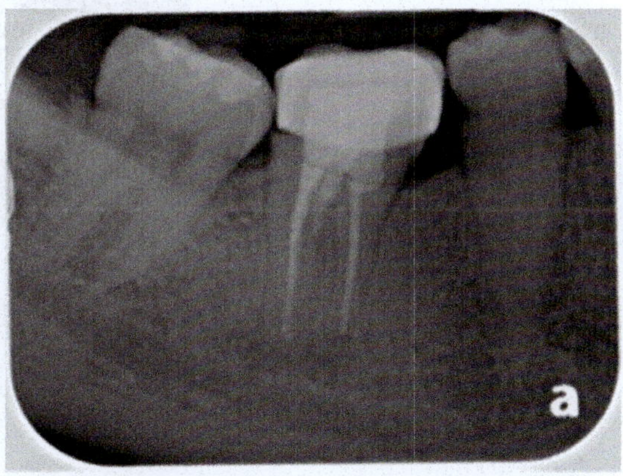

Fig. 12.6 Open margin on the distal of no. 30 may lead to failure of the endodontically treated tooth

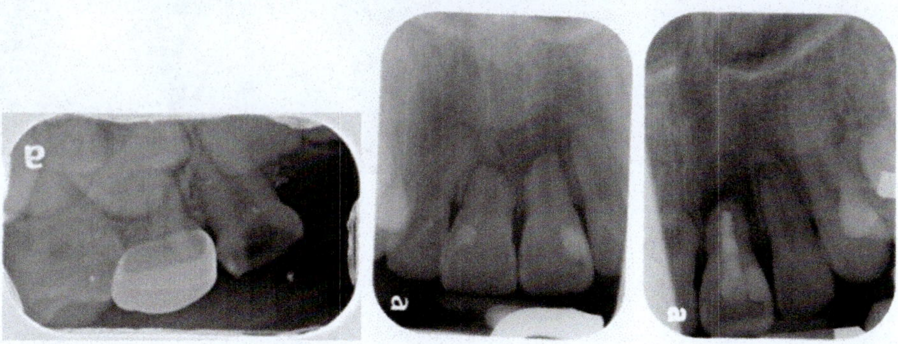

Fig. 12.7 Endodontic treatment on young permanent teeth with possible open apices are good referrals to your specialist (Radiographs by Dr. Jade Rivera)

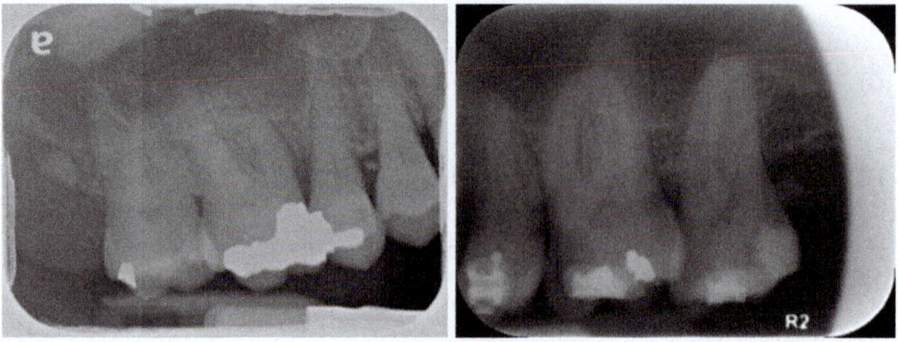

Fig. 12.8 Dilacerated root on no. 3 mesial and no. 14 mesial and distal roots

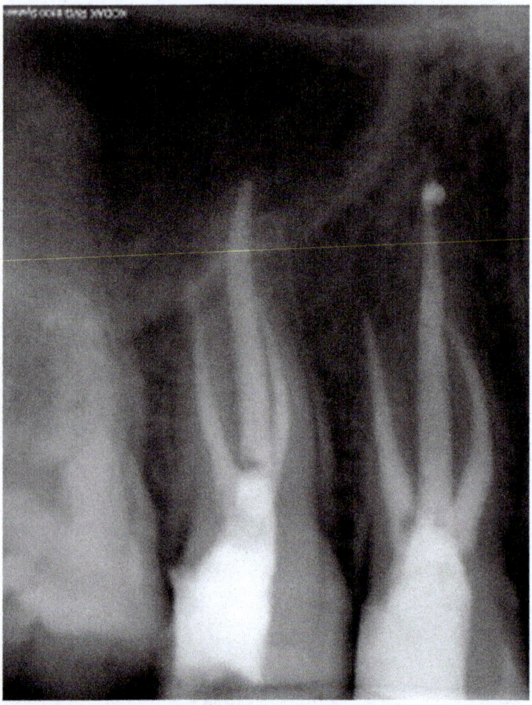

Fig. 12.9 Three canals in maxillary premolars require magnification to detect additional canals

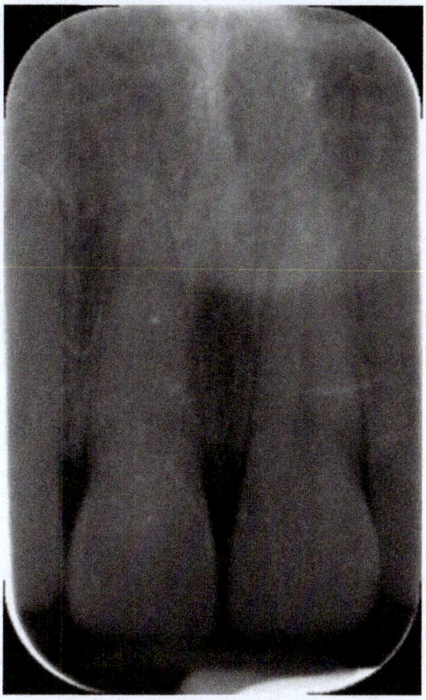

Fig. 12.10 Calcified tooth no. 8 as a result of trauma may render endodontic treatment to be difficult. Referral to endodontist recommended

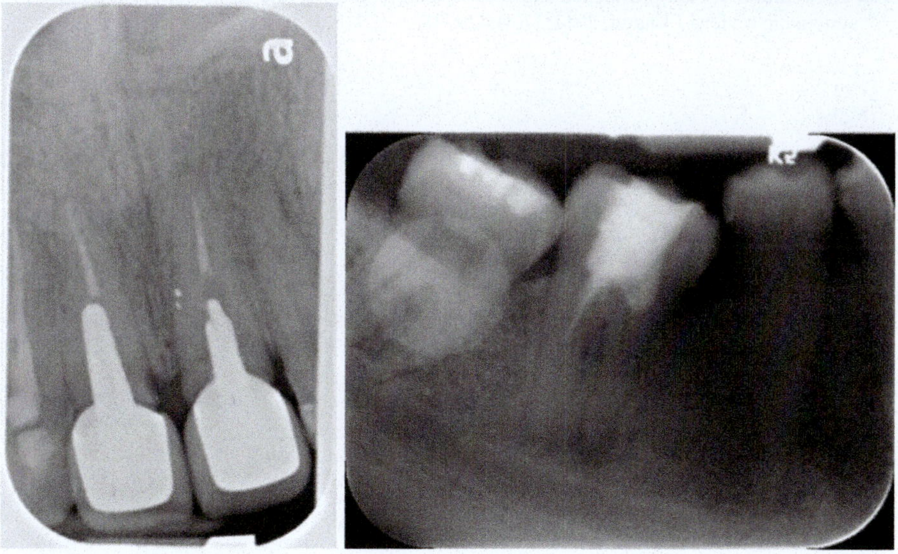

Fig. 12.11 Removal of cemented post and cores may prove to be difficult when re-treating teeth (Radiographs Courtesy of Dr. Daniel Buono)

(d) Unusual number of canals: extra canals and fast breaks (split canals) (Fig. 12.9).
(e) Resorption: external or internal.
(f) Calcifications (Fig. 12.10).
(g) Ease of isolation using rubber dam.
(h) Previous treatment with canal blockage, ledges, or perforations (Fig. 12.11).
(i) Location of the tooth: accessibility issues with position in the mouth, amount of mouth opening, and tooth angulation.
(j) Clinician's skills.
(k) Pain could not be localized to a tooth and endodontic diagnosis could not established. See Chap. 19 The Examination, Differential Diagnosis, and Management of Pain.

References

Aminoshariae A, Kulild JC. Evidence-based recommendations for antibiotic usage to treat endodontic infections and pain: a systematic review of randomized controlled trials. J Am Dent Assoc. 2016;147(3):186–91.

Endodontic Case Difficulty Assessment form: http://www.aae.org/caseassessment/.

Glickman GN. AAE consensus conference on diagnostic terminology: background and perspectives. J Endod. 2009;35:1619.

Pak JG, White SN. Pain prevalence and severity before, during, and after root canal treatment: a systematic review. J Endod. 2011;37(4):429–38.

Periodontics for the General Dental Practitioner

13

Peter Harrison, Eugenia Monaghan, and Karin Schey

Contents

P. Harrison, BDS, MS (✉)
Division of Restorative Dentistry and Periodontology, Dublin Dental University Hospital, Trinity College, Dublin, Ireland
e-mail: peter.harrison@dental.tcd.ie

E. Monaghan, DMD, MS • K. Schey, DMD, MS
Department of Periodontology, University of North Carolina School of Dentistry, Chapel Hill, NC, USA
e-mail: eugenia.monaghan@gmail.com

G.M. Weinstein, M.T. Zientz (eds.), *The Dental Reference Manual*,
DOI 10.1007/978-3-319-39730-6_13

Abstract

Transitioning to clinical care can be difficult for the new practitioner. Didactics provide a great breadth of information and scientific studies; however, this chapter aims to condense this information into an easy-to-use guide for clinical use. Using scientific research and clinical experience, the topics of this chapter will guide a new practitioner through one of the most important foundational aspects of oral health. Beginning with classifying periodontal needs and diagnosing periodontal disease, this chapter outlines steps needed in the clinical evaluation of the patient. Risk factors for periodontal disease and practical aspects of non-surgical periodontal instrumentation are discussed. The text addresses decision-making at periodontal re-evaluation, periodontal maintenance and advanced periodontal needs including surgical therapy. Finally, periodontal emergencies such as abscess and necrotizing ulcerative gingivitis are reviewed with recommended treatment options.

13.1 Epidemiology: Prevalence of Periodontitis

Based on the National Health and Nutrition Examination Survey (NHANES) 2009–2012 data:

45.9% of US adults (≥30 years) have periodontitis. 8.9% have severe periodontitis.

Periodontitis prevalence was elevated among the following groups (Eke et al. 2015):

- Hispanic > African-American > Asian-American > whites
- Male > female
- Smokers

- ≥65 years
- Low income
- Low educational attainment

13.2 Classification

The current classification system is the Armitage classification (1999). This is a detailed and comprehensive classification; based on concerns expressed within the education community about the difficulty of implementing the classification in clinical practice, the American Academy of Periodontology (AAP) commissioned a task force to provide clarity on certain areas of the Armitage classification. In addition, it was announced that the process of developing a new classification system will begin in 2017 (American Academy of Periodontology Task Force Report 2015).

- Diseases of the periodontium are divided into "gingival" and "periodontal" conditions.
- *Gingival conditions* may be plaque-induced (the vast majority) or non-plaque-induced.
- *Periodontal conditions* are subcategorized into seven further areas. Of these, the majority of clinical cases seen by dental practitioners fare addressed within the subcategories chronic periodontitis (the vast majority) and aggressive periodontitis.

13.2.1 Chronic Periodontitis

- The most common form of periodontal disease
- Multifactorial aetiology
  - Biofilm
  - Genetic susceptibility
  - Compromised immune response

For consistency, if the extent of disease varies within the patient, list the most advanced disease first, e.g., "localized severe chronic periodontitis with generalized moderate chronic periodontitis" (Table 13.1).

Table 13.1 Stating a periodontal diagnosis: Think: "Escape (ESC) key"

"*E*xtent" of disease		Localized: <30 % teeth/sites affected
		Generalized: >30 % teeth/sites affected
"*S*everity" of disease	Based on clinical attachment loss noted in the patient	Slight: 1–2 mm CAL
		Moderate: 3–4 mm CAL
		Severe: ≥5 mm CAL
"*C*ondition"		Chronic periodontitis

13.2.2 Aggressive Periodontitis (Lang et al. 1999)

Classification of aggressive periodontitis is not based on the age of the patient. However, the profile of many affected patients is typically younger (usually <30 years).

The following are primary features of aggressive periodontitis:

- Rapid rate of attachment loss and destruction of bone.
- Familial aggregation.
- Patients are otherwise clinically healthy – no systemic disease.

Secondary features (may/may not be present):

- Severity of disease may be disproportionate to amounts of microbial deposits (especially for localized aggressive).
- Increased *Aggregatibacter actinomycetemcomitans* (Aa) (and in some cases *Porphyromonas gingivalis* (Pg)) may be present.
- Cellular: Hyper-responsive macrophage phenotype and abnormal phagocytes.
- Disease (attachment loss and bone loss) may be self-limiting.

13.2.2.1 Localized Aggressive (LAP)

- Diagnosis of "localized" not based on the 30 % rule
- Diagnosis: LAP has a first molar/incisor presentation; interproximal attachment loss on at least two permanent teeth (one of which is a first molar) and not more than two teeth other than first molars/incisors are involved.
- Typical onset around puberty.
- Prevalence: Limited data available; generally estimated to be <1 % adolescents but more prevalent in African-American population.

13.2.2.2 Generalized Aggressive (GAP)

- Diagnosis of "generalized" not based on the 30 % rule (although this is often met; indeed, disease often affects the entire dentition).
- Diagnosis: Interproximal attachment loss on at least three permanent teeth other than first molars/incisors.
- Affected patients usually young (<30 years) but may be older.
- Episodic pattern of destruction.
- Prevalence: Limited data available; estimated at 0.13 % of the US adolescents (Löe and Brown 1991).

13.3 Patient Assessment

A. *Chief Complaint*
   - Periodontal disease can affect different parts of a patient's dentition to varying degrees. Some patients may not even be aware that they have a problem, while others will come to you complaining that their teeth are loose or that their gums bleed.

Table 13.2 Components of periodontal examination

Clinical parameters	Radiographic parameters
Probing depth	Bone height relative to CEJ
Clinical attachment level	Assessment for horizontal/vertical bone loss
Plaque	Presence of intact lamina dura
Bleeding on probing	
Suppuration	
Mobility	
Furcation involvement	
Mucogingival tissue assessment	

B. *Medical and Dental History*
- It is very important to gather an accurate medical history from the patient to help determine possible barriers to treatment as well as possible systemic factors contributing to the presence of disease.

C. *Periodontal Examination* (AAP 2011)

The main objectives of a thorough clinical exam pertain to identifying the main problems and their sources in the patient's mouth. Identify etiologic factors, whether past or present, that will affect the long-term prognosis of all the teeth involved (Table 13.2).

1. *Probing Depth (PD)*
   - Record at six sites per tooth with a calibrated periodontal probe (e.g., UNC-15): distobuccal, buccal, mesiobuccal, mesiolingual, lingual, and distolingual surfaces
2. *Clinical Attachment Level (CAL)*
   - Calculated by adding the probing depth and gingival margin together (PD+GM=CAL).
   - CAL measurements are used in developing a periodontal diagnosis for the patient. Situations of CAL loss are classified as *slight* (CAL 1–2 mm), *moderate* (CAL 3–4 m), or *severe* (5–6 mm).
3. *Bleeding on Probing (BOP)*
   - BOP should be assessed while probing and recorded as "present" or "absent" at each site.
   - The percentage of bleeding sites can be calculated and used during re-evaluations to determine changes in periodontal health.
4. *Suppuration (S)*
   - Similar to BOP, the presence of suppuration indicates a disease process in the periodontium such as infection.
   - If suppuration is suspected, the periodontal probe can be used as a supplemental tool to express the pus by placing the probe flat against the tissue and dragging the probe towards the gingival margin with slight pressure.
5. *Plaque Score*
   - At each periodontal visit for cleaning, nonsurgical therapy, or recall, a plaque score should be calculated, utilizing a plaque disclosing agent.

- Of all the measurements taken during the periodontal charting process, a plaque score is the most visual way to show patients the effects of their home care and oral hygiene.
- Plaque presence is recorded at six surfaces per tooth as a binary "yes" or "no" measurement for the presence of plaque on that particular surface from which a percentage may then be calculated.
- After disclosing the patient and calculating the plaque score percentage, it is important to show the patient with a mirror the sites on their teeth that are not being brushed properly. Effective plaque removal is modelled for the patient. The patient should subsequently be given an opportunity to practice plaque removal at the affected sites.
- The goal is to achieve and maintain a plaque score of *25 % or less*.

6. *Furcations (F)*

	Furcation probe access	Practical assessment
Class I Furcation (F1)	Does not exceed 1/3 of the width of the tooth (<3 mm)	Probe engages furcation slightly but no "catch" present when withdrawn
Class II Furcation Lesion (F2)	Exceeds 1/3 of the tooth width but does encompass the total width of the tooth (>3 mm)	Probe hooks into roof of furcation, "catch" present on attempt to withdraw
Class III Furcation Lesion (F3)	"Through and through" access - probe penetrates through entire width of furcation area	Probe enters furcation (e.g. buccal) and emerges via another furcation site (e.g. lingual) on tooth

- Furcation involvement is assessed using a Nabers (furcation) probe.
- The degree of furcation involvement has implications for individual prognosis of the tooth and for the ability of the patient to successfully maintain this surface devoid of plaque and biofilm.

7. *Mobility (M)*
    - To assess mobility, the blunt end of the explorer and the blunt end of the mirror can be placed on the B and L surfaces of the tooth, respectively, and pressure applied to assess if any pathologic movement is observed. If a gloved finger is used in place of one of these hard objects, a depression in the soft tissue of the finger may incorrectly mimic tooth movement (Fig. 13.1).

- The extent of the mobility is categorized in classes

Class I	Movement of the crown is between 0.2 and 1 mm horizontally in any direction
Class II	Movement of the crown is >1 mm horizontally in any direction
Class III	Movement of the crown in the vertical direction is present in addition to horizontal movement

8. *Mucogingival Assessment*
    - Evaluation gives a descriptive picture of the relative amount of attached, keratinized gingiva.
    - Note the presence of any abnormal attachment of a labial, lingual, or buccal frenum, i.e., close to gingival margin and whose movement impacts on

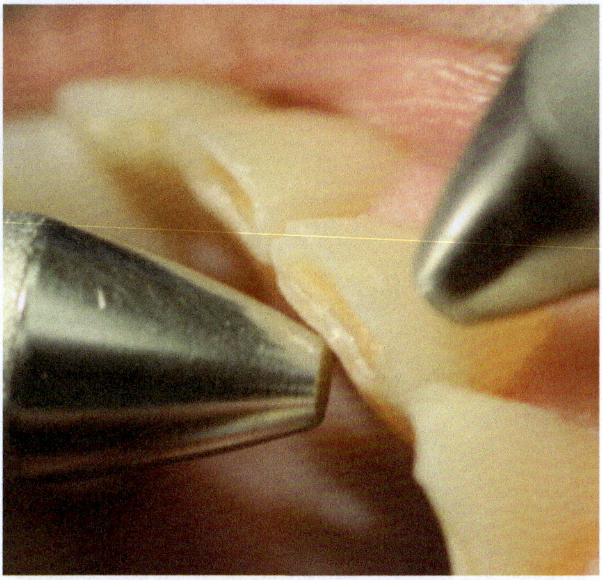

Fig. 13.1 Check for mobility with instruments on either side of the tooth (Photo Courtesy of Dr. Daniel Buono)

Table 13.3 Classification of gingival recession

Class	Marginal tissue recession	Interdental area	Root coverage anticipated
I	Does not extend to MGJ	No periodontal loss	100 %
II	To or beyond MGJ	No periodontal loss	100 %
III	To or beyond MGJ	Loss of tissue or malposition	Partial
IV	To or beyond MGJ	Severe loss of tissue	Not anticipated

gingival tissue. Friel's test involves stretching the lip in the area of a labial/buccal frenum – blanching of the marginal gingival tissue indicates a frenal pull that may be associated with the risk of further gingival recession.

- Stretch the lips gently and note the position of the mucogingival junction (MGJ-where attached gingiva and the alveolar mucosa meet). Note and document the amount of keratinized gingiva present.
- Gingival Recession is categorized using the Miller classification (Miller 1985) (Table 13.3).

9. *Radiographic Analysis*
   - Bitewing radiographs are helpful in determining bone levels both at a single moment in time as well as looking at progression of periodontal disease over time.

- Subgingival calculus can sometimes be visualized as faint radiopaque wisps attached to the tooth usually at the CEJ (Fig. 13.2).
- It is important to remember that radiographs alone are not diagnostic for periodontal issues, and a thorough clinical examination must be conducted.

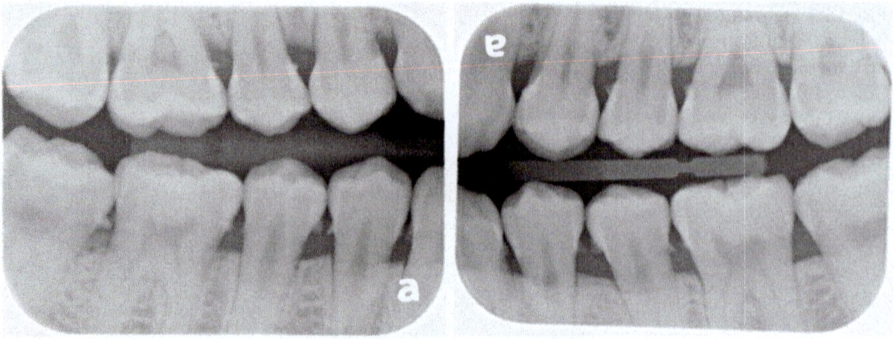

Fig. 13.2 Calculus deposits can be visualized at interproximal surfaces

Table 13.4 Factors associated with periodontal disease risk

	Description	Examples
Risk factor	Exposure to the factor must precede the onset of disease Association confirmed in a prospective longitudinal study	Tobacco smoking Diabetes Plaque deposits/specific pathogenic bacteria
Risk indicator	Potential risk factor – has been identified in a cross-sectional study However, not yet confirmed in a longitudinal study	Osteoporosis HIV/AIDs Stress
Risk marker	Factors that are associated with/predictive of disease but do not cause it	Previous history of periodontal disease
Background characteristic[a]	May sometimes be described as non-modifiable risk factors Evident in epidemiologic studies but causal role difficult to assign	Genetics Age (older) Gender (male) Socio-economic status (lower SES)

[a]Note: These factors may often show associations in epidemiologic studies but may be mediated through more complex means (or due to confounding factors), e.g., higher prevalence of periodontal diseases among males may be a result of poorer OH/dental visit compliance relative to females rather than a direct effect of gender

13.4 Risk Factors

Risk factors, when present, increase the probability that an individual will develop disease. The terminology used to discuss these concepts can be confusing. While many systemic, local, and environmental factors may be associated with disease aetiology, only a few meet the definition of a "true" risk factor (Table 13.4).

13.4.1 Plaque Deposits/Specific Pathogenic Bacteria

- A modifiable risk factor.
- Role as risk factor for gingivitis is clear. Experimental accumulation of plaque deposits results in gingival inflammation; removal of deposits is associated with clinical improvement (Löe et al. 1965).
- Association with periodontitis is not as strong – not all patients with bacterial deposits develop disease and increased plaque does not imply increased disease. However, specific bacterial species have been identified as aetiologic agents for periodontal diseases: *Aggregatibacter actinomycetemcomitans* (Aa), *Porphyromonas gingivalis* (Pg), and *Tannerella forsythia* (Tf) (World Workshop Consensus Report 1996).
- The presence of calculus and local anatomic (e.g., furcations, root concavities, cervical enamel projections) or clinical features (e.g., restoration overhangs, crowding) may contribute to disease risk due to their potential to accumulate/harbour plaque, as well as making plaque removal (patient/professional) more difficult to achieve.

13.4.2 Tobacco Smoking

- A modifiable risk factor strongly associated with periodontal disease and impaired response to therapy.
- Cross-sectional studies indicate smokers have a minimum threefold risk of developing periodontal destruction as measured by attachment loss and bone loss (Grossi et al. 1994; 1995). A dose-related gradient is apparent with the relative risk of disease being further increased among heavier smokers.
- Smoking cessation is associated with improved clinical response to therapy (Grossi et al. 1997).
- Smokers show impaired response to nonsurgical and surgical therapy (Ah et al. 1994), regenerative procedures (Tonetti et al. 1995), and implant procedures (Strietzel et al. 2007).
- Cigarette smokers may still be candidates for periodontal surgery, but the magnitude of beneficial effect is compromised in these patients relative to nonsmokers (Kotsakis et al. 2015).

13.4.2.1 Potential Mechanisms to Mediate Effect on Periodontium

- Effect on microflora
  - Evidence is conflicting – many studies fail to show differences in the amount or composition of plaque. However, increased prevalence of pathogenic species/higher proportion of subjects positive for pathogenic species has been demonstrated in smokers (Zambon et al. 1996).
- Effects on host response:
  - Impaired neutrophil function (reduced chemotaxis/phagocytosis)
  - Altered lymphocyte function

- Effects of nicotine:
  - Altered fibroblast attachment
  - Impact on vascularity of tissues and production of inflammatory mediators

13.4.3 Diabetes

- Strongly associated with periodontal disease.
- Cross-sectional studies indicate that diabetics have approximately a threefold risk of developing periodontal destruction, as measured by bone loss (Emrich et al. 1991).
- Poor glycaemic control has been associated with increased risk of progressive disease, whereas well-controlled diabetics may not have increased risk (Taylor et al. 1998).
- Bidirectional relationship – evidence exists for an association between severe periodontitis and complications of type 2 diabetes (Chapple et al. 2013).
- Advise diabetic patients (i) that risk of periodontal disease is increased by diabetes and (ii) that glycaemic control may be impaired if they have periodontal disease.
- Preventive care and periodontal maintenance strategy should be particularly emphasized.

13.4.3.1 Potential Mechanisms to Mediate Effect on Periodontium (Mealey and Oates 2006)

- Effect on host response
  - Impaired neutrophil function (reduced adherence, chemotaxis/phagocytosis)
  - Hyper-responsiveness of macrophages/monocytes – triggers increase in pro-inflammatory cytokines
- Delayed wound healing (via altered metabolism of connective tissues)
  - Hyperglycaemia affects osteoblasts and fibroblasts – bone formation and collagen turnover affected.
  - Formation of AGEs promotes inflammation and further affects collagen turnover.
  - Interaction of AGEs with specific receptors (AGE-RAGe interactions) on various cells contributes to hyper-inflammatory response.
- Effect on microflora
  - Based on current knowledge, there is insufficient evidence that diabetes significantly modifies the oral microflora (Chapple et al. 2013).
- Hyperglycaemia contributes to an imbalance of free radicals resulting in oxidative stress mediated tissue damage.

13.5 Nonsurgical Periodontal Therapy

13.5.1 Goals

- Remove microbial deposits from tooth surfaces
- Eliminate plaque-retentive irregularities
- Create intra-oral environment that helps in maintenance of gingival tissue health
- Increase effectiveness of patient's self-administered plaque control

13.5.2 Components

- Nonsurgical instrumentation – hand instruments + powered instruments
- Preventive advice – oral hygiene instruction (OHI), tobacco cessation, dietary advice (See Appendix for oral hygiene aids and smoking cessation)
- Address local aetiologic factors – removal of overhangs, replace defective restorations, etc.
- Address other aetiologic factors – systemic disease, habits, etc.

13.5.3 Basic Principles

OH alone is not enough: Some, but limited improvement of gingival conditions may occur in periodontal pockets following improved supragingival plaque control alone (Cercek et al. 1983).

Instrumentation alone is not enough: Instrumentation alone, without improved OH, may result in microbial repopulation of instrumented sites within a short period after therapy (Magnusson et al. 1984).

13.5.4 Expectation Setting for Your Patient

- Explain that periodontal disease is common among the US population and represents a chronic disease. As periodontal disease is frequently asymptomatic, so the dentist has a key role in monitoring progress of disease.
- Address the aetiology of periodontal disease and highlight that only some factors are modifiable – hence, the emphasis on the importance of plaque control and tobacco cessation.
- Advise your patient from the outset if further treatment is likely to be necessary.
- Outline the importance of periodontal maintenance and compliance to longer-term periodontal health.

13.5.4.1 Calculus Detection

- Periodontal explorer
  - Primary instrument for calculus detection.
  - Properties include fine tip and curvature of shank and tip to allow universal use.
  - Used with light grasp, light touch.
  - Example: ODU 11/12.
- Periodontal probe
  - The markings on some manual periodontal probes are inset/grooved, increasing tactile sensation and allowing their use in calculus detection. Example: UNC-12 probe.
- Radiographs
  - Calculus may be detected on radiographic films as a relative opacity on the crown/root surface of a tooth. This may be more easily distinguishable on

  intra-oral radiographic images and may be noted particularly in the root area approximating the CEJ.
  - Not all calculus deposits will be radiographically visible.
- Visual detection
  - Supragingival calculus and some superficial subgingival deposits may be detected by direct vision. This facilitated by drying the teeth, using good lighting and with gentle air deflection of inflamed gingival tissues. In non-pigmented tissues, heavy focal calculus deposits may sometimes be associated with "shadowing" through the gingival tissues and/or localized sites of focal inflammation.

13.5.5 How Do I Know If What I'm Feeling Is Calculus?

- Calculus detection is difficult. Microscopic deposits of calculus may remain undetected in many instances following nonsurgical/surgical therapy, particularly in posterior teeth, interproximal and furcation regions.
- Calculus is most frequently (but not exclusively) detected in the areas at/immediately apical to the CEJ and slightly coronal to the base of the periodontal pocket.

Use light grasp to improve tactile sensation.

- Establish where your explorer position is apico-coronally – can you exclude certain anatomic/tooth-related factors (e.g., CEJ, restoration margins)?
- Explore in several planes (vertical, horizontal, oblique) to distinguish the size and nature of a questionable roughness/deposit (Fig. 13.3).
  - Calculus deposit may take the tactile form of a lump, bump, ledge, ring, or spine; these may be detected as a relative prominence on the root which may be detected in multiple planes. This may assist differentiation from the CEJ.
- Do your radiographs indicate the presence of calculus in the region?

13.5.6 What Else Could It Be?

- CEJ
- Tight contact catching instrument
- Restoration margin
- Tooth anatomy – e.g., root concavity/enamel pearl
- Root roughness

13.5.6.1 Effectiveness of Calculus Removal (Table 13.5)

13.5.6.2 Nonsurgical Therapy: Expected Results

Initial periodontal therapy (instrumentation and effective OH) may be associated with:

- Decreases in BOP/plaque score/probing depths

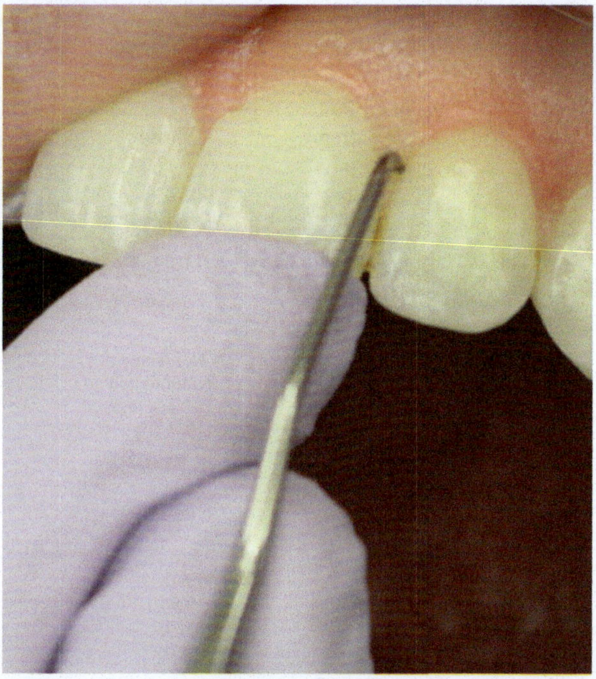

Fig. 13.3 A light grasp of your instrument and a finger rest on the same arch help detection and removal of calculus (Photo courtesy of Mrs. Lorie Primosch)

Table 13.5 Factors influencing effectiveness of calculus removal

Influencing factor	Calculus more likely to be left behind
Tooth type	Molars, especially furcation areas
Tooth surface	Proximal surfaces
Pocket/site features	Deep sites
Operator experience	Inexperienced operators
Instrument type	Hand vs. ultrasonic – similar effectiveness

- Increase in periodontal attachment levels (Badersten et al. 1984)
- Significant improvements in the clinical and microbiologic parameters of periodontal diseases (Haffajee et al. 1997) (Table 13.6) (Fig. 13.4)

13.5.6.3 Nonsurgical Instrumentation

13.6 Hand Instrumentation (Table 13.7)

13.6.1 Working with Gracey Curettes (Table 13.8)

- Modified pen grasp.
- Stable fulcrum – ideally close to tooth being instrumented.

Table 13.6 Mean changes, generally observed in studies in probing depth, probing attachment levels, and gingival recession following a single episode of supra- and sub-gingival instrumentation. (Claffey et al. 2004)

Initial probing depth (mm)	Probing depth (mm)	Probing attachment level (mm)	Gingival recession (mm)
≤3.5	0	−0.5	0.5
4–6.5	1–2	0–1	0–1
≥7	2–3	1–2	1–2

Note: This table is re-used with permission from the publishers (Wiley-Blackwell)

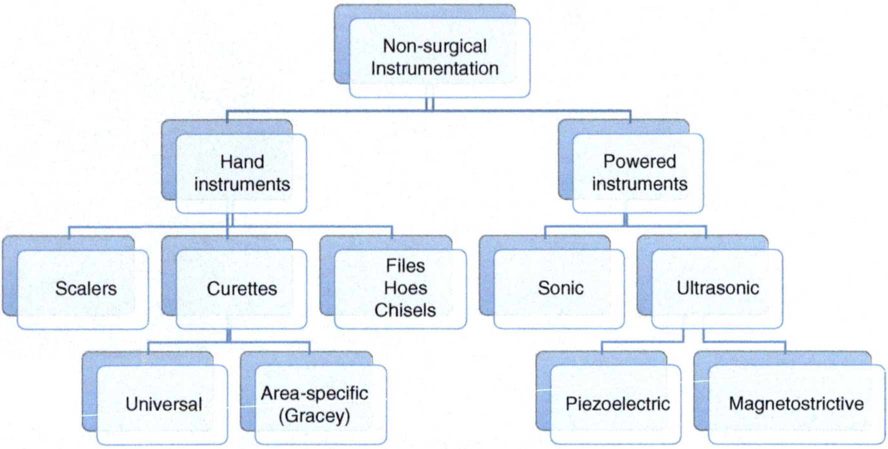

Fig. 13.4 Nonsurgical periodontal therapy – available armamentarium

Table 13.7 Description of hand instrument subclasses

Sickle scaler	Gracey curette	Universal curette
Supragingival instrumentation	Subgingival	Subgingival
Not area-specific	Area-specific	Not area-specific
2 cutting edges	1 cutting edge	2 cutting edges
Pointed toe – may traumatize tissue/tooth if used subgingival	Round toe – decreases risk of tissue laceration/risk of gouging root surface	Round toe
Face at 90° to terminal shank	Face at 70° to terminal shank – offset blade Lower edge = "cutting" edge	Face at 90° to terminal shank

- Correct angulation: when lower shank is parallel to tooth surface being instrumented (Fig. 13.5).
- Apply gentle lateral pressure during instrument strokes to engage calculus deposits.
- Vertical and oblique strokes move in coronal direction – only tip one-third of instrument (i.e., 1–3 mm) is adapted to be in contact with tooth surface.
- Horizontal strokes may be used on buccal/lingual surfaces – these strokes allow more contact between instrument tip and root surface.

Table 13.8 Sample instrumentation kit for provision of nonsurgical therapy in practice

Purpose	Instrument type (and example)	Use	Notes
Diagnostic	*Periodontal probe* UNC-15	Examination/measurement Calculus detection	Inserted parallel to the long axis of the tooth, angled slightly at interproximal Used with "walking stroke"
	Periodontal explorer ODU 11/12	Primary calculus detection instrument	Light touch, light grasp, explore in all directions
	Nabers probe	Furcation assessment	
Ultrasonic instrumentation	*Piezoelectric or Magnetostrictive*	Supra- and subgingival calculus removal	Utilize standard tips for gross supragingival calculus removal Slimline tips for removal of light and subgingival deposits
Hand instrumentation	*Sickle scaler* H5-33	Supragingival calculus removal Especially helpful with lower anteriors	Stay supragingival because this instrument has two cutting edges
	Universal curettes Barnhart 1–2 Barnhart 5–6	Rigid shank for heavy calculus removal	Two cutting edges Used at proximal and flat surface sites
	Gracey curettes 1/2 5/6 9/10 11/12 13/14	1/2: Anteriors 5/6: Premolars 9/10: Buccal and lingual surfaces of posterior teeth 11/12: Mesial surfaces posterior teeth 13/14: Distal surfaces posterior teeth	Single cutting edge Area-specific design Longer shank for deeper pockets Flexible shank for root planing

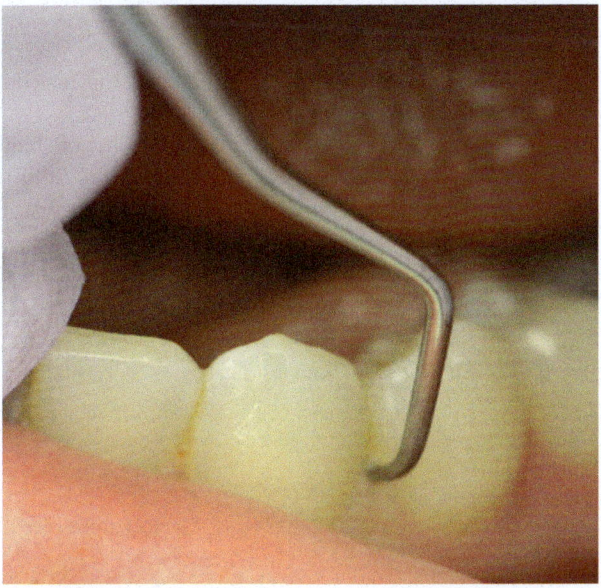

Fig. 13.5 The lower shank should be parallel to the long axis of the tooth that is being scaled (Photo courtesy of Mrs. Lorie Primosch)

13.6.2 Hand Instrument Adaptations

Instrumentation is a repetitive task with the risk of operator fatigue/musculoskeletal injury. Select your instruments carefully – various instrument design features are available to improve ergonomics and enhance the effectiveness of your instrumentation. These include:

- Handles
  - Lightweight handles reduce strain and increase tactile sensitivity.
  - Textured (knurled) handles improve grasp/control and reduce finger fatigue.
- Shank
  - Rigid shanks can increase strength of instrumentation and are helpful for heavy/tenacious deposits.
  - Conversely, flexible shanks enhance tactile sensation and may be more suitable for root debridement.
  - Increased shank lengths allow for access to deep pockets.
- Instrument tip
  - Thinner, shorter blades allow for easier insertion and improved access, particularly in deep pockets (≥5 mm).
  - Tip-coating technology is claimed to maintain instrument sharpness for longer, reducing the need for sharpening.

13.6.3 Guidelines for Sharpening of Hand Instruments

- Inspect hand instruments after each use.
- Sharpen at first sign of dullness.
- Thin/shortened instruments have reduced efficiency and increased risk of fracture – if in doubt, discard.
- Ceramic stones generally used. Lubricate with water (apply damp gauze).
- Keep stone in contact with instrument, always finish on downstroke to remove metal shavings.
- Focus on the terminal (lower) shank of the instrument as your reference point when sharpening (Table 13.9).
  - Establish a "time difference" between lower shank of instrument and sharpening stone (e.g., for a 1-h time difference, hold the instrument with the long axis of its lower shank at a 12 o'clock position while the stone is positioned at the 1 o'clock position) (Fig. 13.6).
- Remember, curettes have a *rounded toe* – this shape must be preserved to avoid modifying the instrument's effectiveness (Fig. 13.7).

Table 13.9 Sharpening of hand instruments

Instrument type	Number of cutting edges	"Time difference" between lower shank and stone	True angle stone-terminal shank desired
Sickle scaler universal curette	2	1 h clock difference	20–30°
Gracey curette	1	2 h clock difference	40–60°

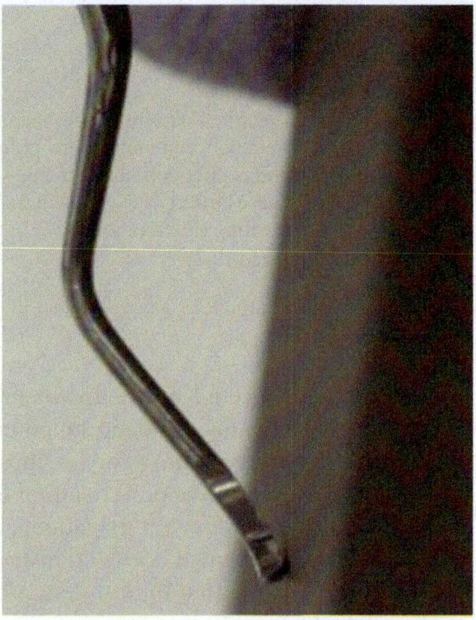

Fig. 13.6 Mastering the sharpening of instruments will prevent premature loss of the cutting edge of a Gracey curette (Photo courtesy of Mrs. Lorie Primosch).

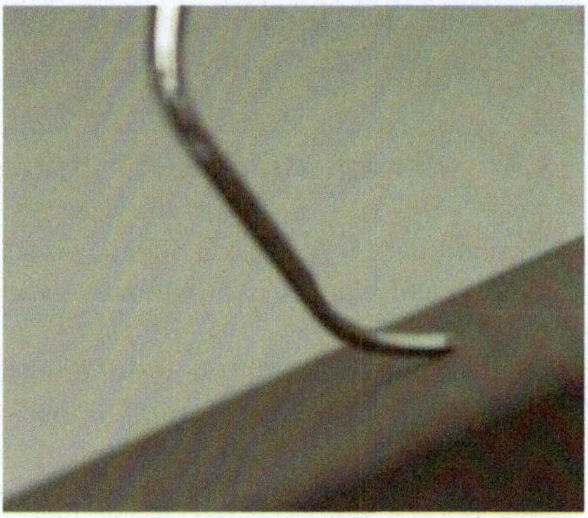

Fig. 13.7 Sharpening around the rounded toe of a Gracey curette (Photo courtesy of Mrs. Lorie Primosch)

13.7 Ultrasonic Instrumentation (Table 13.10)

- An ultrasonic handpiece is effective to remove the majority of plaque and larger pieces of calculus.
- Use is contraindicated in patients with communicable disease, susceptibility to infection, respiratory risks, swallowing difficulty, or a cardiac pacemaker.
- Generally operate at frequency of 18,000–45,000 Hz.

Table 13.10 Ultrasonic instrument types

	Magnetostrictive	Piezoelectric
Tip movement	Elliptical	Linear
Movement generated from:	Electrical current creates magnetic field between metal strips of insert and copper coil in handpiece – causes insert to expand/contract creating tip vibration	Electrical current causes expansion/contraction of ceramic discs in instrument handle creating tip vibration
Example	*Cavitron®*	*Piezon®*

13.7.1 Use

- *Appropriate tip* (e.g., broad tip for heavy calculus deposits; Slimline tips for plaque/light calculus and deep subgingival access).
- *Appropriate power setting* for tip chosen (e.g., low power setting for Slimline tips, minimum *effective* power setting for broader tips).
- *Appropriate water flow* for irrigation, cooling, cavitation effect – generally satisfactory once a fine mist occurs at instrument tip.
- Light grasp, stable (but light) fulcrum/finger rest.
- Angulation of 0–15°.
- Keep tip moving at all times.
- Use overlapping strokes in every direction to cover entirety of root surface.
- All sides of the tip are effective in instrumentation but do not place instrument tip with point against tooth surface.

13.8 Re-evaluation: Key Decisions (Segelnick and Weinberg 2006)

A periodontal re-evaluation should be scheduled for patients with a periodontitis diagnosis and plan for scaling and root planing therapy as part of the initial treatment plan.

Periodontal re-evaluation is not required when a patient is diagnosed with gingivitis, although follow-up may be performed in certain cases at the clinician's discretion. When the periodontal diagnosis is gingivitis, once the initial therapy is completed, the patient should be placed on individualized maintenance therapy.

The re-evaluation appointment typically occurs approximately 6 weeks after the completion of SRP and following elimination of all local contributory factors. While this is not the endpoint of the healing process, this timescale is chosen to allow for initial tissue healing but occurs prior to the time at which the negative consequences of ineffective plaque control might be expected to impact notably on clinical outcome.

This visit should include:

- A complete evaluation of the periodontal status – all clinical measurements recorded
- Certification that urgent dental care and removal of local risk factors have been addressed
- Assessment of patient compliance with preventive care (e.g., OH)/removal of modifiable aetiologic factors such as smoking

- Assessment of outcome of initial therapy (comparison of clinical measurements with pretreatment findings)
- Decision-making for future care

13.8.1 Questions to Ask at Re-evaluation

- Is the patient compliant with OH?
- Has my initial phase treatment been effective?
- Does the patient require further periodontal treatment? If so:
  - Should that be nonsurgical or surgical in nature?
  - Should I do it or should I refer?

13.8.2 Decision-Making at Re-evaluation

- Statement of success of initial therapy: A concise written description of the relative success and areas not responding to initial periodontal care.
- Future periodontal treatment needs: Additional initial periodontal therapy or periodontal surgical needs should be specifically addressed and noted clearly in the written description.
- Relation of periodontal therapy to overall patient treatment plan: The stability of the periodontal situation with regard to proposed restorative treatment should be documented.
- Periodontal maintenance interval: Plans for periodontal maintenance interval and date should be noted. The patient should have a definite maintenance care appointment date scheduled prior to leaving the clinic.
- Establishment of tooth/patient prognosis: The response to initial periodontal therapy, patient compliance, and addressing of local and systemic factors should be utilized to assign a prognosis for maintenance of the dentition.

13.9 Periodontal Maintenance

Periodontal maintenance attempts to prevent recurrence of disease, monitors borderline patients with conditions that must be observed and further evaluated, and tries to slow the progression of disease in patients who cannot or will not consent to corrective periodontal surgery.

Purpose Reassess the patient's overall dental condition, plan future treatment needs, and provide necessary therapy.

The examination involves a comprehensive periodontal assessment. Periodontal parameters must be evaluated and *charted in full at least once per calendar year*, including:

- Probing depths (probe entire mouth): Record depths >4 mm, sites showing BOP, and changes in probing depth from the previous SPT (if sites measured >4 mm previously).

- Location of the gingival margin: Record any changes in gingival margin position and the gingival margin position at all sites with pocket depths >4 mm.
- Assessment of bleeding (BOP)/plaque/furcation/mobility/occlusal stability/calculus deposits/radiographs (as indicated).

13.9.1 Components of Periodontal Maintenance Visit

- Preventive advice (oral hygiene instructions, smoking cessation, etc.) should be addressed/demonstrated/with the possibility for demonstration of capacity for OH by the patient.
- Nonsurgical therapy should be rendered as appropriate.
- A statement of periodontal stability should be recorded and periodontal status/treatment needs should be incorporated into the overall treatment plan.
- Documentation should include recommendations (oral hygiene products/regimens; suggestions for future therapy) and referrals to medical practitioner/dental specialty care, etc.

A 30-year follow-up of patients in a private dental office indicated that a preventive programme involving oral hygiene control and instrumentation could maintain the periodontal health of patients with chronic periodontal disease and was associated with low incidence of periodontal disease and tooth mortality (Axellson et al. 2004).

13.10 Surgical Periodontal Treatment Considerations

Indications for periodontal surgery may include:

- To gain access to address inaccessible/residual calculus deposits
- Pockets ≥6 mm
- Pockets unresponsive to well-administered initial therapy despite compliance/good OH
- Progressive disease (loss of attachment/radiographic evidence of continued bone loss)
- Deep vertical infrabony lesions
- Crown lengthening/aesthetic surgery
- Mucogingival deficiencies/abnormalities (including frenal pull)

13.11 Periodontal Emergencies

13.11.1 Periodontal-Endodontic Lesions

Periodontal-endodontic (perio-endo) lesions may create a dilemma for the dental practitioner.

Various classifications of these lesions have been proposed to reflect the concepts that:

- An endodontic lesion may cause a retrograde periodontitis.
- A periodontal lesion may provoke a pulpal response leading to pathosis/necrosis.
- Lesions may develop independently in the pulp and periodontal tissues.

Establishing the primary cause of a perio-endo lesion may consequently be difficult. The Armitage classification describes only one type of lesion, the "combined periodontal-endodontic lesion" irrespective of cause. See Chap. 12 Endodontics for the diagnosis of a perio-endo lesion.

13.11.1.1 Clinical Findings

- Increased pocket depth at affected tooth.
- Inflamed/necrotic pulp – response to pulpal sensitivity testing may vary/be inconsistent.
- Suppuration/sinus tract may be present.
- Radiographic appearance of "J-shaped lesion" – radiolucency extending at proximal aspect of tooth and extending around apex of root.

13.11.1.2 Treatment

Treatment may vary based on the extent of the lesion, access to the affected tooth/site, and level of residual periodontal support in "unaffected areas" of the tooth.

A systematic review of treatment of periodontal lesions (Schmidt et al. 2014) noted that few well-documented studies exist with notable heterogeneity of treatment protocols. Nevertheless, findings indicated that a reasonable approach might include:

- Nonsurgical endodontic therapy as first treatment step
- Adequate time for tissue healing prior to re-evaluation (most reported studies used a 6–12 month period)

Nonsurgical/surgical periodontal therapy may be indicated as a second step in individual cases.

13.11.2 Gingival Enlargement

13.11.2.1 Clinical Findings

- Lesions typically start as painless enlargement of the interdental papilla area that gradually extend to involve the buccal and lingual marginal gingiva; these areas may coalesce and the enlargement may eventually cover much of the crown.
- Gingival tissue is generally of normal colour, firm, and resilient; it may be lobulated and doesn't tend to bleed. However, as enlargement complicates maintenance of oral hygiene, gingival inflammation may often occur.

- Lesions can occur throughout the mouth but are normally more common in anterior regions.

13.11.2.2 Predisposing Factors

Gingival enlargement occurs as a side effect of using certain medications. Clinical and microscopic features of the hypertrophy induced by the different drugs can be similar. The gingival enlargement may cause aesthetic issues but also practical issues (e.g., may affect speech, occlusion, and mastication, affect tooth eruption, etc.)

13.11.2.3 Associated Drugs

- Anticonvulsants – used to control epileptic seizures, e.g., phenytoin, valproic acid.
- Calcium-channel blockers – used to treat angina and hypertension, e.g., nifedipine, diltiazem, and verapamil.

  Immunosuppressants, e.g., cyclosporine.

13.11.2.4 Treatment

Treatment should be based on the medication being used and the clinical features.

1. Consider discontinuing (usually not possible) or changing the drug – discussion with the physician is necessary.

   If the drug is changed, wait 6–12 months for possible resolution before deciding to proceed with surgery.
2. OHI/preventive care for improved plaque control.
3. Professional debridement to remove any inflammatory stimulus (as needed).
4. For patients in whom enlargement persists, surgical resection may be needed. Classically described using external bevel gingivectomy but frequently location/access and/or considerations regarding the amount of keratinized tissue present may indicate the use of conventional internal bevel incisions and gingivoplasty. In large cases, a flap technique might be considered.

Lesions commonly recur within a short period. Lesions may disappear spontaneously within a few months of stopping the relevant drug, if this is possible.

13.11.3 Necrotizing Ulcerative Gingivitis (NUG)

13.11.3.1 Clinical Findings

NUG may occasionally present in general dental practice as a periodontal "emergency."

An acute infection characterized by necrosis of gingival tissue with the following key clinical features:

- Pain
- Interdental papilla – ulceration/"punched-out" appearance
- Gingival bleeding

The papilla may be covered by a yellow/white/grey slough often referred to as "pseudomembrane."

Bad breath may occur and systemic features (fever, malaise, and lymphadenopathy) are sometimes seen.

Microbiology of affected lesions: dominated by anaerobic bacteria often referred to as the "fusospirochetal complex."

Prevalence Limited data available. Generally estimated at <1 % of the US children with increased prevalence in developing countries (Califano 2003).

Predisposing Factors Include (Khammissa et al. 2014):
- Young age (<25 years)
- Smoking and alcohol use
- Poor diet/malnutrition
- Poor OH
- History of previous NUG
- Stress/illness

13.11.3.2 Treatment (Table 13.11)

13.11.4 Periodontal Abscess

- A periodontal abscess is a localized purulent inflammation in the periodontal tissues adjacent to the periodontal pocket and may lead to destruction of PDL and alveolar bone (Lang et al. 1999).

Table 13.11 Treatment approach for NUG

Control acute phase
Eliminate acute signs
Irrigation (as tolerable for patient) and OHI
Chlorhexidine mouth rinse
± Analgesia
± Systemic antimicrobials (if systemic features present; e.g., metronidazole 250 mg t.i.d.)
Educate
Prevention/Plaque control
Eliminate predisposing factors
Local factors for plaque accumulation
Systemic predisposing factors
Follow-up care
Once patient comfort established, perform further nonsurgical instrumentation (as needed)
Reinforce preventive care/modification of aetiologic factors
Corrective treatment of disease sequela, e.g., gingivoplasty to remove any interproximal craters
Periodontal maintenance

- Periodontal abscess may be acute or chronic in nature and represent a relatively common cause of tooth loss among periodontal patients. Acute periodontal abscesses may be a regularly frequent periodontal "emergency" in general dental practice (Table 13.12).

13.11.4.1 Clinical Findings (Herrera et al. 2014)

- Ovoid swelling in gingiva over lateral aspect of root – usually located apical to mucogingival junction
- Suppuration on gentle pressure/probing – via fistula/through periodontal pocket
- Deeper pocket at site, frequently with BOP
- Pain/gingival tenderness
- Tender to palpation
- Swelling and redness at site
- Tooth mobility/elevation
- ± Radiographic bone loss

Microbiology Usually a polymicrobial infection, not noticeably different to chronic periodontitis lesions. Anaerobic commensal bacteria dominate, in particular *P. gingivalis*.

13.11.4.2 Predisposing Factors

- Untreated periodontal patients – exacerbation of a chronic periodontal lesion
- Following nonsurgical or periodontal maintenance therapy – where instrumentation debris or residual calculus remains deep in tissue/pocket and becomes "trapped" due to healing of more coronal tissues.
- Following surgical therapy – due to residual calculus or infection at foreign material (e.g., membrane)
- Following systemic antibiotic therapy (without subgingival debridement) in a patient with periodontitis

Table 13.12 Differential diagnosis for periodontal abscess (Herrera et al. 2014)

Condition	Possible differences
Gingival abscess	Location (more superficial)
	May have good periodontal health
	Usually associated with foreign objects impacted subgingivally
Pericoronal abscess	Partially erupted tooth involved
	Adjacent teeth vital, no increased probing depths
Root fracture	Fracture may be visible clinically/x-ray
Endodontic perforation/post perforation	Visible on radiograph with multiple exposures
Periapical abscess	Tooth non-vital/questionable vitality
	Probing depth may be "normal"
	Radiographic features (apical radiolucency)

- At previously healthy sites due to impaction of foreign objects (e.g., dental floss, nail-biting) or alteration of the root surface (e.g., cracked tooth, perforation by endodontic instrument)

A. *Acute periodontal abscess*
   - Acute infection from biofilm in a deepened pocket
   - Represents a period of active periodontal destruction (exacerbation)
   - Usually due to marginal closure of a deep pocket and lack of proper drainage, causing extension of infection into tissues

B. *Chronic periodontal abscess*
   - Usually asymptomatic and may be associated with a sinus tract or drainage through an adjacent periodontal pocket. May occasionally "flare-up" to become an acute abscess.
   - See Chap. 12 Endodontics

13.11.4.3 **Treatment Options** (Fig. 13.8)

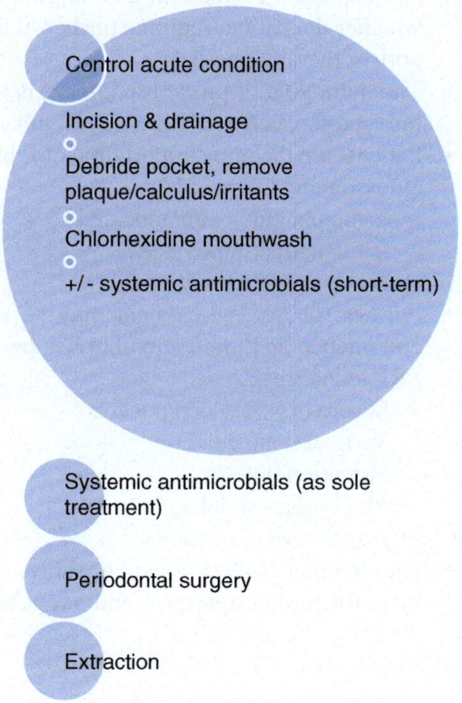

Fig. 13.8 Sequela of treatment options for periodontal abscess

13.12 Periodontal Dilemmas

13.12.1 Gingivitis or Periodontitis?

- Primary difference: Gingivitis is not associated with bone loss.
- A patient with gingivitis will have inflamed gums due to poor plaque control and poor oral hygiene habits.
- *Gingivitis* is reversible once the local factors (such as plaque) are removed and maintained. 90 % of gingivitis is due to poor plaque control; however, other factors such as hormones, medications, and viruses may also play a role.
- *Periodontitis*, on the other hand, is associated with varying degrees of bone loss. There is usually also a history of poor plaque control and poor oral hygiene, and the gingiva will likely also be red and inflamed.
- Quality bitewing radiographs are an essential component to differentiating between gingivitis and periodontitis, as well as thorough clinical examination.
- Treatment for gingivitis involves removal of local factors via a prophy.
- Treatment for periodontitis can be non-surgical or surgical, as discussed in this chapter.

13.12.2 Treat or Maintain?

- At the phase I evaluation, it is important to look at the big picture and determine whether the patient requires further treatment, or can go into a maintenance/supportive therapy phase.
- The main goal of phase I treatment is to control inflammation and its contributing factors, such as plaque, stress, tobacco use, uncontrolled diabetes, etc.
- Patients are the most important factor in determining success of initial treatment: (Jönsson and Öhrn 2014).
  - Is the patient aware/educated?
  - Is the patient motivated?
  - Is the patient *compliant*?
- Further (phase 2) treatment may be recommended if patient shows adequate compliance and motivation but has periodontal issues that are more severe than SRP alone treat.
  - Severe disease/deep pockets
  - Vertical bone defects
  - Furcation defects
  - Mucogingival defects
  - Aggressive perio cases
- On the other hand, if a patient shows poor compliance and motivation, sending them for further treatment will not generate different results.

13.12.3 Antibiotics or Not?

- Systemic antibiotics may be considered in the following instances (Gilliam and Turner 2014):
  - Aggressive periodontitis
  - Refractory or recurrent cases
  - Immunocompromised patients
  - Acute forms of disease (NUG/NUP)
- Antibiotics should be used in conjunction with SRP therapy and not as a stand-alone treatment.

13.13 Appendix: Oral Hygiene and Smoking Cessation

13.13.1 Oral Hygiene and Prevention

The most critical part in treatment is educating our patients to control progression of their disease. Refer to Chap. 3 "Caries Prevention for Caries" risk assessment in conjunction with oral hygiene instructions given to patients. Some of the common oral hygiene aids are listed below. Oral hygiene instructions should be customized for every patient in order to address their specific needs.

Oral hygiene aids	Common uses
Dental floss threaders	Helpful when flossing under a bridge and under orthodontic wires while the patient is in braces
Flossers	Floss is already threaded and may be easier to use with patients who lack dexterity
Superfloss	Same uses as a floss threader but conveniently contains a threader and floss as one unit
Soft picks	Can be inserted between teeth and in difficult to reach recesses of the teeth and gums to clean away plaque and food debris
Stim-U-Dent	Balsa wood picks to remove plaque and to gently massage gingival tissues
End-tufted brush	Cleans surfaces not accessible by a toothbrush of floss
Interdental/Proxabrushes	May be used in large embrasure spaces, root furcation areas, orthodontic appliances, and bridges. Interchangeable brushes come in a variety of sizes
Gauze	In large edentulous areas bordered by teeth, gauze can be rolled and used to clean the proximal surfaces of teeth that border these edentulous spaces
Oral irrigator	Oral irrigation unit for flushing debris from the oral cavity and delivering antimicrobial rinses to specific tissues within the mouth. This is not a substitute for flossing

13.13.2 Smoking Cessation: The 5 As

There are many resources to assist patients in smoking cessation. For patients and healthcare workers, the Unites States Department of Health and Human Services has a comprehensive website on this topic: http:///www.ahrq.gov/professionals/clinicians-providers/guidelines-recommendations/tobacco/index.html.

13.13.2.1 Ask

- Ask *all* patients about smoking status and tobacco use and record in the chart. For current smokers, this should be done at every visit.
- Questions: "What do you smoke?" "How many per day?" "How long have you been a smoker?" "How long after waking do you take your first cigarette?" "Have you ever tried to quit?"

13.13.2.2 Advice

- Advise all smokers to quit.
- Using simple language, explain the oral health effects of tobacco and benefits of quitting.
- For those not ready to quit: advice that you would like to help when patient is willing.
- Provide motivational literature.

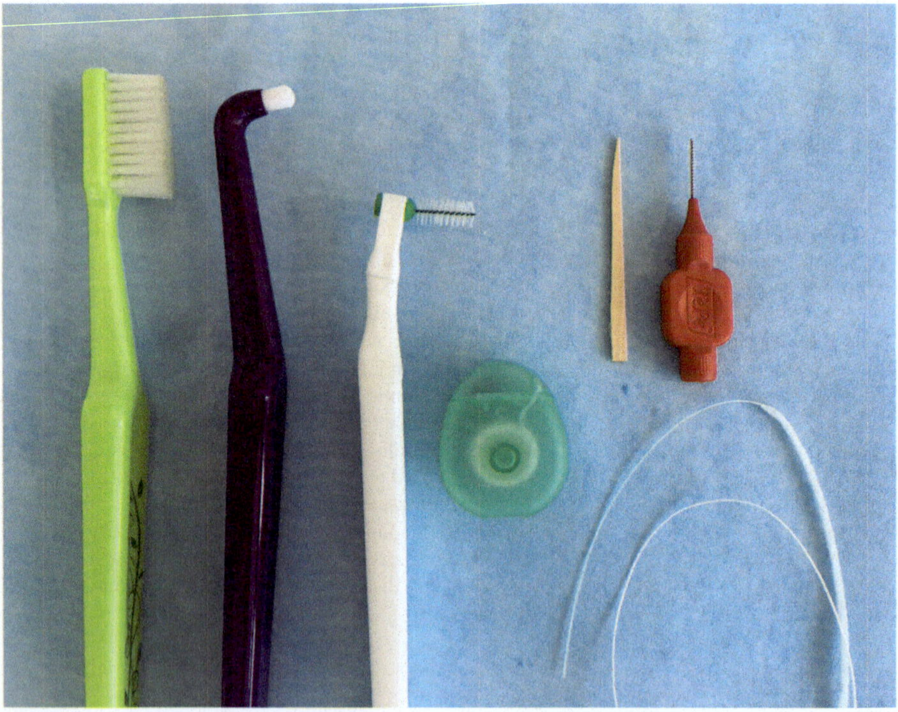

Fig. 13.9 A Selection of hygiene aids used to provide individualized oral hygiene instruction to patients

13.13.2.3 Assess

- Assess readiness to quit. Ask the patient simply if they want to quit and record the reply.
- If not, help motivate the patient to quit:
  - Identify patient's reasons to quit (health, costs, children, etc.). Help build confidence to quit. Make note to ask again at the next visit.
- If yes, provide resources and assist!

13.13.2.4 Assist

- Reinforce the reasons to quit (patient motivations) and benefits.
- Discuss any past attempts and why patient feels they may have failed.
- Help patient to set a quit date (soon – ideally within 2 weeks). Write this down.
- Recommend patient to utilize a support structure (family/friends/colleagues) and avoid factors that stimulate tobacco use from their environment.
- Provide resources (self-help and information regarding nicotine-replacement therapy).

13.13.2.5 Arrange

- Review progress at follow-up visits.
- If relapse, review reasons for failure and plan for next quit attempt.
- Refer for help from quit line/smoking cessation programme.

References

Ah MK, Johnson GK, Kaldahl WB. The effect of smoking on the response to periodontal therapy. J Clin Periodontol. 1994;21:91–7.

American Academy of Periodontology Task Force Report on the update to the 1999 classification of periodontal diseases and conditions. J Periodontol 2015;86(7):835–8.

American Academy of Periodontology (AAP). Comprehensive periodontal therapy: a statement of the American Academy of Periodontology. J Periodontol. 2011;82(7):943–9.

Armitage GC. Development of a classification system for periodontal diseases and conditions. Ann Periodontol. 1999;4:1–6.

Axellson P, Nyström B, Lindhe J. The long-term effect of a plaque control program on tooth mortality, caries and periodontal disease in adults. Results after 30 years of maintenance. J Clin Periodontol. 2004;31:749–57.

Badersten A, Nilveus R, Egelberg J. Effect of nonsurgical periodontal therapy. II. Severely advanced periodontitis. J Clin Periodontol. 1984;11(1):63–76.

Califano JV. Research, Science and Therapy Committee American Academy of Periodontology. Position paper: periodontal diseases of children and adolescents. J Periodontol. 2003;74:1696–704.

Cercek JF, Kiger RD, Garrett S, Egelberg J. Relative effects of plaque control and instrumentation on the clinical parameters of human periodontal disease. J Clin Periodontol. 1983;10(1):46–56.

Chapple IL, Genco R, Working group 2 of joint EFP/AAP workshop. Diabetes and periodontal diseases: consensus report of the joint EFP/AAP workshop on periodontitis and systemic diseases. J Periodontol. 2013;84(4 Suppl):S106–12.

Claffey N, Polyzois I, Ziaka P. An overview of nonsurgical and surgical therapy. Periodontol 2000. 2004;36:35–44.

Consensus report. Periodontal diseases: pathogenesis and microbial factors. Ann Periodontol 1996;1(1): 926–32.
Eke PI, Dye BA, Wei L, et al. Update on prevalence of periodontitis in adults in the United States: NHANEs 2009 to 2012. J Periodontol. 2015;86:611–22.
Emrich LJ, Shlossman S, Genco RJ. Periodontal disease in non-insulin-dependent diabetes mellitus. J Periodontol. 1991;62:123–30.
Fonseca D, Cortelli J, et al. Clinical and microbiologic evaluation of scaling and root planing per quadrant and one-stage full-mouth disinfection associated with Azithromycin or Chlorhexidine: a clinical randomized controlled trial. J Periodontol. 2015;86(12):1340–51.
Gilliam D, Turner W. Antibiotics in the treatment of periodontal disease: a guide for the general dental practitioner. Prim Dent J. 2014;3(3):43–7.
Grossi SG, Zambon JJ, Ho AW, et al. Assessment of risk for periodontal disease. II. Risk indicators for attachment loss. J Periodontol. 1994;65:260–7.
Grossi SG, Genco RJ, Machtei EE, et al. Assessment of risk for periodontal disease. II. Risk indicators for alveolar bone loss. J Periodontol. 1995;66:23–9.
Grossi SG, Zambon J, Machtei EE, et al. Effects of smoking and smoking cessation on healing after mechanical periodontal therapy. J Am Dent Assoc. 1997;128:599–607.
Haffajee AD, Cugini MA, Dibart S, et al. The effect of SRP on the clinical and microbiological parameters of periodontal diseases. J Clin Periodontol. 1997;24(5):324–34.
Herrera D, Alonso B, De Arriba L, et al. Acute periodontal lesions. Periodontol 2000. 2014;65:149–77.
Jönsson B, Öhrn K. Evaluation of the effect of nonsurgical periodontal treatment on oral health-related quality of life: estimation of minimal important differences 1 year after treatment. J Clin Periodontol. 2014;41(3):275–82.
Khammissa RA, Ciya R, et al. Oral Medicine Case Book 65: necrotising stomatitis. SADJ. 2014;69(10):468–70.
Kotsakis GA, Javed F, Hinrichs JE. Impact of cigarette smoking on clinical outcomes of periodontal flap surgical procedures: a systematic review and meta-analysis. J Periodontol. 2015;86: 254–63.
Lang NP, Bartold PM, Cullinan M, et al. Consensus report: aggressive periodontitis. Ann Periodontol. 1999;4:53.
Löe H, Brown LJ. Early onset periodontitis in the United States of America. J Periodontol. 1991;62:608–16.
Löe H, Theilade E, Jensen SB. Experimental gingivitis in man. J Periodontol. 1965;36:177–87.
Magnusson I, Lindhe J, Yoneyama T, Liljenberg B. Recolonization of a subgingival microbiota following scaling in deep pockets. J Clin Periodontol. 1984;11(3):193–207.
Mealey BL, Oates TW. Diabetes mellitus and periodontal diseases. J Periodontol. 2006;77: 1289–303.
Miller PD. A classification of marginal tissue recession. Int J Periodontics Restorative Dent. 1985;2:9–13.
Schmidt JC, Walter C, Amato M, Weiger R. Treatment of periodontal-endodontic lesions – a systematic review. J Clin Periodontol. 2014;41:779–90.
Segelnick S, Weinberg M. Reevaluation of initial therapy: when is the appropriate time? J Periodontol. 2006;77(9):1598–601.
Strietzel FP, Reichart PA, Kale A, et al. Smoking interferes with the prognosis of dental implant treatment: a systematic review and meta-analysis. J Clin Periodontol. 2007;34:523–44.
Taylor GW, Burt BA, Becker MP, et al. Non-insulin-dependent diabetes mellitus and alveolar bone loss progression over 2 years. J Periodontol. 1998;69:76–83.
Tonetti MS, Pini-Prato G, Cortellini P. Effect of cigarette smoking on periodontal healing following GTR in infrabony defects. A preliminary retrospective study. J Clin Periodontol. 1995;22:229–34.
Zambon JJ, Grossi SG, Machtei EE, et al. Cigarette smoking increases the risk for subgingival infection with periodontal pathogens. J Periodontol. 1996;67(Suppl):1050–4.

Common Lesions in Oral Pathology for the General Dentist

14

Indraneel Bhattacharyya, Hardeep K. Chehal, and Mohammed N. Islam

Contents

I. Bhattacharyya, DDS, MSD (✉) • M.N. Islam, DDS
Oral Pathology, University of Florida College of Dentistry, Gainesville, FL, USA
e-mail: IBHATTACHARYYA@dental.ufl.edu

H.K. Chehal, DDS
Oral Pathology, Creighton University School of Dentistry, Omaha, NE, USA

G.M. Weinstein, M.T. Zientz (eds.), *The Dental Reference Manual*,
DOI 10.1007/978-3-319-39730-6_14

14.1 Introduction

Some of the most common lesions that patients present with are organized based on their presentation. In attempting to simplify this very complex array of possible diagnoses, they are organized as follows. In each of the lesions, their demographics, differential diagnosis, and treatments are described and pictured with examples (Tables 14.1 and 14.2).

Table 14.1 Soft tissue lesions

White	Red	Ulcers	Raised soft tissue (bumps)	Pigmented
1. Leukoplakia	1. Geographic tongue	1. Squamous carcinoma	1. Pyogenic granuloma	1. Varicosity
2. Lichen planus	2. Desquamative gingivitis	2. Aphthous stomatitis	2. Peripheral giant cell granuloma	2. Amalgam tattoo
3. Leukoedema	3. Candidiasis	3. Herpetic stomatitis	3. Fibroma	3. Macule
4. Cheek/tongue chewing	4. Erythroplakia	4. Traumatic	4. Peripheral ossifying fibroma	
5. Candidiasis			5. Mucocele	
			6. Papilloma	
			7. Lymphoepithelial cyst	

Table 14.2 Hard tissue lesions

Radiolucent	Radiopaque
1. Periapical granuloma	1. Odontoma
2. Periapical cyst 3. Dentigerous cyst	2. Cemento-osseous dysplasia
4. Odontogenic keratocyst (keratocystic odontogenic tumor)	3. Idiopathic osteosclerosis
5. Lateral periodontal cyst 6. Ameloblastoma 7. Simple bone cyst (traumatic bone cyst) 8. Nasopalatine duct cyst	4. Condensing osteitis

14.2 White Soft Tissue Lesions

14.2.1 Leukoplakia

14.2.1.1 Synonyms

- Leukokeratosis; erythroleukoplakia

14.2.1.2 Introduction

- A white lesion of unknown cause which is considered precancerous (Warnakulasuriya 2007).
- It is a common premalignant lesion of the oral mucosa.
- Risk factors include consumption of alcohol and tobacco, microorganisms, and trauma.
- Malignancy transformation rate is 4–6 % (Petti 2003, Axéll 1996).
- All leukoplakias should be assessed histopathologically and treated vigorously if dysplasia is prominent.

14.2.1.3 Demographics

- Strong male predilection
- Female predilection in regional populations where women use tobacco products more than men
- Seen more frequently in older individuals (average age 60 year)

14.2.1.4 Appearance (Fig. 14.1a–d)

- A clinical term defined as a predominantly white lesion of the oral mucosa that cannot be characterized clinically and pathologically as any other disease; a diagnosis of exclusion.
- The lip vermillion, gingiva, and buccal mucosa are the sites of predilection; the tongue, lip vermillion, and floor of the mouth lesion account for 90% of leukoplakia dysplasia/carcinoma.
- Classified as homogenous, nodular (speckled), verruciform, and proliferative verrucous leukoplakia (van der Waal 2010).
- Homogenous: well-demarcated uniform white plaques with or without fissuring.
- Nonhomogeneous are predominantly mixed red and white lesions in which keratotic white nodules or patches are distributed over an atrophic erythematous background.
- Verruciform: presence of thick white lesions with papillary surface; lesions are heavily keratinized and are seen mostly in older adults.
- Proliferative verrucous: special type of leukoplakia with extensive papillary or verrucous white plaques that tend to slowly involve extensive mucous surfaces with an invariable transformation into squamous cell carcinoma or verrucous carcinoma over a period of several years.

14.2.1.5 Clinical Differential Diagnosis

- Lichen planus
- Candidiasis

14.2.1.6 Treatment and Prognosis

- No current consensus.
- Repeat follow-up visits and biopsies are essential.
- Each clinical appearance or phase of leukoplakia has a different potential for malignant transformation.
- Speckled leukoplakia carries the highest average transformation potential, followed by verrucous leukoplakia.
- Homogeneous leukoplakia carries the lowest risk.
- For dysplastic leukoplakia, the clinician must consider the histologic grade when planning treatment and follow-up.
- In general, the greater the degree of dysplasia, the greater the potential for malignant change.

- Additionally, multiple factors play a role in determining the optimum management procedure. These factors include the persistence of the lesion over many years, the development of leukoplakia in a nonsmoker, and the lesion's occurrence on high-risk areas such as the floor of the mouth, the soft palate, the oropharynx, or the ventral surface of the tongue.
- Non-surgical: carotenoids (beta-carotene, lycopene), vitamins A, C, and K, fenretinide, bleomycin, and photodynamic therapy (Ribeiro 2010).
- Surgical: conventional surgery, electrocauterization, laser ablation, or cryosurgery.

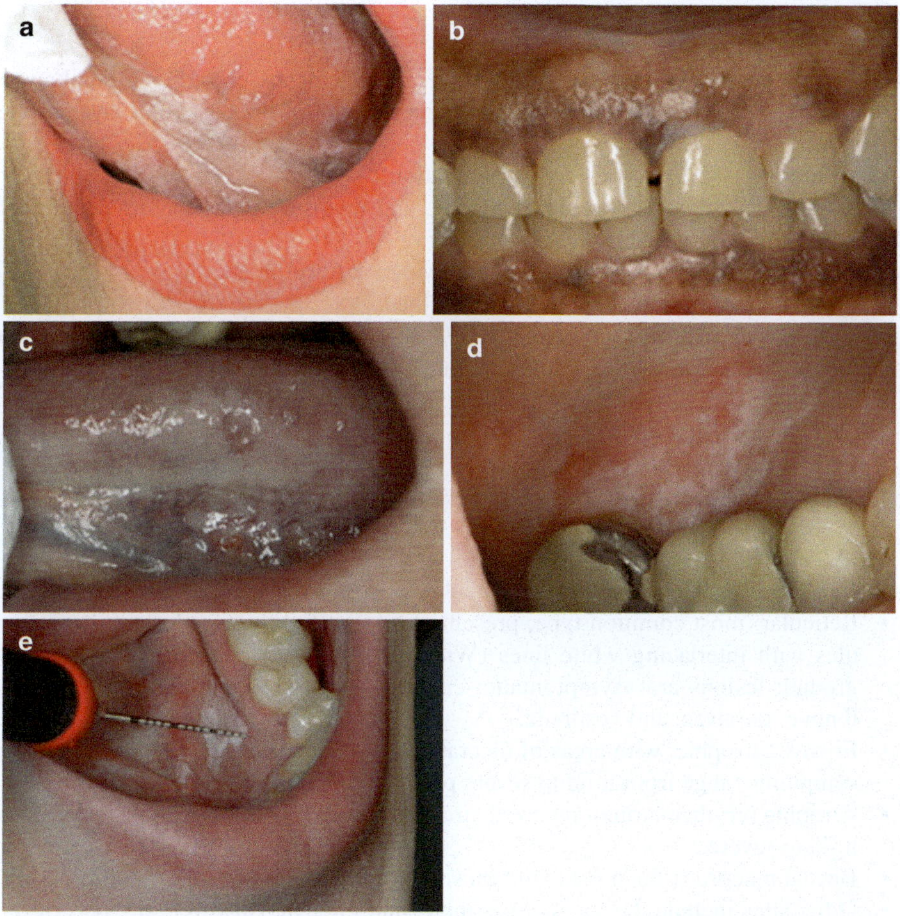

Fig. 14.1 (**a**) Thick extensive leukoplakia of ventral tongue and floor of mouth in a nonsmoker. Biopsy revealed significant epithelial dysplasia. (**b**) Small area of somewhat verrucous leukoplakia on the maxillary facial gingiva. Patient is a smoker. No dysplasia detected upon microscopic examination. (**c**) Thin leukoplakia on the lateral/ventral border of the tongue. Biopsy revealed mild epithelial dysplasia. (**d**) Irregular erythroleukoplakia of the palatal mucosa. Biopsy revealed epithelial dysplasia. (**e**) An irregular bordered rough (verrucous) surfaced distinct leukoplakic lesion on the floor of the mouth in a heavy smoker

- Presence of epithelial dysplasia is the strongest predictor of future malignant transformation (Warnakulasuriya 2007, Petti 2003).
- Histopathologic evaluation for dysplasia/carcinoma should be done for nonhomogeneous lesion.

14.2.2 Lichen Planus (LP)

14.2.2.1 Synonyms

- Lichenoid mucositis

14.2.2.2 Introduction

- A chronic immunologically mediated mucocutaneous condition of unknown cause resulting from a cell-mediated degeneration of the basal cell layer of the epithelium (Au 2013).
- Affects 0.1–4.0 % of the general population.
- Oral lesions may be chronic, remitting, and relapsing with varying degrees of morbidity (Giunta 2001).
- Lesions range from asymptomatic to severely painful in nature.
- Genetic involvement is yet to be determined.
- The World Health Organization's (WHO) criteria describe lichen planus as a condition predisposed to malignant transformation.

14.2.2.3 Demographics

- Female predominance seen
- Most patients between 30 and 60 years of age

14.2.2.4 Appearance (Fig. 14.2a–e)

- Classified into three main forms: reticular, erosive, and atrophic (or erythematous).
- Reticular: most common type; present as white, slightly raised plaques or papules with interlacing white lines (Wickham striae) on an erythematous background; lesions are asymptomatic; common sites include the buccal mucosa, tongue, gingivae, and vestibule.
- Erosive: atrophic, with areas of ulceration, erythema, and keratotic white striae; symptoms range from mild to severe pain.
- Atrophic (erythematous): mucosal atrophy; red, diffuse lesion; pain ranges from mild to severe.
- Buccal mucosa is the most common sites where lesions are usually bilateral.
- Other sites include the tongue, vestibule, and gingiva. However, any part of the oral mucosa maybe involved.
- Lichen planus on the dorsum of the tongue often appears plaque-like.
- Direct immunofluorescence demonstrates a shaggy band of fibrinogen in the basement membrane zone in 90–100 % of cases.
- Malignant transformation of lichen planus is highly controversial; malignant transformation is more likely in erosive lesions.
- The reported incidence of malignant transformation is anywhere from as low as 0.4 % to as high as 1.5 % (Fitzpatrick et al. 2014).

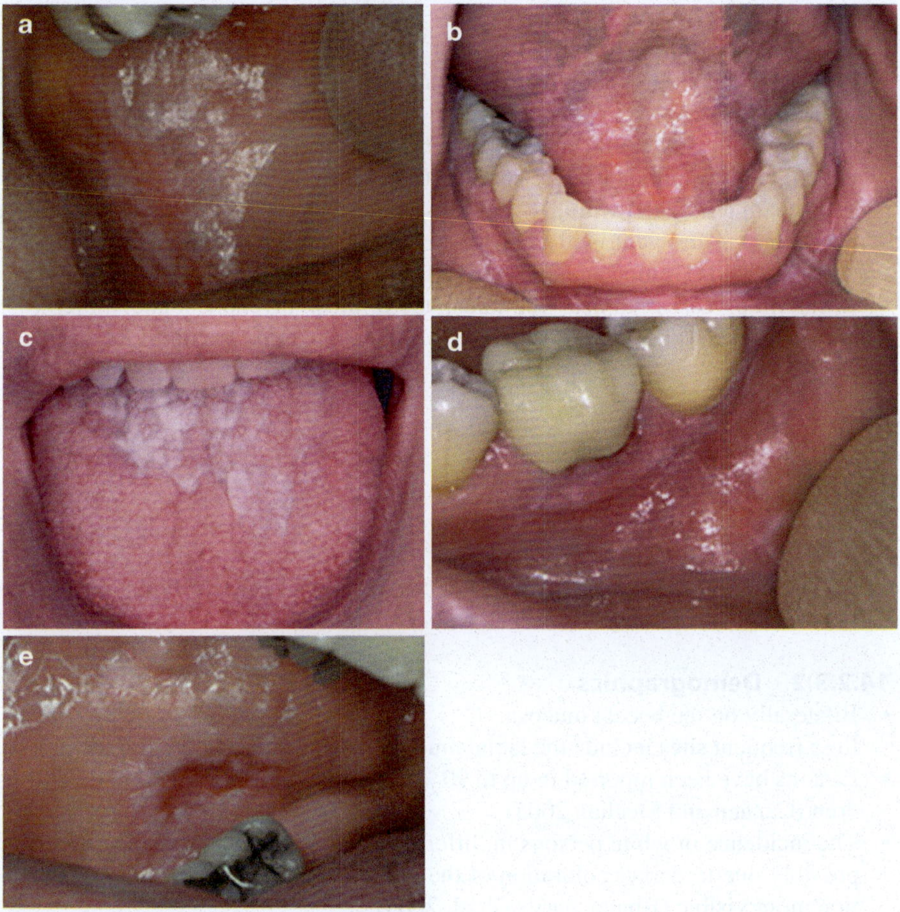

Fig. 14.2 (**a**) Classic reticular LP on the buccal mucosa. (**b**) Reticular LP on the buccal vestibule as well as the floor of the mouth. (**c**) Plaque-like LP on the dorsum of the tongue. (**d**) Erosive erythematous involvement of the posterior mandibular gingiva with striations is typical of LP. (**e**) Central ulcerative lesion of the posterior buccal mucosa rimmed by white striations typical of erosive LP

14.2.2.5 Clinical Differential Diagnosis

- Drug-induced lichenoid reaction
- Contact mercury hypersensitivity
- Chronic graft-versus-host disease
- Erythema multiforme
- Lupus erythematosus
- Candidiasis
- Mucous membrane pemphigoid
- Squamous cell carcinoma
- Granulomatous lichenoid mucositis (affects upper lip)
- Leukoplakia resembling keratotic lichen planus
- Desquamative gingivitis (erosive LP)

14.2.2.6 Treatment and Prognosis

- May be difficult to treat.
- Lesions tend to regress and reappear in an unpredictable fashion.
- Reticular lesions: No treatment needed.
- Symptomatic erosive and atrophic lesions: corticosteroids recommended; strong topical corticosteroids usually sufficient (fluocinonide, betamethasone, clobetasol); healing induced within 1–2 weeks; systemic corticosteroids generally not necessary; insufficient evidence that to support the superiority of any specific corticosteroid (Usatine and Tinitigan 2011, Lodi et al. 2012).
- Recalcitrant cases: topical retinoids, tacrolimus, mycophenolate mofetil, or cyclosporine has been used; side effects and cost may be prohibitive.

14.2.3 Leukoedema

Synonyms: None

14.2.3.1 Introduction

- A development alteration, of unknown cause, which is considered to be a variation of normal anatomy rather than a disease (Martin and Crump 1972)

14.2.3.2 Demographics

- Bilaterally on the buccal mucosa.
- Less frequent sites include the labial mucosa, soft palate, and floor of the mouth.
- Lesions have been reported in up to 90 % of black adults and 50 % of black children (Canaan and Meehan 2005).
- The incidence in white persons in different studies is highly variable (10–80 %) possibly due to darker coloration of the mucosa in blacks, rendering the alteration more visible (Bhattacharyya et al. 2003).
- Similar changes have also been reported on the vaginal and laryngeal mucosa.

14.2.3.3 Appearance (Fig. 14.3)

- Buccal lesions are poorly defined diffuse, gray-white, opalescent macules which cannot be rubbed off.
- Occasionally, the lesion may present as fine grooves or folds.
- Mucosal changes are not usually noticeable until adolescence.
- Some studies relate the severity of the lesion to smoking.
- Clinical diagnosis is made easily because the lesion disappears or fades upon stretching the mucosa.

14.2.3.4 Clinical Differences Diagnosis

- Frictional keratosis
- Snuff dippers keratosis
- White sponge nevus
- Witkop's disease
- Clinical stretch test helps distinguish leukoedema from other lesions

14.2.3.5 Treatment and Prognosis

- No treatment required; it is a benign condition.
- Does not change significantly even after 20–30 years.

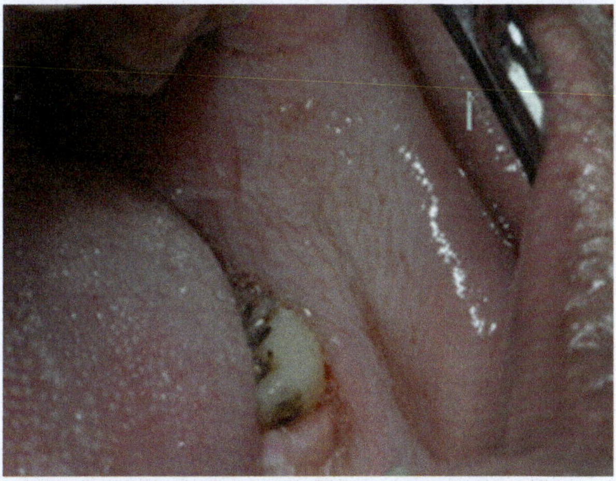

Fig. 14.3 Diffuse pale gray-white change of the buccal mucosa in a middle-aged male patient

14.2.4 Cheek/Tongue Chewing

14.2.4.1 Synonyms

- Morsicatio mucosae oris; morsicatio buccarum; morsicatio labiorum; morsicatio linguarum

14.2.4.2 Introduction

- "Morsicatio" represents changes in the mucosa covering the tongue, buccal mucosa, or lips caused by chronic tissue irritation, such as biting, sucking, or friction (Glass and Maize 1991).
- Etiology unknown (Allen and Camisa 2008).
- Self-induced injury which may be associated with stress or mental illness (Scully and Hegarty 2010).

14.2.4.3 Demographics

- Can be seen in any age and gender
- Increased prevalence in women older than 35 years of age (Woo and Lin 2009)
- Known occupational association in glassblowers

14.2.4.4 Appearance (Fig. 14.4a, b)

- Thick rough white asymptomatic areas intermixed with red and ulcerated zones of oral mucosa (Woo 2010).

- Superficial areas may be peeled off or removed by patient.
- Anterior buccal mucosa is affected most frequently; unilaterally or bilaterally.
- Lateral border or tongue and lips may also be involved.

14.2.4.5 Clinical Differential Diagnosis

- Leukoedema
- White sponge nevus
- Snuff dipper's keratosis
- Chemical keratosis
- Oral hairy leukoplakia (Tomás Carmona et al. 2000)

14.2.4.6 Treatment and Prognosis

- If other conditions mentioned above are in consideration, an incisional biopsy may be required.
- No treatment required, other than mitigation of trauma.
- Complete resolution takes place upon resolution of chronic trauma.
- No malignant potential.

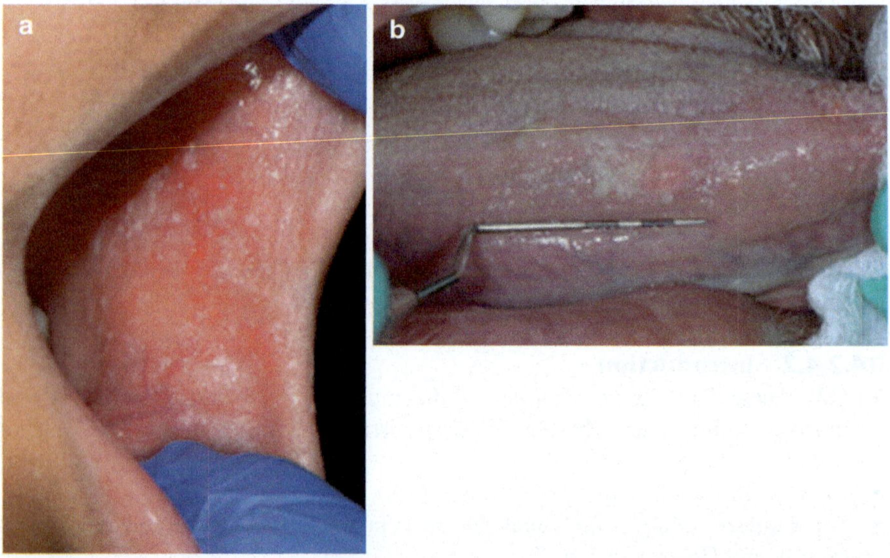

Fig. 14.4 (**a**) CK Chg. Typical "shredded" appearance of the cheek mucosa in a 10-year-old girl. (**b**) CK Chg. White rough area on the lateral border of the tongue in a 65-year-old male

14.2.5 Candidiasis (See Candidiasis in Red Lesions)

- Condensing osteitis presents as a radiopaque/radiolucent lesion between the apex of teeth #29 and 30.
- Large condensing osteitis between the apex of teeth #30 and 31.

14.3 Red Soft Tissue Lesions

14.3.1 Geographic Tongue

14.3.1.1 Synonyms

- Erythema migrans; benign migratory glossitis; wandering rash of the tongue; erythema areata migrans; stomatitis areata migrans

14.3.1.2 Introduction

- A common benign condition seen in 1–2 % of the population (Jainkittivong and Langlais 2005).
- Often an incidental finding.
- Cause and pathogenesis are still elusive (Femiano 2001).
- No statistically significant association with atopic individuals noted.

14.3.1.3 Demographics

- Affects all ages
- No gender predilection noted

14.3.1.4 Appearance (Fig. 14.5a, b)

- Multiple well-demarcated asymptomatic erythematous areas surrounded partially or completely by a yellow-white slightly raised serpentine line seen.
- The erythematous zones on tongue represent atrophy of the filiform papillae.
- Anterior two-thirds of dorsal surface of the tongue most frequent site.
- Lesions may also involve the lateral and ventral surfaces of the tongue (Menni et al. 2004).
- Other oral mucosal surfaces such as labial, buccal, floor of mouth, and palatal areas may be involved in rare cases (Assimakopoulos et al. 2002).
- Lesions develop in one area, heal in days to weeks, and then develop in a different area,

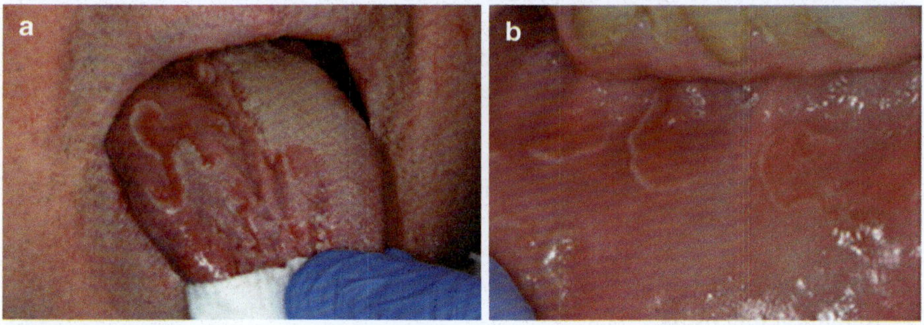

Fig. 14.5 (a) Erythematous zones surrounded by whitish-yellow circinate borders. (b) Patient with erythema migrans of the labial mucosa. He also has classic tongue lesions

14.3.1.5 Clinical Differential Diagnosis

- Pyostomatitis vegetans
- Stomatitis herpetiformis

14.3.1.6 Treatment and Prognosis

- No treatment required
- Symptomatic lesions treated with topical steroids (Menni et al. 2004)

14.3.2 Desquamative Gingivitis

14.3.2.1 Synonyms

- None

14.3.2.2 Introduction

- A clinical term common to a wide number of disorders characterized by erythema, desquamation, erosion, and blistering of attached and marginal gingiva (Rees 2011).
- Most common conditions include lichen planus, mucous membrane pemphigoid, and pemphigus (Endo et al. 2008).
- Lichen planus and mucous membrane pemphigoid constitute 80 % of cases.
- Histopathological examination and direct immunofluorescence testing essential to establish a definitive diagnosis.

14.3.2.3 Demographics

- Seen in adults
- Greater frequency in women
- Can affect gingiva anywhere in the oral cavity (Nisengard and Neiders 1981)

14.3.2.4 Appearance (Fig. 14.6a, b)

- Usually involved gingiva appears erythematous and inflamed and exhibits sloughing (Scully and Porter 1997).
- Pain and discomfort often noted with the condition.
- Nikolsky sign is often positive (separation of intact superficial epithelium under firm lateral pressure).

14.3.2.5 Clinical Differential Diagnosis

- Traumatic lesions
- Thermal burns
- Plasma cell gingivitis
- Radiation mucositis
- Erythroplakia

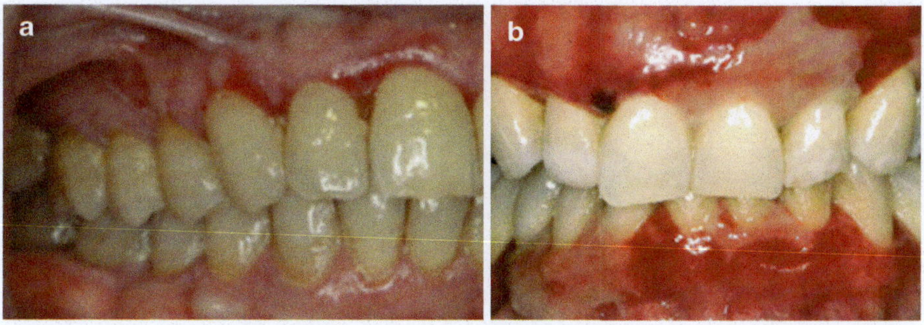

Fig. 14.6 (**a**) Ulcerative and erythematous areas of the facial gingiva in a 62-year-old male. Biopsy revealed erosive lichen planus. (**b**) Extensive desquamation of the gingiva on both arches with areas of bloody blisters in a patient with benign mucous membrane pemphigoid

14.3.2.6 Treatment and Prognosis

- A definitive diagnosis of the specific disease or disorder is needed to provide adequate treatment (Guiglia et al. 2007).
- Requires elimination or control of local irritants
- Many cases respond to topical corticosteroids and plaque control.
- Lesions tend to wax and wane and may go into remission.
- Periodic follow-up and long-term care of patients are essential.

14.3.3 Candidiasis

14.3.3.1 Synonyms

- Moniliasis; yeast infection; thrush

14.3.3.2 Introduction

- Yeastlike fungal organisms of the genus *Candida* of which *Candida albicans* is the most prevalent species in both health and disease (Barnett 2008).
- Among the most common human pathogens.
- Infection is more common when individual becomes immunocompromised.
- Systemic infections are rare but serious when they do occur.

14.3.3.3 Demographics

- Commensal carriage of this species occurs in approximately 50% of individuals.
- Predisposing factors for infection include local host factors (denture use, steroid inhaler use, reduced salivary flow, nutritional deficiencies) and systemic host factors (infants and elderly, diabetes mellitus, immunosuppression, broad-spectrum antibiotics) (Samaranayake et al. 2009, Soysa et al. 2006).
- Seen across all ages from newborn to older adults.

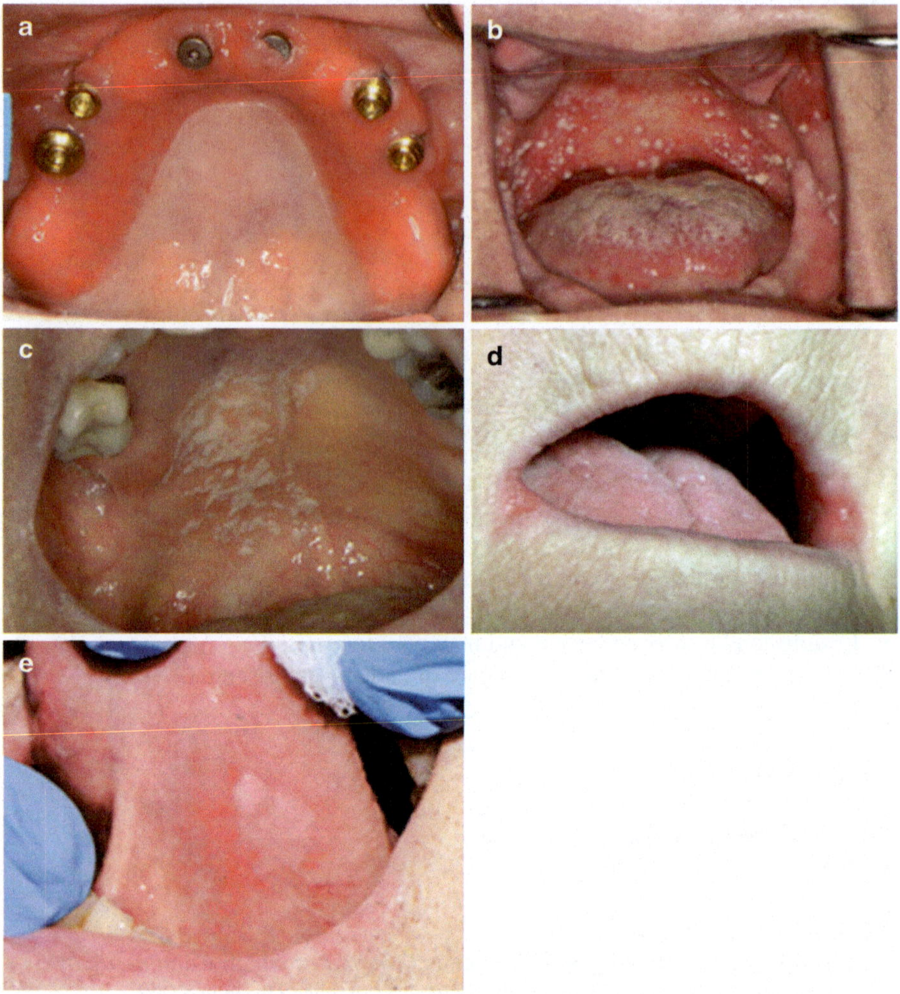

Fig. 14.7 (**a**) Denture sore mouth. (**b**) Pseudomembranous candidiasis in an elderly patient with recent history of using antibiotics. (**c**) Pseudomembranous candidiasis. (**d**) Angular cheilitis. (**e**) Hyperplastic candidiasis on the ventral tongue with associated traumatic keratosis

14.3.3.4 Appearance (Fig.14.7a–e)

- Presents clinically in four forms: pseudomembranous, acute erythematous, chronic erythematous, and chronic hyperplastic.
- Pseudomembranous: characterized by superficial white plaques that are easily removed by gentle rubbing of the lesion (diagnostic feature), leaving a erythematous base; seen in neonates and the elderly at rates of 5–10 % (Rüping et al. 2008).
- Acute erythematous: aka "antibiotic sore mouth"; results from broad-spectrum antibiotics use; painful lesion.

- Chronic erythematous: aka "denture stomatitis"; causes include wearing dentures 27/7, ill-fitting dentures, and poor oral hygiene; usually asymptomatic (Webb et al. 2005).
- Hyperplastic: characterized by white plaques; do not rub off; histological examination needed for a definitive diagnosis; potential for the development of squamous cell carcinoma at lesional sites is of concern; cause of change unclear.
- Angular cheilitis: commissural erythema; candida along with bacterial infection implicated.
- Median rhomboid glossitis: erythematous candidiasis involving the dorsal tongue.

14.3.3.5 Clinical Differential Diagnosis

- Leukoplakia
- Erythroplakia
- Traumatic erythema

14.3.3.6 Treatment and Prognosis

- Traditional antifungal agents: topical (nystatin, amphotericin, miconazole, clotrimazole) and systemic (ketoconazole, fluconazole, itraconazole).
- Denture care: remove during sleep and immerse in a suitable antimicrobial cleansing agent; hot water-immersed dentures have been of benefit in the treatment of denture stomatitis.

14.3.4 Erythroplakia

14.3.4.1 Synonyms

- Erythroplasia; erythroplasia of Queyrat

14.3.4.2 Introduction

- A red lesion of unknown cause which is considered premalignant.
- Has the highest rate of malignant transformation as compared to other oral premalignant conditions; in one study, 91 % of lesional biopsies showed dysplasia, carcinoma in situ, or carcinoma (Shafer and Waldron 1975).
- Far less common than leukoplakia (van der Waal 2011).
- Lesions are frequently overlooked (Reichart and Philipsen 2005).

14.3.4.3 Demographics

- Typically occurs in the middle aged and the elderly.
- Most commonly involves the floor of the mouth, ventral tongue, soft palate, and tonsillar fauces (Villa et al. 2011).
- Etiology is poorly understood (van der Wall 2009).
- Predisposing factors include tobacco and alcohol.
- *Candida albicans* has often been demonstrated as secondary infection; positive correlation between the presence of dysplastic epithelium and candidal hyphae has not been shown.
- Role of human papilloma virus is controversial.

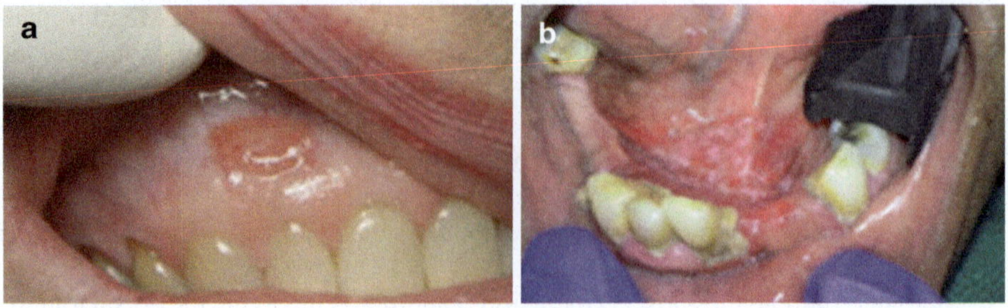

Fig. 14.8 (**a**) Distinct erythroplakic patch on the maxillary gingiva in a 65-year-old female. Patient is a nonsmoker. Biopsy revealed squamous cell carcinoma. (**b**) Speckled red and white lesion on the floor of the mouth in a 72-year-old male. Patient is a heavy smoker. Biopsy revealed squamous cell carcinoma

14.3.4.4 Appearance (Fig.14.8a, b)

- A clinical term defined as any lesion of the oral mucosa that presents as bright red velvety plaques which cannot be characterized clinically or pathologically as any other recognizable condition; a diagnosis of exclusion.
- Classified as homogenous, erythroplakia interspersed with patches of leukoplakia and granular or speckled.
- Homogenous: smooth and velvety surface.
- Erythroplakia interspersed with patches of leukoplakia: numerous, small irregular foci of leukoplakia dispersed in the erythroplakic patch.
- Granular or speckled: irregular, red granular surface interspersed with white or yellow foci.
- May be multicentric; rarely covers extensive areas of the mouth.
- Patients in whom carcinoma in situ has been diagnosed generally aware of an alteration in the involved site for at least 2.7 years prior to biopsy.

14.3.4.5 Clinical Differential Diagnosis

- Fungal infections (oral candidiasis, histoplasmosis)
- Bacterial infections (tuberculosis)
- Atrophic lichen planus
- Lupus erythematosus
- Pemphigus
- Pemphigoid

14.3.4.6 Treatment and Prognosis

- Due to high malignant transformation rate, early detection and treatment are of utmost importance (Yang et al. 2015).
- Observation for 1–2 weeks following the elimination of suspected irritants is acceptable.
- Thereafter, prompt biopsy is mandatory for lesions that persist.
- Epithelial dysplasia or carcinoma in situ warrants complete removal of lesion.
- Due to high recurrence rates and multifocal involvement, follow-up is mandatory.

14.4 Ulcers in the Soft Tissue

14.4.1 Squamous Cell Carcinoma

14.4.1.1 Synonyms

- None

14.4.1.2 Introduction

- It is the most common malignancy of the oral cavity; accounts for more than 90 % of all oral cancers (Chaturvedi 2012).
- A recent increase in tongue cancer in young females seen (20–44 years); frequently without alcohol or tobacco exposure (Deschler et al. 2014 and Muller et al. 2008).
- Major risk factors: tobacco, alcohol, combined alcohol and tobacco (synergistic effect), betel quid, and high-risk human papilloma virus (HPV-16).
- Other risk factors: *Candida*, *Neisseria*, and streptococci (role still controversial), dietary factors (vitamin D deficiency implicated), immune status, environmental pollutants (arsenic, chromium, nickel), occupational exposures (construction, painting, carpentry, metalworking), and heritable conditions (Fanconi anemia, dyskeratosis congenita, and Bloom syndrome)

14.4.1.3 Demographics

- Most often seen in older population (average age 62 years); duration of change approximately of 4–8 months
- Slight predilection for males in the USA and significant male predominance worldwide
- HPV-positive tumors
  - Younger white male predilection.
  - Patients approximately 10 years younger than HPV-negative tumors.
  - Patients tend to be in higher socioeconomic group.

14.4.1.4 Appearance (Figs. 14.9a–e and 14.10)

- Often preceded or accompanied by leukoplakia, erythroplakia, erythroleukoplakia, or proliferative verrucous leukoplakia.
- Most common sites: tongue; accounts for 40–50 % of all cases; majority of cases seen on the lateral or ventrolateral surfaces, rare on the dorsum.
- The floor of the mouth is the second most common site (35 %); other less common sites include buccal mucosa, gingiva, and palate.
- Presents as an indurated mass or ulcer.
- Minimal pain during early growth years.
- Varied clinical presentations: exophytic, endophytic, leukoplakic, erythroplakic, and erythroleukoplakic.
- Destruction of underlying bone, if present, may be painless or painful.

14.4.1.5 Clinical Differential Diagnosis

- Chronic traumatic ulcer
- Epithelial dysplasia

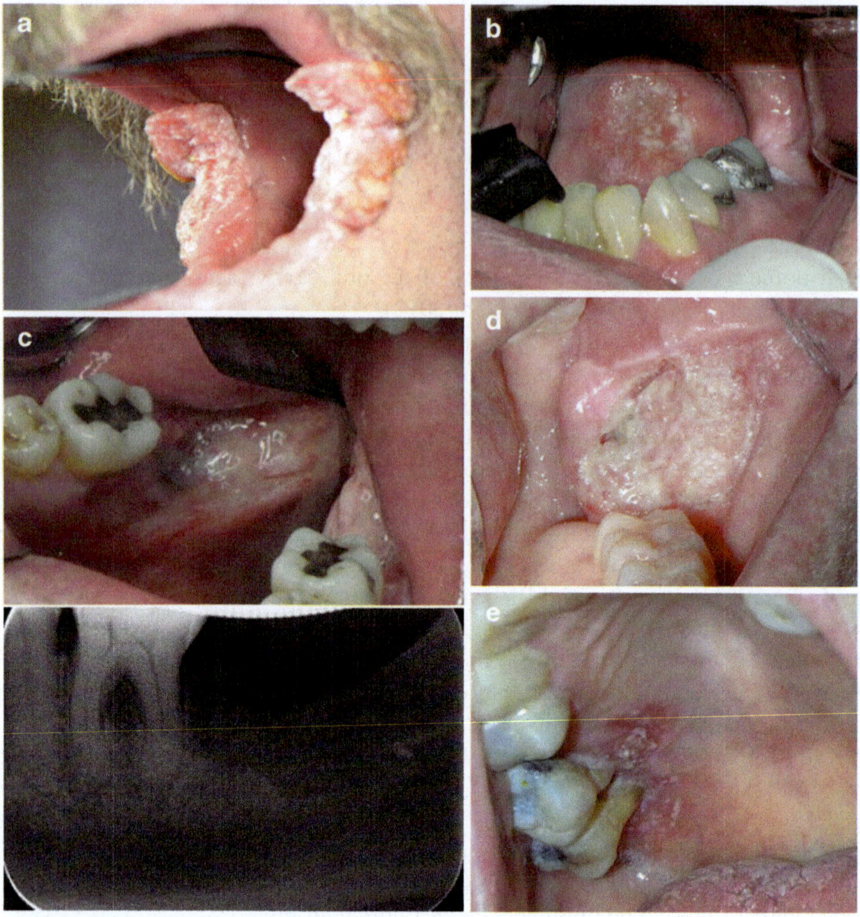

Fig. 14.9 (**a**) Large fungating exophytic carcinoma of the commissure of mouth encroaching upon the skin. (**b**) A Large endophytic ulcer with raised borders on the lateral/ventral tongue surface. Biopsy showed a moderately differentiated squamous cell carcinoma. (**c**) Carcinoma of the alveolar ridge with involvement of the underlying bone. Radiograph demonstrating erosion and irregular radiolucency of the bone. (**d**) Large fungating exophytic carcinoma of the buccal mucosa. (**e**) Carcinoma of the palatal gingiva and mucosa resulting in gingival recession. Carcinoma simulating periodontal disease. Destructive ulcerative carcinoma of the mandibular gingiva in 68-year-old female

- Carcinoma in situ
- Deep fungal infection
- Chronic bacterial ulcers

14.4.1.6 Radiographic Features

- Most oral tumors are favorable to visual examination; imaging is done for tumors that are palpable but not visible.
- Soft tissue tumors: computerized tomographic (CT) scans, magnetic resonance imaging (MRI), and positron emission tomography (PET) most commonly used;

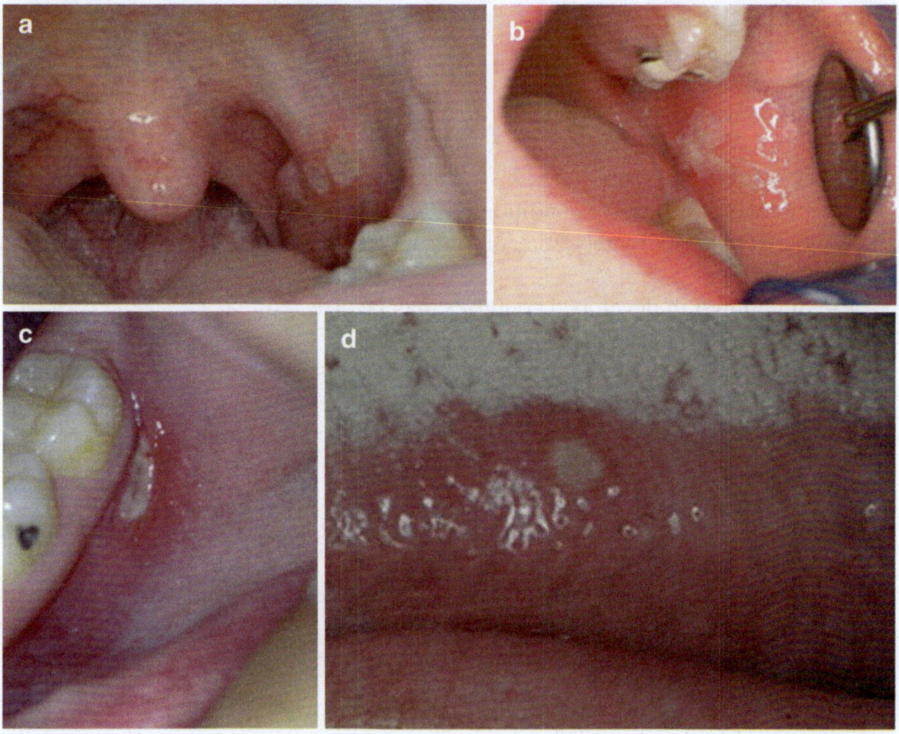

Fig. 14.10 (**a**) Major aphthous ulcerations on the tonsillar fauces in a 38-year-old female. (**b**) Major aphthous ulceration on the posterior buccal mucosa. (**c**) Minor aphthous ulceration on the posterior buccal vestibule in an 18-year-old female. (**d**) Minor aphthous ulceration on the lateral border of the tongue in a 26-year-old male

however, stage I tumors (less than 2 cm in size) are not visible on these scans; recently, intraoral ultrasound has been an alternative to MRI in assessing tongue tumor thickness.

- Tumors invading bone: panoramic and periapical images are of help in assessing mandibular or maxillary invasion. Radioactive isotope-labeled scans also useful in determining extent of tumor.

14.4.1.7 Treatment and Prognosis

- Almost always requires a multidisciplinary approach (Haddad 2008).
- Most early and late stage tumors are treated surgically with clear margins (1–2 cm) (Yesuratnam et al. 2014).
- Neck dissection done when lymph nodes are involved.
- Apart from surgery, stage III-IV tumors with adjuvant radiation and/or chemotherapy therapy.
- HPV-positive tumors have a better prognosis than HPV-negative tumors; HPV tumor status should be assessed in appropriate settings.
- HPV vaccination for prevention of oral carcinomas has not been approved by the US Food and Drug Administration.
- 5-year survival rate is approximately 63 %.

14.4.2 Aphthous Stomatitis

14.4.2.1 Synonyms

Aphthous stomatitis

14.4.2.2 Introduction

- Most common ulcerative condition of the oral mucosa.
- They affect approximately 20 % of the population (Porter et al. 2000, Scully and Porter 2008).
- 1 % of children in developed countries may be affected.
- Etiology still obscure.
- Multiple predisposing factors: positive family history, local trauma, nutritional deficiency (iron, folic acid and vitamin, food hypersensitivity (gluten)), immune disturbances, smoking cessation, psychological stress, and others.

14.4.2.3 Demographics

- Lesions most commonly seen in young adults; 80 % of affected patients report their first ulceration before the age of 30 years.
- Hereditary is a well-documented predisposing factor; positive family history is seen in 30–40 % of patients (Chavan et al. 2012).
- Higher prevalence in higher socioeconomic class.

14.4.2.4 Appearance (Fig. 14.11a–d)

- Lesions characterized by recurrent bouts of single or multiple rounded, flat, painful oral ulcers.
- Associated with prodromal symptoms of burning, itching, and stinging.
- Ulcers typically appear with gray-white pseudomembranes surrounded by thin erythematous halos.
- Occur in the nonkeratinized mobile oral mucosa; keratinized mucosa may be involved in immunocompromised patients.
- Depending on the size, number, and appearance, they are classified into three clinical forms: minor, major, and herpetiform.
- Minor aphthous ulcerations: up to 1 cm in diameter; show a variable recurrence rate and heal without scarring in 10–14 days.
- Major aphthous ulcerations: 1–3 cm in diameter; demonstrate the longest duration per episode; heal in 2–6 weeks and may cause scarring.
- Herpetiform aphthous ulcerations: 1–3 mm in diameter; numerous lesions; heal within 7–10 days; recurrences closely spaced.

14.4.2.5 Clinical Differential Diagnosis

- Viral stomatitis
- Traumatic ulcer
- Pemphigus

14.4.2.6 Treatment and Prognosis

- No specific diagnostic test exists.

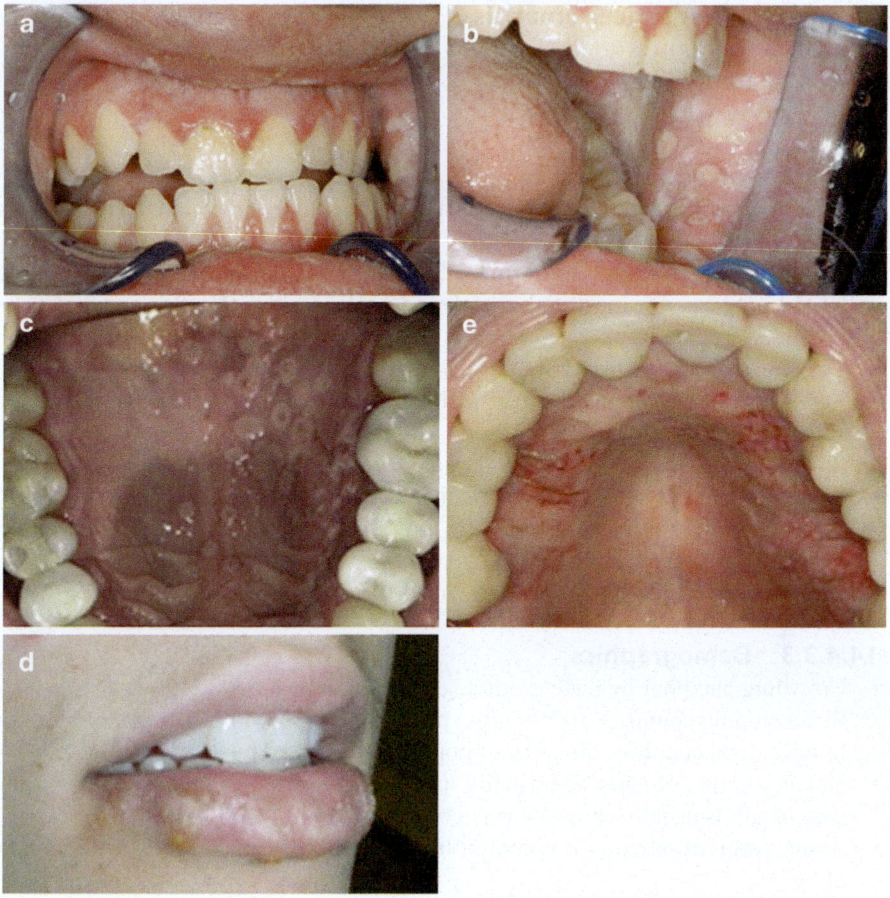

Fig. 14.11 (**a**) Gingival involvement is evident with enlargement and ulceration. (**b**) Same patient as Fig. 14.1 exhibiting buccal mucosal involvement. (**c**) Secondary multiple discrete ulcerations of the palatal mucosa in a 46-year-old. (**d**) Herpes labialis in a 26-year-old with multiple crusted ulcers and generalized swelling of the lower lip. (**e**) Secondary herpes on the palatal mucosa in a 76-year-old male. Lesions started within 3–4 days following significant periodontal surgery

- In order to discard the underlying systemic causes, a complete series of laboratory tests should be evaluated (complete blood count, iron, vitamin B12, and folic acid) (Belenguer-Guallar et al. 2014).
- Biopsy of the lesion is only recommended in the case of diagnostic uncertainty, since the findings only indicate a simple nonspecific inflammatory lesion (Belenguer-Guallar et al. 2014).
- Refer patient to internist (to rule out malabsorption syndrome, food allergies, gluten sensitivity.
- Majority of patients spontaneously enter remission.
- Most common therapy: topical corticosteroids; decreases pain and duration but has no effect on future occurrence of new lesions.

14.4.3 Oral Herpetic Stomatitis

14.4.3.1 Synonyms

- Cold sore

14.4.3.2 Introduction

- HSV is a double-stranded DNA virus and is a member of the human herpes virus (HHV) family.
- Though the virus exists in 2 forms, HSV-1 (or HHV-1) and HSV-2 (or HHV-2), HSV-1 accounts for most oral, facial, and ocular lesions (Usatine and Tinitigan 2010).
- Transmission occurs primarily through infected saliva or active perioral lesions.
- The virus must come into contact with a break in the integrity of the mucosa or skin of a susceptible host.
- Infection includes primary infection, latency, and recurrent infection.
- Primary infection: initial exposure of an individual without antibodies to the virus.
- Latent infection: virus is taken up by the sensory nerves and transported to the associated sensory ganglion.
- Recurrent infection: reactivation of virus.

14.4.3.3 Demographics

- Crowding and poor hygiene promote exposure to HSV.
- In developing countries 100 % of the population exposed by 30 years of age.
- In developed countries 50–60 % of population exposed by 30 years of age.
- Primary herpes at early age usually results in gingivostomatitis, whereas exposure in adults usually causes pharyngotonsillitis.
- Acute gingivostomatitis is common in children between 6 months and 5 years of age.

14.4.3.4 Appearance (Fig. 14.12a–e)

- Age of initial infection affects clinical presentation of primary HSV-1 infection.
- Primary herpes: early age exposure: gingivostomatitis; late age exposure: pharyngotonsillitis.
- Acute gingivostomatitis: has an abrupt onset of symptoms and is accompanied by constitutional symptoms such as cervical lymphadenopathy, fever, chills, anorexia, irritability, and sore mouth. Numerous small vesicles that eventually rupture to form ulcers are noted on both attached and movable mucosa affected. The gingiva may be enlarged, erythematous, and extremely painful.
- Pharyngotonsillitis presents with sore throat, headache, fever, and malaise, and oral lesions are similar to those noted above usually on the tonsils and posterior pharynx.
- Recurrent infection (secondary herpes) occurs in a healthy host at or near the site of primary infection almost always involving bound down or keratinized mucosa such as lip vermillion and adjacent skin (herpes labialis) and hard palate and attached gingiva.

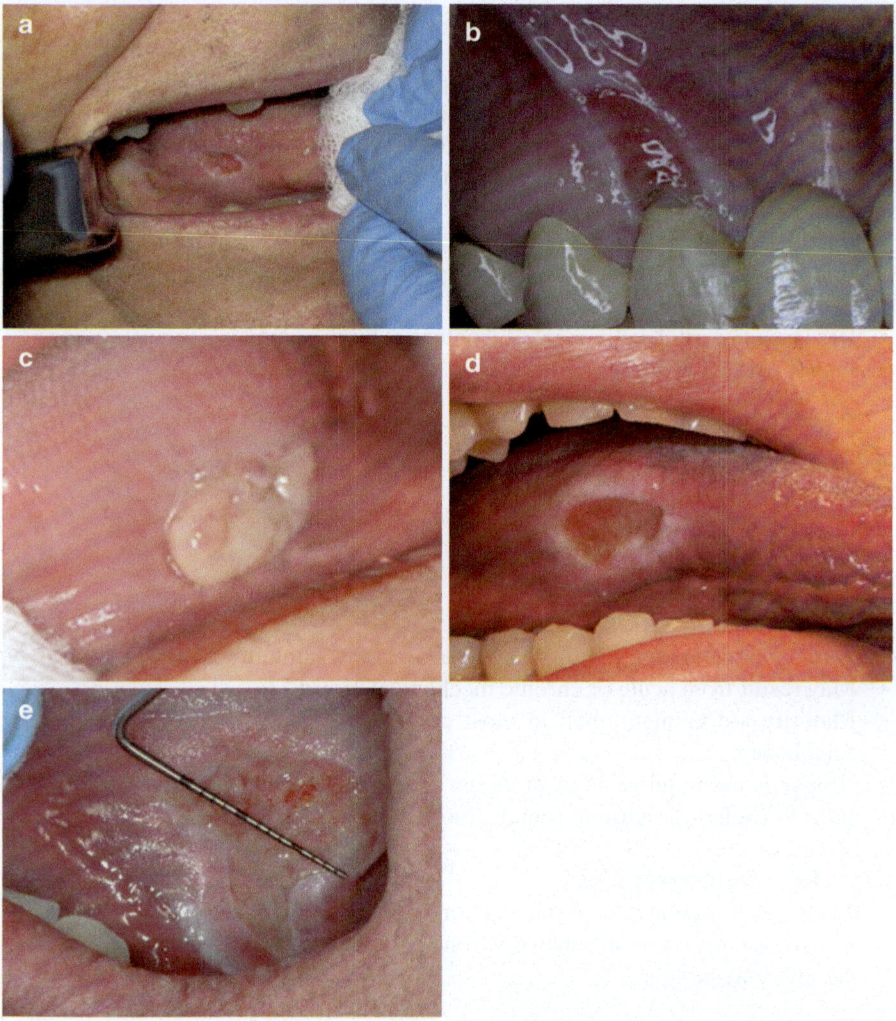

Fig. 14.12 (**a**) Ulceration of tongue associated with chronic trauma from maxillary molar in a partially edentulous elderly patient. (**b**) Linear ulcer on the maxillary gingiva associated with tooth brushing trauma. (**c**) TUGSE on the lateral tongue in a 72-year-old female. The lesion is present for about 3 months. (**d**) Long-standing ulceration of the lateral tongue. Note thick white borders. (**e**) Large painful long-standing ulcer of tongue simulating carcinoma. Patient reports chronic trauma. Note thick white borders

- Prodromal signs (tingling, burning, or pain) appear before onset of lesions.
- In an immunocompromised host, recurrent ulcers appear anywhere on the oral mucosa and may resemble aphthous ulcers when on nonkeratinized mucosa.

14.4.3.5 Clinical Differential Diagnosis

- Aphthous ulcers
- Traumatic ulcers

14.4.3.6 Treatment and Prognosis

- Healing occurs within 7–10 days.
- Primary infection: Symptomatic support (hydration, pain control, supportive care); antiviral medications are beneficial if administered early (acyclovir suspension, acyclovir or valacyclovir tablets initiated during the first 3 days of symptoms) (Woo and Challacombe 2007; Rahimi et al. 2012; Arduino and Porter 2006).
- Recurrent infection: best result if antiviral medication administered during the first 3 days of symptoms (acyclovir; penciclovir cream or ointment for herpes labialis) (Woo and Challacombe 2007).
- Research toward development of a potential herpes simplex vaccination is ongoing (Rahimi et al. 2012).

14.4.4 Traumatic Ulcers

14.4.4.1 Synonyms

- None

14.4.4.2 Introduction

- A relatively common finding (Parlak et al. 2006; Jainkittivosng et al. 2002)
- May result from acute or chronic mechanical injury
- Majority are unintentional; in most cases cause and effect relationship easily established
- Biopsy is not required in most cases; some may warrant histological investigations to exclude conditions which clinically mimic traumatic lesions

14.4.4.3 Demographics

- Mechanical trauma related: may occur at any age; no gender predilection
- Usually occurs on tissues that are prone to accidental biting such as tongue, buccal mucosa and lips

14.4.4.4 Appearance (Fig. 14.13a–e)

- Vary significantly; depending on cause.
- Acute mechanical trauma: caused by accidental mucosal biting: ulcerated lesion on an erythematous background, covered by a removable, yellowish fibrinopurulent exudate; heal uneventfully with few days.
- Chronic mechanical trauma: from sharp edges of teeth, restorations and ill-fitting dentures; present as a solitary shallow or deep ulcer with varying degrees of peripheral keratosis; borders of ulcer is indurated in most cases, and the floor is covered by a white or yellowish fibrin clot; may be asymptomatic or painful; common sites include the lips, tongue, and buccal mucosa.
- Traumatic ulcerative granuloma with stromal eosinophilia (TUGSE) is usually a large ulcer associated with tumefaction; most common site is the tongue; gingiva, the buccal mucosa, alveolar mucosa, and lips may also be affected (Hirshberg et al. 2006).

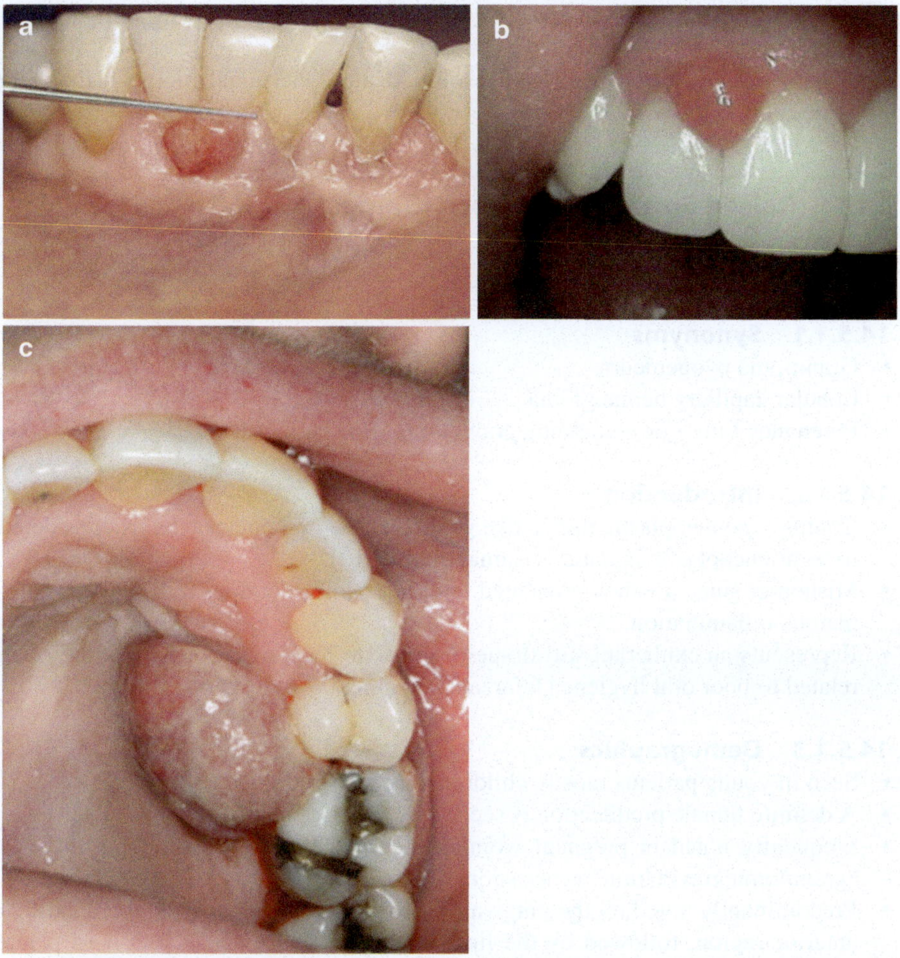

Fig. 14.13 (**a**) Ulcerated sessile gingival mass. (**b**) Anterior maxillary gingival mass. (**c**) Large growth on gingiva that exhibited rapid growth

14.4.4.5 Clinical Differential Diagnosis

- Squamous cell carcinoma
- Aphthous ulcers
- Neutropenic ulcers
- Medication-induced ulcers
- Infectious diseases ulcers
- Autoimmune diseases ulcers

14.4.4.6 Treatment and Prognosis

- Removal of causative factor is critically important. In addition application of topical anesthetic or protective film provides temporary relief; acute ulcers heal within 1–2 weeks without scarring; recurrence not expected.

- Biopsy of lesions that do not resolve after 2–4 weeks following mitigation of trauma.
- TUGSE: many lesions undergo resolution after incisional biopsy (Hirshberg et al. 2006).

14.5 Raised Soft Tissue Lesions (Bumps)

14.5.1 Pyogenic Granuloma

14.5.1.1 Synonyms

- Granuloma pyogenicum
- Lobular capillary hemangioma
- Pregnancy tumor or granuloma gravidarum

14.5.1.2 Introduction

- Common nonneoplastic tumor-like growth of the oral mucosa that is considered to be nonneoplastic in nature (Kamal et al. 2012).
- Misnomer since it is not associated with infections, nor does it display granulomatous inflammation.
- Represents an exuberant soft tissue response to local irritation or trauma; often related to poor oral hygiene (Jafarzadeh et al. 2006).

14.5.1.3 Demographics

- Seen in young patients mostly children and young adults.
- A definite female predilection is seen.
- Frequently noted in pregnant women; hence, the term "pregnancy tumor" or "granuloma gravidarum" is occasionally used.
- Predominantly noted on the gingiva (three quarters) especially on the maxillary anterior region, followed by the lips, tongue, buccal mucosa, and hard palate (Jafarzadeh et al. 2006) (Insert Figures PG1, PG2).

14.5.1.4 Appearance (Fig. 14.14a–c)

- Varied clinical appearances but typically reddish sessile or pedunculated smooth-surfaced or lobulated mass.
- The surface is invariably ulcerated.
- May range in size from few millimeters to several centimeters.
- Typically, painless though bleeding is common on slightest provocation.
- Has a tendency to exhibit rapid growth which may be clinically worrisome (Jafarzadeh et al. 2006) (Asha et al. 2014) (Insert Figure PG3).

14.5.1.5 Clinical Differential Diagnosis

- Includes the classic "bump on the gum" differential peripheral giant cell granuloma and peripheral ossifying fibroma

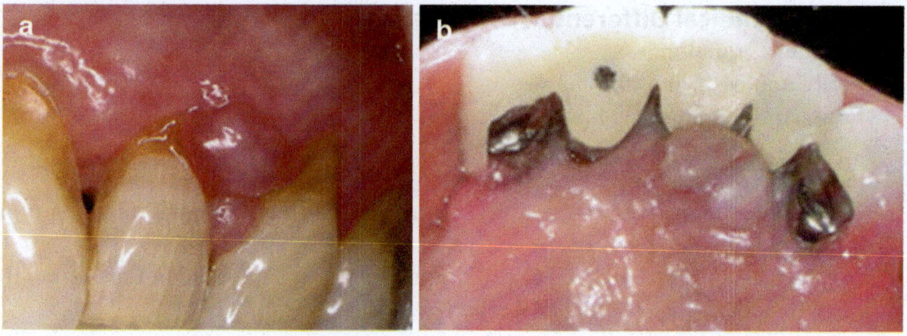

Fig. 14.14 (**a**) Small sessile mass in the maxillary canine region. (**b**) Small sessile lobular mass in the mandibular anterior lingual aspect

14.5.1.6 Treatment and Prognosis

- Removal is important as it can grow to large sizes and even move adjacent teeth, and maintenance of oral hygiene may be compromised.
- Conservative surgical excision down to periosteum prevents recurrences.
- Scaling of associated teeth helps in reducing recurrences.
- Long-term follow-up is not required.

14.5.2 Peripheral Giant Cell Granuloma

14.5.2.1 Synonyms

- Giant cell epulis; osteoclastoma; giant cell reparative granuloma

14.5.2.2 Introduction

- Most common giant cell lesion of the oral cavity.
- Etiology is unknown.
- Not a true neoplasm but is considered reactive in nature possibly related to local irritation or trauma (Rodrigues et al. 2015).
- Unique microscopic appearance with abundant cellularity, multinucleated giant cells and inflammatory cells.

14.5.2.3 Demographics

- Can be found in all age groups, with a relative predilection in 40–60 years range.
- Noted exclusively on the gingiva or tooth-bearing areas such as the edentulous ridges.
- The mandible is more commonly affected especially in the incisor-canine region (Insert figures PGCG 1 and PGCG 2).
- Females are more frequently affected than males with a ratio estimated to be 2:1.
- Lesions are usually around 1–2 cm in diameter.

14.5.2.4 Appearance (Fig. 14.15a, b)

- Sessile or pedunculated lobular or smooth-surfaced mass
- Surface often demonstrating ulceration
- Reddish to reddish purple in color

14.5.2.5 Clinical Differential Diagnosis

- Pyogenic granuloma
- Peripheral ossifying fibroma
- Peripheral odontogenic fibroma

14.5.2.6 Radiographic Features

- Not applicable in most cases; however, it may cause a "cupping" resorption of the underlying alveolar bone.
- In larger lesions, a central giant cell granuloma should be ruled out radiographically (Gandara-Rey et al. 2002).

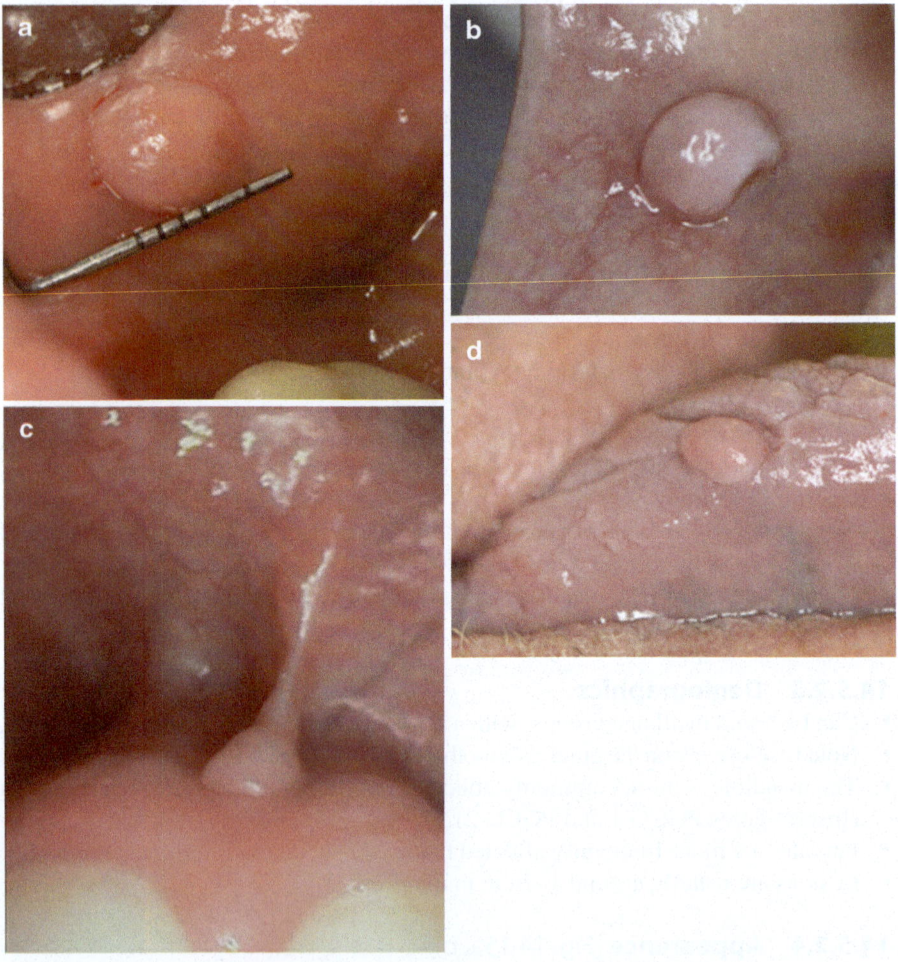

Fig. 14.15 (**a**) Sessile fibrous hyperplasia on the buccal mucosa along the bite line. (**b**) Fibroma of the buccal mucosa with hyperkeratosis. (**c**) Fibroma on the maxillary frenum. (**d**) Fibroma on the lateral tongue

14.5.2.7 Treatment

- May cause mobility or displacement of associated teeth if left untreated (Brown et al. 2015).
- Conservative surgical excision down to the underlying bone.
- Removal of local factors or irritants.
- An estimated recurrence rate of 10% has been reported.
- Laser excision may also be considered.
- May arise around a dental implant.

14.5.3 Fibroma

14.5.3.1 Synonyms

- Focal fibrous hyperplasia, irritation Fibroma, traumatic fibroma, fibrous nodule

14.5.3.2 Introduction

- The most common soft tissue lesion of the oral cavity
- Not considered a true neoplasm but represents a localized hyperplasia of fibrous connective tissue in response to irritation or trauma (Gonsalves et al. 2007)

14.5.3.3 Demographics

- More common in individuals in the fourth to sixth decades of life (Esmeili et al. 2005).
- A slight female predominance has been reported.
- Most common on the buccal mucosa along the occlusal plane but may occur anywhere in the oral cavity.
- Small fibrous nodules of the maxillary frenum are also commonly seen.
- Usually less than one centimeter in size but much large lesions have been reported.
- Usually asymptomatic.

14.5.3.4 Appearance (Fig. 14.16a–d)

- Typically appears as a smooth-surfaced pink sessile nodular growth similar in color to the surrounding mucosa.
- Ulceration or increased keratinization of the surface is common due to chronic trauma.

14.5.3.5 Clinical Differential Diagnosis

- A wide range of "bumps" may be included in the differential including lipoma.
- Fibrosed pyogenic granulomas.
- Other benign mesenchymal neoplasms (Esmelli 2005).

14.5.3.6 Treatment and Prognosis

- Simple complete excision is considered the best treatment.
- Recurrence is rare.
- Biopsy is recommended in order to rule out other tumors that may resemble the fibroma.

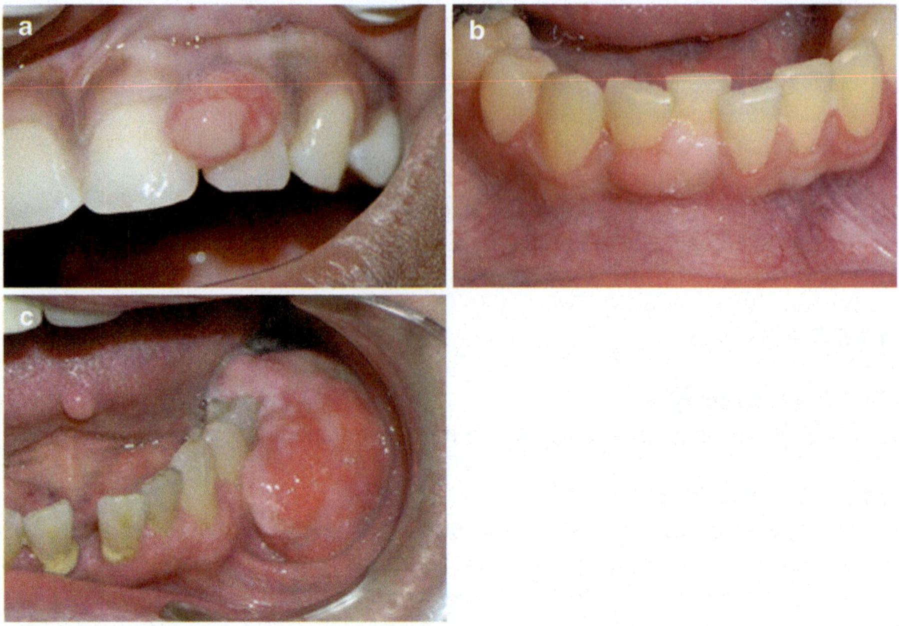

Fig. 14.16 (a) Ulcerated and pedunculated mass on the maxillary facial gingiva in a 16-year-old female. (b) Sessile mass in the anterior mandibular gingiva in a 17-year-old female. (c) A peripheral ossifying fibroma measuring >4 cm in diameter involving the entire posterior mandibular gingiva. The lesion has loosened associated teeth and encroaches on the occlusal surface

14.5.4 Peripheral Ossifying Fibroma

14.5.4.1 Synonyms

- Peripheral fibroma with calcification; Ossifying Fibroid Epulis

14.5.4.2 Introduction

- Common gingival lesion that is considered to be reactive rather than a true tumor
- The lesion is believed to arise from the periodontal ligament, hence the potential to produce calcification (Bodner and Dayan 1987)

14.5.4.3 Demographics

- Predominantly seen in teenagers and young adults (Cuisia and Brannon 2001)
- Predilection for females, up to two-thirds of the cases reported are in women
- Occurs exclusively on the gingiva, more common on the maxillary anterior facial gingiva in the incisor-canine region

14.5.4.4 Appearance (Fig. 14.17a–c)

- Nodular pink gingival mass that may be pedunculated or sessile.
- Ulceration of the surface epithelium is common.
- Arises from the interdental papilla.

- Usually less than a centimeter in size but larger lesions have been reported.
- May cause migration and loosening of adjacent teeth.

14.5.4.5 Radiographic Features

- Not applicable in most cases since it is not required for diagnosis. The amount of calcification within a lesion is usually insufficient to reflect on a radiograph.
- However, in rare cases with extensive calcification, radiographic evidence is noted.

14.5.4.6 Treatment and Prognosis

- Local surgical excision down to periosteum to prevent recurrence.
- 15–20 % recurrence rate is reported (Buduneli et al. 2001).
- Submission of tissue for microscopic examination is recommended in order to rule out other entities and continued growth.

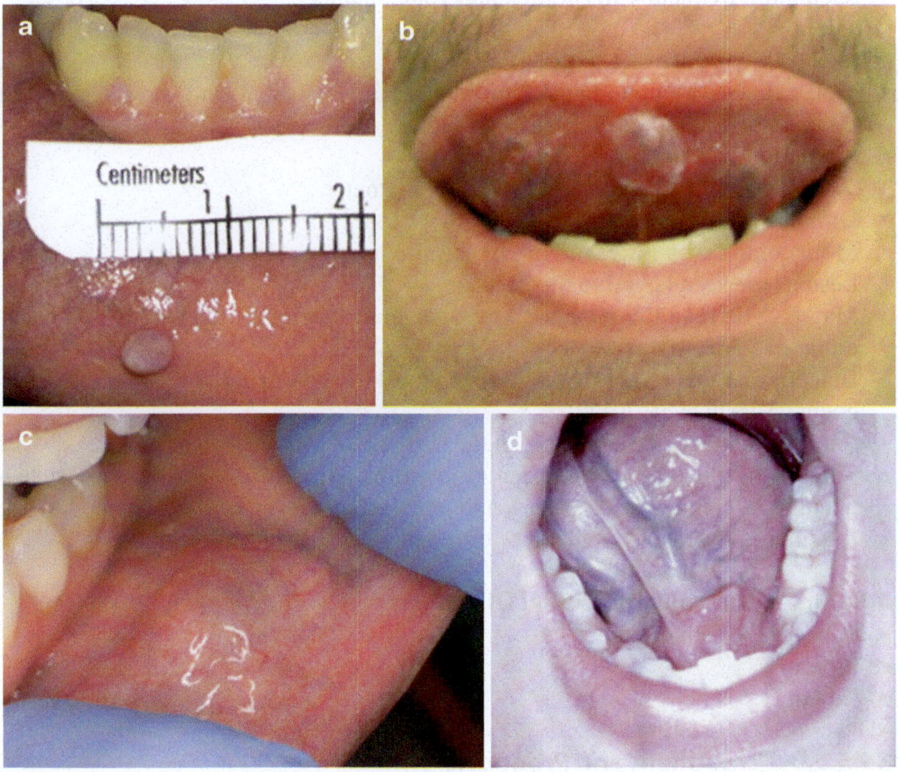

Fig. 14.17 (**a**) The mucocele presenting as a small pedunculated lesion on the lower lip. (**b**) Mucocele of the ventral tongue tends to exhibit a higher recurrence. (**c**) Large sessile dome-shaped swelling of the lower lip in a 12-year-old male. (**d**) A ranula is a mucocele of the floor of the mouth

- Thorough debridement of involved teeth to eliminate possible irritants is recommended.
- Periodontal surgery may be required to restore aesthetics.

14.5.5 Mucocele

14.5.5.1 Synonyms

Mucus extravasation phenomenon; mucus escape reaction

14.5.5.2 Introduction

- A well-defined lesion due to the accumulation and retention of saliva in the connective tissue
- Caused by trauma to the minor salivary gland duct

14.5.5.3 Demographics

- Seen more frequently in children and young adults

14.5.5.4 Appearance (Fig. 14.18a–d)

- Well-defined, asymptomatic, bluish lesion, translucent and slowly growing lesions.
- Asymptomatic and fluctuant.
- Vary in size from 1 mm to several cm in diameter.
- Duration varies from few days to many years.
- More common on lower lip; rarely develop on upper lip.
- Lesions are seen lateral to the lip line.
- May also be found in the buccal mucosa, tongue, floor of the mouth, and retromolar pad area.
- Blandin and Nuhn mucoceles in the ventral portion of the tongue are less frequent (Adachi et al. 2011).
- Superficial mucoceles are seen on the soft palate and retromolar pad areas.
- Superficial mucoceles have been reported to occur in association with lichen planus, lichenoid drug eruptions, and graft-versus-host disease (Mandel 2001).
- Ranula is a mucocele on the floor of the mouth (Baurmash 2003).

14.5.5.5 Clinical Differential Diagnosis

- Salivary duct cyst
- Fibroma
- Lipoma

14.5.5.6 Treatment and Prognosis

- Some disappear spontaneously.
- Chronic lesions require removal of the feeding gland and/or marsupialization (Bahadure et al. 2012).

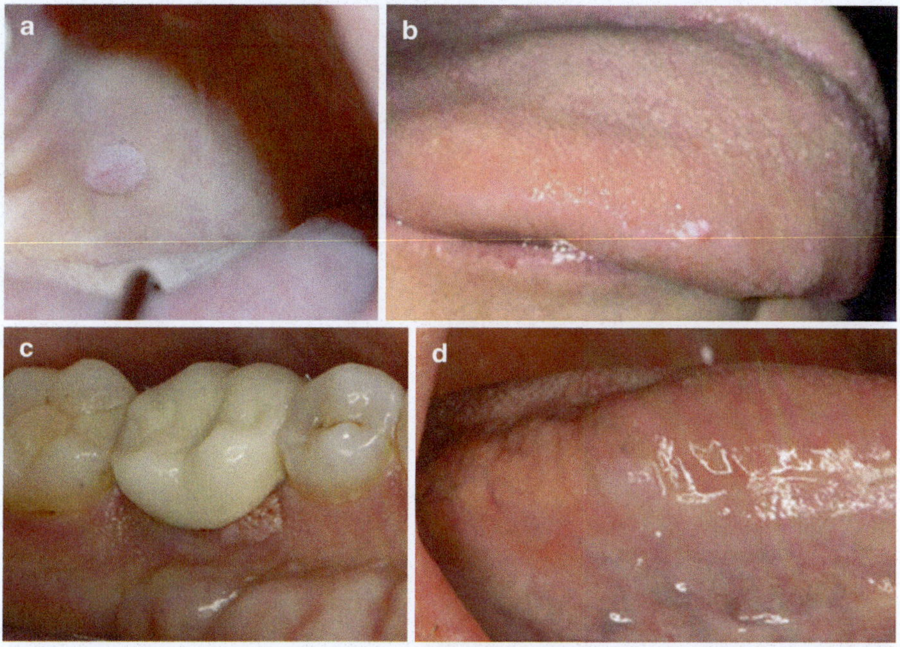

Fig. 14.18 (**a**) Large papilloma of the soft palate; the lesion was present for at least four years. (**b**) Small white papillary lesion on the lateral dorsal tongue. (**c**) Papilloma of the mandibular lingual gingiva with fingerlike projections that is evident. (**d**) "Flat" papilloma of the tongue. The lesion is sessile but demonstrates a papillary surface

14.5.6 Papilloma

14.5.6.1 Synonyms

- Squamous papilloma

14.5.6.2 Introduction

- Epithelial proliferation caused by HPV 6 and HPV 11 (Abbey et al. 1980, Syrjanen 2003)

14.5.6.3 Demographics

- Commonly seen in 30–50 years of age (Carniero et al. 2009)
- No gender predilection

14.5.6.4 Appearance (Fig. 14.19a–d)

- Sessile or pedunculated lesion
- Multiple fingerlike projections
- Color varies from normal color to red to white
- Usually solitary
- Commonly seen on the soft palate or tongue (Bao et al. 2012)

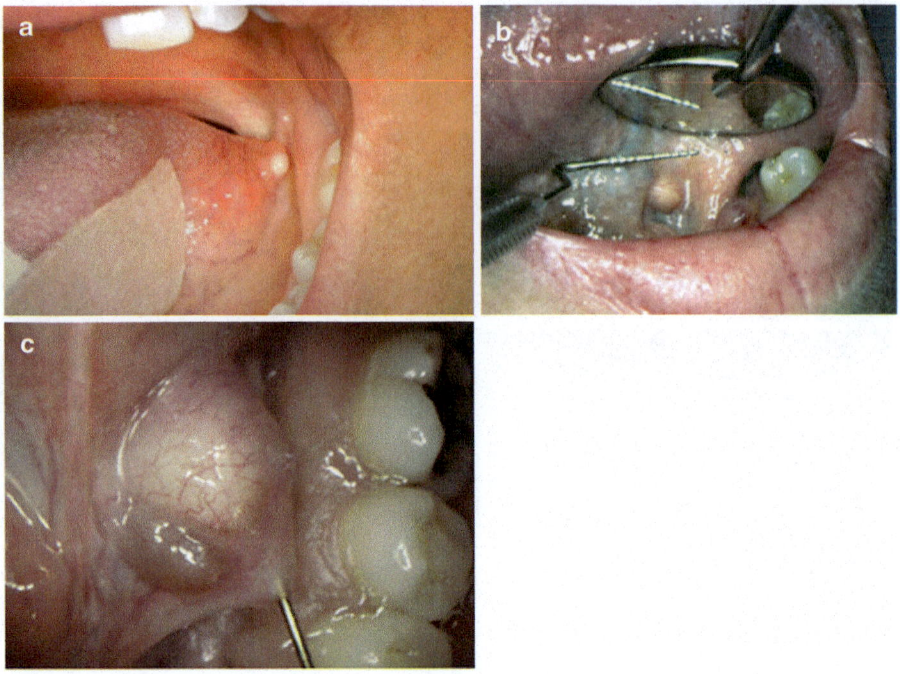

Fig. 14.19 (**a**) This is a typical lymphoepithelial cyst appearing as a yellowish-white sessile nodule on the posterior lateral tongue. (**b**) A fairly common location for this entity; lymphoepithelial cyst on the floor of the mouth. (**c**) A large lymphoepithelial cyst on the floor of the mouth in a 58-year-old male

14.5.6.5 Clinical Differential Diagnosis

- Verruca vulgaris
- Condyloma acuminatum
- Verruciform xanthoma

14.5.6.6 Treatment and Prognosis

- Conservative surgical excision

14.5.7 Lymphoepithelial Cyst

14.5.7.1 Synonyms

- Benign lymphoepithelial cyst

14.5.7.2 Introduction

- A cyst with lymphoid tissue in its wall
- May be acquired or developmental (Yang et al. 2012)
- Acquired: Pinching off or obstruction of epithelial tissue of tonsillar crypts; leads to keratin-filled cyst within the lymphoid tissue

- Developmental: Cyst arising from entrapped epithelial or salivary tissue in lymphoid tissue during embryogenesis

14.5.7.3 Demographics

- Occurs at any age; more frequent in young adults

14.5.7.4 Appearance (Fig. 14.20a–c)

- Small, well-demarcated, yellow or white submucosal nodule
- May be firm or soft
- Asymptomatic; pain secondary to trauma
- Frequently reported on the floor of the mouth, ventral tongue, posterior lateral borders of the tongue, palatine tonsils, or soft palate (Buchner and Hansen 1980a, Khelemsky and Mandel 2010)

14.5.7.5 Clinical Differential Diagnosis

- Lymphoid hyperplasia
- Salivary duct cyst
- Epithelial inclusion cyst

14.5.7.6 Treatment and Prognosis

- Surgical excision

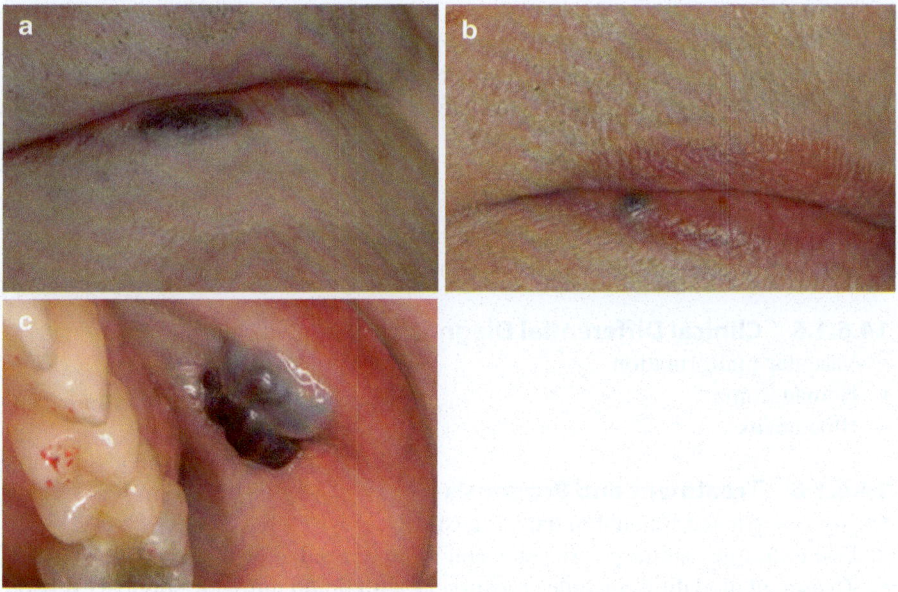

Fig. 14.20 (**a**) A large varicosity on the lower lip of a 72-year-old male. (**b**) Small varicosity of the lower lip in a 78-year-old female. (**c**) A large varicosity on the buccal mucosa. Biopsy revealed organizing thrombus within the lesion

14.6 Pigmented Soft Tissue Lesions

14.6.1 Varicosity

14.6.1.1 Synonyms

- Varices

14.6.1.2 Introduction

- Abnormally dilated and tortuous vein.
- Results from a loss of tone of the connective tissue supporting the vein as a result of loss of elasticity of the elastic fibers or by the weakening of the venous wall.
- Focal and acquired vascular malformation.
- Exact cause unknown.
- Considered to be related to the process of ageing, smoking, and/or cardiovascular disease (Hedström and Bergh 2010).
- Lesions are asymptomatic.

14.6.1.3 Demographics

- Seen in adults.
- Rarely seen in infants.
- Males and females are affected equally.

14.6.1.4 Appearance (Fig. 14.21a–c)

- Present either as multiple blue-purple blebs or ridges or as solitary nodules.
- Ventral surface of the tongue is the site of predilection (Ettinger and Manderson 1974).
- Multiple lesions are seen on the lateral or ventral surface of the tongue and floor of the mouth.
- Solitary lesions are seen typically on the lips and buccal mucosa.
- Lips and buccal mucosa are less common sites.

14.6.1.5 Clinical Differential Diagnosis

- Vascular malformation
- Hemangioma
- Blue nevus

14.6.1.6 Treatment and Prognosis

- None warranted for sublingual varicosities.
- Due to trauma, solitary varicosities on lip may need to be treated.
- Treatment modalities include cryosurgery with liquid nitrogen, surgical excision, sclerosing agents, infrared coagulation, and laser photocoagulation (Azevedo et al. 2003, Gomes et al. 2006).

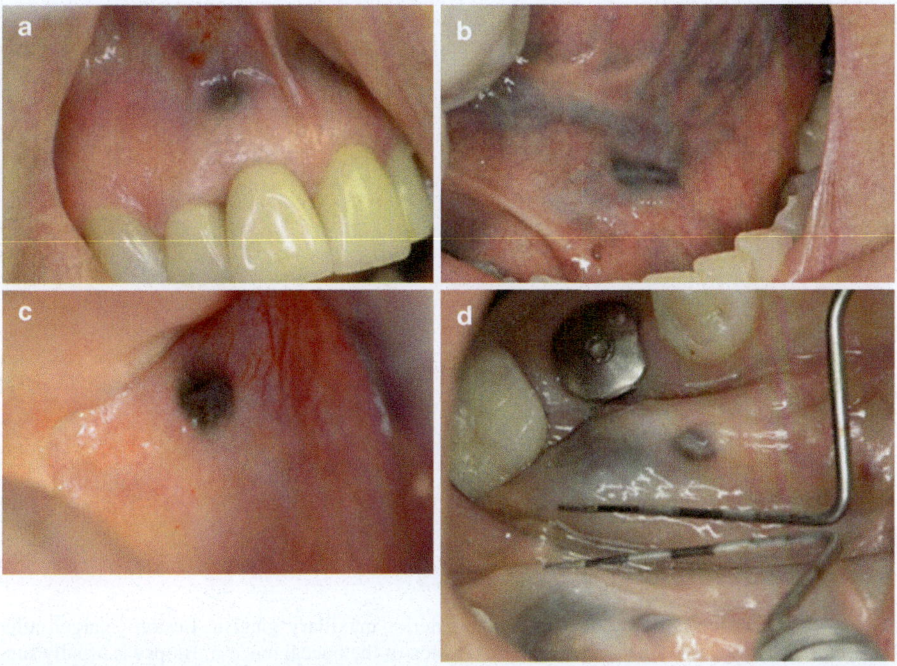

Fig. 14.21 (**a**) Typical amalgam tattoo on the attached tissue in the anterior maxilla. (**b**) Tattooing of the floor of the mouth. (**c**) Large area of deep pigmentation on the posterior buccal mucosa in an edentulous patient. (**d**) Extensive tattooing of the floor of the mouth. Patient extraction of mandibular molar which had large amalgam restoration

14.6.2 Amalgam Tattoo

14.6.2.1 Synonyms

- Focal argyrosis

14.6.2.2 Introduction

- Implantation of amalgam particles into oral mucosa
- Causes: iatrogenic, chronic friction of mucosa against an amalgam restoration, a new amalgam restoration incorporated into dental floss during flossing, high-speed air turbines driving amalgam particles into the oral mucosa or accidental dropping of amalgam pieces into extraction sockets (Buchner and Hansen 1980b)

14.6.2.3 Demographics

- Any mucosal surface adjacent to an amalgam filling may be affected (gingiva, buccal mucosa, palate, and tongue).
- Most common pigmented lesion of the oral cavity.

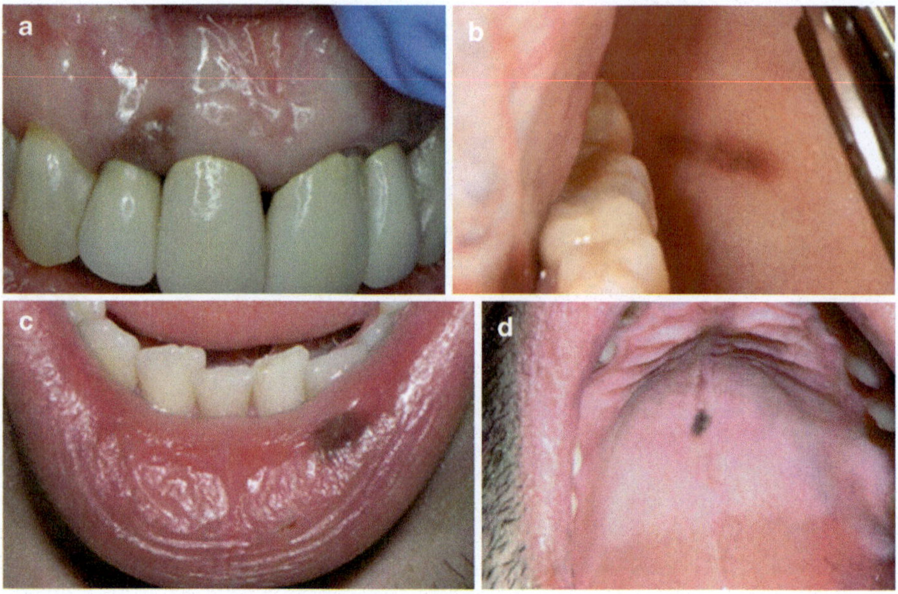

Fig. 14.22 (a) Unusual large macule in the anterior maxillary gingiva. Lesion enlarged after restorations were placed. (b) Large pigmented lesion of the buccal mucosa. Biopsy is usually suggested for such lesions. (c) Macule of the lower lip in a 28-year-old male. (d) Deeply pigmented macule on the hard palate in a 46-year-old male

14.6.2.4 Appearance (Fig. 14.22a–d)

- Blue, black, or gray macules.
- Borders are well-defined or diffuse.
- A slight lateral spread may be seen in early lesions.
- Asymptomatic.

14.6.2.5 Clinical Differential Diagnosis

- Nevi
- Early melanoma
- Medicament-induced pigmentation

14.6.2.6 Radiographic Features

- Amalgam particles may be visible on radiographs if they are sufficiently large.
- Appear as densely radiopaque particles of variable sizes.
- Seen in soft tissue, in areas correlated with the clinical discoloration (Buchner 2004).

14.6.2.7 Treatment and Prognosis

- A strong presumptive clinical diagnosis does not warrant a biopsy or treatment.
- A biopsy may be obtained in cases of doubt.
- Conservative surgical excision, if aesthetics is at stake (Shah and Alster 2002).

14.6.3 Oral Melanotic Macule

14.6.3.1 Synonyms

- Focal melanosis

14.6.3.2 Introduction

- Common focal oral pigmentation
- No malignant potential
- Result from an increase in melanin in the basal or parabasal cells of the epithelium (Buchner et al. 2004)

14.6.3.3 Demographics

- One of the most common melanotic lesions seen in oral cavity (80 % of melanotic lesions)
- Seen more frequently in adults; wide age range
- Female predilection

14.6.3.4 Appearance (Fig. 14.23a–d)

- Appears as an asymptomatic well-demarcated brown lesion.
- The lip is the most common location; other sites of predilection include the buccal mucosa, gingiva, and palate (Lerman et al. 2009).
- Uniformly pigmented lesion.
- Solitary in majority of cases; multiple lesions seen in relation to some syndromes.

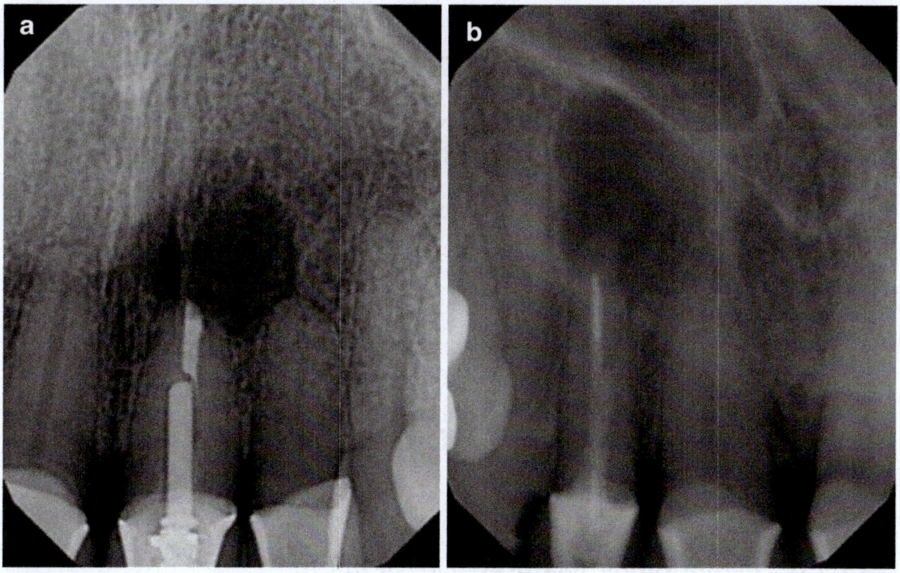

Fig. 14.23 (**a**) Radiolucent lesion involving the apex of teeth #8. (**b**) Radiolucent lesion involving the apex of teeth #8 and #9

- Syndromic multiple macules seen in Peutz-Jeghers syndrome, McCune Albright syndrome, Carney syndrome complex, Bannayan-Ruvalcaba-Riley syndrome, and Laugier- Hunziker syndrome.
- After rapidly reaching their size, they remain constant.
- They do not darken with exposure to sun.

14.6.3.5 Clinical Differential Diagnosis

- Post-inflammatory hyperpigmentation (Lima et al. 2010)
- Medication-induced oral pigmentation (Lima et al. 2010)
- Addison disease
- Early superficial melanoma

14.6.3.6 Treatment and Prognosis

- No treatment needed
- Biopsy recommended in case of doubt (Shen et al. 2011)

14.7 Radiolucent Lesions of the Oral Cavity

14.7.1 Periapical Granuloma/Abscess

14.7.1.1 Synonyms

Chronic apical periodontitis, periapical inflammatory disease (abscess: acute apical periodontitis)

14.7.1.2 Introduction

- Mass of chronically/acutely inflamed granulation tissue at the apex of a non-vital tooth (Bhaskar 1966).
- These can transform into periapical cysts or may undergo acute exacerbations with abscess formation (Estrela et al. 2008).

14.7.1.3 Demographics

Not applicable

14.7.1.4 Appearance

- Usually asymptomatic, but pain and sensitivity can develop.
- Almost, always seen in association with non-vital teeth.

14.7.1.5 Clinical/Radiographic Differential

- Periapical cyst
- Periapical abscess

14.7.1.6 Radiographic Features: (Fig. 14.24a, b)

- A radiolucency of variable size is noted (Estrela et al. 2008).
- It may be associated with root resorption.

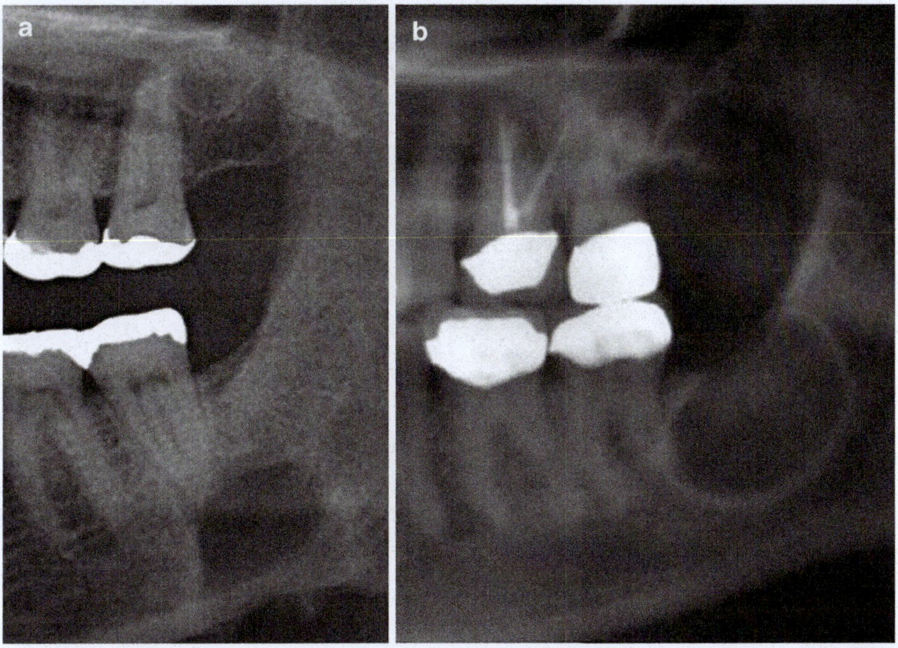

Fig. 14.24 (**a**) Periapical cyst with well-defined radiolucency at the apex of tooth #18. (**b**) Well-defined radiolucency with a sclerotic border distal to the roots of tooth #18

14.7.1.7 Treatment and Prognosis
- If restorable, the tooth is treated with root canal therapy.
- Non-restorable teeth have to be sacrificed.

14.7.2 Periapical Cyst

14.7.2.1 Synonyms
Radicular cyst, apical periodontal cyst, periapical cyst, lateral radicular cyst

14.7.2.2 Introduction
- These arise from the stimulated cell rests of Malassez at the apex of a non-vital tooth resulting in the formation of a true epithelium-lined cyst (Nair 1998).
- Not uncommon and tends to grow slowly without attaining a large size.
- Spontaneous resolution of small lesions is possible (Rosenberg et al. 2010).

14.7.2.3 Demographics
Not applicable

14.7.2.4 Appearance
- Asymptomatic usually.
- Large cysts may exhibit swelling and mild sensitivity (Nair 1998).

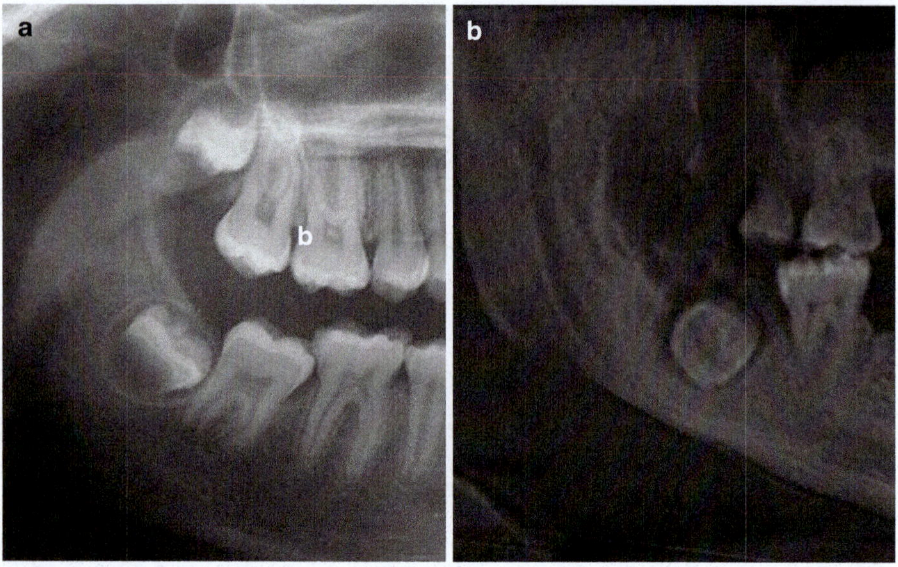

Fig. 14.25 (**a**) Small dentigerous cyst lesion involving tooth #32. (**b**) DC 2 larger dentigerous cyst involving tooth #32

- The involved tooth usually does not respond to thermal and electric pulp testing.

14.7.2.5 Clinical/Radiographic Differential

- Periapical granuloma and periapical abscess
- Odontogenic cyst or tumor
- Mesenchymal lesion
- Rarely metastatic lesions

14.7.2.6 Radiographic Features: (Fig. 14.25a, b)

- Rounded radiolucency around the apex of a non-vital tooth (Nair 1998).
- Loss of the lamina dura is possible (Rosenberg et al. 2010).
- Root resorption is common.

14.7.2.7 Treatment and Prognosis

- Enucleation of the cyst followed with appropriate management similar to periapical granuloma/abscess (Rosenberg et al. 2010).
- It usually does not recur.
- If required submission of tissue for examination is important.

Pearl: lateral radicular cyst

- Similar to the apical periodontal cyst but arising from the aberrant lateral canals

14.7.3 Dentigerous Cyst

14.7.3.1 Synonyms

- Follicular Cyst

14.7.3.2 Introduction

- It is formed by the separation of the follicle from around the crown of an unerupted tooth (Aher et al. 2013).
- It is the most common type of developmental odontogenic cyst (Gonzalez et al. 2011).
- May be attached to the tooth at the cementoenamel junction.

14.7.3.3 Demographics

- They are seen mostly in patients between 10 and 30 years of age.
- Most common location is the mandibular third molars followed by the maxillary canines (Aher et al. 2013).

14.7.3.4 Appearance

- Small dentigerous cysts are generally asymptomatic.
- It may grow to a considerable size, with associated painless expansion and displacement of the involved tooth (Gonzalez et al. 2011).

14.7.3.5 Clinical/Radiographic Differential

- Odontogenic keratocyst
- Unicystic ameloblastoma
- Glandular odontogenic cyst

14.7.3.6 Radiographic Features: (Fig. 14.26a, b)

- A unilocular radiolucent area in association with crown of an unerupted tooth.
- Usually well defined with sclerotic border, but infected cyst may have ill-defined borders.
- Almost 50 % cases exhibit root resorption adjacent teeth if cyst is large in size (Gonzalez et al. 2011).
- Radiographic distinction is that the radiolucent area should be at least 3–4 mm in diameter.

14.7.3.7 Treatment and Prognosis

- Careful enucleation of the cyst together with removal of the unerupted tooth is the treatment of choice (Tamgadge et al. 2011).
- Large cysts may be treated by marsupialization.
- The prognosis is excellent and recurrence is seldom noted.
- Complications associated with dentigerous cysts include ameloblastomatous transformation, squamous cell carcinoma arising within the lining epithelium, or even a mucoepidermoid carcinoma arising within the lining epithelium.

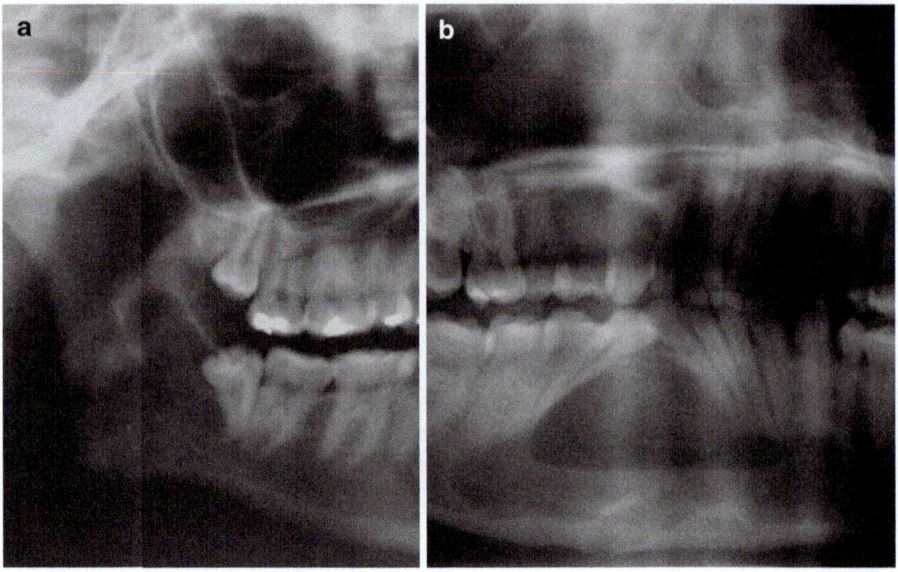

Fig. 14.26 (**a**) Large odontogenic keratocyst involving tooth #32. (**b**) Odontogenic keratocyst involving the anterior mandible with significant root divergence

14.7.4 Odontogenic Keratocyst

14.7.4.1 Synonyms

Keratocystic odontogenic tumor (KOT)

14.7.4.2 Introduction

- A developmental odontogenic cyst unique for its histopathologic features and clinical behavior (Islam and Bhattacharyya 2015).
- It is thought to be a neoplasm due to its different growth mechanism and biologic behavior (Ramesh et al. 2015).

14.7.4.3 Demographics

- 60 % are diagnosed in people between 10 and 40 years (Ramesh et al. 2015).
- Mandible is involved in 60–80 % cases, usually the posterior body and ascending ramus areas.
- It grows in an anteroposterior direction within the medullary cavity of the bone causing little or no expansion.
- Patients with multiple keratocysts or with one cyst below the age of 20 years should be evaluated for the nevoid basal cell carcinoma (Gorlin-Goltz) syndrome (Ramesh et al. 2015).

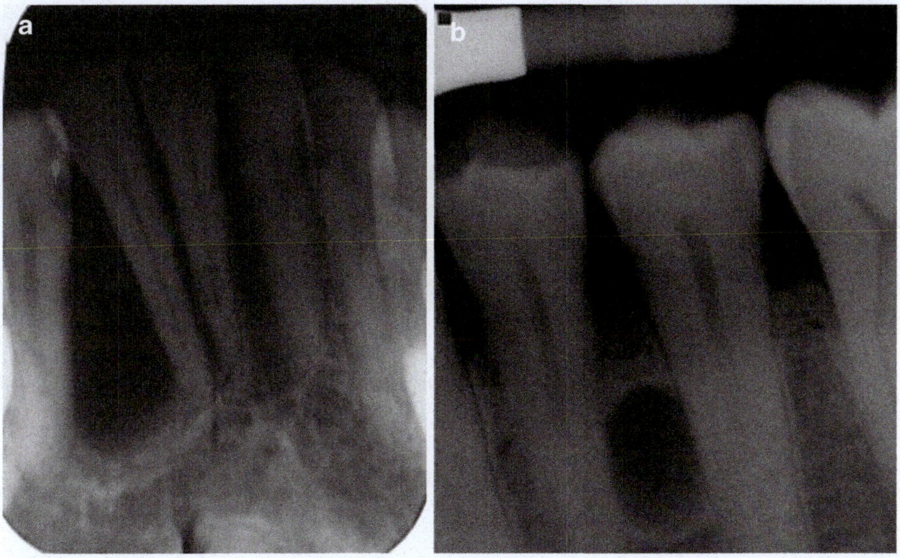

Fig. 14.27 (**a**) Lateral periodontal cyst involving the interradicular aspect of teeth # 23 and 24 with divergence. (**b**) Lateral periodontal cyst involving the interradicular aspect of teeth # 20 and 21

14.7.4.4 Appearance

Not applicable unless completely a soft tissue variant

14.7.4.5 Clinical/Radiographic Differential

- Radicular cyst
- Dentigerous cyst
- Lateral periodontal cyst
- Glandular odontogenic cyst
- Ameloblastoma

14.7.4.6 Radiographic Features: (Fig. 14.27a, b)

- Mostly a well-defined uni- or multilocular radiolucent area with smooth corticated margins (Madras and Lapointe 2008).
- Seen in the posterior body and ascending ramus of the mandible.
- Unerupted tooth associated in 25–40 % of cases.

14.7.4.7 Treatment and Prognosis

- Commonly treated by enucleation and curettage (Madras and Lapointe 2008).
- Tends to recur with a rate of approximately 30 % (Li 2011).
- Patients are not considered disease-free even up to/after 10 years of initial diagnoses.

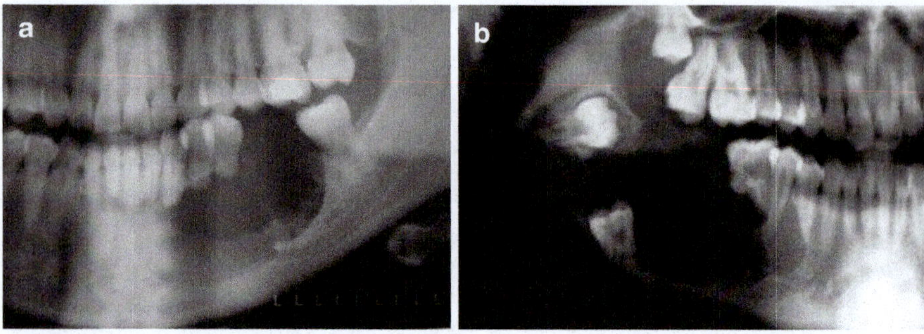

Fig. 14.28 (a) Ameloblastoma exhibiting root resorption. (b) Ameloblastoma exhibiting multilocular radiolucency with impacted tooth pushed to the lower border of the mandible and associated root resorption

14.7.5 Lateral Periodontal Cyst (LPC)

14.7.5.1 Synonyms

- Botryoid odontogenic cysts (multilocular variant)

14.7.5.2 Introduction

- LPC account for less than 2% of the developmental odontogenic cysts of the jaws (Friedrich et al. 2014).
- This diagnosis is reserved only when the cyst is noted in the lateral periodontal region of a vital tooth.

14.7.5.3 Demographics

- 65% are seen in the mandibular canine-premolar area as well as the maxillary lateral incisor region.
- Usually an asymptomatic lesion detected on routine radiographs.

14.7.5.4 Appearance

- Not applicable

14.7.5.5 Clinical/Radiographic Differential

- Lateral radicular cyst
- Glandular odontogenic cyst
- Odontogenic keratocyst
- Ameloblastoma

14.7.5.6 Radiographic Features: (Fig. 14.28a, b)

- LPCs commonly present as a well-circumscribed radiolucent area located laterally to the roots.
- These lesions have a multilocular appearance occasionally, and in those cases the term "botryoid odontogenic cyst" is used (Frei et al. 2014).

14.7.5.7 Treatment and Prognosis

- Conservative enucleation is the treatment of choice. Recurrence is unusual.

14.7.6 Ameloblastoma

14.7.6.1 Synonyms

None

14.7.6.2 Introduction

- Ameloblastomas are the most common clinically significant odontogenic tumor (Masthan et al. 2015).
- These are slow-growing, locally invasive tumors that run a benign course in most cases.
- Ameloblastomas may be of three different clinical radiologic types:
  - Conventional solid or multicystic (about 86 % of all cases)
  - Unicystic (about 13 % of all cases)
  - Peripheral (extra osseous) (about 1 % of all cases)

14.7.6.3 Demographics

- Ameloblastomas tend to occur in adults (third to seventh decades) (Masthan et al. 2015).
- These are often asymptomatic tumors and may not be seen in children or teenagers.
- A painless swelling or expansion of the jaw is the usual clinical presentation.
- About 85 % of conventional ameloblastomas occur in the mandible, most often in the molar-ascending ramus area (Reichart et al. 1995).

14.7.6.4 Appearance

If expansive and large, may be clinically appreciated as a jaw swelling

14.7.6.5 Clinical/Radiographic Differential

- Large-sized dentigerous cysts
- Central giant cell granuloma
- Odontogenic keratocyst
- Odontogenic myxoma

14.7.6.6 Radiographic Features: (Fig. 14.29a, b)

- Typical radiographic feature is a multilocular radiolucent lesion that may present with a "soap bubble" appearance (Philipsen and Reichart 1998).
- Buccal and lingual cortical expansion with resorption of the roots of adjacent teeth.
- An unerupted tooth, most often a mandibular third molar, is associated with the radiolucent defect (Junquera et al. 2003).

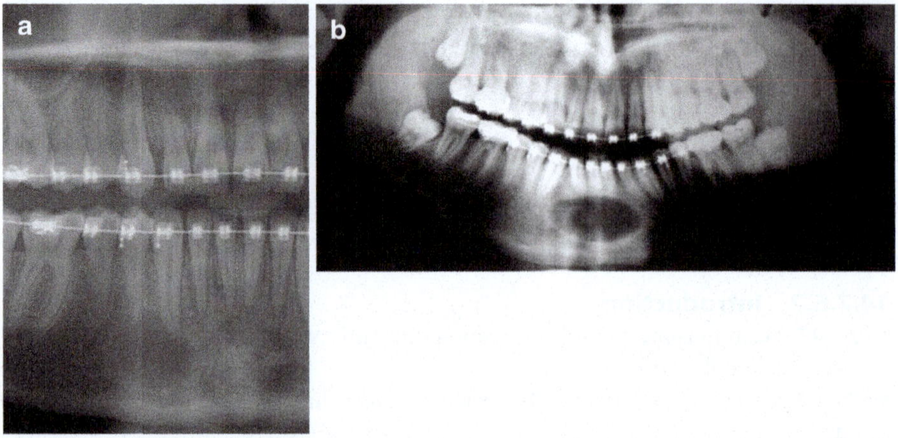

Fig. 14.29 (**a**) Simple bone cyst appears as a well-defined radiolucency with mild scalloping. (**b**) The well-defined corticated radiolucency on the anterior of the mandible is a simple bone cyst

14.7.6.7 Treatment and Prognosis

- The treatment is simple enucleation and curettage to en bloc resection.
- Recurrence rates of 55–90 % have been reported, and patients may not be considered free of disease after 20 years from initial diagnosis (Reichart et al. 1995).
- Unicystic ameloblastoma: has a relatively unique presentation including conservative treatment with enucleation and curettage, and a recurrence rate of 10–20 % has been reported (Philipsen and Reichart 1998).

14.7.7 Simple Bone Cyst

14.7.7.1 Synonyms

- Traumatic bone Cyst and hemorrhagic bone cyst

14.7.7.2 Introduction

- The cause and pathogenesis remain uncertain and controversial (Curran et al. 1973).

14.7.7.3 Demographics

- Usually asymptomatic and seen in patients between 10 and 20 years of age.
- Common location is mandible, especially in the premolar and molar areas (Kaugars and Cale 1987).

14.7.7.4 Appearance

- Not applicable

14.7.7.5 Clinical/Radiographic Differential

- If seen in proximity to teeth: Lateral radicular cyst
- Glandular odontogenic cyst

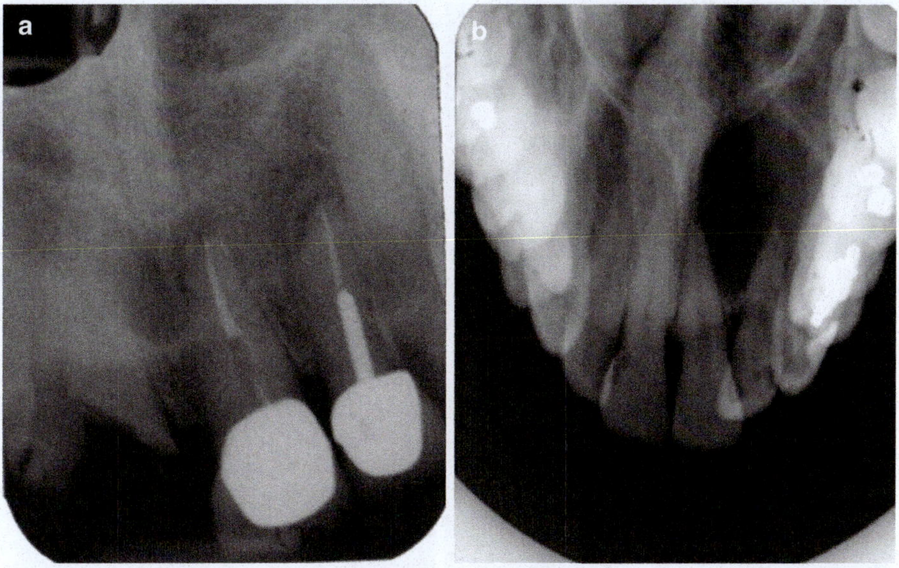

Fig. 14.30 (**a**) Nasopalatine duct cyst is seen as a radiolucency involving the root of tooth #9. (**b**) Nasopalatine duct cyst causing divergence of roots between teeth # 7 and 8

- Odontogenic keratocyst
- Unicystic ameloblastoma

14.7.7.6 Radiographic Features: (Fig. 14.30a, b)

- Well-delineated radiolucent defect with scalloping upward between the roots.

14.7.7.7 Treatment and Prognosis

- Surgical exploration to establish the diagnosis usually proves curative (Bhattacharyya et al. 2014).

14.7.8 Nasopalatine Duct Cyst

14.7.8.1 Synonyms

- Incisive Canal Cyst

14.7.8.2 Introduction

- Most common non-odontogenic cyst, occurring in about 1 % of the population.
- It is believed to arise from remnants of the nasopalatine duct (Bains et al. 2016).

14.7.8.3 Demographics

- Symptoms include swelling of the anterior palate, drainage, and pain (Aparna et al. 2014).

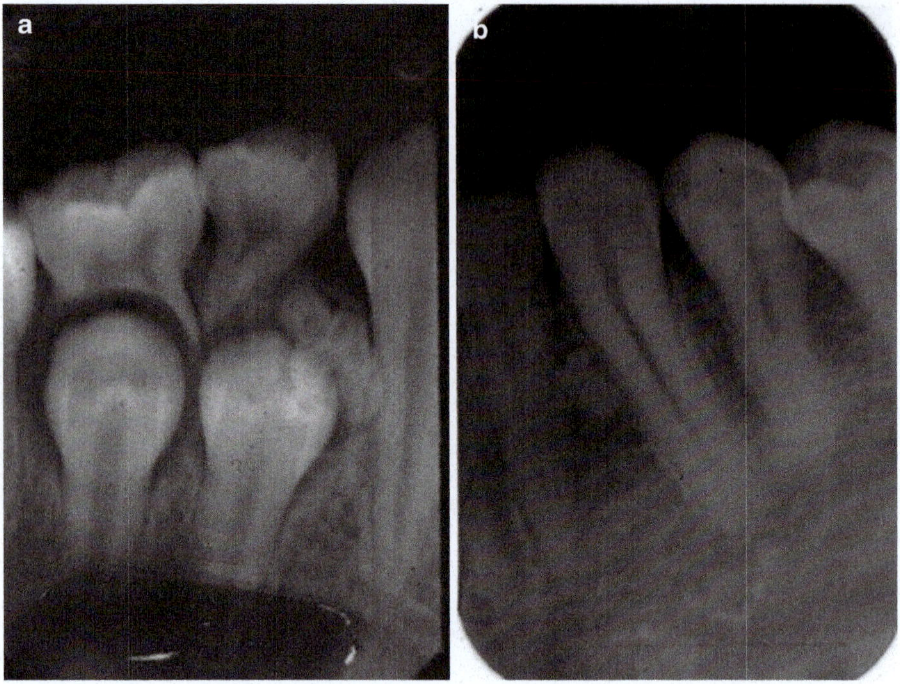

Fig. 14.31 (**a**) Odontoma presents as a radiopaque lesion preventing eruption of the premolar tooth. (**b**) The odontoma lesion is found in the interradicular aspect of teeth# 26 and 27

14.7.8.4 Appearance

- If large, may be appreciated clinically as an anterior maxillary swelling (Aparna et al. 2014)

14.7.8.5 Clinical/Radiographic Differential

- Large incisive foramen
- Median palatal cyst
- Lateral periodontal cyst
- Odontogenic keratocyst

14.7.8.6 Radiographic Features: (Fig. 14.31a, b)

- A well-circumscribed (occasionally resembling an "inverted pear") radiolucency in or near the midline of the anterior maxilla between and apical to the central incisor teeth.
- Most cysts range from 1.0 to 2.5 cm diameter.

14.7.8.7 Treatment and Prognosis

- Nasopalatine duct cysts are treated by surgical enucleation.

14.8 Radiopaque Lesions

14.8.1 Odontoma

14.8.1.1 Synonyms
Not applicable

14.8.1.2 Introduction
- Most common odontogenic tumor.
- Odontomas are considered hamartomas rather than true neoplasms.
- These may be compound and complex types.
- The compound odontoma is composed of multiple, small toothlike structures (De Oliveira et al. 2001).
- The complex odontoma consists of a conglomerate mass of enamel and dentin, which bears no anatomic resemblance to a tooth.
- Some may show features of both types.

14.8.1.3 Demographics
- Most odontomas are detected during the first two decades of life, and the mean age at the time of diagnosis is 14 years.
- Odontomas occur somewhat more frequently in the maxilla than in the mandible.
- The compound type is more often seen in the anterior maxilla (Kulkarni et al. 2012).
- Complex odontomas occur more often in the molar regions of either jaw.

14.8.1.4 Appearance
Lack of and/or delayed eruption most commonly encountered clinical problem.

14.8.1.5 Clinical/Radiographic Differential Diagnosis
- Supernumerary tooth
- Retained radicular fragments
- Idiopathic osteosclerosis
- Condensing osteitis

14.8.1.6 Radiographic Features: (Fig. 14.32a, b)
- These present as a collection of toothlike structures of varying size (Kulkarni et al. 2012).
- The complex odontoma presents as a calcified mass with the radiodensity of tooth structure.
- An unerupted tooth is frequently associated with the odontoma, and the odontoma prevents eruption of the tooth (Verma et al. 2015).

14.8.1.7 Treatment and Prognosis
- Odontomas are treated by simple local excision, and the prognosis is excellent.

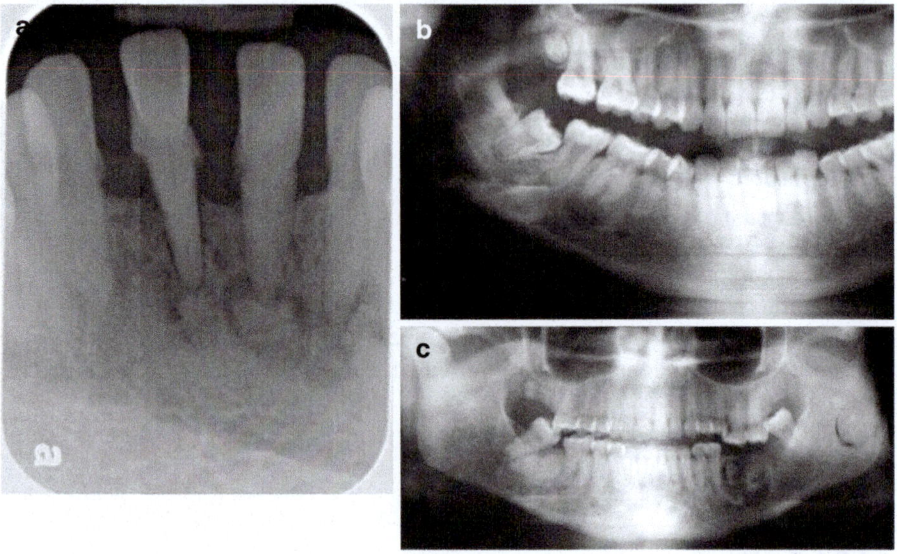

Fig. 14.32 (a) Periapical cemento-osseous dysplasia appears as mixed radiopaque and radiolucent lesions at apex of anterior teeth. (b) A radiolucent periapical cemento-osseous dysplasia lesion associated with tooth #30. (c) Mixed radiopaque and radiolucent lesions involving the entire lower jaw with periapical cemento-osseous dysplasia lesions

14.8.2 Cemento-Osseous Dysplasias

14.8.2.1 Synonyms

- Cemental dysplasia and benign fibro-osseous lesions

14.8.2.2 Introduction

- These are limited to the tooth-bearing areas of the jaws. Cemento-osseous dysplasia is the most common type of fibro-osseous lesion in day-to-day dental practice (Bhattacharyya and Islam 2015).
- On the basis of their clinical and radiologic features, it is prudent to separate these into three groups (Ryan et al. 2014; Islam et al. 2008):
  - Periapical cemento-osseous dysplasia
  - Focal cemento-osseous dysplasia
  - Florid cemento-osseous dysplasia

14.8.2.3 Demographics

- Periapical cemento-osseous dysplasias (Islam et al. 2008).
  - Predominantly involves the lower anterior periapical region.
  - May be multiple in presentation.
  - There is a marked predilection for female patients (14:1) and for blacks.
- Focal cemento-osseous dysplasia (Ryan et al. 2014).
  - These lesions are more commonly seen in whites and young to middle-aged females.
  - The posterior mandible (i.e., premolar/molar region) is the predominant site.

- Florid cemento-osseous dysplasia (Islam et al. 2008)
  - These show a striking predilection for adult black women.
  - The lesions tend to be bilateral with often quite symmetric involvement.
  - Rarely these may present with dull pain, especially with intervention.
- Generally, cemento-osseous dysplasia is seen between ages 30 and 50 (Islam et al. 2008).
- Teeth are invariably vital and seldom have restorations.

14.8.2.4 Appearance

- Not applicable

14.8.2.5 Clinical/Radiographic Differential Diagnosis

- Periapical granuloma
- Cyst and abscess
- Idiopathic osteosclerosis
- Condensing osteitis

14.8.2.6 Radiographic Features: (Fig. 14.33a–c)

- Asymptomatic, usually discovered incidentally (Bhattacharyya and Islam 2015).
- Most lesions tend to have a mixed radiolucent and radiopaque appearance.
- The end-stage lesions tend to show circumscribed dense calcifications with a narrow radiolucent rim (Islam et al. 2008).

14.8.2.7 Treatment and Prognosis

- Do not require treatment and biopsy is not indicated

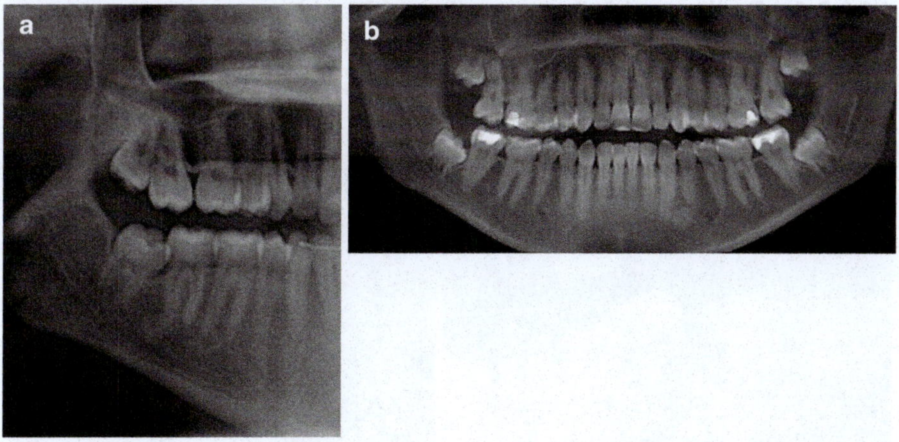

Fig. 14.33 (**a**) Idiopathic osteosclerosis presents as a radio-opacity at the apex of tooth # 31. (**b**) Isolated radiopacity between the apex of vital teeth # 21 and 22 was diagnosed as idiopathic osteosclerosis

14.8.3 Idiopathic Osteosclerosis

14.8.3.1 Synonyms

- Dense bone island and bone scar

14.8.3.2 Introduction

- These are isolated, asymptomatic, uniformly radiopaque foci of dense bone often noted on routine dental radiographs (Moshfeghi et al. 2014).
- Commonly seen in the periapical areas of teeth with vital pulps (Yonetsu et al. 1997)

14.8.3.3 Demographics

- Invariably asymptomatic (Moshfeghi et al. 2014).
- It is most commonly seen between 20 and 40 years of age (Yonetsu et al. 1997).
- About 90 % of examples are seen in the mandible, most often in the first molar area.

14.8.3.4 Appearance

Not applicable

14.8.3.5 Clinical/Radiographic Differential Diagnosis

- Condensing osteitis
- Focal chronic sclerosing osteomyelitis
- Cemento-osseous dysplasia
- Osteoblastoma

14.8.3.6 Radiographic Features: (Fig. 14.34a, b)

- A well-defined, round or elliptical radiodense mass usually varying from 3 mm to 2 cm.

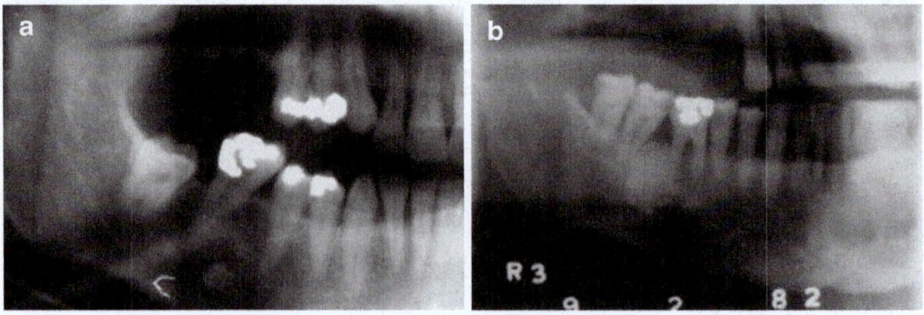

Fig. 14.34 (**a**) Condensing osteitis presents as a radiopaque/radiolucent lesion between the apex of teeth # 29 and 30. (**b**) Large condensing osteitis between the apex of teeth # 30 and 31

- The radiodense area is not surrounded by a radiolucent rim (Moshfeghi et al. 2014).
- Mostly associated with the root apex of vital/asymptomatic teeth (Yonetsu et al. 1997).

14.8.3.7 Treatment and Prognosis

- No treatment is indicated.

14.8.4 Condensing Osteitis

14.8.4.1 Synonyms

Focal sclerosing osteomyelitis

14.8.4.2 Introduction

- Localized areas of bone sclerosis associated with pulpitis (from large carious lesions or deep coronal restorations) or pulpal necrosis (Verzak et al. 2012; Holly et al. 2009).

14.8.4.3 Demographics

- This is seen most frequently in children and young adults (Holly et al. 2009).
- Most cases occur in the premolar and molar areas of the mandible commonly associated with non-vital teeth (Verzak et al. 2012).

14.8.4.4 Appearance

- Not applicable

14.8.4.5 Clinical/Radiographic Differential Diagnosis

- Condensing osteitis
- Focal chronic sclerosing osteomyelitis
- Cemento-osseous dysplasia
- Osteoblastoma

14.8.4.6 Radiographic Features

- A localized, usually uniform, zone of increased radiodensity adjacent to the apex of an involved or symptomatic tooth (Verzak et al. 2012).

14.8.4.7 Treatment and Prognosis

- Treatment consists of resolution of the odontogenic focus of infection either by extracting the tooth or endodontic treatment if lesions are active (Holly et al. 2009).
- 85 % of cases of condensing osteitis will regress spontaneously, mostly completely or partially (Mainville et al. 2016).

References

White Soft Tissue Lesions

Axéll T, Pindborg JJ, Smith CJ, van der Waal I. Oral white lesions with special reference to precancerous and tobacco-related lesions: conclusions of an international symposium held in Uppsala, Sweden May18–21 1994. An International Collaborative Group on Oral White Lesions. J Oral Pathol Med. 1996;25:49–54.

Petti S. Pooled estimate of world leukoplakia prevalence: a systematic review. Oral Oncol. 2003;39:770–80.

Ribeiro AS, Salles PR, da Silva TA, Mesquita RA. A review of the nonsurgical treatment of oral leukoplakia. Int J Dent. 2010;2010:186018.

van der Waal I. Potentially malignant disorders of the oral and oropharyngeal mucosa: present concepts of management. Oral Oncol. 2010;46:423–5.

Warnakulasuriya S, Johnson NW, van der Waal I. Nomenclature and classification of potentially malignant disorders of the oral mucosa. J Oral Pathol Med. 2007;36:575–80.

Lichen Planus (LP)

Au J, Patel D, Campbell JH. Oral lichen planus. Oral Maxillofac Surg Clin N Am. 2013;25:93–100.

Fitzpatrick SJ, Hirsch SA, Gordon SC. The malignant transformation of oral lichen planus and oral lichenoid lesions: a systematic review. J Am Dent Assoc. 2014;145(1):45–56.

Giunta JL. Oral lichenoid reactions versus lichen planus. J Mass Dent Soc. 2001;50(2):22–5.

Lodi G, Carrozzo M, Furness S, Thongprasom K. Interventions for treating oral lichen planus: a systemic review. Be J Dermatol. 2012;66:938–47.

Usatine RP, Tinitigan M. Diagnosis and treatment of lichen planus. Am Fam Physician. 2011;84:53–60.

Leukoedema

Bhattacharyya I, Cohen D, Silverman Jr S. Red and white lesions of the oral mucosa. In: Greenberg MS, Glick M, editors. Burket's oral medicine: diagnosis and treatment. 10th ed. Hamilton: BC Decker; 2003. p. 85–125.

Canaan TJ, Meehan SC. Variation of structure and appearance of the oral mucosa. Derm Clin N Am. 2005;49:1–14.

Martin JL, Crump EP. Leukoedema of the buccal mucosa in Negro children and youth. Oral Surg Oral Med Oral Pathol. 1972;34:49–58.

Cheek/Tongue Chewing

Allen AM, Camisa C. Oral disease. In: Callen JP, Horn TD, Mancini AJ, Salasche SJ, Schaffer JV, Schwarz T, editors. Dermatology. 2nd ed. Spain: Mosby Elsevier; 2008. p. 1044.

Glass LF, Maize JC. Morsicatio buccarum et labiorum (excessive cheek and lip biting). Am J Dermatopathol. 1991;13:271–4.

Scully C, Hegarty A. The oral cavity and lips. In: Burns T, Breathnach S, Cox N, Griffiths C, editors. Rook's textbook of dermatology, vol. 69. 8th ed. Massachusetts: Blackwell; 2010. p. 87–8.
Tomás Carmona I, Cameselle Tejeiro J, Diz Dios P, Seoane Lestón J, Castro Ferreiro M, Limeres Posses J. Morsicatio linguarum versus oral hairy leukoplakia. Dermatology. 2000;201:281–2.
Woo SB, Lin D. Morsicatio mucosae oris–a chronic oral frictional keratosis, not a leukoplakia. J Oral Maxillofac Surg. 2009;67:140–6.

Geographic Tongue

Assimakopoulos D, Patrikakos G, Fotika C, Elisaf M. Benign migratory glossitis or geographic tongue: an enigmatic oral lesion. Am J Med. 2002;113:751–5.
Femiano F. Geographic tongue (migrant glossitis) and psoriasis. Minerva Stomatol. 2001;50:213–7.
Jainkittivong A, Langlais RP. Geographic tongue: clinical characteristics of 188 cases. J Contemp Dent Pract. 2005;6:123–35.
Menni S, Boccardi D, Crosti C. Painful geographic tongue (benign migratory glossitis) in a child. J Eur Acad Dermatol Venereol. 2004;18:737–8.

Desquamative Gingivitis

Endo H, Rees TD, Hallmon WW, Kuyama K, Nakadai M, Kato T, et al. Disease progression from mucosal to mucocutaneous involvement in a patient with desquamative gingivitis associated with pemphigus vulgaris. J Periodontol. 2008;79(2):369–75.
Guiglia R, Di Liberto C, Pizzo G, Picone L, Lo Muzio L, Gallo PD, et al. A combined treatment regimen for desquamative gingivitis in patients with oral lichen planus. J Oral Pathol Med. 2007;36(2):110–6.
Nisengard RJ, Neiders M. Desquamative lesions of the gingiva. J Periodontol. 1981;52: 500–10.
Rees TD. Desquamative gingivitis/mucocutaneous diseases commonly affecting the gingiva. In: Hall's critical decisions in periodontology. 5th ed, Harpenau LA, Kao RT, Lundergan WP, Sanz M. China: People's Medical Publishing House; 2011.
Scully C, Porter SR. The clinical spectrum of desquamative gingivitis. Semin Cutan Med Surg. 1997;16:308–13.

Candidiasis

Barnett JA. A history of research on yeasts 12: medical yeasts part 1, Candida albicans. Yeast. 2008;25:385–417.
Rüping MJ, Vehreschild JJ, Cornely OA. Patients at high risk of invasive fungal infections: when and how to treat. Drugs. 2008;68:1941–62.
Samaranayake LP, Keung Leung W, Jin L. Oral mucosal fungal infections. Periodontol. 2009;49:39–59.
Soysa NS, Samaranayake LP, Ellepola AN. Diabetes mellitus as a contributory factor in oral candidosis. Diabet Med. 2006;23:455–9.
Webb BC, Thomas CJ, Whittle T. A 2-year study of Candida associated denture stomatitis treatment in aged care subjects. Gerodontology. 2005;22:168–76.

Erythroplakia

Reichart PA, Philipsen HP. Oral leukoplakia-a review. Oral Oncol. 2005;41:551–6.
Shafer WG, Waldron CA. Erythroplakia of the oral cavity. Cancer. 1975;36:1021–8.
Van der Waal I. Potentially malignant disorders of the oral and oropharyngeal mucosa: terminology, classification, and present concepts of management. Oral Oncol. 2009;45(4–5): 317–23.
Villa A, Villa C, Abati S. Oral cancer and oral erythroplakia: an update and implication for clinicians. Aus Dent J. 2011;56:253–6.
Yang SW, Lee YS, Chang LC, Hwang CC, Luo CM, Chen TA. Clinical characteristics of narrow-band imaging of oral erythroplakia and its correlation with pathology. BMC Cancer. 2001; 5:406.

Squamous Cell Carcinoma

Chaturvedi AK. Epidemiology and clinical aspects of HPV in head and neck cancers. Head Neck Pathol. 2012;6 Suppl 1:S16–24.
Deschler DG, Richmon JD, Khariwala SS, Ferris RL, Wang MB. The "new" head and neck cancer patient-young, nonsmoker, nondrinker, and HPV positive: evaluation. Otolaryngol Head Neck Surg. 2014;151:375–80.
Haddad R, Annino D, Tishler RB. Multidisciplinary approach to cancer treatment: focus on head and neck cancer. Dent Clin N Am. 2008;52(1–17):vii.
Muller S, Pan Y, Li R, Chi AC. Changing trends in oral squamous cell carcinoma with particular reference to young patients: 1971–2006. The Emory University experience. Head Neck Pathol. 2008;2:60–6.
Yesuratnam A, Wiesenfeld D, Tsui A, Iseli TA, Hoorn SV, Ang MT. Preoperative evaluation of oral tongue squamous cell carcinoma with intraoral ultrasound and magnetic resonance imaging-comparison with histopathological tumour thickness and accuracy in guiding patient management. Int J Oral Maxillofac Surg. 2014;43:787–94.

Apthous Stomatitis

Belenguer-Guallar I, Jiménez-Soriano Y, Claramunt-Lozano A. Treatment of recurrent aphthous stomatitis. A literature review. J Clin Exp Dent. 2014;6(2):e168–74.
Chavan M, Jain H, Diwan N, Khedkar S, Shete A, Durkar S. Recurrent aphthous stomatitis: a review. J Oral Pathol Med. 2012;41(8):577–83.
Porter SR, Hegarty A, Kaliakatsou F, Hodgson TA, Scully C. Recurrent aphthous stomatitis. Clin Dermatol. 2000;18(5):569–78.
Scully C, Porter S. Oral mucosal disease: recurrent aphthous stomatitis. Br J Oral Maxillofac Surg. 2008;46(3):198–206.

Oral Herpetic Stomatitis

Arduino PG, Porter SR. Oral and perioral herpes simplex virus type 1 (HSV-1) infection: review of its management. Oral Dis. 2006;12:254–70.
Rahimi H, Mara T, Costella J, Speechley M, Bohay R. Effectiveness of antiviral agents for the prevention of recurrent herpes labialis: a systemic review and meta-analysis. Oral Surg Oral Med Oral Pathol Oral Radiol Endod. 2012;113:618–27.
Usatine RP, Tinitigan R. Nongenital herpes simplex virus. Am Fam Physician. 2010;82:1075–82.

Woo SB, Challacombe SJ. Management of recurrent oral herpes simplex infections. Oral Surg Oral Med Oral Pathol Oral Radiol Endod. 2007;103(Suppl):S12.e1–18.

Traumatic Ulcers

Hirshberg A, Amariglo N, Akrish S, Yahalom R, Rosenbaum H, et al. Traumatic ulcerative granuloma with stromal eosinophilia: a reactive lesion of the oral mucosa. Am J Clin Pathol. 2006;126:522–9.

Jainkittivosng A, Aneksuk V, Langlias RP. Oral mucosal conditions in elderly dental patients. Oral Dis. 2002;8:218–23.

Parlak AH, Koybasi S, Yavuz T, Yesildal N, Aydogan I, et al. Prevalence of oral lesions in 13 to 16 year old students in Duzce. Turkey Oral Dis. 2006;12:552–8.

Pyogenic Granuloma

Asha V, Dhanya M, Patil BA, Revanna G. An unusual presentation of pyogenic granuloma of the lower lip. Contemp Clin Dent. 2014;5(4):524–6.

Jafarzadeh H, Sanatkhani M, Mohtasham N. Oral pyogenic granuloma: a review. J Oral Sci. 2006;48(4):167–75.

Kamal R, Dahiya P, Puri A. Oral pyogenic granuloma: various concepts of etiopathogenesis. J Oral Maxillofac Pathol. 2012;16(1):79–82.

Peripheral Giant Cell Granuloma

Brown AL, Camargo de Moraes P, Sperandio M, Borges Soares A, Araújo VC, Passador-Santos F. Peripheral giant cell granuloma associated with a dental implant: a case report and review of the literature. Case Rep Dent. 2015. doi:10.1155/2015/697673.

Gandara-Rey JM, Pacheco Martins Carneiro JL, Gandara-Vila P, Blanco-Carrion A, García-García A, Madriñán-Graña P, Martín MS. Peripheral giant-cell granuloma. Review of 13 cases. Med Oral. 2002;7(4):254–9.

Rodrigues SV, Mitra DK, Pawar SD, Vijayakar HN. Peripheral giant cell granuloma: this enormity is a rarity. J Indian Soc Periodontol. 2015;19(4):466–9.

Fibroma

Esmeili T, Lozada-Nur F, Epstein J. Common benign oral soft tissue masses. Dent Clin N Am. 2005;49(1):223–40.

Gonsalves WC, Chi AA, Neville BW. Common oral lesions: part II. Masses and neoplasia. Am Fam Physician. 2007;75:509–12.

Peripheral Ossifying Fibroma

Bodner L, Dayan D. Growth potential of peripheral ossifying fibroma. J Clin Periodontol. 1987;14:551–4.

Buduneli E, Buduneli N, Unal T. Long-term follow-up of peripheral ossifying fibroma: report of three cases. Periodontol Clin Invest. 2001;23(1):11–4.

Cuisia ZE, Brannon RB. Peripheral ossifying fibroma—a clinical evaluation of 134 pediatric cases. Pediatr Dent. 2001;23(3):245–8.

Mucocele

Adachi P, Pires-Soubhia AM, Horikawa FK, Shinohara EH. Mucocele of the glands of Blandin–Nuhn. Clinical, pathological, and therapeutical aspects. Oral Maxillofac Surg. 2011;15:11–3.

Bahadure RN, Fulzele P, Thosar N, Badole G, Baliga S. Conventional surgical treatment of oral mucocele: a series of 23 cases. Eur J Paediatr Dent. 2012;13:143–6.

Baurmash HD. Mucoceles and ranulas. J Oral Maxillofac Surg. 2003;61:369–78.

Mandel L. Multiple superficial oral mucoceles: case report. J Oral Maxillofac Surg. 2001;59:928–30.

Papilloma

Abbey LM, Page DG, Sawyer DR. The clinical and histopathologic features of a series of 464 oral squamous papillomas. Oral Surg Oral Med Oral Pathol. 1980;49:419–28.

Bao Z, Yang X, Shi L, Feng J, Liu W, Zhou Z. Clinicopathologic features of oral squamous papilloma and papillary squamous cell carcinoma: a study of 197 patients from eastern China. Ann Diagn Pathol. 2012;16(6):454–8.

Carniero TE, Marinho SA, Verli FD, Mesquita AT, Lima NL, Miranda JL. Oral squamous papilloma: clinical, histologic and immunohistochemical analyses. J Oral Sci. 2009;151(3):367–72.

Syrjanen S. Human papillomavirus infections and oral tumors. Med Microbiol Immunol. 2003;192:123–8.

Lymphoepithelial Cyst

Buchner A, Hansen LS. Lymphoepithelial cyst of the oral cavity. Oral Med Oral Pathol. 1980a;50:441–9.

Khelemsky R, Mandel L. Lymphoepithelial cyst of floor of the mouth. J Oral Maxillofac Surg. 2010;68:3055–7.

Yang X, Ow A, Zhang C-P, Yang WJ, Hu YJ, Zhong LP. Clinical analysis of 120 cases of intraoral lymphoepithelial cyst. Oral Surg Oral Med Oral Pathol Oral Radiol Endod. 2012;113:448–52.

Varicosity

Azevedo LH, Del Vechio A, Nakajima E, Galletto V, Migliari DA. Lip and oral venous varices treated by photocoagulation and high intensity diode laser. Quintessence Int. 2003;44(2):171–4.

Ettinger RL, Manderson RD. A clinical study of sublingual varices. Oral Surg Oral Med Oral Path. 1974;38:540–5.

Gomes CC, Gomez RS, Vieira do Carmo MA MA, Castro WH, Gala-Garcia A, Mesquita RA. Mucosal varicosities: case report treated with monoethanolamine oleate. Med Oral Patol Oral Cir Bucal. 2006;11:E44–6.

Hedström L, Bergh H. Sublingual varices in relation to smoking and cardiovascular diseases. Br J Oral Maxillofac Surg. 2010;48:136–8.

Amalgam Tattoo

Buchner A. Amalgam tattoo (amalgam pigmentation) of the oral mucosa: clinical manifestations, diagnosis, and treatment. Refuat Hapeh Vehashinayim. 2004;21:25–8.
Buchner A, Hansen LS. Amalgam pigmentation (amalgam tattoo) of the oral mucosa: a clinicopathologic study of 268 cases. Oral Surg Oral Med Oral Pathol. 1980b;49:139–47.
Shah G, Alster TS. Treatment of an amalgam tattoo with a Q-switched alexandrite 9755 nm) laser. Dermatol Surg. 2002;28:1180–1.

Oral Melanotic Macule

Buchner A, Merrell PW, Carpenter WM. Relative frequency of solitary melanocytic lesions of the oral mucosa. J Oral Pathol Med. 2004;33:550–7.
Lerman MA, Karimbux N, Guze KA, Woo SB. Pigmentation of the hard palate. Oral Surg Oral Med Oral Pathol Oral Radiol Endod. 2009;107:8–12.
Lima B, Najarian DJ, Lee M, Miller C. Numerous hyperpigmented macules of the oral mucosa. J Am Acad Dermatol. 2010;62:171–3.
Shen ZY, Liu W, Bao ZX, Zhou ZT, Wang LZ. Oral melanotic macule and primary oral malignant melanoma: epidemiology, location involved, and clinical implications. Surg Oral Med Oral Pathol Oral Radiol Endod. 2011;112:e21–5.

Periapical Granuloma/Abscess

Bhaskar SN. Oral surgery-oral pathology conference No. 17, Walter Reed Army Medical Center. Periapical lesions-types, incidence, and clinical features. Oral Surg Oral Med Oral Pathol. 1966;21:657–71.
Estrela C, Leles CR, Hollanda AC, Moura MS, Pécora JD. Prevalence and risk factors of apical periodontitis in endodontically treated teeth in a selected population of Brazilian adults. Braz Dent J. 2008;19:34–9.

Periapical Cyst

Nair PN. New perspectives on radicular cysts: do they heal? Int Endod J. 1998;31:155–60.
Rosenberg PA, Frisbie J, Lee J, Lee K, Frommer H, Kottal S, et al. Evaluation of pathologists (histopathology) and radiologists (cone beam computed tomography) differentiating radicular cysts from granulomas. J Endod. 2010;36:423–8.

Dentigerous Cyst

Aher V, Chander PM, Chikkalingaiah RG, Ali FM. Dentigerous cysts in four quadrants: a rare and first reported case. J Surg Tech Case Rep. 2013;5:21–6.
Gonzalez SM, Spalding PM, Payne JB, Giannini PJ. A dentigerous cyst associated with bilaterally impacted mandibular canines in a girl: a case report. J Med Case Rep. 2011;23(5):230.
Tamgadge A, Tamgadge S, Bhatt D, Bhalerao S, Pereira T, Padhye M. Bilateral dentigerous cyst in a non-syndromic patient: report of an unusual case with review of the literature. J Oral Maxillofac Pathol. 2011;15:91–5.

Odontogenic Keratocyst

Islam NM, Bhattacharyya I. Diagnostic discussion. Odontogenic keratocyst. Todays FDA. 2015;27:75–8.
Li TJ. The odontogenic keratocyst: a cyst, or a cystic neoplasm? J Dent Res. 2011;90:133–42.
Madras J, Lapointe H. Keratocystic odontogenic tumour: reclassification of the odontogenic keratocyst from cyst to tumour. J Can Dent Assoc. 2008;74:165–165h.
Ramesh M, Krishnan R, Chalakkal P, et al. Gorlin-Goltz Syndrome: case report and literature review. J Oral Maxillofac Pathol. 2015;19:267.

Lateral Periodontal Cyst (LPC)

Frei M, Buettner M, Perren A, Reichart PA, Bornstein MM. Diagnosis and interdisciplinary treatment of a botryoid odontogenic cyst in the posterior mandible: report of a case. Quintessence Int. 2014;45(3):233–7.
Friedrich RE, Scheuer HA, Zustin J. Lateral periodontal cyst. In Vivo. 2014;28:595–8.

Ameloblastoma

Junquera L, Ascani G, Vicente JC, García-Consuegra L, Roig P. Ameloblastoma revisited. Ann Otol Rhinol Laryngol. 2003;112:1034–9.
Masthan KM, Anitha N, Krupaa J, et al. Ameloblastoma. J Pharm Bioallied Sci. 2015;7:167–70.
Philipsen HP, Reichart PA. Unicystic ameloblastoma. A review of 193 cases from the literature. Oral Oncol. 1998;34:317–25.
Reichart PA, Philipsen HP, Sonner S. Ameloblastoma: biological profile of 3677 cases. Eur J Cancer B Oral Oncol. 1995;31:86–99.

Simple Bone Cyst

Bhattacharyya I, Islam MN, Chehal HK, et al. Unusually large and aggressive traumatic bone cysts of the jaws- a series of five cases. Oral Surg. 2014;7:40–7.
Curran J, Kennett S, Young A. Traumatic (haemorrhagic) bone cyst of the mandible: report of an unusual case. J Can Dent Assoc. 1973;39:853–5.
Kaugars G, Cale A. Traumatic bone cyst. Oral Surg. 1987;63:318–23.

Nasopalatine Duct Cyst

Aparna M, Chakravarthy A, Acharya SR, et al. A clinical report demonstrating the significance of distinguishing a nasopalatine duct cyst from a radicular cyst. BMJ Case Rep. 2014;18:2014.
Bains R, Verma P, Chandra A, Tikku AP, Singh N. Nasopalatine duct cyst mimicking an endodontic periapical lesion: a case report. Gen Dent. 2016;64:63–6.

Odontoma

De Oliveira BH, Campos V, Marçal S. Compound odontoma-diagnosis and treatment: three case reports. Pediatr Dent. 2001;23:151–7.

Kulkarni VK, Deshmukh J, Banda NR, et al. Odontomas-silent tormentors of teeth eruption, shedding and occlusion. BMJ Case Rep. 2012;14:2012.

Verma S, Arul AS, Arul AS, et al. Erupted complex odontoma of the posterior maxilla: a rarity. J Nat Sci Biol Med. 2015;6:167–9.

Cemento-Osseous Dysplasias

Bhattacharyya I, Islam N. Diagnostic discussion. Periapical cemento-osseous dysplasia. Todays FDA. 2015;27:52–7.

Islam MN, Cohen DM, Kanter KG, Stewart CM, Katz J, Bhattacharyya I. Florid cemento-osseous dysplasia mimicking multiple periapical pathology-an endodontic dilemma. Gen Dent. 2008;56:559–62.

Ryan M, Powers DB, Puscas L. Mandibular mass. Focal Cemento-Osseous Dysplasia (FCOD). JAMA Otolaryngol Head Neck Surg. 2014;140:985–6.

Idiopathic Osteosclerosis

Moshfeghi M, Azimi F, Anvari M. Radiologic assessment and frequency of idiopathic osteosclerosis of jawbones: an interpopulation comparison. Acta Radiol. 2014;55:1239–44.

Yonetsu K, Yuasa K, Kanda S. Idiopathic osteosclerosis of the jaws: panoramic radiographic and computed tomographic findings. Oral Surg Oral Med Oral Pathol Oral Radiol Endod. 1997;83:517–21.

Condensing Osteitis

Holly D, Jurkovic R, Mracna J. Condensing osteitis in oral region. Bratisl Lek Listy. 2009;110:713–5.

Mainville GN, Lalumière C, Turgeon D, Kauzman A. Asymptomatic, non-expansile radio-opacity of the jaw associated with external root resorption: a diagnostic dilemma. Gen Dent. 2016;64:32–5.

Verzak Z, Celap B, Modrić VE, et al. The prevalence of idiopathic osteosclerosis and condensing osteitis in Zagreb population. Acta Clin Croat. 2012;51:573–7.

Oral and Maxillofacial Surgery 15

Stacey Nedrud and John Hardeman

Contents

S. Nedrud, DMD (✉)
Oral and Maxillofacial Surgery Resident, University of Florida Health – Jacksonville, University of Florida College of Medicine, Jacksonville, FL, USA
e-mail: stacey.nedrud@jax.ufl.edu

J. Hardeman, DDS, MD
Oral and Maxillofacial Surgery, University of Florida College of Dentistry, Gainesville, FL, USA

G.M. Weinstein, M.T. Zientz (eds.), *The Dental Reference Manual*,
DOI 10.1007/978-3-319-39730-6_15

Abstract

Oral and Maxillofacial Surgery encompasses so much more than just extractions. This chapter outlines the basic principles of atraumatic extractions, bone preservation, pre-prosthetic surgery, and basic oral pathology procedures. It would be prudent for a general dentist to also be familiar with the basic management of acute facial swellings and abscesses.

15.1 Exodontia

15.1.1 Diagnosis and Treatment Planning

- Simple extractions
  - Indications for dental extraction include decay, periodontal disease, tooth fracture, pre-prosthetic, pathology, adverse effects of chemotherapy and radiation therapy, and orthodontics (Sakar et al. 2008; Ness and Peterson 2004).
  - Factors determining complexity include caries, previous root canal treatment, bulbous, curved, or long roots, ankylosis, and proximity to the maxillary sinus or the inferior alveolar nerve (Sakar et al. 2008; Ness and Peterson 2004).
  - Evaluate radiographically for impaction, root morphology, hypercementosis, or ankylosis (Sakar et al. 2008). Currently, conventional panoramic radiographs provide a sufficient screening tool for the dentoalveolar region (Monaco et al. 2004; Juodzbalys and Daugela 2013). Cone beam CT technology allows a more accurate three-dimensional image, but at a higher dose of radiation (Monaco et al. 2004; Juodzbalys and Daugela 2013; Li 2013). The operator needs a clear visualization of adjacent structures such as the maxillary sinus, the inferior alveolar nerve, and the mental foramen. It is also important to evaluate root curvature, root length, and evidence of prior endodontic treatment (Ness and Peterson 2004; Juodzbalys and Daugela 2013) (Fig. 15.1).
- Complex extractions of third molars
  - Indications to extract impacted dentition include pericoronitis, cystic formation from a retained follicle (e.g., dentigerous cyst or keratocyst), facilitating orthodontic treatment and arch length, dentition in the line of a fracture, tumors, caries, and periodontal disease of adjacent teeth (Sakar et al. 2008; Rafetto 2012).
  - Factors determining complexity in order of increasing degree of difficulty include mesioangular impaction, vertical impaction and horizontal impaction, and distoangular impaction (Ness and Peterson 2004; Juodzbalys and Daugela 2013).

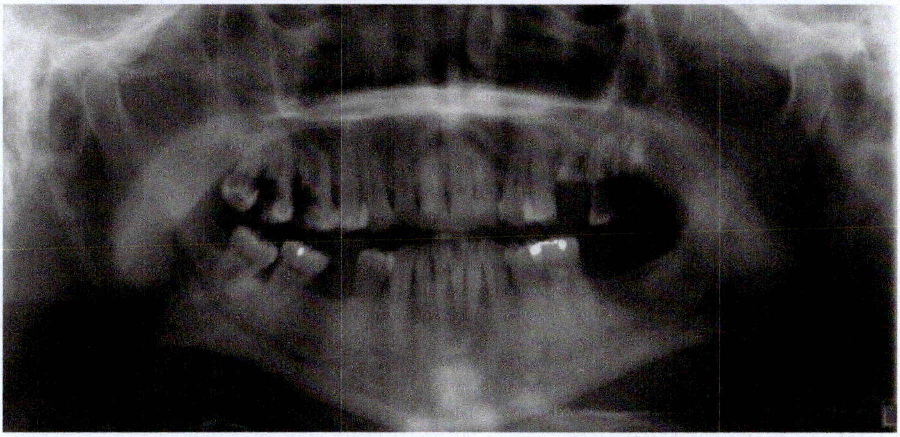

Fig. 15.1 Panoramic radiographs are an excellent screening tool to determine anatomic landmarks and the degree of difficulty of the extraction

- In addition, the level of complexity is compounded by soft tissue impaction, partial bony impaction, or complete bony impaction (Ness and Peterson 2004).
- Impacted third molars buried in the ramus of the mandible are more difficult to remove (Pell and Gregory Classification) (Ness and Peterson 2004; Juodzbalys and Daugela 2013).
- Conical roots are easier to extract than divergent roots. Roots that are only 1/3–2/3 formed are much less difficult to extract, at an average age of 16–18 years old (Ness and Peterson 2004).
- Palatally or lingually positioned teeth are more difficult to extract (Ness and Peterson 2004).
- A large follicular sac around the crown makes the tooth easier to extract (Ness and Peterson 2004).
- Extracting teeth prior to 20 years of age makes the surgery less difficult (Ness and Peterson 2004).

15.1.2 Armamentarium

- Practice universal precautions; every patient should be treated as though they have a communicable disease.
- Place a gauze throat screen at all times to prevent accidental aspiration.
- Use a bite block for access and to decrease temporomandibular joint (TMJ) pain from rotational torquing forces.
- Position the patient nearly upright in the dental chair to extract mandibular teeth, and position the dental chair in a supine position to extract maxillary teeth (Sakar et al. 2008).
- Small and large elevators are used as a wedge and a rotational force. Elevators separate alveolar bone from the tooth surface, in addition to rotating the tooth out of the socket (Sakar et al. 2008).

- A #9 Periosteal elevator or Woodson instrument expands the periodontal ligament (PDL) space to facilitate extraction without excessive bony or soft tissue destruction.
- Forceps can be used in multiple vectors, to remove the tooth: apical, buccal, lingual, rotational, and tractional vectors. The tooth is usually delivered buccally and coronally (Sakar et al. 2008).
- Rongeurs are useful to extract root tips and to remove minimal surrounding bone.
- East-West elevators are used for leverage against bone, often through the radicular bone, to extract root tips.
- A surgical drill and bur with irrigation is crucial for surgical extractions and pre-prosthetic surgery.

15.1.3 Simple Exodontia

- Local anesthesia
  - Profound anesthesia must be administered to the tooth as well as the adjacent tissues. Although analgesia is achieved, pressure sensation persists. Be cognizant of the amount of local anesthetic needed in the presence of a local infection.
  - Be aware of the maximum recommended dosing levels of local anesthetic in an adult (Table 15.1).
  - Cardiac patients: limit the amount of epinephrine to 0.04 mg which is equivalent to two cartridges of local anesthetic with 1:100,000 epinephrine (Malamed 1997).
  - Pregnant patients: note that lidocaine is a Category B drug (Massoomi 2008).
  - Have a thorough knowledge of anatomical innervations when providing local anesthetic. Periodontal ligament (PDL) and intraosseous injections can help in difficult situations.
- Utilize the small straight elevator in the PDL space as a means of alveolar bone expansion and separation, in addition to luxation of the tooth. Luxating the tooth with an elevator will prevent root fracture at the time of extraction (be cognizant of inadvertent adjacent tooth luxation).
- Forceps use
  - Excessive force is a poor substitute for proper technique.
  - #150 maxillary forceps are used for extraction of maxillary anterior and posterior teeth (Sakar et al. 2008).
  - Asch forceps are used for extraction of mandibular anterior teeth (Sakar et al. 2008).

Table 15.1 Maximum dosage of local anesthetic (Cummings et al. 2011; Massoomi 2008)

Local anesthetic	Vasoconstrictor	Maximum recommended dosage (mg/lb)
2 % lidocaine	1:100,000 epinephrine	3.2
2 % mepivacaine	1:20,000 levonordefrin	2.4
3 % mepivacaine	Plain	2.4
4 % articaine	1:100,000 epinephrine	3.2

  - Seat the forceps as apically as possible. Apply careful buccal and lingual forces slowly to expand the alveolar bone. Conical roots can be rotated in screwdriver or figure-eight motions (Sakar et al. 2008).
  - #151 mandibular forceps or #23 cowhorn forceps are used for extraction of mandibular posterior teeth (Sakar et al. 2008).
  - Cowhorn forceps placed in the interradicular furca will luxate the tooth coronally. If the tooth is grossly decayed and consequently fractures at the furca, each root can be delivered separately (Sakar et al. 2008).
  - Placing the operator's opposing hand over the alveolus surrounding the tooth being luxated allows the operator to protect adjacent teeth, while gauging the amount of force placed on the surgical site (Sakar et al. 2008).
- Surgical extraction of a complex tooth is often less invasive than nonsurgical techniques.

15.1.4 Bone and Site Preservation

- Maximize the use of elevators, such as a #9 Periosteal elevator, Woodson instrument, or surgical osteotome, to expand the periodontal ligament (PDL) space. Use apical pressure to further expand the alveolar bone prior to any forceps use. Preserving a four-wall socket prevents collapse of the alveolar ridge (Moy 2004; Bartee and Lignelli 2008).
- Ensure adequate mobility of the tooth prior to the extraction in order to prevent root and alveolar wall fracture. Minimize twisting motions when extracting the roots to reduce the propensity for alveolar wall fracture (Moy 2004).
- If a surgical bur is needed, remove periradicular and interradicular bone by troughing around the perimeter of the tooth and between the roots and apply forceps to facilitate removal of the tooth. If this is not successful, use the surgical bur to section the tooth, and an East-West elevator as a rotational force to remove each root separately. Another useful technique is to create a purchase point in the tooth with a surgical bur to aid elevation and extraction. #702 crosscut tapered or straight fissure burs work well for surgical extractions, as do #6 or #8 round burs. Copious irrigation while using the surgical hand piece lessens the incidence of thermal trauma and bone necrosis (Sakar et al. 2008).
- Bone augmentation may be necessary after extraction in anticipation of future implant or bridge placement or for other aesthetic, functional, and structural reasons. A less traumatic extraction process, coupled with socket augmentation, significantly reduces alveolar ridge dimensional changes (Moy 2004; McAllister and Haghighat 2007; Camargo et al. 2004).
  - The treatment modality will vary according to the morphology of each defect; the defect may be horizontal, vertical, or both. Bone resorption also varies between the maxilla and the mandible (Moy 2004; McAllister and Haghighat 2007).
  - The number of resulting walls in the defect may determine the type of graft (e.g., particulate socket graft vs. block grafting and augmentation) (Bartee and Lignelli 2008; Block 2006).

- Careful consideration of the soft tissue volume and quality is necessary to improve aesthetic and functional results. A wide band of keratinized mucosa ameliorates the overall health of the tissue and results in fewer complications (Geurs et al. 2010).
- Bone augmentation modalities include the use of biologic growth factors (e.g., platelet-rich plasma (PRP), bone morphogenetic protein (BMP), leukocyte- and platelet-rich fibrin (L-PRF)), particulate and block grafting, distraction osteogenesis, and guided bone regeneration (GBR), with and without membrane barriers (McAllister and Haghighat 2007; Wikesjo et al. 2007). Several GBR approaches have been studied to be effective: ePTFE membranes, bioresorbable membranes, freeze-dried bone allograft, bone autograft, bone xenograft, alloplastic materials, and others (McAllister and Haghighat 2007; Camargo et al. 2004; Block 2006; Moy 2004). When selecting the augmentation material, consider biocompatibility, bioresorbability, functional and structural stability, and ease of use (Moy 2004; McAllister and Haghighat 2007; Block 2006). Studies have shown freeze-dried bone allograft to lack adequate bioresorbability as compared to bioglass material and bovine bone materials (Moy 2004) (Figs. 15.2 and 15.3).
- Immediate implant placement, often with bone augmentation, has shown comparable success to the traditional delayed implant placement, but this will not be further discussed in this chapter (McAllister and Haghighat 2007).
- When augmenting and grafting early in the practitioner's experience, it is important to release the soft tissue adequately to allow for primary soft tissue closure and to completely cover the graft site. Management of graft sites where

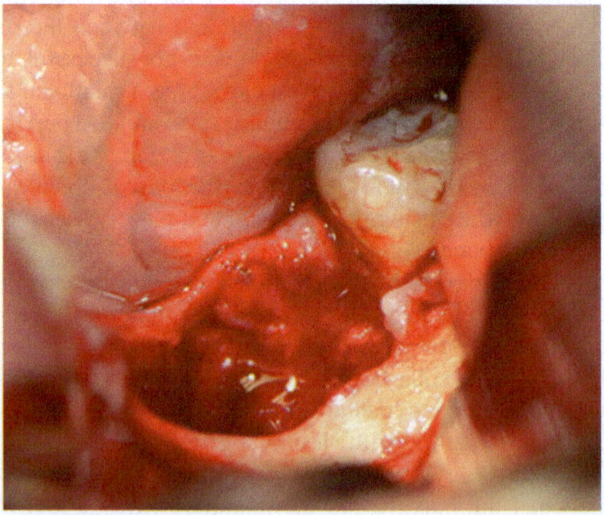

Fig. 15.2 This photo illustrates an extraction surgical site, utilizing bone preservation techniques. This patient had severe horizontal and vertical bone loss prior to extraction, and thus the case warranted a particulate bone graft to reconstruct the alveolar ridge

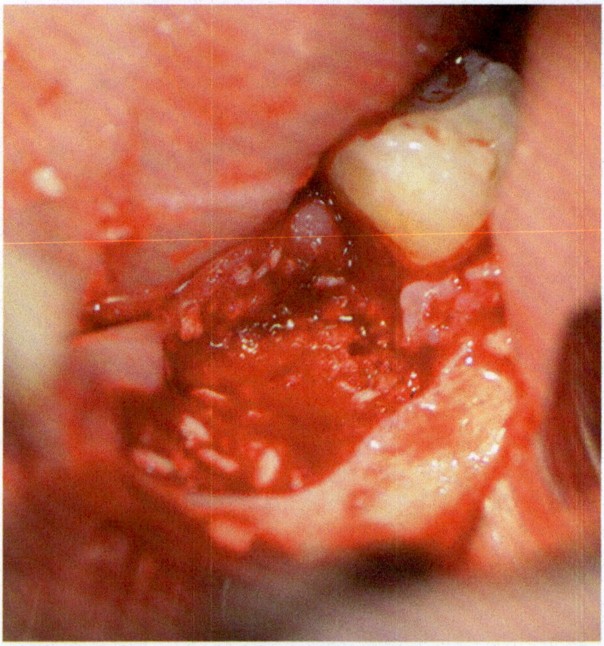

Fig. 15.3 This photo illustrates the mineralized particulate bone graft in place immediately after extraction of the tooth of the same patient as in Fig. 15.2, with healthy bleeding tissue at the site. The site will then be closed primarily to prevent complications such as dehiscence, infection, and failure of the graft

secondary healing is necessary requires a higher level of experience and soft tissue management skills. Membrane exposure is associated with higher bone resorption and other complications. Maintenance of primary wound closure is critical to prevent dehiscence with membrane exposure and infection (McAllister and Haghighat 2007; Camargo et al. 2004; Block 2006; Misch 2008).

– Alveolar ridge resorption after bone augmentation should be considered, especially if implant placement is the treatment goal; resorption usually occurs in the first 6–8 months but varies according to the GBR technique used (Moy 2004; Bartee and Lignelli 2008; Block 2006).

15.1.5 Complex Exodontia

- Simple flap design
  – Envelope flap: Incise the gingival sulcus at the cervical margin of the teeth, through the periosteum, two to three teeth anterior and one to two teeth posterior to the tooth in question. Apically reflect the full-thickness mucoperiosteal flap. If a vertical releasing incision is necessary for visualization, a posterior vertical releasing incision is more aesthetic. Two releasing incisions, an anterior and a posterior, may be necessary in rare cases (Peterson 2002).

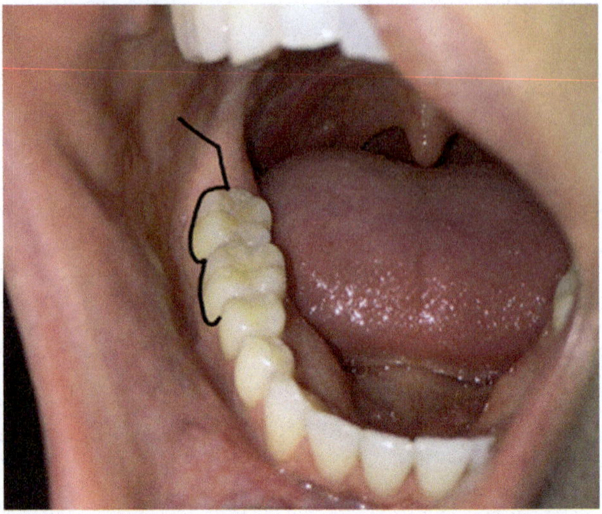

Fig. 15.4 The overlay illustrates an example of an impacted mandibular third molar incision utilizing the "hockey stick incision"

 - Mandibular third molars: Incise the gingiva two to three teeth anterior to the extraction site, scalloping around the gingival sulcus. Then, continue the incision to the central groove on the distal of the second molar. Turn the blade and cut 1–1.5 cm distal through soft tissue, and then turn to incise an obtuse angle toward the buccal, about 1 cm, to create a vertical release (the hockey stick incision) (Sakar et al. 2008; Ness and Peterson 2004; Peterson 2002) (Fig. 15.4).
 - Maxillary third molars: Cut two to three teeth anterior, scalloping around the gingival sulcus. Distal to the second molar, cut a C-shaped incision, hugging the maxillary tuberosity toward the buccal. Retract the gingiva superiorly enough to be able to fully view the third molar. You may need to use a #9 Periosteal Elevator to flake away maxillary bone anterior to the third molar (Sakar et al. 2008; Ness and Peterson 2004; Peterson 2002) (Fig. 15.5).
 - The flap should always be a full-thickness mucoperiosteal flap. Ensure all tissue retractors are only resting on bone, deep to periosteum (Peterson 2002).
 - The base of any flap must be wider than the apex (free margin) to prevent ischemia of the flap (Peterson 2002).
- Surgical extraction
  - The guiding principle is to create a space in the alveolar bone surrounding the tooth root.
  - Sectioning a tooth to facilitate individual root extraction:
    - Section a molar parallel to the roots at the bifurcations: perpendicular to buccal bone for mandibular molars and in a "Y" formation for maxillary molars. Always use radiographs to understand the root morphology to know the vector in which to section the tooth (Sakar et al. 2008).
    - Section and remove a molar crown to create better access to the roots in order to simplify the sectioning of the roots, as above (Sakar et al. 2008).

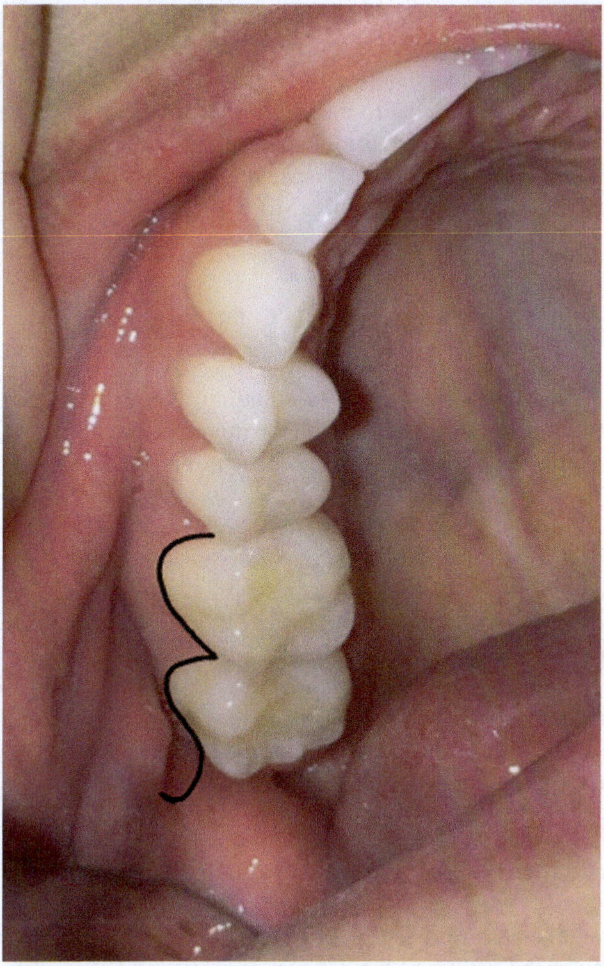

Fig. 15.5 The overlay illustrates an example of an impacted maxillary third molar incision utilizing the "C-shaped incision"

- Be sure to remove adequate bone covering the impacted third molar, and to create a deep buccal trough, with a distal component. However, avoid using the drill to trough the lingual bone of mandibular teeth. Be cognizant of the depth of the surgical cut (Sakar et al. 2008).
- When using surgical burs, know the exact measurements of the bur being used. Below is an example of the specifications for a #702 crosscut Extra Long/Surgical Bur from Patterson Dental (Patterson Dental surgical burs 2016):
  - Head length: 4.5 mm
  - Head diameter: 1.6 mm
  - Numeric shank length: 25 mm

- Utilize radiographs to know the distance to the vital structures, such as the inferior alveolar nerve, maxillary sinus, and inferior border of the mandible.
- Have a thorough understanding of all pertinent anatomy to avoid complications, especially pertaining to the inferior alveolar and lingual nerves.
- Coronectomies of impacted third molars are a valid treatment option when the risk of nerve damage is highly suspected. Ensure the tooth has not been elevated, and the roots are not mobile (Monaco et al. 2012; Auyong and Le 2011; Miloro and Kolokythas 2011).

15.1.6 Debridement and Closure

- Use a bone file or rasp to smooth all surrounding alveolar bone (Sakar et al. 2008).
- Irrigate all extraction sites and beneath the mucoperiosteal flaps. Curette the follicle unless curetting presents a danger to the inferior alveolar nerve (Sakar et al. 2008).
- Intraorally, chromic gut suture is commonly used. Vicryl suture often lasts too long and may have to be removed at a subsequent appointment. 3-0 or 4-0 size sutures are commonly used sizes for intraoral suturing. A study by Otten et al. shows resorbable sutures aggregate fewer colonies of bacteria than nonresorbable sutures (Otten et al. 2005).
- Place one to two interrupted sutures to reapproximate the mandibular flap sites. Watertight closure is not advised (Sakar et al. 2008).
- Often, maxillary posterior incisions do not need to be sutured unless the tissue does not reapproximate well or if there are buccal gingival tears.

15.1.7 Medications

- Common analgesics are listed in Table 15.2 (see also Chap. 22: Prescriptions)
- Always inform the patient of the dangers of pain medication use:
  - Addiction
  - Tolerance
  - Alcohol use in conjunction with narcotics
  - The possibility of respiratory depression
  - Driving while impaired

Table 15.2 Common analgesics (Sakar et al. 2008; Fletcher and Spera 2002)

Analgesic, generic name	Common brand name	Common dosage	Common sig
Ibuprofen	Motrin	600–800 mg	q8h
Codeine, acetaminophen	Tylenol #3	30 mg codeine/300 mg acetaminophen	q6h
Hydrocodone, acetaminophen	Norco	5 mg hydrocodone/325 mg acetaminophen	q4-6h
Oxycodone, acetaminophen	Percocet	5 mg oxycodone/325 mg acetaminophen	q4-6h

15.1.8 Informed Consent

- One must obtain an informed consent for any and all possible procedures in most states (Curley 2011).
- Be sure to indicate and explain the risks, among them "pain, bleeding, swelling, infection, damage to teeth and/or adjacent structures, temporary and permanent paresthesia" (Curley 2011).
- Include the benefits of the procedure and the medical alternatives. Add "any other indicated procedures" to the consent to account for alternative plans (Curley 2011).
- Always document risks, benefits, and rationale for surgery, as well as the alternatives to surgery, in the chart. Document that the patient (or other legal representative) voices understanding of the discussion presented to them. Imaging and models used in the consent should also be documented. Informed refusal should also be documented (Curley 2011).
- A witness, such as an assistant, should sign confirmation of the verbal and written consent.

15.1.9 Complications

- Extraction of the wrong tooth:
  - Confirm the patient and procedure with a pre-procedural surgical time out before starting.
  - Always count the teeth and cross reference with the medical records and dental assistants (Lee et al. 2007).
- Damage to adjacent teeth or structures (Juodzbalys and Daugela 2013):
  - Protecting adjacent teeth with the operator's opposite hand allows the surgeon to control the force, as well as gauge the force being placed on adjacent structures.
  - Inform the patient of the risk of damage to adjacent prosthetics, including crowns, bridges, and orthodontic appliances.
- Management of uncontrolled bleeding:
  - Ensure adequate pressure with gauze for 30 minutes or longer (Malmquist 2011).
  - Silver nitrate sticks provide chemical hemostasis.
  - Place hemostatic materials, such as Gelfoam, Collatape, bone wax, or other hemostatic agents in the extraction site. Chitosan-derived hemostatic bandages, such as HemCon bandages, are recently being used to control excessive bleeding (Malmquist 2011).
  - Suturing provides a means of hemostasis as well, although this is not effective with an extraction site that is not a watertight closure.
- Damage to the inferior alveolar or lingual nerve:
  - The most important risk factor is the anatomic proximity of the tooth to the nerve in question (Auyong and Le 2011).
  - Avoid complications with a thorough and well-documented examination radiographically (Miloro and Kolokythas 2011).

- Have the patient return when the local anesthesia has dissipated, for further clinical examination (Sakar et al. 2008), dermatome mapping, and evaluation of deficits in pain, temperature, pressure, light touch, direction sense, and two-point discrimination (Auyong and Le 2011).
- Refer to Oral and Maxillofacial Surgery early for evaluation and further mapping.

- Dry socket (alveolar osteitis):
  - Diagnosed clinically: continued radiating pain past the 72 hour mark, halitosis, and an exposed socket with no clot or tissue (Sakar et al. 2008; Krakowiak 2011). Tobacco use, preexisting infection, poor oral hygiene, and increased age, among other factors, increase the risk of alveolar osteitis (Krakowiak 2011).
  - Irrigate the site copiously with Peridex 0.12 % and a Monoject syringe. Give the patient a prescription for Peridex and advise q4h rinses with a Monoject syringe (Sakar et al. 2008). Moist warm heat compresses are helpful (Krakowiak 2011).
  - Pack the extraction site with dry socket paste (ingredients include various combinations of medications, but most often include eugenol, iodoform, and benzocaine) and gauze ribbon or a resorbable carrier vehicle. The packing should be replaced every 2 days if the pain persists, to prevent further infection (Sakar et al. 2008; Krakowiak 2011).
  - Remove any granulation tissue if the patient presents with continued pain.
  - Refer to Oral and Maxillofacial Surgery if the problem persists.

15.1.10 Indications for Referral to Oral and Maxillofacial Surgery

- Complex extractions:
  - Referral is warranted if there are any concerns for the proximity of the inferior alveolar and/or lingual nerve, and possible detrimental involvement.
  - Do not hesitate to refer if the general dentist does not possess the comfort level in surgically removing bone for impacted teeth and/or an adequate level of comfort with flap surgery. Please see the previous sections on factors in determining the difficulty of third molar extractions.
  - If the patient requires or desires sedation, for comfort, anxiety, or medical reasons, referral is warranted.
- Pericoronitis and facial space infections: symptoms may be severe and may cause facial space infections, trismus and fever, among other symptoms. The patient should go to the emergency department for IV fluids and IV antibiotics and to monitor the airway. The patient may require an incision and drainage (Osborn et al. 2008).
- Exposure and bond/bracketing for pre-orthodontic care, for bony impacted teeth (Felsenfeld and Aghaloo 2002).
- Patients undergoing dentoalveolar surgery with a history of oral or IV bisphosphonate medication use or with a previous history of head and neck radiation therapy (Chaudhry and Ruggiero 2007; Ruggiero et al. 2014).

15.2 Pre-prosthetic Surgery

15.2.1 Alveoloplasty

- Ensure all the extraction sites and alveolar bone are smooth and free of loose bone fragments (Spagnoli et al. 2004).
- If there are sharp or irregular areas, use either a rasp/bone file or Rongeurs to smooth the bone. Remove all loose bone. Surgical burs may be used but can facilitate over-reduction (Spagnoli et al. 2004).
- Remove all bony undercuts (Spagnoli et al. 2004).
- Minimize bone removal pre-prosthetically, to ensure an adequate ridge remains for retention of prosthetics (Spagnoli et al. 2004).
- Ensure proper irrigation of all surgical sites (Sakar et al. 2008).

15.2.2 Labial Frenectomy

- Surgical removal is warranted if the patient presents with difficulty speaking or for pre-prosthetically reasons (Digman et al. 2008).
- The operator should retract the upper lip anteriorly and superiorly, and then incise down to periosteum and along the attachment of the labial mucosa (Digman et al. 2008).
- Undermine and close the labial mucosa and allow the alveolar mucosa to secondarily granulate (Digman et al. 2008).
- Completely excise the frenum to prevent recurrence (Digman et al. 2008).

15.2.3 Lingual Frenectomy

- Removal is warranted most commonly if the patient presents with limited tongue mobility, denture instability, periodontal and aesthetic concerns, or oral hygiene problems (Spagnoli et al. 2004; Digman et al. 2008).
- It is advised to make the patient comfortable. Nitrous oxide gas often suffices for children, but sedation and general anesthesia have been suggested by Digman et al. (Spagnoli et al. 2004; Digman et al. 2008).
- Inject local anesthetic. Often, infiltration is preferred over a block (Spagnoli et al. 2004; Digman et al. 2008).
- The operator may choose to retract the tongue with gauze, skin hooks, or a midline placed suture (Spagnoli et al. 2004; Digman et al. 2008; Wlodawsky and Strauss 2004).
- Using either an electrocautery or a laser (CO_2 is suggested here, set at 5 W), incise the frenum vertically along the ventral surface of the tongue, taking care to avoid Wharton's duct. If the frenum also creates tension on the lingual mandibular gingiva, the frenum may also be released here (Spagnoli et al. 2004; Digman et al. 2008; Wlodawsky and Strauss 2004).

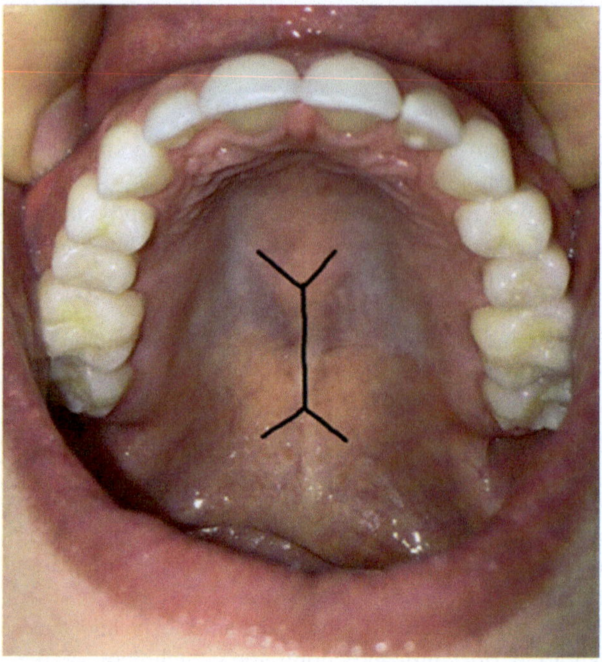

Fig. 15.6 The overlay illustrates an example of a palatal torus incision utilizing the "double reverse arrowhead incision"

- If the CO_2 laser technique is used and hemostasis is achieved, closure is not necessary (Sosovicka 2008; White et al. 1998).
- Of note, following laser frenectomy procedures, wound healing is often delayed, but postoperative pain is decreased (Sosovicka 2008; White et al. 1998).

15.2.4 Tori Removal

- Flap Design
  - Hydro-dissect the mucosal tissue with local anesthetic to release the tissue from the torus prior to incision (Spagnoli et al. 2004).
  - Mandibular tori: if the patient is dentate, use a scallop incision in the gingival sulcus along the lingual surfaces of the teeth, from molar to molar. If the patient is edentulous, make a mid-crestal incision from the regions of the molar to molar. Carefully retract the tissue over the tori, beneath the periosteum.
  - Maxillary tori: Create a double reverse arrowhead incision. This allows for good visibility and simplifies postsurgical closure (Spagnoli et al. 2004) (Fig. 15.6).
- Tori Removal
  - Mandibular tori: score between each bony protuberance with a #702 fissure bur, or similar, reverse cutting bur, perpendicular to the mandible. Either chisel the remaining tori with an osteotome or remove the bony protuberances

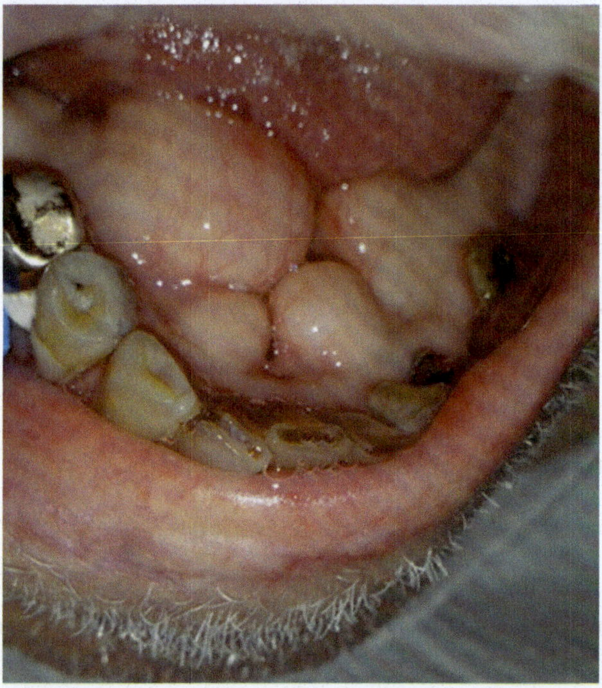

Fig. 15.7 This middle-aged patient complained of speech difficulties due to his large bilateral "kissing" mandibular tori. This patient was referred to an Oral and Maxillofacial Surgeon for surgical removal

with an egg bur parallel to the mandible. Smooth all surfaces with a pineapple or egg bur (Spagnoli et al. 2004) (Fig. 15.7).
  - Maxillary tori: score between each bony protuberance with a #702 fissure bur, or similar, reverse cutting bur, perpendicular to the maxilla. Either chisel the remaining tori with an osteotome or remove the bony protuberances with an egg bur (Spagnoli et al. 2004).
  - At all times, protect all soft tissue with a larger retractor, such as a Seldin #23 retractor.
  - Irrigate copiously after complete removal of the torus.
- Closure
  - Mandibular incisions can easily be closed with any continuous suturing technique, if the patient is edentulous. Dentate incisions can often be closed with multiple interrupted sutures (Spagnoli et al. 2004).
  - For mandibular tori removal, once the incision is closed, place a rolled 4 × 4 gauze in the anterior floor of the mouth and have the patient compress the gauze packing with the patient's tongue anteriorly, to help prevent hematoma formation (Spagnoli et al. 2004).
  - Maxillary tori incisions are difficult to close due to the thinner gingiva overlying the palatal tori. Continuous suturing is often successful. Presurgical fabrication of stents with the bony defect removed eliminates dead space and facilitates healing (Spagnoli et al. 2004).

15.2.5 Complications

- The anatomical path of the lingual nerve varies, but traverses the floor of mouth, often only protected by a layer of oral mucosa (Ziccardi 2011). Take great care when reflecting the mandibular lingual gingival tissue and when surgically removing the tori.
- The local tissue can be friable and is prone to dehiscence and wound breakdown. Protect all soft tissue with a large retractor, such as a Seldin #23, during the surgery (Spagnoli et al. 2004).
- A hematoma may form in the floor of the mouth. Place gauze pressure packings under the tongue to prevent a collection of blood for 1 day postoperatively (Spagnoli et al. 2004).

15.3 Management of Infections

15.3.1 Diagnosis and Treatment Planning

- Radiographic evaluation:
  - Dentoalveolar infections often originate from periapical granulomas from pulpal necrosis or from a periodontal source (Lypka and Hammoudeh 2011).
  - CT scans are widely used and effective in identifying drainable collections. Ultrasounds aid in differentiating a cellulitis from an abscess (Osborn et al. 2008).
- Clinical evaluation:
  - Patients often present with fluctuant, erythematous swellings that are warm to touch, with a rapid progression. The swelling is often extremely painful (Flynn 2004) (Table 15.3).
  - The patient can present with systemic signs of infection such as fever, chills, malaise, and loss of appetite (Osborn et al. 2008).
  - Patients often present with odynophagia, dysphagia, neck pain, neck swelling, and trismus (Osborn et al. 2008).
  - Ludwig's Angina, commonly secondary to dental infection, must be addressed with prompt diagnosis and surgical intervention (Osborn et al. 2008).

15.3.2 Antibiotics

- If indicated, IV fluids and IV antibiotics are appropriate medical management in a hospital setting (Osborn et al. 2008).
- Antibiotic therapy should initially be empiric. The best treatment would then tailor the antibiotic regimen to the microbes obtained from the culture and sensitivity results gathered during the incision and drainage (Osborn et al. 2008; Flynn 2004).
- Empiric oral antibiotics of choice are described in Table 15.4.

Table 15.3 Differentiating cellulitis from abscess clinically (Flynn 2004)

Cellulitis	Abscess
Acute onset	Delayed onset
Diffuse borders	Well-circumscribed borders
Soft or indurated to palpation	Fluctuant to palpation

Table 15.4 Prescriptions for common antibiotics (Osborn et al. 2008; Flynn 2011)

Antibiotic, generic name	Common dosage	Common sig
Penicillin V	500 mg	q6h
Amoxicillin	500 mg	q8h
Amoxicillin/clavulanic acid	875 mg/125 mg	q12h
Clindamycin	300 mg	q6h

15.3.3 Incision and Drainage

- Sites of odontogenic infection are notoriously difficult to anesthetize (Johri and Piecuch 2011). The provider should attempt an anesthetic block of the site.
- The aim is to establish primary drainage of the infection, as well as to remove the source of infection. The earlier the tooth can be extracted, the more favorable the outcome (Johri and Piecuch 2011).
- Primary drainage can be established via the tooth socket alone when significant soft tissue involvement is not present (Johri and Piecuch 2011).
- Incision and Drainage Technique
  - Incise over the dependent area of fluctuance, intraorally, with a 1-cm incision. Be aware of pertinent anatomy.
  - If the incision appears to require an extraoral approach, it is recommended to refer the patient to an Oral and Maxillofacial Surgeon or to the emergency department.
  - Insert a closed hemostat into the incision and spread the hemostats upon exiting the incision site. Never blindly close the hemostats in the surgical wound (Flynn 2004).
  - Place a Penrose drain in the site, and suture the drain in place with resorbable sutures.
  - Keep the drain in place, ideally approximately 72 hours.

15.3.4 Indications for Referral to Oral and Maxillofacial Surgery or to Emergency Department

- Airway issues: shortness of breath or stridor (Osborn et al. 2008; Flynn 2004).
- Fluctuant, erythematous swelling that has progressed rapidly (Osborn et al. 2008; Flynn 2004) (Figs. 15.8 and 15.9).
- Odynophagia, dysphagia, neck swelling, and trismus (Osborn et al. 2008).
- Patient is septic, dehydrated, febrile (Osborn et al. 2008).
- Ludwig's Angina (Osborn et al. 2008).
- Necrotizing fasciitis (Flynn 2004).

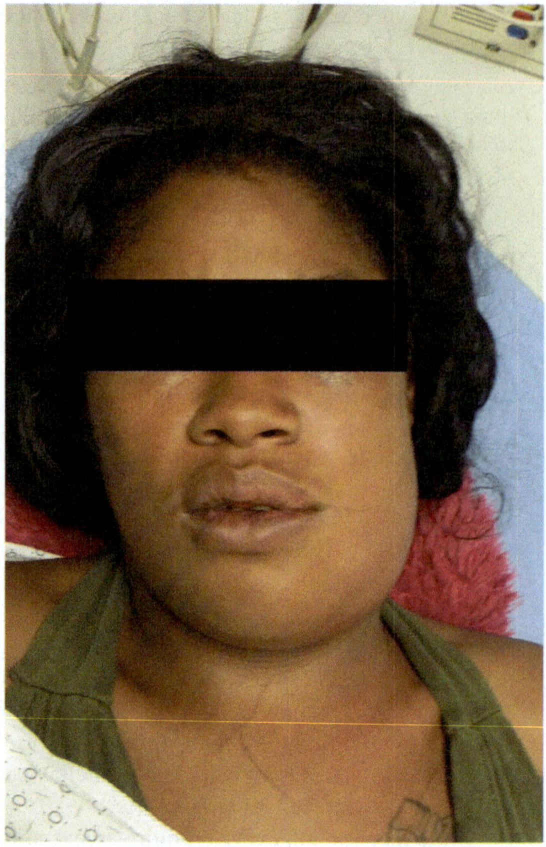

Fig. 15.8 This patient shows a large facial asymmetry, found to be a fluctuant abscess. Note the erythema extending to the neck and chest, outlined with a marking pen. This patient must be monitored carefully for rapid progression of the abscess and airway involvement. This patient presented with severe trismus and was taken to the operating room for an incision and drainage procedure

15.4 Oral Pathology

15.4.1 Indications to Biopsy

- Ninety percent of individuals with oral cancer have a smoking history (Ghali and Scott Connor 2004). Alcohol in combination with tobacco can be a risk factor, with studies showing a 35-fold increase in risk of oropharyngeal cancer in those that smoked tobacco and consumed daily alcohol (Blot et al. 1988; Ghali and Scott Connor 2004; Rothman and Keller 1972). Chewing betel nut is also a risk factor for oral squamous cell carcinoma in patients predominantly from India and Southeast Asia (Ghali and Scott Connor 2004).
- Biopsy intraoral abnormalities and lesions, especially erythroplakic lesions, leukoplakic lesions, and erythroleukoplakia that cannot be scraped off, and especially lesions that do not resolve after a 2-week trial of treatment or watching (Ghali and Scott Connor 2004).
- Pay special attention during a thorough oral cancer screening to examine the floor of mouth, lateral surfaces of the tongue, retromolar trigone, and hard and

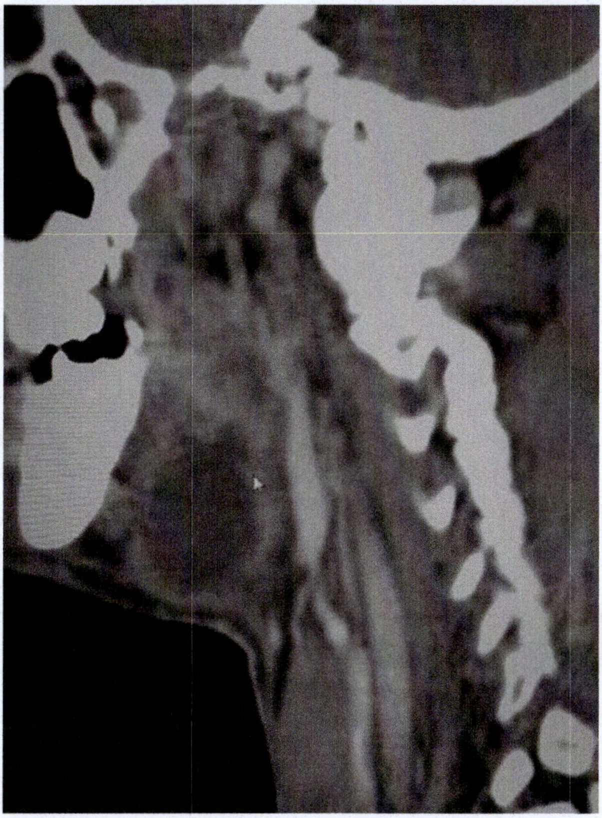

Fig. 15.9 This well-demarcated submandibular/parapharyngeal space abscess also warranted an incision and drainage in the operating room. This abscess could rapidly turn into an airway emergency

soft palate, which are common sites of malignancy (Ghali and Scott Connor 2004). Make sure to palpate the base of the tongue as well (Ghali and Scott Connor 2004). Palpation of the neck is critical to detect the presence of cervical nodal involvement (Broumand et al. 2006).

- Remember the areas of high transformation to malignancy, especially the minor salivary glands in the labial vestibule and mucosal lip (Ghali and Scott Connor 2004).

15.4.2 Biopsy Procedure

- Punch biopsies are useful for smaller, intraoral lesions (Neitzel 2005).
- A biconvex or elliptical excision with a Bard-Parker scalpel can remove a lesion, with appropriate surgical margins, and still provide good aesthetic closure (Ghali and Scott Connor 2004; Neitzel 2005).

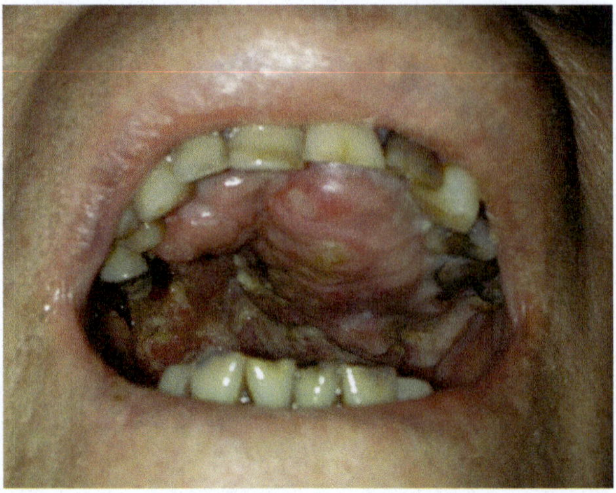

Fig. 15.10 This middle-aged patient presented very late with a large, nonresectable squamous cell carcinoma

- Controlling bleeding
  - Silver nitrate sticks for chemical hemostasis
  - Gauze pressure and time
  - Often, suturing the incision closed will prevent further bleeding.

15.4.3 Indications for Referral to Oral and Maxillofacial Surgery

- Biopsies:
  - Highly vascular regions with concerns for bleeding, such as deep neck and scalp
  - High patient anxiety levels
  - Need for sedation or general anesthesia
  - Outside the dentist's comfort or skill level
- Concern for pathology:
  - Clinical abnormalities found on a thorough oral cancer screening are described above (Ghali and Scott Connor 2004). Areas of leukoplakia or erythroplakia, especially if ulcerated, firm, or fixed, may be suspicious for a malignancy (Broumand et al. 2006) (Fig. 15.10).
  - Referral is necessary if radiographic evidence shows a bony pathology, notably radiolucencies or radiopacities that cannot be treated with routine dental procedures. Plain films are not useful for routine screening, as they only show later signs of cortical breakdown (Broumand et al. 2006).
  - Pain abnormalities or paresthesia/dysesthesia (perineural invasion) that cannot be routinely diagnosed (Broumand et al. 2006).

References

Auyong TG, Le A. Dentoalveolar nerve injury. Oral Maxillofac Surg Clin North Am. 2011;23(3):395–400. Print.

Bartee BK, Lignelli JL. Guided tissue regeneration in dentistry: techniques for management of localized bone defects. In: Raymond F, Marciani R, Turvey T, editors. Oral and maxillofacial surgery, vol. 1. 2nd ed. St. Louis: Saunders; 2008. p. 428–57. Print.

Block MS. Horizontal ridge augmentation using, particulate bone. Atlas Oral Maxillofac Surg Clin North Am. 2006;14(1):27–38. Print.

Blot WJ, et al. Smoking and drinking in relation to oral and pharyngeal cancer. Cancer Res. 1988;48(11):3282–7. Print.

Broumand V, Lozano TE, Gomez JA. Evaluation and staging of oral cancer. Oral Maxillofac Surg Clin North Am. 2006;18(4):435–44. Print.

Camargo PM, et al. Alveolar bone preservation following tooth extraction: a perspective of clinical trials utilizing osseous grafting and guided bone regeneration. Oral Maxillofac Surg Clin North Am. 2004;16(1):9–18, v. Print.

Chaudhry AN, Ruggiero SL. Osteonecrosis and bisphosphonates in oral and maxillofacial surgery. Oral Maxillofac Surg Clin North Am. 2007;19(2):199–206, vi. Print.

Cummings DR, Yamashita DD, McAndrews JP. Complications of local anesthesia used in oral and maxillofacial surgery. Oral Maxillofac Surg Clin North Am. 2011;23(3):369–77. Print.

Curley AW. The law and dentoalveolar complications: trends and controversies. Oral Maxillofac Surg Clin North Am. 2011;23(3):475–84. Print.

Digman SW, Hayes SL, Niel J-LG. Pediatric dentoalveolar surgery. In: Fonseca R, Robert M, Timothy T, editors. Oral and maxillofacial surgery, vol. 1. 2nd ed. St. Louis: Saunders, Elsevier; 2008. p. 165–84. Print.

Felsenfeld AL, Aghaloo T. Surgical exposure of impacted teeth. Oral Maxillofac Surg Clin North Am. 2002;14(2):187–99. Print.

Fletcher MC, Spera JF. Pre-emptive and postoperative analgesia for dentoalveolar surgery. Oral Maxillofac Surg Clin North Am. 2002;14(2):137–51. Print.

Flynn TR. Principles of management of odontogenic infections. In: Miloro M et al., editors. Peterson's principles of oral and maxillofacial surgery. 2nd ed. Hamilton: BC Decker Inc; 2004. p. 277–93. Print.

Flynn TR. What are the antibiotics of choice for odontogenic infections, and how long should the treatment course last? Oral Maxillofac Surg Clin North Am. 2011;23(4):519–36, v–vi. Print.

Geurs NC, Vassilopoulos PJ, Reddy MS. Soft tissue considerations in implant site development. Oral Maxillofac Surg Clin North Am. 2010;22(3):387–405, vi–vii. Print.

Ghali GE, Scott Connor M. Oral cancer: classification, staging, and diagnosis. In: Miloro M et al., editors. Peterson's principles of oral and maxillofacial surgery. 2nd ed. Hamilton: BC Decker Inc; 2004. p. 617–30. Print.

Johri A, Piecuch JF. Should teeth be extracted immediately in the presence of acute infection? Oral Maxillofac Surg Clin North Am. 2011;23(4):507–11, v. Print.

Juodzbalys G, Daugela P. Mandibular third molar impaction: review of literature and a proposal of a classification. J Oral Maxillofac Res. 2013;4(2):e1. Print.

Krakowiak PA. Alveolar osteitis and osteomyelitis of the jaws. Oral Maxillofac Surg Clin North Am. 2011;23(3):401–13. Print.

Lee JS, et al. Prevention of wrong-site tooth extraction: clinical guidelines. J Oral Maxillofac Surg. 2007;65(9):1793–9. Print.

Li G. Patient radiation dose and protection from cone-beam computed tomography. Imaging Sci Dent. 2013;43(2):63–9. Print.

Lypka M, Hammoudeh J. Dentoalveolar infections. Oral Maxillofac Surg Clin North Am. 2011;23(3):415–24. Print.

Malamed SF. Handbook of local anesthesia. 4th ed. St. Louis: Mosby; 1997. Print.

Malmquist JP. Complications in oral and maxillofacial surgery: management of hemostasis and bleeding disorders in surgical procedures. Oral Maxillofac Surg Clin North Am. 2011;23(3):387–94. Print.

Massoomi NS. Local anesthetics. In: Fonseca R, Robert M, Timothy T, editors. Oral and maxillofacial surgery, vol. 1. 2nd ed. St. Louis: Saunders, Elsevier; 2008. p. 35–55. Print.

McAllister BS, Haghighat K. Bone augmentation techniques. J Periodontol. 2007;78(3):377–96. Print.

Miloro M, Kolokythas A. Inferior alveolar and lingual nerve imaging. Atlas Oral Maxillofac Surg Clin North Am. 2011;19(1):35–46. Print.

Misch CM. Autogenous bone grafting for dental implants. In: Fonseca R, Robert M, Timothy T, editors. Oral and maxillofacial surgery, vol. 1. 2nd ed. St. Louis: Saunders; 2008. p. 406–27. Print.

Monaco G, et al. Reliability of panoramic radiography in evaluating the topographic relationship between the mandibular canal and impacted third molars. J Am Dent Assoc. 2004;135(3):312–8. Print.

Monaco G, et al. Coronectomy: a surgical option for impacted third molars in close proximity to the inferior alveolar nerve. J Am Dent Assoc. 2012;143(4):363–9. Print.

Moy PK. Alveolar ridge reconstruction with preprosthetic surgery: a precursor to site preservation following extraction of natural dentition. Oral Maxillofac Surg Clin North Am. 2004;16(1):1–7. v. Print.

Neitzel CD. Biopsy techniques for skin disease and skin cancer. Oral Maxillofac Surg Clin North Am. 2005;17(2):143–6. v. Print.

Ness GM, Peterson LJ. Impacted teeth. In: Miloro M, editor. Peterson's principles of oral and maxillofacial surgery. 2nd ed. Hamilton: BC Decker Inc; 2004. p. 139–55. Print.

Osborn TM, Assael LA, Bell RB. Deep space neck infection: principles of surgical management. Oral Maxillofac Surg Clin North Am. 2008;20(3):353–65. Print.

Otten JE, et al. Bacterial colonization on different suture materials – a potential risk for intraoral dentoalveolar surgery. J Biomed Mater Res B Appl Biomater. 2005;74b(1):627–35. Print.

Patterson Dental surgical burs. 2016. Web. 12/23/2015 2016.

Peterson LJ. Principles of complicated exodontia. In: Peterson LJ, Hupp JR, Tucker MR, editors. Contemporary oral and maxillofacial surgery. 4th ed. St. Louis: Elsevier; 2002. p. 156–83. Print.

Rafetto LK. Controversy, evidence, and third molar management. Atlas Oral Maxillofac Surg Clin North Am. 2012;20(2):253–61. Print.

Rothman K, Keller A. The effect of joint exposure to alcohol and tobacco on risk of cancer of the mouth and pharynx. J Chronic Dis. 1972;25(12):711–6. Print.

Ruggiero SL, et al. American Association of Oral and Maxillofacial Surgeons position paper on medication-related osteonecrosis of the jaw-2014 update. J Oral Maxillofac Surg. 2014;72(10):1938–56. Print.

Sakar M, Ogle OE, Harry D. Basic and complex exodontia and surgical management of impacted teeth. In: Fonseca RJ, Robert M, Timothy T, editors. Oral and maxillofacial surgery, vol. 1. 2nd ed. St. Louis: Saunders, Elsevier; 2008. p. 185–211. Print.

Sosovicka MF. Lasers in oral and maxillofacial surgery. In: Fonseca R, Robert M, Timothy T, editors. Oral and maxillofacial surgery, vol. 1. 2nd ed. St. Louis: Saunders, Elsevier; 2008. p. 237–58. Print.

Spagnoli DB, Gallehon SG, Misiek DJ. Preprosthetic and reconstructive surgery. In: Miloro M et al., editors. Peterson's principles of oral and maxillofacial surgery. 2nd ed. Hamilton: DC Becker Inc; 2004. p. 156–86. Print.

White JM, et al. Nd : Yag and Co2 laser therapy of oral mucosal lesions. J Clin Laser Med Surg. 1998;16(6):299–304. Print.

Wikesjo UM, et al. Bone morphogenetic proteins: a realistic alternative to bone grafting for alveolar reconstruction. Oral Maxillofac Surg Clin North Am. 2007;19(4):535–51, vi-vii. Print.

Wlodawsky RN, Strauss RA. Intraoral laser surgery. Oral Maxillofac Surg Clin North Am. 2004;16(2):149–63. Print.
Ziccardi VB. Microsurgical techniques for repair of the inferior alveolar and lingual nerves. Atlas Oral Maxillofac Surg Clin North Am. 2011;19(1):79–90. Print.

Suggested Reading

Atlas of Human Anatomy, by Frank H. Netter.
Peterson's Principles of Oral and Maxillofacial Surgery, by Michael Miloro, GE Ghali, Peter Larsen, and Peter Waite.
Oral and Maxillofacial Surgery Volume 1, by Raymond Fonseca, Robert Marciani, and Timothy Turvey.

Pediatric Dentistry for the General Practitioners

16

Dennis Bear, Maggie Wang, and Abimbola Adewumi

Contents

D. Bear, DMD (✉)
Pediatric Dentistry Resident, University of Minnesota School of Dentistry, Minneapolis, MN, USA
e-mail: dbear.dental@gmail.com

M. Wang, DMD, MS
Private practice Orthodontist, M.S. from the University of Washington (Seattle), Minneapolis, MN, USA

A. Adewumi, BDS, MS
University of Florida Pediatric dentistry, University of Florida College of Dentistry, Gainesville, FL, USA

G.M. Weinstein, M.T. Zientz (eds.), *The Dental Reference Manual*,
DOI 10.1007/978-3-319-39730-6_16

Abstract

The American Dental Association and the American Academy of Pediatric Dentistry recommend establishment of a dental home by a child's first birthday. However, many children's first encounter with a dentist is when they are 3–4 years and older at a general practitioner's office, where their parents visit. During the child's first visit, it is important for the general dentist to build a positive first impression of the dental profession. In this chapter, we will discuss tooth development and eruption, behavioral guidance techniques including pharmacological consideration in pediatric patients, preventive and restorative, common pediatric dental emergencies, orthodontic considerations, clinical pearls, and when to refer to a pediatric specialist.

16.1 Tooth Development and Eruption

A very important task a general dentist faces when meeting a pediatric patient for the first time and during subsequent periodic visits is to evaluate the child's eruption pattern as well as identify any delayed, ectopic eruption or disrupted eruption sequence. The eruption charts are provided by American Dental Association to use as a general guideline. However, individual variances exist, and it is important for a general dentist to look for symmetry (Tables 16.1 and 16.2).

Table 16.1 Primary teeth eruption table

	Enamel completion	Eruption	Root completion	Exfoliation
Mandibular centrals	2.5 months	6 months	1.5 years	6–7 years
Mandibular laterals	3 months	7 months	1.5 years	7–8 years
Maxillary centrals	1.5 months	7.5 months	1.5 years	6–7 years
Maxillary laterals	2.5 months	9 months	2 years	7–8 years
Mandibular 1st molars	5.5 months	12 months	2.5 years	9–11 years
Maxillary 1st molars	6 months	14 months	2.5 years	9–11 years
Mandibular canines	9 months	16 months	3 ¼ years	9–12 years
Maxillary canines	9 months	18 months	3 ¼ years	10–12 years
Mandibular 2nd molars	10 months	20 months	3 years	10–12 years
Maxillary 2nd molars	11 months	24 months	3 years	10–12 years

Table 16.2 Permanent teeth eruption table (AAPD 2014a, b, c, d, e, f)

	Enamel completion	Eruption	Root completion
Mandibular 1st molars	2.5–3 years	6–7 years	9–10 years
Maxillary 1st molars	2.5–3 years	6–7 years	9–10 years
Mandibular centrals	4–5 years	6–7 years	9 years
Maxillary centrals	4–5 years	7–8 years	10 years
Mandibular laterals	4–5 years	7–8 years	10 years
Maxillary laterals	4–5 years	8–9 years	11 years
Mandibular canines	6–7 years	9–10 years	12–14 years
Maxillary 1st premolars	5–6 years	10–11 years	12–13 years
Mandibular 1st premolar	5–6 years	10–12 years	12–13 years
Maxillary 2nd premolars	6–7 years	10–12 years	12–14 years
Mandibular 2nd premolars	6–7 years	11–12 years	13–14 years
Maxillary canines	6–7 years	11–12 years	13–14 years
Mandibular 2nd premolars	7–8 years	11–13 years	14–15 years
Maxillary 2nd premolars	7–8 years	12–13 years	14–16 years
Mandibular 3d molars	–	17–21 years	–
Maxillary 3rd molars	–	17–21 years	–

Some general trends of eruption include: (AAPD 2014a)

- "Rule of 4's" for primary teeth eruption: four teeth erupt every 4 months beginning with four teeth at age 7 months.
- The eruption of teeth usually occurs symmetrically in each arch.
- There may be ethnic and gender variations with respect to eruption times, e.g., African American children and girls may generally experience earlier eruption times.
- Variation of 6 months of either side of the usual eruption age may be considered normal for a given child.
- Mandibular teeth occur before the maxilla, except permanent premolars.

- Formation of all permanent teeth begins between birth and 2.5 years.
- Look for missing teeth, supernumerary teeth, submerged teeth (ankyloses), and malformed teeth. Inform parents and treatment plan for the future.
- Be aware that children with certain medical conditions such as Down's syndrome or cleft lip and palate may experience generalized delayed eruption of teeth.

16.2 Behavioral Management Consideration

16.2.1 First Meeting with the Dentist

For most general dentists, especially the recent graduate, the idea of treating children can create a certain level of stress and anxiety. Although most practitioners may have received some didactic training during their dental school experience with regards to principles of tooth eruption, space maintenance, and management of children, their clinical experience is limited. This often creates a feeling of intimidation when asked to provide dental care to the pediatric population. The best way for young practitioners to gain experience in working with children is to be open minded and being familiar with AAPD policies and guidelines. In addition, reaching out to local pediatric dental faculty could be an additional resource when faced with particularly challenging cases.

A general dentist has one chance to create a good first impression of dentistry to a child (Fig. 16.1). The success of this interaction usually determines the outcomes of subsequent dental visits. For example, children can sense if their dentist is uncomfortable and this may inadvertently create mistrust between the child and the dentist. Depending on the age and cognitive development of the child, this distrust can manifest in the form of a refusal to cooperate, crying, and an adverse behavioral pattern, even with the simplest procedures. The authors recommend that the new practitioner review the AAPD policy guidelines on behavioral modification techniques. This can be accessed on ISSN: http://www.aapd.org/media/policies_guidelines/g_behavguide.pdf (Accessed on March 30, 2016).

Be confident when you speak to kids and remember that you are the adult and authority figure at that appointment. It is important to understand that not all children are the same nor will they behave the same. Greet them in a friendly manner and asses what type of child is sitting in your dental chair. Also try to engage the parents early to enquire about their child's past dental experience. Some practitioners categorize children by the level of fear and their response to fear.

16.2.2 Types of Children (Casamassimo et al. 2013)

1. *The fearless child.* This is a happy and confident child. They are open to strangers and are willing to try anything once. These children typically have some dental exposure or good coaching/examples from parental figures. These children usually trust the dentist, and it is important to recognize and respect this trust so as not to break it.

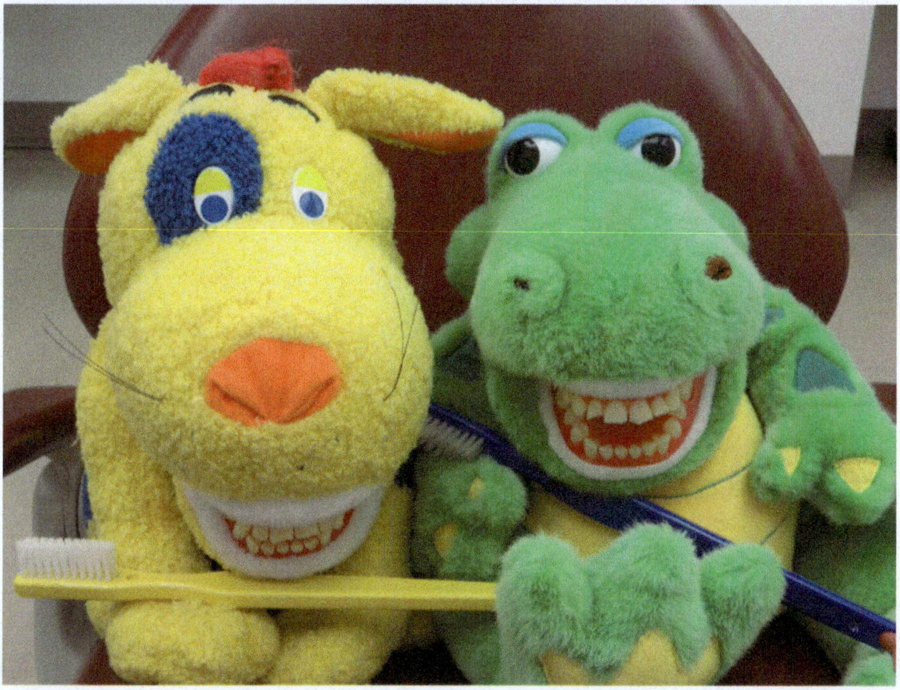

Fig. 16.1 For younger children, the use of puppets is a helpful tool for many reasons (Photo courtesy of Dr. Khiem Truong)

2. *The cautious child.* This child may or may not have had any dental exposure. They are not quick to warm up to strangers. The cautious child will participate in treatment but may need some coaching from the parent. Tell-show-do works extremely well with these children. These children can be reasoned with and can easily be behaviorally managed.
3. *The fearful child.* These children may not seem afraid at first when talking to them and even act "macho" but may scream in terror at the sight of an exam mirror. They may have had a bad past dental experience or fearful parents who have reinforced bad behaviors in the chair. It is very important to educate the parent that their dental experience is not indicative of their child's experience. When performing treatments, several behavioral techniques may need to be adopted. Chemical anxiolytics such as nitrous oxide gas or benzodiazepines may also need to be considered.
4. *The scared-out-of-their-mind child.* A completely terrified child. These children are very difficult or impossible to be reasoned with. They do not want to try anything new and do not trust anyone. These children may have had one or a few bad encounters with the dentist. Their parental figures may be also terrified of the dentist and impose this fear on the child. It is recommended to refer these children to pediatric dentist for sedation or more advanced behavioral modification modalities.

Table 16.3 Substituting dental terms for "kids' language"

Dental terms	Kid's terms	Dental terms	Kid's terms	Dental terms	Kid's terms
Cotton roll	Tooth pillow	Handpiece	Water whistle	Rubber dam	Tooth raincoat
Rubber dam clamp	Tooth ring	Saliva ejector	Mr. Thirsty	Local anesthetic	Sleepy juice
Explorer	Tooth counter	Etch	Blue shampoo	Sealant	Tooth face painting
Caries	Sugar bugs	X-rays	Tooth picture	Cleaning/prophy	Tickling teeth
Fluoride	Tooth vitamins	Fillings	White play-doh	Silver crowns	Tooth jewelry
Extraction	Wiggle a tooth	Extraction forceps	Mr. Wiggle	Nitrous oxide	Ice cream air
Bite blocks	Tooth chair	Dentist's loupes	Binoculars	Impression	Tooth print with play-doh

16.2.3 Kids' Language

When speaking with children about impending dental treatment, a general dentist should be careful to use language that creates a positive mind-set. The dentist must gauge the child's cognition and use "kids-friendly" words to convey their "dental" message in order to build and maintain trust. Depending on the age of the child, using words like needle, shot, drill, pull, or yank teeth or any other word that suggest unpleasantness and invoke fear must be avoided. Here are some suggestions (Table 16.3).

16.2.4 Tell-Show-Do

This behavior-shaping tool is well accepted and very popular with children and adult patients (Fig. 16.2).

Tell – The dentist informs the child in age-appropriate terms what is going to happen.

Show –This is then followed by demonstrating to the child, in a nonthreatening way either on themselves, the parent, or the child.

Do – Then without deviating from the demonstration, continue with the procedure that is to be performed.

16.2.5 Desensitization

This is considered an expansion of the Tell-Show-Do technique. Here stimuli with the least anxiety are presented first. Higher anxiety evokers are presented as the

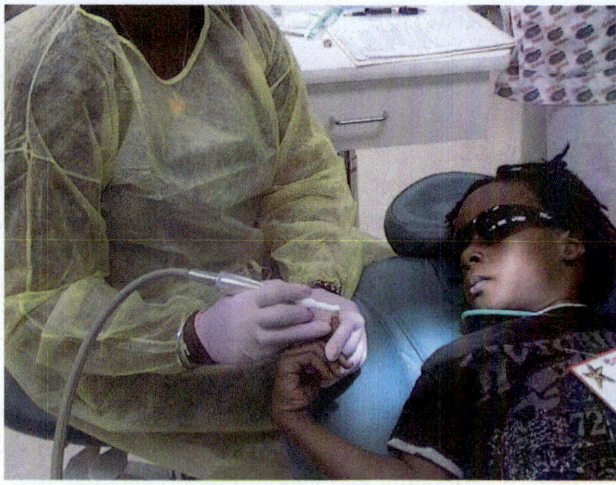

Fig. 16.2 The dentist demonstrating the prophylaxis cup on the child's finger before using it to clean his teeth

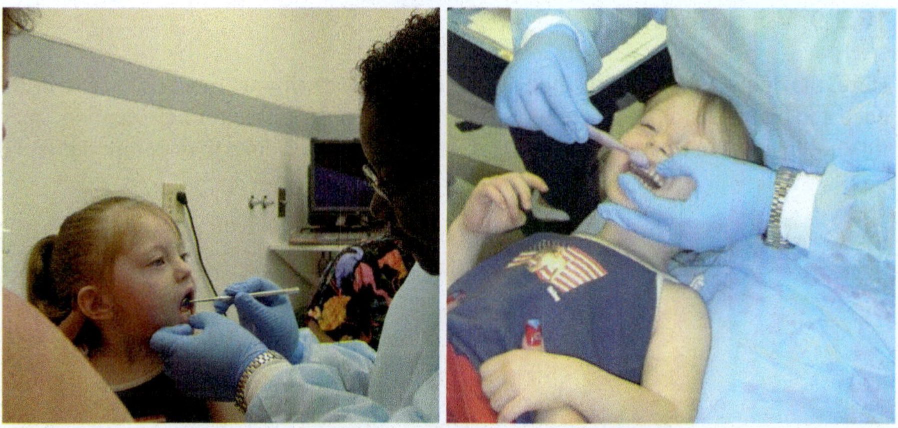

Fig. 16.3 The dentist begins by using the mirror while the young child sits on her mother's lap before proceeding to do a toothbrush cleaning using a lap exam

child is able to tolerate them, e.g., using a prophylaxis cup before using a high speed handpiece (Fig. 16.3).

16.2.6 Positive Reinforcement

This is a technique used to reward desirable positive behavior by praising the child or providing a reward and this further strengthens the recurrence of such behavior in future. Many dental offices have small prizes to give to pediatric patients at the end of the visit such as stickers and simple toys. Other social reenforcers include positive voice modulation, e.g., being "goofy," facial expression, verbal praise, and appropriate physical demonstrations of affection by all members of the dental team.

16.2.7 Distraction

This is a technique of diverting the patient's attention from what may be perceived as an unpleasant procedure or sensation by focusing their thoughts on something other than what is being done. Examples include asking patient to wiggle his or her toes during impression taking; giggle the cheeks during local anesthetic injection; and giving patient storytelling, animated voices, or even a short break during a stressful procedure.

16.2.8 Modeling

This technique is very effective in families that have two or more children. A younger, inexperienced, or apprehensive child learns to stay calm and how to act properly by watching an older sibling or someone they look up to (Fig. 16.4),

16.2.9 Voice Control

Here, the dentist uses a controlled alteration of voice volume, tone, or pace to influence and direct the child's behavior. It may be uncomfortable for new dentists since it is not learned in dental school. It takes time and experience to develop; the facial

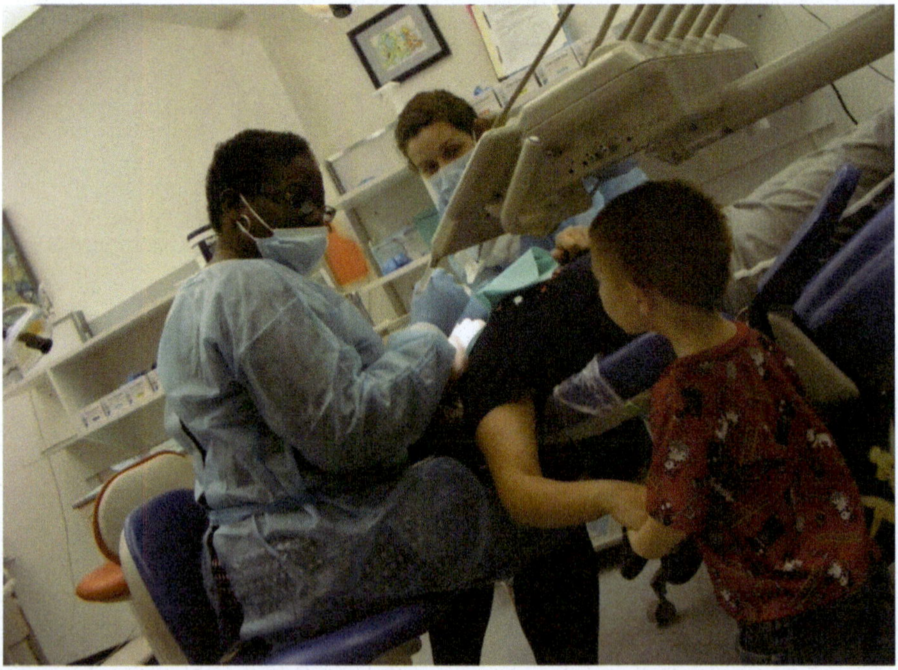

Fig. 16.4 While the older sibling receives treatment, her younger brother holds her hand and watches on. This process usually reassures the younger sibling that there is nothing to fear

expression is as important as voice, and it is important to explain this technique to parents beforehand to prevent misunderstanding the dentist or assistants for being "mean" to their child.

16.2.10 Parental Presence or Absence

There must be a discussion and agreement between the dentist and parent before the child sits in the chair. Parents of children >3 years that come into the operatory must be prepared to leave if/when child shows undesirable behavior. Generally children under 36–40 months do better with parents present. The behavior and attitude of a parent can be directly related to a good or a bad dental visit for their child. Children can sense their parents' fear and parents can unintentionally transfer fear to their child by their body language or nonverbal cues. It cannot be perceived by either the parent or child as punitive. Sometimes, a dentist can use parents as leverage to obtain appropriate behavior response. First, explain the procedure to the parents separately. During the procedure, if the child shows negative or undesirable behavior, the parents are asked to leave the operatory immediately. Once the child's behavior improves, the parents can return to the room.

16.3 Pharmacologic Considerations

Please always refer to a dental drug reference guide for the proper dosage to give your pediatric patients. There are numerous sources online that offer up-to-date dosages and precautions. One example is http://www.epocrates.com/marketing/products/rx/index.html.

16.3.1 Fluoride

Using fluoride for the prevention and control of dental caries is proven to be both safe and effective when dosed appropriately (AAPD 2014b). The frequency of fluoride exposure from various sources should be identified when formulating a dental plan for the patient. Fluoride sources could include water, dietary supplements, mouth rinses, and toothpaste. Prior to prescribing supplemental fluoride to any child, initial testing of the drinking water should be performed. A caries risk assessment is also essential in order for proper parental counseling to reduce the child's caries risk (See Chap. 3 Caries Prevention) (Table 16.4, Fig. 16.5).

16.3.1.1 Topical Fluoride

Topical fluoride application is available via professionally applied topical fluoride treatment, over-the-counter rinses for home use, prescription rinses and gels for home use, and fluoride-containing toothpastes. Over-the-counter fluoride mouth rinses are not recommended for preschool-aged children. Toothpaste

Table 16.4 Dietary fluoride supplementation schedule (AAPD 2014a, b, c, d, e, f)

	Concentration of fluoride		
Age	<0.3 ppm F	0.3–0.6 ppm F	>0.6 ppm F
Birth–6 months	0	0	0
6 months–3 year	0.25 mg	0	0
3–6 year	0.50 mg	0.25 mg	0
6–16 year	1.00 mg	0.50 mg	0

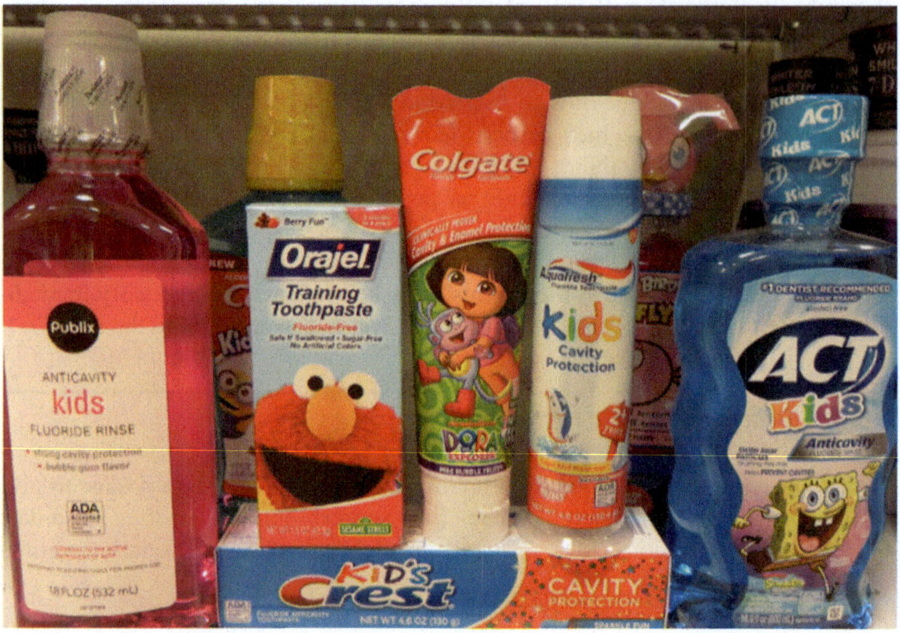

Fig. 16.5 Commercially available fluoride comes in various “child-friendly” packages

usage should be always supervised by parents in young children. American Academy of Pediatric Dentistry recommends for children under 3 years old a smear or rice-size amount of fluoridated toothpaste twice a day. A small amount of toothpaste equal to the size of a pea should be wiped onto the toothbrush by the caretaker for children between ages 3–6 years old twice a day. Caution should be taken by the parents and prescribing dentists to not create fluoride overdose during critical periods of enamel formation and fluorosis (AAPD 2014a, b, c, d, e, f).

16.3.2 Local Analgesics

Dosage of local anesthetic in pediatric patients should be measure by the child's body weight. Children do not have fully developed livers which slow down

Table 16.5 Local anesthetic efficacious dosage for pediatrics (AAPD 2015b)

Anesthetic	Maximum dosage Mg/kg	Maximum dosage Mg/lb	Maximum total dosage (mg)	Mg/ cartridge (mg)	Duration of action in minutes: Pulp	Duration of action in minutes: Soft tissue
Lidocaine 2 % 1:000,000 epi	4.4	2.0	300	36	60	180–240
Mepivacaine 3 % plain	4.4	2.0	300	54	5–10	90–120
Articaine 4 % 1:100,000 epi	7.0	3.2	500	68	60–75	180–300
Prilocaine 4 % plain	8.0	3.6	600	72	10–15 (infiltration) 60–120 (block)	40–60 (infiltration) 120–240 (block)

Bupivacaine is not recommended in pediatric patients due prolonged numbness and postoperative Trauma (AAPD 2015a, b)

metabolism of certain anesthetics. Use caution in the amount of anesthetic you give and never exceed the maximum total dosage based on the child's weight (Table 16.5).

To calculate the maximum amount of lidocaine 2 % with 1:100,000 epinephrine and the number of cartridges that can be safely administered to a 30-lb patient, perform the calculations below (AAPD 2015a, b):

Maximum dosage (mg/lbs) × patients weight (lbs) = Maximum total dosage (mg) $2.0 \times 30 = 60$ *mgs*

Maximum total dosage (mg) ÷ mg/cartidge = Maximum # cartridges $60 \div 36 = 1.67$ *cartridges*

Clinical tips in administering local anesthesia (LA):

- Consider having an assistant place his/hers arms lightly across the child's chest or hold their hands during the injection to protect the child from reaching up and grabbing the syringe.
- Use a bite block or a mouth prop during LA administration to prevent the child from suddenly closing their mouth; this is sometimes a reflex reaction to the LA "stab."
- Use distraction techniques, like wiggling the cheek or lip when giving local anesthesia.
- For upper infiltration, insert a 30-gauge needle 1 mm or less into the tissue and very slowly infiltrate a quarter of a carpule. Wait a couple seconds and then proceed with normal injection protocol to give the rest of the carpule.
- After buccal anesthesia is achieved, you may give buccal intrapapillary injection numbing the palatal through the buccal. This is due to the porous nature of the maxilla. Then give normal palatal injection. This procedure may take longer but is a good way to reduce discomfort and introduce kids to dental procedures.

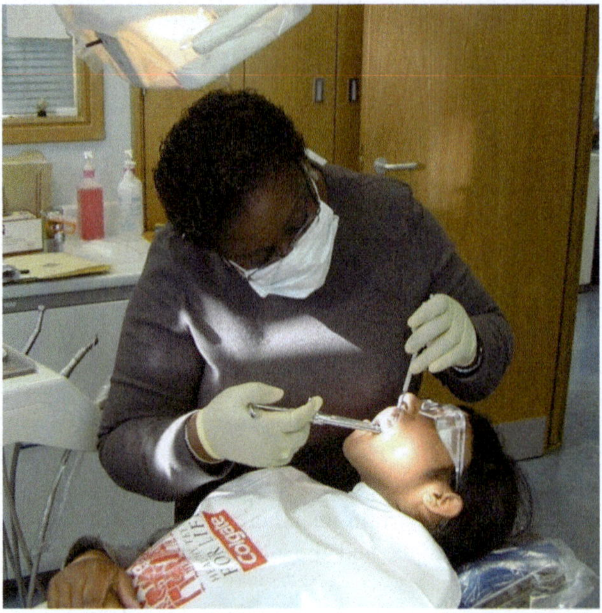

Fig. 16.6 Local anesthesia should not be a problem in older well-behaved children

- Remember that pain is how you feel and a child in pain is an uncooperative child so it is important to try and achieve profound anesthesia as much as possible. Always test your LA *subjectively* by asking child if the area feels "heavy, weird, different, or swollen" compared to the contralateral side. Remember most children may not know what numb means especially if this is their first LA experience. You can also test LA *objectively* by using an explorer to gently touch the mucosa around the tooth and watch for signs of pain such as "wincing, raised, or hunched shoulders, withdrawal from injection site". You can also ask the child to raise their hand, as a stop sign if they feel a sharp pain (Fig. 16.6).

16.3.3 Postoperative Pain Control in Pediatric Patients

Pain management in children requires careful consideration. Anxiety also reduces the pain threshold so the dentist must take care to perform a behavioral evaluation ahead of time so as to plan for pain as well as anxiety management. If at all possible, it should be done by planning preoperative strategies to control and minimize physical and mental trauma to the child. A careful review of a patient's medical history is necessary to identify allergies and contraindications to prescribed analgesics (Table 16.6).

16.3.4 Common Antibiotics for Odontogenic Infection in Children

Following careful examination of the patient and determination that the infection is bacterial in nature, consideration of antibiotic prescription can be considered. A careful review of the medical history is also necessary to avoid contraindications.

Table 16.6 Dosage for pediatric pain management (Mosby 2014)

Medication	Recommended dosage (oral)	Benefits	Disadvantage/ contraindication	Dispensed
Acetaminophen	Under 44 kg: 10–15 mg/kg every 4–6 h max = 2.6 g/day Over 44 kg: 325 mg–650 mg/ dose every 4–6 h max = 4 g/day	Antipyretic agent Safe record of use	No anti-inflammatory action Mild pain relief Caution on patient with liver disorders	Drops: 80 mg/0.8 ml Suspension: 160 mg/5 ml Chewable tabs: 80 mg/tabs Tablets: 325 mg, 500 mg
Ibuprofen	4–10 mg/kg every 6–8 h 40 mg/kg/day	Antipyretic anti-inflammatory properties relieves moderate to severe pain	Gastric irritant Impair clotting May be contraindicated in some asthmatic children	Suspension: 40 mg/1 ml (oral drops) 100 mg/5 ml (oral) Chewable: 50 mg and 100 mg tabs Tablets: 200 mg, 400 mg, 600 mg, 800 mg
Aspirin	Oral, rectal: 10–15 mg/kg/ dose every 4–6 h up to a total of 80–100 mg/kg/ day	Antipyretic anti-inflammatory properties	Gastric irritant Impair clotting Reye's syndrome – especially in children who take aspirin when experiencing fever or other symptoms of viral illness Allergies in children (last choice for children)	Chewable tabs: 81 mg Caplets, tablets: 325 mg, 500 mg Suppository, rectal: 300 mg, 600 mg
Acetaminophen w/codeine	Under 44 kg: Codeine: 0.5–1 mg/kg every 4–6 h Over 44 kg: Codeine: 30–60 mg/dose every 4–6 h. See acetaminophen table for consideration	Codeine acts at central site of pain Acetaminophen at peripheral site for enhanced analgesia	Acute dosing (3 days or less). Codeine can cause nausea, sedation, constipation, and dependency. Use acetaminophen with caution in patients with liver disorders	Suspension: acetaminophen 120 mg and codeine phosphate 12 mg per 5 ml Tablets: #3: Acetaminophen 300 mg and codeine phosphate 30 mg #4: Acetaminophen 300 mg and codeine phosphate 60 mg

Table 16.7 Antibiotic dosage (AAPD 2014a, b, c, d, e, f; Wynn et al. 2015)

Antibiotics	Dosage Children	Adults	Contraindication	Warnings/ precautions
Penicillin VK	≤12 years; 25–50 mg/kg q6-8h for at least 7 days; max dose 3 g/day	>12 years: 500 mg q6h for at least 7 days	0.7–10 % allergy rate Around 85 % of allergic reaction is delayed and take greater than 2 days to develop	Severe renal impairment (modify dosage), history of seizure, hypersensitivity to cephalosporins
Clindamycin	<12 years: 10–25 mg/kg/ day for 10 days >12 years: 600–1800 mg/ day for 10 days; Max dose 2–3 g/day	150–450 mg q6h for at least 7 days; max dose 1.8 g/day	Hypersensitivity to clindamycin; previous pseudomembranous colitis, regional enteritis, ulcerative colitis	Liver dysfunction (modify dosage); discontinue drug if significant diarrhea, cramps, or blood and mucus passage occurs
Cephalexin (Keflex)	25–50 mg/kg/ day q6h; Severe infection: 50–100 mg/kg/ day q6h; max dose 3 g/ day	250–1000 mg q6h; max dose 4 g/day	Allergy to the cephalosporin group of antibiotics	Inflammation of the large intestine, kidney disease, colitis
Amoxicillin	<40 kg: 20–40 mg/kg/ day q8h; >40 kg: 250–500 mg q8h or 875 mg q12h for at least 7 days; max dose 2 g/day	>40 kg: 250–500 mg q8h or 875 mg q12h for at least 7 days; max dose 2 g/day	Hypersensitivity to amoxicillin, penicillin	Severe renal impairment (modify dosage); low incidence of cross-allergy with other beta-lactams and cephalosporins exists

The most common side effects of antibiotics include mild diarrhea, abdominal pain, nausea, and vomiting. In teenage patients, precautions should be given to patients that antibiotics can affect effectiveness of oral contraceptives (Table 16.7).

16.3.5 Nitrous Oxide (Laughing Gas)

A general dentist needs to be certified by an institution after receiving proper education and clinical training hours prior to administering nitrous oxide in his or her own practice (Fig. 16.7).

Characteristics of nitrous oxide:

1. Reduces or eliminates anxiety, promotes analgesia, and potentiates the effects of sedatives
2. Reduces the gag reflex but not the cough reflex
3. Minimal or nonexistent toxicity when used on healthy patients properly

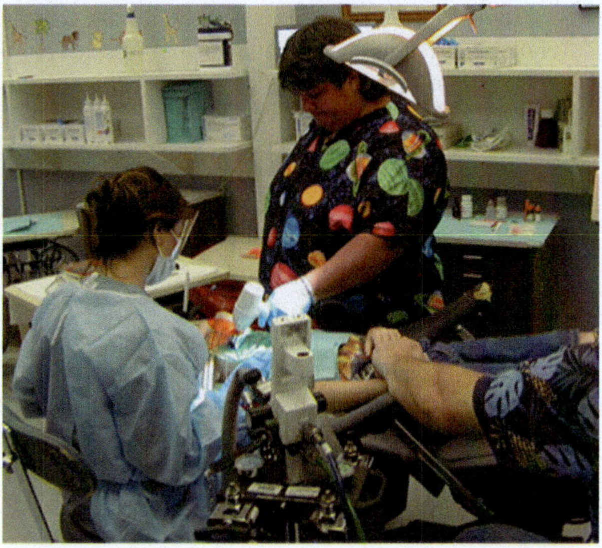

Fig. 16.7 Nitrous oxide patients should be attended to by the provider and an assistant to monitor the patient through the whole procedure

4. Highly insoluble in blood and water; therefore quick absorption and elimination
5. Mostly (99 %) eliminated from the body through the lungs without significant biotransformation, which makes it have minimal effect on other organ systems
6. Not metabolized through the liver
7. Reduces untoward movement and reaction to dental treatment
8. Enhances communication and patient cooperation. More effective when used in conjunction with hypnotic suggestions and other simple behavioral modification techniques
9. Raises the patient's pain reaction threshold
10. Increases tolerance for longer appointments

Nitrous oxide is not indicated for every pediatric patient. The key to a successful dental appointment with the help of nitrous oxide lies in dentist's patient selection. Here are the types of patients who could benefit from nitrous oxide:

1. The fearful and anxious, yet cooperative patients
2. Patients with a strong gag reflex
3. Patient who is fearful of specific procedures, such as the "shot" or the drill
4. A cooperative child undergoing a lengthy dental procedure

Nitrous oxide will not help in treatment with these types of children by a general dentist without other sedative measures:

1. Chronologically immature child
2. The cognitively impaired child

The success and effectiveness of nitrous oxide is largely dependent on psychological reassurance. This can only be accomplished if the patient has the ability to understand verbal communication.

3. Defiant child

   This is the child that behaves poorly for dental treatment, not because of excessive fear or anxiety or a physical or mental disability, but because he or she just doesn't want to. A general dentist should attempt behavior modification techniques or refer the child to a pediatric specialist.

16.3.5.1 Contraindications

- *Absolute*: Pregnancy (may cause spontaneous abortion in chronic exposure especially in the first trimester of pregnancy), otitis media, congenital pulmonary blebs, sinus blockage, bowel obstruction, nasal obstruction, cystic fibrosis, and COPD.
- *Relative*: URI, extreme phobias, hysterical behavior to dentistry, and patients with a previous bad experience with nitrous oxide and children who have no respect for authority, do not follow instructions, or are naturally defiant must be assessed with caution.
- Note: Nitrous oxide is not contraindicated in patients with asthma. It is nonirritating to the mucous membranes, and since anxiety can trigger an asthmatic episode, nitrous oxide usage can reduce the possibility of an attack in the dental chair.

16.3.5.2 Nitrous Oxide Dosage (AAPD 2013)

- Low = 33 % N_2O (children) – 2 L/min N_2O to 4 L/min O_2.
- Medium = 50 % N_2O (most adults, max children) – 3 L/min N_2O to 3 L/min O_2.
- High = 62.5 % N_2O (some adults) – 5 L/min N_2O to 3 L/min O_2.
- Maximum = 70 % – 7 L/min N_2O to 3 L/min O_2.
- Oxygen must always keep flowing at the rate of at least 3 L/min.

16.3.5.3 Delivery Protocol (AAPD 2013)

1. Give verbal instruction to the patient. Describe to child floating sensation (will be flying like Superman or Batman) and they may feel warm and tingly (ants are climbing on them).
2. Place monitors: pulse oximeter and BP cuff if available.
3. Turn on 5 L/min oxygen (100 %) before placing the mask on the patient.
4. Place mask on patient – ensure snug fit (no breeze in eyes).
5. Adjust scavenging system valve to green zone.
6. Two delivery methods:
   (a) The standard titration process begins by decreasing the oxygen flow and increasing the nitrous oxide flow to obtain a concentration of 20 % nitrous oxide and 80 % oxygen. Then slowly increasing N_2O and decreasing O_2 until desired level is reached.
   (b) Rapid titration (useful for nervous patients) administration is initiated with a 50 % oxygen/50 % nitrous oxide concentration prior to seating of the nasal hood.

7. When finishing procedure, turn off the nitrous and leave the patient on 100 % oxygen for 5 min.
8. The dentist must remember to document the amount and rate of nitrous oxide administered during the procedure along with the 100 % at the end of treatment.

16.3.5.4 Clinical Tips (Rappaport et al. 2011)

1. Nitrous too low: no effect.
2. Nitrous too high: oppression, unpleasant, nausea, sleepiness, sweating.
3. Quick onset in 2–3 min.
4. Total flow = 5–6 L/min = respiratory minute ventilation = tidal volume x respiratory rate = 500 mL × 12.
5. Fluctuating amounts during treatment may result in nausea and vomiting.

16.4 Treatment Considerations

16.4.1 Medical History: The Exam and Caries Risk Assessment

Before performing a clinical exam, a dentist should discuss past and present medical history with the parents and the children. Review any medical conditions and medications the child may be taking. If the medical history is too complicated for your practice, consult with the patient's pediatrician or refer to a pediatric dentist. The general must know their limitations with respect to treating or managing medically compromised children in their office.

The actual exam is a great way for the dentist to access a child's behavior and level of anxiety as well as gauge whether a child can be treated successfully with simple behavioral management techniques or requires sedation. A child's caries risk assessment should be completed in order to determine the customized plan for the patient's needs. There are many forms online that can be utilized such as those on the American Dental Association site: http://www.ada.org/~/media/ADA/Member%20Center/FIles/topics_caries_under6.ashx.

16.4.2 Sealants

Sealants play a very important role in preventive dentistry and have proven to reduce the occurrence of pit and fissure caries. Prior to treatment planning for sealants, a general dentist needs to perform a thorough caries risk assessment. Sealants should be placed based upon the patient's caries risk, and not the age or time elapsed since tooth eruption (AAPD 2014a, b, c, d, e, f).

Once treatment is planned, the key to clinical success is isolation. Rubber dam placement is highly recommended. The current sealant material of choice is resin based. Sealant placement method should include cleaning of the pits and fissures with pumice and without removal of any appreciable enamel. In some circumstances, preventive resin restoration (PRR) is indicated, where the dentist cleans out the pits and grooves with a small bur. The dentist needs to monitor existing sealants for incipient lesion progression and sealant retention.

Important Tip When sealing mandibular permanent molar, it is important to seal the occlusal as well as buccal surfaces, whereas for the maxillary molars, the lingual surface must be sealed in addition to the occlusal surface.

16.4.3 Restorations Consideration in Primary Teeth (Casamassimo et al. 2013)

In primary teeth, considerations of the anatomical characteristics should be taken to ensure the success of restorations.

1. Mesiodistal dimension of a primary molar crown is greater than the cervico-occlusal dimension.
2. Buccal and lingual surfaces converge toward the occlusal.
3. Enamel and dentin are thinner.
4. The pulp chambers of primary teeth are proportionally larger and closer to the surface.
5. Primary teeth contacts are broader and flatter.
6. Shorter clinical crown height.

16.4.3.1 Composite Restorations

Composite is recommended for primary teeth in pit-and-fissure caries, class II lesions that the preparations do not extend beyond the proximal line angles, and class III, IV, and V lesions. Avoid using composite as the material of choice when:

1. Isolation is a problem.
2. Carious lesions involve multiple surfaces.
3. High-risk patients present with extensive rampant decay or with poor oral hygiene.

16.4.3.2 Amalgam Restorations

Amalgam is recommended for primary teeth in class I lesions, class II lesions where the preparation does not extend beyond the proximal line angles, and class V lesions.

In primary molars, 3-surfaced amalgam restorations can be placed, although full coverage with a stainless steel crown may be a better treatment option.

16.4.4 Pulp Therapies (Table 16.8)

Generally, stainless steel crowns (SSCs) are recommended for primary teeth having received pulp therapy. However, in a tooth with conservative pulpal access, intact walls, and less than 2 years to exfoliation, amalgam or resin restorations can also be considered.

Table 16.8 A summary of pulp therapy in primary teeth (AAPD 2014a, b, c, d, e, f)

Pulp therapy	Indication	Pulpal diagnosis	Radiographic diagnosis	Technique	Prognosis
Indirect pulp cap	When the deepest carious dentin is not removed to avoid a pulp exposure	Normal pulp or reversible pulpitis	No radiographic evidence of external or internal root resorption	A liner such as a resin-modified glass ionizer, calcium hydroxide, zinc oxide/eugenol, or glass ionomer cement is placed over the remaining carious dentin to stimulate healing and repair	As long as the tooth remains sealed from bacterial contamination, the prognosis is good for caries to arrest and reparative dentin to form. Normal exfoliation time of the primary tooth
Direct pulp cap	Pinpoint mechanical (noncarious) exposure of the pulp during cavity preparation or traumatic injury	Normal pulp	No radiographic evidence of external or internal root resorption	A biocompatible base such as TMA or calcium hydroxide may be placed in contact with the exposed pulp tissue	No posttreatment signs or symptoms such as sensitivity, pain, or swelling should be evident. Pulp healing and reparative dentin formation should result. No harm to the succedaneous tooth
Pulpotomy	Pulp exposure in primary tooth during caries removal	Normal pulp or reversible pulpitis	No evidence of radicular pathology. No radiographic evidence of external or internal root resorption	Coronal pulpal tissue is amputated, and the remaining radicular tissue is judged to be vital without suppuration, purulence, necrosis, or excessive hemorrhage that cannot be controlled by a damp cotton pellet after several minutes	Radicular pulp remains asymptomatic without clinical signs and symptoms such as sensitivity, pain, or swelling. No external root resorption. Internal root resorption may be self-limiting and stable
Pulpectomy	Primary tooth exhibits clinical signs of irreversible pulpitis or necrosis	Irreversible pulpitis or necrotic pulp	May or may not have radicular pathology	Root canals are debrided and shaped with files. Irrigate with 1 % NaOCl and/or chlorhexidine. After the canals are dried, a resorbable materials such as zinc oxide eugenol, and iodoform-based paste are used to fill the canals	Clinical signs and symptoms should resolve within a few weeks. Radiographic evidence should resolve in 6 months. Normal resorption of the primary tooth root and filling material. Normal eruption of the succedaneous tooth
Root canal treatment	Permanent teeth	Irreversible pulpitis or necrotic pulp	May or may not have radicular pathology	Follow the normal RCT protocol. Note that in young permanent teeth when apex is fully formed and apexification needs to be initiated prior to root canal filling	

16.4.5 Stainless Steel Crowns (SSCs)

Most of the general dentists' offices do not routinely use stainless steel crowns. If your office is located in a relatively remote or rural area, or the nearest pediatric dentist is far away, you should consider stocking up stainless steel crowns in the office. It is the standard of care with many indications for use in pediatric patients. If a general dentist cannot provide stainless steel crowns, the patient should be referred to a pediatric specialist.

16.4.5.1 Indications for SSC (Casamassimo et al. 2013):

1. Following a pulpotomy or pulpectomy
2. Teeth with developmental defects such as molar incisor hypomineralization (MIH), dentinogenesis, or amelogenesis imperfecta
3. Extensive carious lesions, with multiple surfaces where an amalgam restoration is likely to fail.
4. Fractured teeth
5. Extensive tooth surface loss due to attrition, abrasion, or erosion
6. Children with high caries risk and rampant decay
7. Primary molars in children under 4 years old

16.5 Pediatric Emergencies

The most common pediatric dental emergencies involve:

- Odontogenic infections (OIs)
- Facial cellulitis from odontogenic infections
- Dental and facial trauma to the primary or permanent teeth
- Loose teeth
- Bleeding or pain following extractions

A general dentist should strive to provide emergency treatment as needed, stabilize the condition, and refer to related specialists as soon as possible.

16.5.1 Assess the Emergency

For emergency patients, a quick yet thorough soft and hard tissue exam followed by an extraoral and intraoral exam. Take periapical radiographs to evaluate dental damage, such as fracture of the crown or root. Take a panoramic radiograph to rule out possible alveolar, condylar, and jaw fractures. Look for subjects that may be dislodged inside the soft tissue of the lip or cheeks, such as pieces of a tooth, orthodontic brackets and wire, and foreign objects (Tables 16.9 and 16.10).

Table 16.9 Types of injuries to teeth (Diangelis et al 2012)

Type of injury	Signs and symptoms	Treatment	Prognosis/ follow-up
Concussion – injury to tooth supporting structures with no mobility or displacement but tender to palpation/ percussion no gingival bleeding	No mobility or displacement but tender to palpation/ percussion	None. Observe and follow-up	1-year follow-up on pulpal condition
Subluxation – an injury to the tooth supporting structures without displacement of the tooth	Gingival bleeding Tender to percussion Increased mobility (±) Pulp sensitivity	No treatment is often needed The child may want to eat soft food for 2 weeks Flexible splint may be used if child has discomfort	Long-term prognosis is generally good Monitor 2 weeks, 4 weeks, 6–8 weeks, and 1 year Use clinical and radiographic control
Lateral luxation – a displacement injury to the tooth in any direction other than axially. Fracture of the buccal and palatal alveolar plate may be present	Tooth is often displaced palatally or buccally Rigid nonmobile Metallic sound upon percussion Radiographs show a widened PDL	(Primary teeth) No occlusal interference: observe allowing for spontaneous repositioning If occlusal interference: use local anesthesia and reposition with combined labial/palatal pressure Severe displacement: extract (permanent teeth) Give anesthesia Clean exposed root with saline Reposition tooth with digitation Stabilize tooth with flexible splint for 4 weeks	(Primary teeth) monitor (Permanent teeth) Tooth may revascularize or go through pulpal necrosis Monitor 2 weeks, 4 weeks, 6–8 weeks, and 1 year If necrosis then RCT
Intrusion – a displacement injury of the tooth into the alveolar bone. There can be a comminution or fracture of the alveolar socket	Tooth is often intruded in the alveolar socket Tooth is immobile PDL may be absent from radiograph The CEJ of intruded tooth is more apical than adjacent teeth	Spontaneous eruption (primary teeth) apex displaced toward or through labial bone plate: observe for spontaneous repositioning (2–4 months) If apex displaced into developing tooth germ, extract (permanent teeth) Orthodontic repositioning Surgical repositioning RCT 3–4 weeks posttrauma permanent teeth	High incidence for (primary teeth) Monitor 2 weeks, 4 weeks, 6–8 weeks, and 1 year (Permanent teeth) ankylosis and pulpal necrosis in permanent teeth Monitor 2 weeks, 4 weeks, 6–8 weeks, and 1 year

(continued)

Table 16.9 (continued)

Type of injury	Signs and symptoms	Treatment	Prognosis/ follow-up
Avulsion (primary teeth) – tooth is completely displaced out of socket	Tooth is missing from the socket X-ray to confirm tooth was not intruded	(Primary teeth) During examination make sure that all avulsed teeth are accounted for. For unaccounted teeth take X-rays of site in order to ensure no primary teeth were intruded or root fracture with loss of the coronal fragment. If the avulsed tooth has not been found, refer the child to the pediatrician to exclude aspiration	(Primary teeth) It is not recommended to reimplant primary teeth. (Permanent teeth) See avulsion chart below for permanent teeth

16.6 Pediatric Pearls

- *Do not plan for more procedures in one visit than you or the child can handle.* With deep sedation, a pediatric dentist may be able to do eight stainless steel crowns and pulpotomies in one visit. With only behavioral management or nitrous sedation, a general dentist may be able to do only one or two fillings in one setting. Keep in mind of children's low pain tolerance and short attention span.
- Always warn children not to bite the "numb" check or lips post anesthetics.
- Teach parents to start flossing their children's teeth around age 3–4, when contacts start to develop between the primary teeth.
- Bruxing is common and perfectly normal in the primary dentition.

16.7 Miscellaneous Pediatric/Orthodontic Considerations

The American Association of Orthodontists recommends that every child should first visit an orthodontist no later than age 7. Although comprehensive orthodontic treatment does not start at age 7, interceptive treatment may be appropriate in children with specific problems, such as anterior crossbite, posterior crossbite, open bite, ectopic eruption, complete skeletal Class III, and oral habits.

A general dentist is often the first dental professional to see a patient and first to recognize that the patient may have an orthodontic problem. It is important to refer to the orthodontist in a timely manner, so the most appropriate treatment can be produced at the most appropriate time. From age 6 and older, there are a few different types of treatment approaches an orthodontist can provide: space maintainers, orthodontic appliances, guiding general dentists for serial extractions, and phase I or full orthodontic treatment.

Table 16.10 Management of avulsed permanent teeth (Andreasen et al. 2012; Lambert 2015)

Avulsed permanent teeth	Condition	Treatment recommendation
Closed apex	Extra oral dry Time <60 mins	1. Clean the area with saline or chlorhexidine. Make sure no alveolar wall fracture 2. Verify normal position of avulsed tooth both clinically and radiographically
		3. Replant and place a flexible splint for up to 2 weeks. Use systemic antibiotics doxycycline, penVk, or amoxicillin. RCT 2 weeks after
	Extraoral dry Time >60 mins	1. Clean the area with saline, or chlorhexidine. Make sure no alveolar wall fracture 2. Clean necrotic PDL off with gauze. Soak tooth in 2 % sodium fluoride 3. Verify normal position of avulsed tooth both clinically and radiographically 4. Replant and place a flexible splint for up to 4 weeks. Use systemic antibiotics doxycycline, penVk, or amoxicillin. RCT 7–10 days after or RCT in hand before reimplantation. Expect ankylosis
Open Apex	Extra oral dry Time <60 mins	1. Make sure no alveolar wall fracture exists. Soak tooth in doxycycline for 5 min. Rinse debris with saline 2. Verify normal position of avulsed tooth both clinically and radiographically 3. Replant and place a flexible splint for up to 2 weeks. Use systemic antibiotics doxycycline, penVk, or amoxicillin. RCT need only if no signs of revascularization
	Extra oral dry Time >60 mins	1. Make sure no alveolar wall fracture. Irrigate tooth with saline. Clean necrotic tissue off with gauze 2. Verify normal position of avulsed tooth both clinically and radiographically 3. Replant and place a flexible splint for up to 2 weeks. Use systemic antibiotics doxycycline, penVk, or amoxicillin. RCT 1 week later consider no reimplantation due to poor prognosis of revascularization. Expect ankylosis

16.7.1 Common Space Maintainers

Space maintainers are known by many parents are "spacers." They are generally indicated in early loss of primary teeth, prior to ½–2/3 of root formation of the succedaneous teeth. In some children, space maintainers need to stay for 2 years or more. Therefore, it is important for the general dentist to perform periodic checkups on the health of the banded teeth and oral hygiene (Tables 16.11 and 16.12).

16.7.2 Common Orthodontic Appliances

Many orthodontic appliances can be used with or without braces to facilitate habit cessation, correct functional shift, and deliver minor orthodontic correction.

Table 16.11 Space maintainers and their indications

Types	Indication
Lingual holding arch	Early loss of primary mandibular molars bilaterally
Nance	Early loss of primary maxillary molars bilaterally
Band-and-loop	Early loss of a single tooth such as 2nd primary molar, after eruption of the 1st permanent molar
Distal shoe	Early loss of the most distal primary molar, such as 2nd primary molar, prior to eruption of the 1st permanent molar

Table 16.12 Correctional orthodontic appliances (Proffit et al. 2012; AAPD 2014a, b, c, d, e, f)

Types	Indication	Duration	Follow-up observation
Thumb crib	Thumb or finger sucking habit	6 months	Anterior open bite closes slightly without any fixed orthodontic treatment. Depends on the malocclusion, the orthodontist will decide the following treatment
Tongue crib	Tongue thrusting habit	6 months	Anterior open bite closes slightly without any fixed orthodontic treatment. Depends on the malocclusion, the orthodontist will decide the following treatment
Bluegrass tongue trainer	Tongue thrusting habit	6 months	Anterior open bite closes slightly without any fixed orthodontic treatment. Depends on the malocclusion, the orthodontist will decide the following treatment
Palatal expander	Unilateral or bilateral posterior functional or skeletal crossbite	Leave in the mouth for 4–6 months post expansion at orthodontist's discretion	Multiple types of expander can be used by an orthodontist such as Quad-helix and Hyrax. Expander can be used with or without fixed appliances (braces)
Spring aligners	Singer tooth anterior crossbite	Patient needs to be seen by orthodontist monthly for adjustment on the aligner	Spring aligners are very effective in tipping a maxillary anterior tooth out of crossbite, when space is available. It is often recommended in young children who are not ready for phase I orthodontic treatment. Patient compliance is required

16.7.3 Extraction Under Orthodontic Guidance

After a child has seen an orthodontist for a consultation, sometimes the orthodontist will refer the patient back to the general dentist for extraction of primary or permanent teeth. Early extraction of primary teeth can lead to arch length deficiency, midline shifting, and impaction of permanent teeth. Extraction of carious permanent teeth can lead to shifting of the rest of the permanent teeth and not enough space available for future tooth replacement.

Serial extraction is a planned extraction of specific primary teeth and permanent teeth in a timely manner due to foreseen crowding. If done at the right time, serial extraction can facilitate eruption, prevent canine impaction, and reduce the complexity of future orthodontic treatment (Proffit et al. 2012).

16.7.4 Phase I Orthodontic Treatment

Phase I orthodontic treatment is also limited treatment, designed with specific goals to correct early skeletal discrepancies and functional occlusion shift and provide early esthetic corrections. Most children who received phase I orthodontic treatment eventually end up choosing to go through phase II treatment for esthetic concerns.

16.7.5 Full Orthodontic Treatment (Proffit et al. 2012)

The average time for a simple full orthodontic treatment is between 18 and 24 months. During this time, it is important for the general dentist and orthodontist to maintain frequent conversation about patient's oral hygiene and restorative needs. The general dentist should be actively involved in the orthodontic treatment planning when there is restorative needs post orthodontic treatment such as build up for peg lateral incisors, veneers/crowns for transposed teeth, flippers, or Maryland bridges for missing teeth.

16.7.6 Orthodontic Myths Among General Dentists (Proffit et al. 2012)

- *A child is too young to get braces until he or she has all permanent teeth.* Endlessly waiting for all permanent teeth to erupt prior having an orthodontic consultation can lead to missing the golden timing for interceptive or phase I treatment. Growth modification in hope to guide skeletal development sometimes needs to start at the transitional dentition age, in order to catch the peak of growth.
- *Wisdom teeth need to be extracted prior to start of braces. Teeth will shift and get crocked again when wisdom teeth come in.* Many research studies have shown that late mandibular incisor crowding is multifactorial. Relapse after orthodontic treatment happens to anyone at anytime, regardless of whether wisdom teeth were extracted. Just like the rest of human body, teeth and occlusion are constantly evolving as we mature. The key to prevent relapse is excellent retainer wear.

- *All cavities need to be filled prior to an orthodontic consultation. Orthodontic* treatment should not be started without a patient first completing all restorations and has a good oral hygiene. However, a general dentist should recognize a child's orthodontic needs and refer for consultation prior to starting extensive restorations, noting that sometimes posterior permanent teeth can be extracted instead of filled.

16.8 When to Refer to a Pediatric Dentist

Being the first professional for many children, the general dentists have an important responsibility to build the best first impression possible for the generations to come. The dentists should always keep the patients' best interests in mind. The bottom line is "Do no harm." If you cannot provide the best care or feel uncomfortable treating a child, refer. Build the best first impression of dental professionals. Here are a few examples when you should refer.

1. Unmanageable children and/or their parents, after several attempts of behavioral management.
2. The patient has extensive needs that may be better treated under sedation or general anesthetic, i.e., rampant decay.
3. The office is not equipped with the armamentarium needed for the procedures, i.e., SSCs and nitrous oxide.
4. Developmentally or physically disabled patients who the dentist cannot communicate well with.
5. The dentist and/or the staff do not have the kids' friendly personality and patience. It is ok to admit that you are not good with children. That is why we have the specialists. Instead of putting the children and yourself through the suffering, please refer them to someone who will give them a much better experience and care that they deserve.

References

Andreasen JO, Ebeleseder KA, Kenny DJ, Trope M, Sigurdsson A, Andersson L, Bourguignon C, Flores MT, Hicks ML, Lenzi AR, Malmgren B, Moule AJ, Pohl Y, Tsukiboshi M. International Association of Dental Traumatology guidelines for the management of traumatic dental injuries: 1. Fractures and luxations of permanent teeth. Dent Traumatol. 2012;28:66–71. Erratum in Dent Traumatol. 2012;28: 499.

American Academy of Pediatric Dentistry (AAPD). Guideline on use of nitrous oxide for the pediatric dental patient. Chicago: American Academy of Pediatric Dentistry (AAPD); 2013. p. 5 [40 references].

American Academy of Pediatric Dentistry (AAPD). Dental growth and development. Chicago: American Academy of Pediatric Dentistry (AAPD); 2014a. p. 1 [1 reference].

American Academy of Pediatric Dentistry (AAPD). Guideline on fluoride therapy. Chicago: American Academy of Pediatric Dentistry (AAPD); 2014b. p. 4 [37 references].

American Academy of Pediatric Dentistry(AAPD). Guideline on use of antibiotic therapy for pediatric patients. reference manual revised. 2014c;37(6):289–91.

American Academy of Pediatric Dentistry (AAPD). Guideline on management of the developing dentition and occlusion in the pediatric dental patient. Chicago: American Academy of Pediatric Dentistry (AAPD); 2014d. p. 13 [138 references].

American Academy of Pediatric Dentistry (AAPD). Guideline on pulp therapy for primary and immature permanent teeth. Chicago: American Academy of Pediatric Dentistry (AAPD); 2014e. p. 9 [109 references].

American Academy of Pediatric Dentistry (AAPD). Guideline on restorative dentistry. Chicago: American Academy of Pediatric Dentistry (AAPD); 2014f. p. 12. [135 references].

American Academy of Pediatric Dentistry (AAPD). Guideline on behavior guidance for the pediatric dental patient. Chicago: American Academy of Pediatric Dentistry (AAPD); 2015a. p. 14 [95 references].

American Academy of Pediatric Dentistry (AAPD). Guideline on use of local anesthesia for pediatric dental patients. Chicago: American Academy of Pediatric Dentistry (AAPD); 2015b. p. 7 [36 references].

Casamassimo PS, et al. Pediatric dentistry: infancy through adolescence. 5th ed. St. Louis: Elsevier/Sanders; 2013.

DiAngelis AJ, Andreasen JO, Ebeleseder KA, Kenny DJ, Trope M. International Association of Dental Traumatology guidelines for the management of traumatic dental injuries: 1. Fractures and luxations of permanent teeth. Dent Traumatol. 2012;28:2–12.

Lambert D. Splinting rationale and contemporary treatment options for luxated and avulsed permanent teeth. Gen Dent. 2015;63(6):56–60.

Proffit WR, et al. Contemporary orthodontics. 5th ed. St. Louis: Mosby; 2012.

Rappaport B, Mellon RD, Simone A, Woodcock J. Defining safe use of anesthesia in children. N Engl J Med. 2011;364(15):1387–90.

Wynn RL, Meiller TF, Crossley HL. Drug information handbook for dentistry. 21st ed. Hudson: Lexicomp; 2015.

Orthodontics

17

Eddy J. Sedeño III, Melissa Alfonso, and Calogero Dolce

Contents

Abstract

Orthodontics consists of the manipulation of teeth and bones using external forces, biological processes, and growth. Appliances to help correct the position of the teeth can be found dating back to 1000 B.C. and ancient Egypt. One of the first textbooks describing orthodontic treatment was written by Norman Kingsley in 1879. Edward H. Angle, known as the "father of modern orthodontics," established the Angle School of Orthodontia in 1900 and made orthodontics the first specialty in dentistry. In addition, he also established many of the tenets by which we classify normal occlusion today (Asbell 1990).

Orthodontics has evolved in many ways in the past century from banding of teeth to preadjusted brackets and clear aligner treatment, such as Invisalign®. People seek treatment for various reasons including craniofacial abnormalities,

E.J. Sedeño III, DMD, MS (✉) • M. Alfonso, DMD, MS • C. Dolce, DMD, MS
Department of Orthodontics, University of Florida, College of Dentistry, Gainesville, FL, USA
e-mail: Ejsedeno@gmail.com

G.M. Weinstein, M.T. Zientz (eds.), *The Dental Reference Manual*,
DOI 10.1007/978-3-319-39730-6_17

protrusive teeth, crowding, and difficulty maintaining healthy teeth, speech issues, and esthetics. The American Association of Orthodontists believes that 75 % of the population would benefit from some sort of orthodontic treatment and recommends that children have an evaluation by an orthodontist by age 7. The purpose of this chapter is to provide the general dentist with the basic diagnostic principles in orthodontics, reasons to refer a patient to an orthodontist, the use of orthodontics in restorative treatment, and recommendations for simple Invisalign® cases. This chapter is not intended to be a comprehensive overview of orthodontic diagnosis or treatment; rather it is a condensed description of important factors for general practitioners to be aware of.

17.1 Diagnosis

17.1.1 Medical and Dental History

Determining a patient's orthodontic needs begins with an orthodontic evaluation. The first and most important aspect of this is the patient's chief complaint, which provides the dentist and orthodontist with an idea of the patient's perception of the malocclusion and expectations from orthodontic treatment. Whether or not the patient's personality is affected by the chief complaint may also provide insight. A medical and dental history is obtained to determine if certain aspects of the medical history may affect a patient's ability to have orthodontic treatment or the prognosis of orthodontic treatment. Some medical conditions affecting orthodontics are diabetes, asthma, and cardiovascular or joint replacements that necessitate the need for antibiotic prophylaxis. The chronic use of certain medications can also affect the movement of teeth. This includes medicines that affect the inflammatory pathway such as nonsteroidal anti-inflammatory medicines and corticosteroids, as well as drugs that target the bone remodeling pathway (i.e., bisphosphonates) (Bartzela et al. 2009). Since there are a number of ways that medical history, medications, and allergies can affect orthodontic treatment, it is important to ensure that the patient is fully disclosing this information. The most significant allergies include those to nickel, contained in several orthodontic wires and brackets, and latex, contained in rubber bands and elastomeric ties.

Obtaining the dental history begins with ensuring that the patient has a dental home and is in good oral health. In most cases, orthodontic treatment should not begin until this is confirmed. Another important aspect of the dental history is trauma to the face, which can affect condylar growth, or to the teeth, which can affect tooth development, resulting in loss of vitality, root resorption, and/or ankylosis. A history of early extractions with or without space maintenance can provide the orthodontist with a perspective on the etiology of the malocclusion. Other aspects of dental history that can help to provide further information are history of orthodontic treatment, caries risk, and past habits such as thumb sucking or mouth breathing. Refer to Chap. 3, Caries Prevention, which contains caries risk assessments for adults and children.

17.1.2 Orthodontic Evaluation and Records

Full orthodontic records consist of:

1. Extraoral and intraoral clinical exam (Fig. 17.7)
2. Study models
3. Extraoral and intraoral photographs
4. Radiographs

17.1.2.1 Clinical Exam

Facial balance and symmetry is assessed during the extraoral examination. In the frontal view, the vertical dimensions are assessed by dividing the face into thirds, with variations from normal including short or long middle or lower thirds of the face. Asymmetries can be noted by assessing the relationship between the nose, mouth, chin, and dental midlines. The amount of tooth and gingiva show on smile should also be noted from the frontal view. Esthetic smiles typically have full tooth show plus 1–2 mm of gingiva. Excessive gingival show is termed a "gummy smile" and can be indicative of a hyperactive maxillary lip or excessive vertical growth of the maxilla. From the smile view, an occlusal cant can be detected if present by comparing the plane of the occlusion with a line drawn between the pupils of the eyes. From the profile view, the relationship between the maxilla and mandible is assessed. In a normal, Class I relationship of the jaws, the mandible is slightly posterior to the maxilla, resulting in a straight to slightly convex profile. When the profile is overly convex, the patient's soft tissue is assessed as Class II. When it is concave the patient is classified as Class III. (Fig. 17.1)

The clinical exam consists of an extraoral and intraoral evaluation. The extraoral evaluation includes an assessment of the patient's temporomandibular joint (TMJ), including presence of popping, clicking, pain, or locking. In patients with TMJ pain, orthodontics should not be started until the pain is controlled. The effects of orthodontics on the TMJ are varied and not widely understood. Orthodontics is not a proper treatment for TMJ joint pain, generally. The muscles of mastication, opening, and closing should be palpated for the presence of myofascial pain. Range of motion should be evaluated for normalcy of maximum opening, protrusion, and excursive movements.

The intraoral evaluation begins with evaluating the health of the teeth and periodontium, as well as the level of oral hygiene. These can be categorized as poor, good, or excellent. Full periodontal probing should be done in all patients over the age of 18. Some orthodontists may also advocate periodontal probing of younger patients to screen for subgingival calculus, deep pockets, and aggressive periodontitis.

Molar classification is determined based on the relationship of the first molars, as originally described by Edward H. Angle (Angle 1899). Normal, Class I, relationship is defined as the mesiobuccal cusp tip of the maxillary first molar lining up with the buccal groove of the mandibular first molar. (Fig. 17.2) Class I relationship of

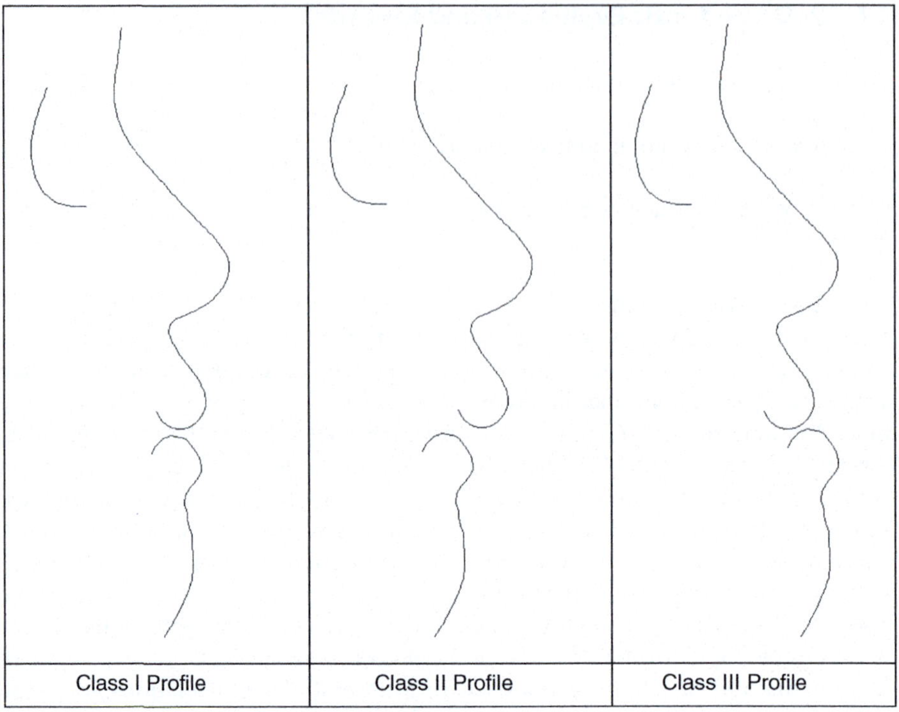

Fig. 17.1 Example of Class I, II, and III profiles

the canine is defined as the cusp tip of the maxillary canine positioned directly interproximal between the mandibular canine and first premolar. (Fig. 17.3) Any deviation of the maxillary teeth anterior to the mandibular teeth is classified as Class II molar and/or canine. (Fig. 17.4 and 17.5) Posterior deviations are classified as Class III. (Fig. 17.6) The extent to which a patient is Class II or III is defined by the amount of cusps from the Class I position (¼, ½, full cusp, or more than a full cusp). Class II malocclusions are further classified into Division 1 (Fig. 17.4) or Division 2. Class II Division 2 malocclusions typically demonstrate retroclination of the upper central incisors, a deep overbite, and proclination of the upper lateral incisors. (Fig. 17.5) If Class II or III occlusion appears unilaterally with the opposing side being Class I, the occlusion would be defined as being a subdivision on that side. For example, a patient that is Class I on the right, but Class II, Division 1 on the left would be classified as Class II, Division 2, subdivision left.

Overjet is measured, in millimeters, from the incisal edge of the maxillary incisor to the most labial point of the opposing mandibular incisor. A relationship where the maxillary incisors lie anterior to the mandibular teeth results in positive overjet. When the maxillary teeth are posterior to the mandibular incisors, the overjet is recorded as negative. Overbite is recorded as the measurement from the incisal edge of the maxillary incisor to the incisal edge of the opposing mandibular incisor. Teeth

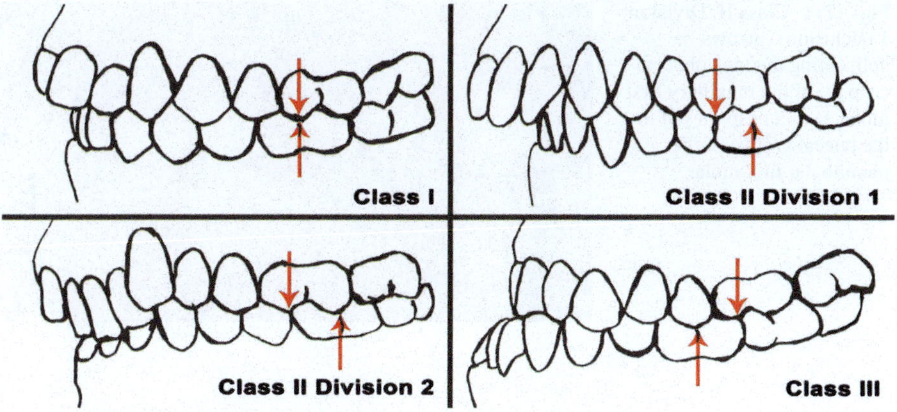

Fig. 17.2 Examples of molar classification with arrows illustrating position of mesiobuccal cusp of maxillary first molar and buccal groove of the mandibular first molar. The relationship of these is used to determine the molar classification

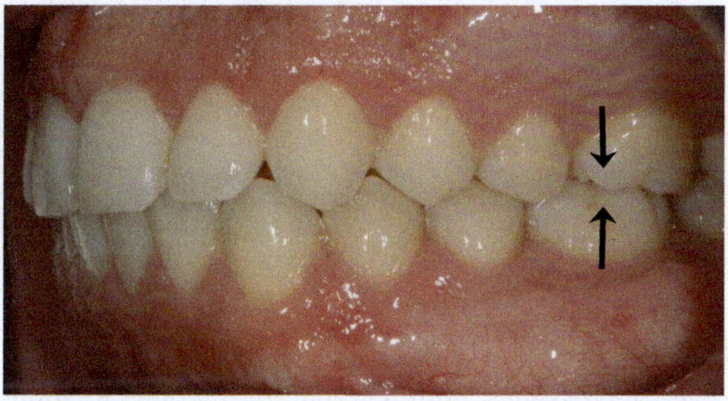

Fig. 17.3 Class I occlusion – arrows delineating the mesiobuccal cusp tip of the maxillary first molar lining up with the buccal groove of the mandibular first molar

with overlap are recorded as having positive overbite, while those without are edge to edge or cases with space between the incisors there is negative overbite (i.e., open bite). The overall overjet and overbite should both be recorded based on the teeth with the worst relationship (Cangialosi et al. 2004). If the patient's lower incisors are touching the palatal tissues, this is termed an impinging overbite and can sometimes result in loss of gingival tissue or palatal inflammation. The midlines of both the upper and the lower jaw should also be recorded in relationship to the face and to each other. Crossbites in the anterior and posterior should be noted. Posterior crossbites presenting with maxillary tooth completely buccal to the mandibular tooth is termed a Brodie crossbite.

Every patient should be evaluated for a slide or shift from centric relation (CR) into maximum intercuspation (MI). Slides are caused by interferences which prevent the patient from biting where the proper mandibular position is. Classification,

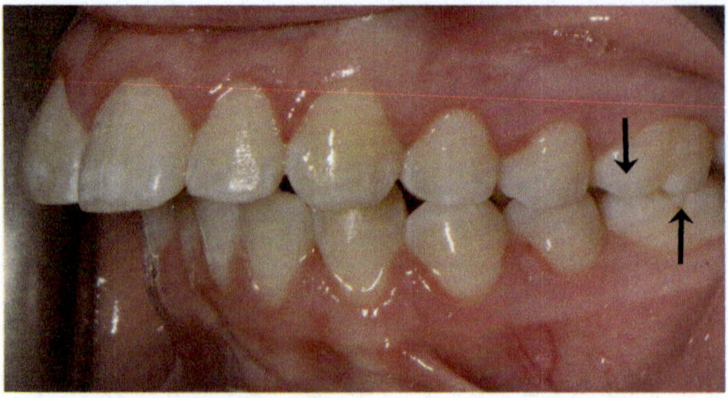

Fig. 17.4 Class II, Division 1 occlusion – arrows delineating the mesiobuccal cusp tip of the maxillary first molar ¾ of a cusp mesial to the buccal groove of the mandibular first molar

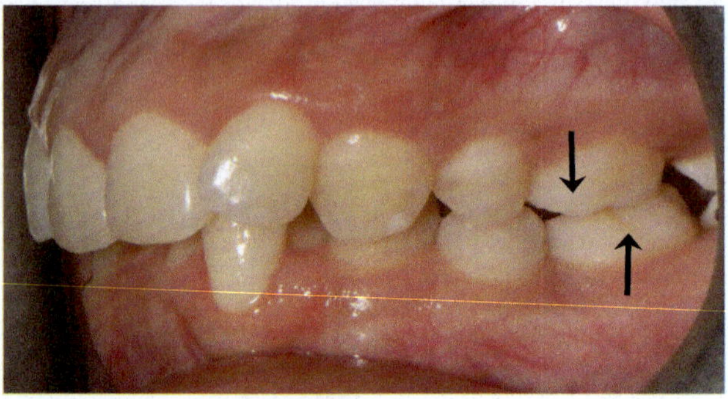

Fig. 17.5 Class II, Division 2 occlusion – arrows delineating the mesiobuccal cusp tip of the maxillary first molar ¾ of a cusp mesial to the buccal groove of the mandibular first molar. Note the lateral incisor overlapping the retroclined central incisor and deep bite, typical of this malocclusion

overjet, crossbites, midlines, and several other relationships may be different in CR and should be recorded in both relationships. When orthodontic treatment begins, oftentimes the shift is eliminated, and the mandible settles in the CR position. For this reason, malocclusions should be treated to the assessment in CR.

17.1.2.2 Study Models

Stone or digital models are used to study the occlusal relationships from several angles and to generate a space analysis. In order to perform a space analysis, the widths of all of the teeth are measured and recorded. The arch length is recorded from mesial of one permanent first molar to the mesial of the contralateral molar. If the arch length is greater than the sum of the tooth widths of the second premolar to the contralateral second premolar, there is spacing. If it is smaller, there is crowding. In the mixed dentition, the lower permanent incisors can be used to predict the width of the canine and premolars. The Moyers and Tanaka-Johnston analyses are the most commonly used methods for this. The Moyers analysis provides a table with prediction values based on the cumulative width of the lower incisors. The

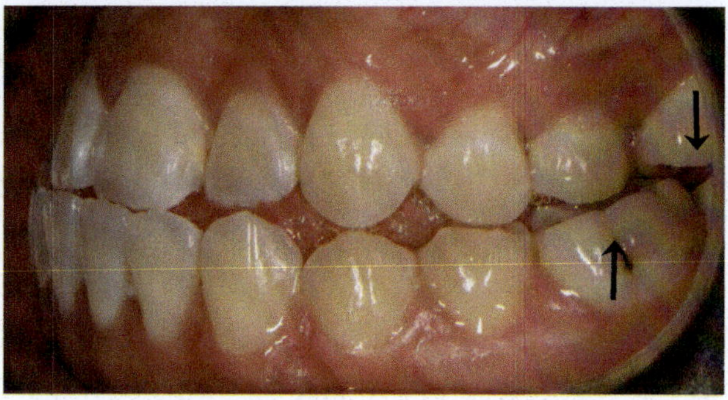

Fig. 17.6 Class III occlusion – arrows delineating the mesiobuccal cusp tip of the maxillary first molar a full cusp distal to the buccal groove of the mandibular first molar

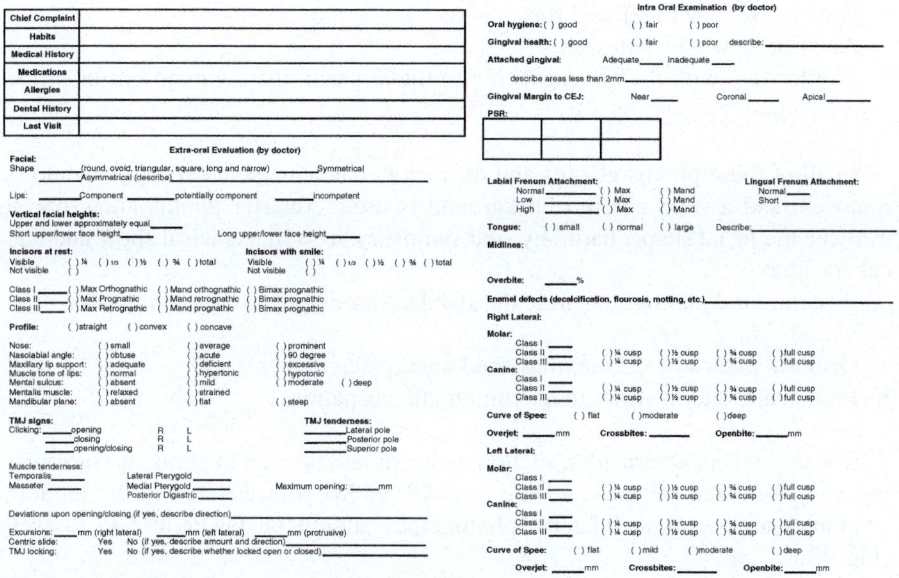

Chief Complaint	
Habits	
Medical History	
Medications	
Allergies	
Dental History	
Last Visit	

Extra-oral Evaluation (by doctor)

Facial:
Shape ____(round, ovoid, triangular, square, long and narrow) ____Symmetrical
____Asymmetrical (describe)____

Lips: ____Component ____potentially component ____incompetent

Vertical facial heights:
Upper and lower approximately equal____
Short upper/lower face height____ Long upper/lower face height____

Incisors at rest:
Visible ( ) ¼ ( ) 1/3 ( ) ½ ( ) ¾ ( ) total
Not visible ( )

Incisors with smile:
Visible ( ) ¼ ( ) 1/3 ( ) ½ ( ) ¾ ( ) total
Not visible ( )

Class I ____( ) Max Orthognathic ( ) Mand orthognathic ( ) Bimax prognathic
Class II____( ) Max Prognathic ( ) Mand retrognathic ( ) Bimax prognathic
Class III____( ) Max Retrognathic ( ) Mand prognathic ( ) Bimax prognathic

Profile: ( )straight ( ) convex ( ) concave

Nose: ( ) small ( ) average ( ) prominent
Nasolabial angle: ( ) obtuse ( ) acute ( ) 90 degree
Maxillary lip support: ( ) adequate ( ) deficient ( ) excessive
Muscle tone of lips: ( ) normal ( ) hypertonic ( ) hypotonic
Mental sulcus: ( ) absent ( ) mild ( ) moderate ( ) deep
Mentalis muscle: ( ) relaxed ( ) strained
Mandibular plane: ( ) absent ( ) flat ( ) steep

TMJ signs:
Clicking: ____opening R L
____closing R L
____opening/closing R L

TMJ tenderness:
____Lateral pole
____Posterior pole
____Superior pole

Muscle tenderness:
Temporalis____ Lateral Pterygold____
Masseter ____ Medial Pterygold____ Maximum opening: ____mm
Posterior Digastric____

Deviations upon opening/closing (if yes, describe direction)____

Excursions: ____mm (right lateral) ____mm (left lateral) ____mm (protrusive)
Centric slide: Yes No (if yes, describe amount and direction)____
TMJ locking: Yes No (if yes, describe whether locked open or closed)____

Intra Oral Examination (by doctor)

Oral hygiene: ( ) good ( ) fair ( ) poor
Gingival health: ( ) good ( ) fair ( ) poor describe:____
Attached gingival: Adequate____ Inadequate ____
describe areas less than 2mm____
Gingival Margin to CEJ: Near____ Coronal____ Apical____
PSR:

Labial Frenum Attachment:
Normal____ ( ) Max ( ) Mand
Low ____ ( ) Max ( ) Mand
High ____ ( ) Max ( ) Mand

Lingual Frenum Attachment:
Normal____
Short ____

Tongue: ( ) small ( ) normal ( ) large Describe:____

Midlines:

Overbite: ____%

Enamel defects (decalcification, flourosis, motting, etc.)____

Right Lateral:

Molar:
Class I ____
Class II ____ ( ) ¼ cusp ( ) ½ cusp ( ) ¾ cusp ( ) full cusp
Class III____ ( ) ¼ cusp ( ) ½ cusp ( ) ¾ cusp ( ) full cusp
Canine:
Class I ____
Class II ____ ( ) ¼ cusp ( ) ½ cusp ( ) ¾ cusp ( ) full cusp
Class III____ ( ) ¼ cusp ( ) ½ cusp ( ) ¾ cusp ( ) full cusp

Curve of Spee: ( ) flat ( ) moderate ( ) deep

Overjet: ____mm **Crossbites:** ____ **Openbite:** ____mm

Left Lateral:

Molar:
Class I ____
Class II ____ ( ) ¼ cusp ( ) ½ cusp ( ) ¾ cusp ( ) full cusp
Class III ____ ( ) ¼ cusp ( ) ½ cusp ( ) ¾ cusp ( ) full cusp
Canine:
Class I ____
Class II ____ ( ) ¼ cusp ( ) ½ cusp ( ) ¾ cusp ( ) full cusp
Class III ____ ( ) ¼ cusp ( ) ½ cusp ( ) ¾ cusp ( ) full cusp

Curve of Spee: ( ) flat ( ) mild ( ) moderate ( ) deep

Overjet: ____mm **Crossbites:** ____ **Openbite:** ____mm

Fig. 17.7 Example of a comprehensive records form

Tanaka-Johnston analysis determines the width of the canine and premolars by calculating one-half of the sum of the mandibular incisors and adding 10.5 mm to determine the width of the mandibular teeth on one side and 11 mm for the maxillary teeth. Adding the predicted values to the incisors and comparing that to the arch length provides the amount of spacing or crowding that is expected.

The width of the teeth can also be used to determine if a tooth-size discrepancy exists. Based on Bolton's tooth-size analysis (Bolton 1962), the ratio of the tooth widths, first molar to first molar, of the mandible to the maxilla, should ideally be 0.91. The mandible to maxilla ratio of canine to canine widths should be 0.77. Ratios greater than the norm indicate mandibular excess or maxillary deficiency.

Less than the norm indicates maxillary excess or mandibular deficiency. If a tooth-size discrepancy goes undetected, there may be difficulty in finishing with a Class I molar and canine relationship.

In addition to the information obtained in the intraoral examination, models can provide a way to help treatment plan. The models can be moved in all planes of space to determine what treatment options may serve to correct the malocclusion. They can also be used to create tooth setups for treatment planning and presenting to the patient.

17.1.2.3 Photographs

The American Board of Orthodontics advocates the use of three extraoral photos consisting of:

- Anterior view with relaxed lips
- Anterior view with full smile
- Profile view with the patient facing to the left with the ear exposed for proper orientation

In all of these photos glasses and distractors (such as large earrings) should be removed, and a solid colored background is used. Anterior photos allow one to evaluate the facial shape, harmony, and symmetry, as well as incisal show and buccal corridors.

Five intraoral photos constitute the standard for diagnosis. These include:

- Occlusal photos of the maxillary and mandibular arches
- Frontal and lateral views in maximum intercuspation

The use of cheek retractors, suction, or air should be used to eliminate surrounding soft tissue and saliva. If a slide from CR to MI is discovered in the intraoral examination, frontal and lateral photographs should be taken in CR as well. (Fig. 17.8)

17.1.2.4 Radiographs

Radiographs serve an important role in treatment planning. Most general dentists readily have access to panoramic radiographs. These serve to assess tooth eruption, development, root parallelism, and pathology. In patients that are 18 years old or older, vertical bitewings should be taken to assess bone levels around the teeth and to detect the presence of bone loss.

Lateral cephalometric radiographs help in the skeletal assessment (Steiner 1960). These radiographs are typically traced. (Fig. 17.9) A number of skeletal points are marked and serve as the basis for several linear and angular measurements. Some basic points for skeletal evaluation are:

- Sella (S): the middle of the sella turcica
- Nasion (N): the most anterior point of the nasofrontal suture

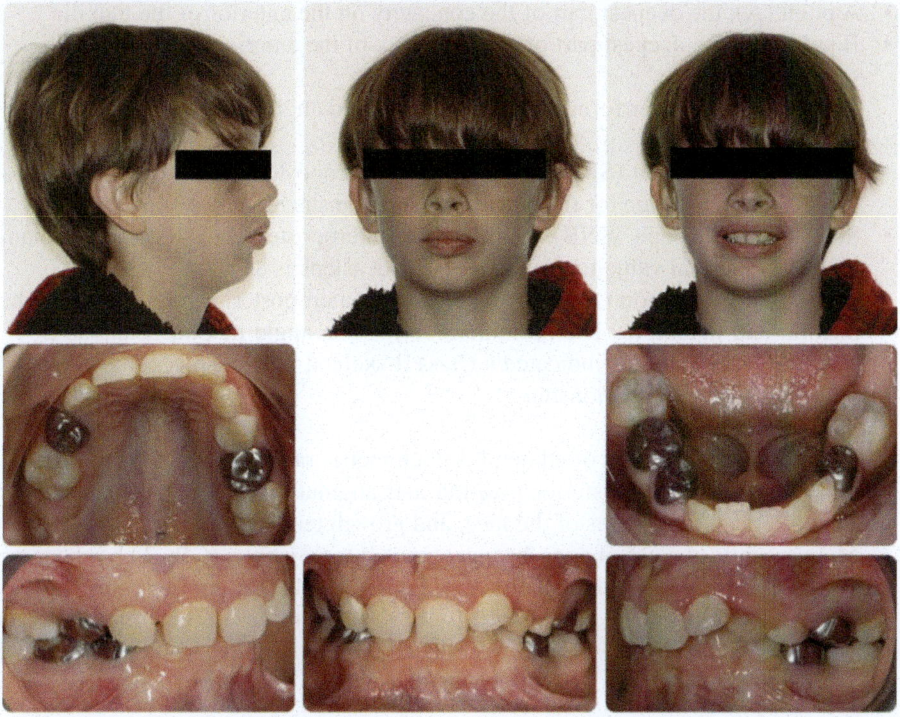

Fig. 17.8 Example of photo composite

Fig. 17.9 Lateral cephalometric radiograph with key landmarks labeled

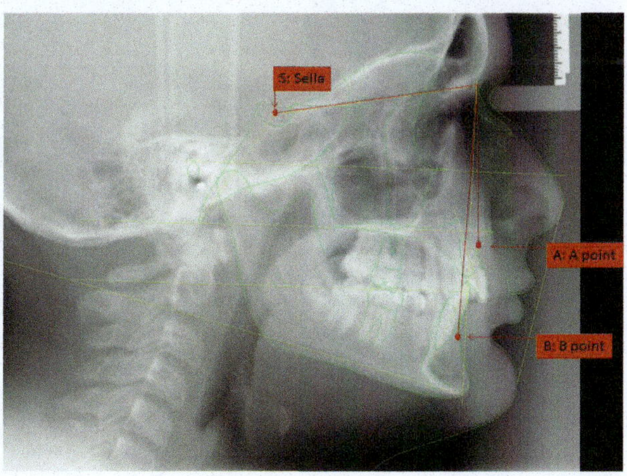

- A point (A): the deepest part of the concavity on the anterior of the maxilla
- B point (B): the deepest part of the concavity of the anterior of the mandible

These points together form a number of lines and angle:

- Sella-Nasion-A point (SNA): Indicates the anteroposterior position of the maxilla. The normal value for this angle in Caucasians is 82°.
- Sella-Nasion-B point (SNB): Indicates the anteroposterior position of the mandible. The normal value for this angle in Caucasians is 80°.
- A point-Nasion-B point (ANB): Indicates the anteroposterior relationship of the maxilla and mandible. The normal value for this angle in Caucasians is 2–4°. Values greater than this indicated a Class II skeletal relationship. Smaller values indicate a Class III relationship.

More advanced analysis of a lateral cephalometric radiograph can provide information about the anteroposterior position and angulation of the upper and lower incisors, vertical dimensions of the face, and growth tendencies.

More recently, the use of cone-beam computed tomography (CBCT) has become more popular in the field of orthodontics. (Fig. 17.10) Full or limited view CBCTs can be used when skeletal asymmetries, impacted teeth, or cleft lip and palate is suspected. CBCTs can also be used to extract digital models, panoramic, and lateral cephalometric radiographs. In cases where a CBCT is indicated, the radiation

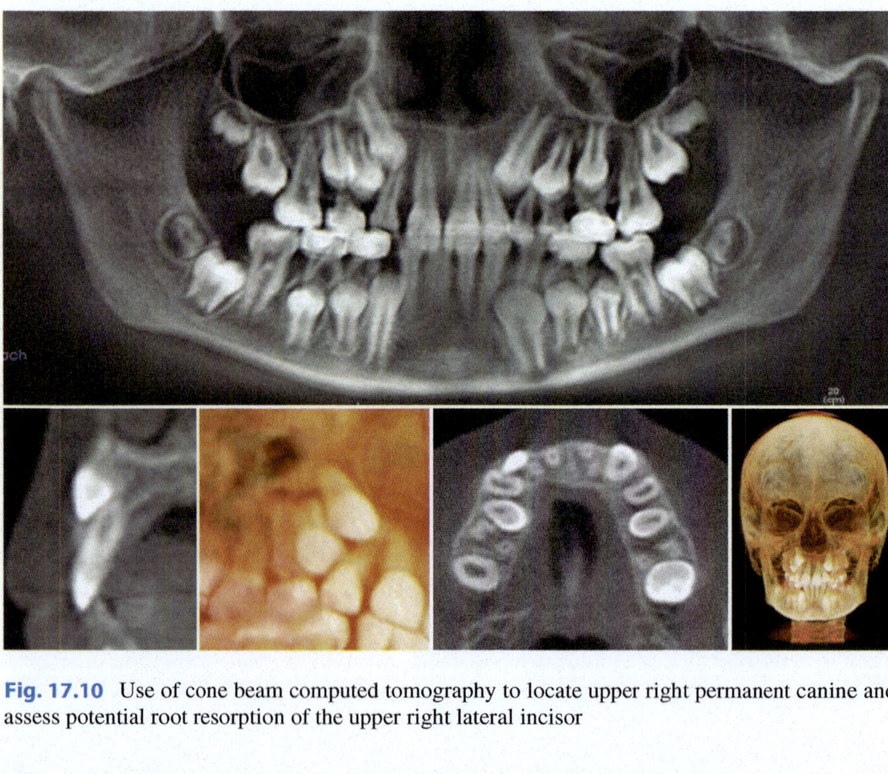

Fig. 17.10 Use of cone beam computed tomography to locate upper right permanent canine and assess potential root resorption of the upper right lateral incisor

exposure to the patient should be considered to determine which combination of radiographs would keep it as low as possible in accordance with the as low as reasonably achievable (ALARA) principle for dentistry (ADA 2012).

17.1.3 Creating the Orthodontic Problem List and Objectives

17.1.3.1 Ideal Soft Tissue, Skeletal, and Occlusal Features

Before determining a problem list or objectives, it is important for dental practitioners to recognize what ideal soft tissue, skeletal, and occlusal features are. Soft tissue profiles are ideally Class I with a 90° or slightly obtuse nasolabial angle. The upper and lower lip should have adequate support and lip curl. From the frontal perspective the face should be symmetric. When smiling, the upper and lower midlines should be on with the facial midline. Ideal tooth show is full maxillary incisor plus 1–2 mm of gingival show as previously discussed. Esthetically gingival margin heights should be at the proper heights in relationship to one another and symmetrical. The shape of the smile from canine to canine based on the incisal edges should follow the shape lower lip. In the vertical dimension, the facial thirds should be about equal. Skeletal ideals are based off of the lateral cephalometric radiograph. The ideal skeletal evaluation would reveal a Class I relationship of the maxilla and mandible in good anteroposterior relationship to the rest of the face. SNA, SNB, and ANB are used to determine this and are described above.

"Ideal" occlusion has been described by a number of authors. Angle was responsible for developing the first classification system for molar relationships as Class I, II, or III as described above. Andrews developed six occlusal features consistent in a series of "ideal" occlusions which has since been used to develop what is considered the norm for objectives (Andrews 1972). The first is molar relationship, similar to the Angle's classification; Class I molar relationship is ideal. Other features of the ideal occlusion are proper mesiodistal and buccolingual tip of the crowns of the teeth, no rotations, no spacing, and a flat curve of Spee. The mesiodistal tip of teeth can be evaluated on a panoramic radiograph. The buccolingual tip, also known as torque, of the incisors is evaluated on a lateral cephalometric radiograph, while the torque of molars is evaluated on study models. Other ideal aspects of occlusion are 1–2 mm of overjet, 20% overbite, lack of crossbites, no crowding, and Class I canine. Ideal functional aspects of occlusion are incisor guidance in protrusion and canine guidance in excursive movements. Some patients may require group function for guidance when the canines are worn down significantly. Contacts on all of the teeth should be even in maximum intercuspation, and no slide from CR to MI should exist.

17.1.3.2 Developing the Problem List

Based on the known ideal features and the information collected during the exam, a problem list is developed. This list can then be used in determining objectives, assessing the difficulty of a case, or in communicating information in a referral to an orthodontic specialist. The most important problem that should be included in the list is the patient's chief complaint. Inability to address this in orthodontic treatment would result in an overall failure of treatment.

Ackerman and Proffit developed a system of categorizing problems into five main groups (Ackerman et al. 2007). The first is the dentofacial appearance, which includes symmetry, facial proportions, incisor display, lip support, and soft tissue profile. The second category includes the teeth and arch form including alignment, symmetry of the jaws, and spacing or crowding. The next three categories include the skeletal and dental problems in the transverse, anteroposterior (sagittal), and vertical planes of space. In the transverse problems include posterior crossbites, torque of the posterior dentition, and asymmetries of the maxilla and/ or mandible. In the sagittal plane, classification of the molar, canine, and skeleton are noted, as well as anterior crossbites and overjet. A slide or shift forward from CR to MI would also constitute a problem in the sagittal plane. Lastly, the dental deviations in the vertical category would include overbite which would result in a deep or open bite. Skeletally, vertical problems would include vertical maxillary excess or a steep or flat mandibular plane. Some traits in malocclusions may not be easily categorized. For example, open bites can have both skeletal and dental etiologies. Cases such as this and other skeletal issues are more complex and should be referred to the orthodontist for comprehensive orthodontic treatment. Some problems do not meet the qualifications for any of these categories. Such examples are periodontal health and maxillary frenum attachments.

When treating orthodontic cases, the Ackerman-Proffit analysis can be used to develop soft tissue, skeletal, and dental objectives. Objectives are then used to determine optimal treatment options for the patient. Every patient presents with a unique set of problems and diagnoses and therefore a unique treatment plan should be developed for every patient to properly treat them.

The five categories of the Ackerman-Proffit analysis are also useful in referring a patient to orthodontics. A list of concerns that the general dentist has in regard to the patient can be listed simply as:

1. Soft tissue frontal and profile
2. Arch form, space analysis, and symmetry
3. Transverse dimension
4. Anteroposterior dimension
5. Vertical dimension

Use of this concise method helps streamline the referral process and alerts the orthodontist to the potential complexity of a case.

17.2 Orthodontic Treatment in the Primary and Mixed Dentition

17.2.1 Timing and Goals of Treatment

Malocclusions in younger patients can lead to functional issues, psychological problems, or dental disease, including increased susceptibility to caries, periodontal disease, and traumatic injury (Proffit et al. 2013). While many of these patients may benefit from orthodontic treatment, it is not an immediate need for all. Orthodontic treatment typically begins between the ages of 9 and 14, but some malocclusions can benefit from earlier treatment. The American Dental Association recommends that children visit the dentist by age one. In addition to maintaining regular dental care and oral hygiene, it is the responsibility of the general or pediatric dentist to monitor the child's dental and craniofacial development during these critical years. If any abnormalities in the development of the dentition or craniofacial complex are noted, parents should be informed and a referral to an orthodontist should be made.

Distinguishing the complexity of orthodontic problems is a crucial skill for the dentist to attain (Proffit et al. 2013). Intervention at the appropriate time allows the practitioner the opportunity to guide jaw growth, lower the risk of trauma to protruded teeth, correct harmful oral habits, improve appearance and self-esteem, guide permanent teeth into a more favorable position, improve the way lips meet, and maintain or develop space for erupting teeth. The decision to treat a patient or refer to a specialist depends on the experience of the general dentist and the severity of the malocclusion. Unless earlier treatment is indicated, the American Association of Orthodontists recommends that a child has a complete orthodontic evaluation and/or referral no later than age 7 to determine treatment needs and timing (Suresh et al. 2015). Prior to this time, close monitoring of radiographs, eruption sequence, space analysis, and jaw relation should be integrated by the general or pediatric dentist from much earlier in life.

It is known that skeletal patterns and malocclusions are established in early childhood. Early treatment may consist of intraoral and extraoral appliances to exert the greatest control over dentoskeletal form and function. Proper orthodontic evaluations and treatment of children can prevent the development of more serious problems and may result in shorter or less complicated treatment at a later age. While the literature provides some conflicting evidence, there are some indications that some correctable dental discrepancies left untreated can turn into permanent skeletal discrepancies and even worsen. The rationale for early orthodontic treatment is to eliminate skeletal or dental disharmonies and enhance occlusal development to promote normal growth and development, improve function, and avoid psychosocial distress during the formative years (Bahreman 2013).

17.2.2 Indications for Early Orthodontic Referral and Treatment

It is of utmost importance for primary care dentists to be able to distinguish problems that need to be treated soon and those that can wait for later comprehensive orthodontic care. Indications for early orthodontic referral and treatment can be broadly categorized into the following ten signs seen in a child's or young adolescent's dentition:

1. Severe overjet
2. Deep impinging bite
3. Posterior crossbites

4. Anterior crossbites
5. Parafunctional habits
6. Severe crowding
7. Ectopic eruption
8. Delayed eruption and impacted teeth
9. Psychological factors
10. Growth discrepancies

These characteristics should be kept in mind while evaluating children at each regular visit. If identified involving permanent teeth, appropriate measures to prevent, maintain, or correct should be attempted without delay.

17.2.2.1 Severe Overjet

Young patients can present with severe overjet due to maxillary skeletal or dental protrusion or mandibular retrusion which may indicate a skeletal growth discrepancy or parafunctional habit. Many practitioners believe that excessive overjet predisposes the maxillary incisors to traumatic injury, like fractures or avulsions. Recent studies have found similar rates of incidence regardless of the amount of protrusion of the maxillary incisors (Wieslander 1975; Chen et al. 2011). The patient may also encounter psychological distress due to teasing or low self-esteem. The etiology of the overjet should first be identified, and treatment should target the teeth or jaw at fault by using removable or fixed appliances to retract the incisors or functional appliances to promote growth (i.e., Herbst appliance) when indicated.

17.2.2.2 Deep Impinging Bite

The lower anterior teeth erupt until they are in contact with the lingual surface of the maxillary incisors. If they are positioned too far posterior they can over-erupt into the palate instead resulting in a deep impinging bite. Constant trauma can cause inflammation of palatal tissue and damage to periodontal tissues. Locking the mandible posteriorly can inhibit its maximum growth potential. Indentations of the lower incisors on palatal gingiva are a common finding. A fixed or removable bite plane may be indicated to reduce trauma to palatal tissue, allow posterior teeth to extrude, and restrict eruption of the anterior teeth until orthodontic treatment can be provided.

17.2.2.3 Posterior Crossbites

Posterior crossbites can present as unilateral or bilateral (Fig. 17.11) and can include a single tooth or multiple teeth. Bilateral crossbites are much more common than unilateral crossbites, but the latter can be more damaging and challenging to treat. Left untreated, a unilateral posterior crossbite can cause asymmetric growth of the condyles, which can manifest as a permanent skeletal problem such as an occlusal cant, a deviated chin, or temporomandibular joint disorder. It is important to note that a patient with a bilateral crossbite and a shift from CR to MI due to an occlusal interference can mimic a true unilateral crossbite. It is crucial to have the patient in CR when assessing the transverse relationships of the posterior segments.

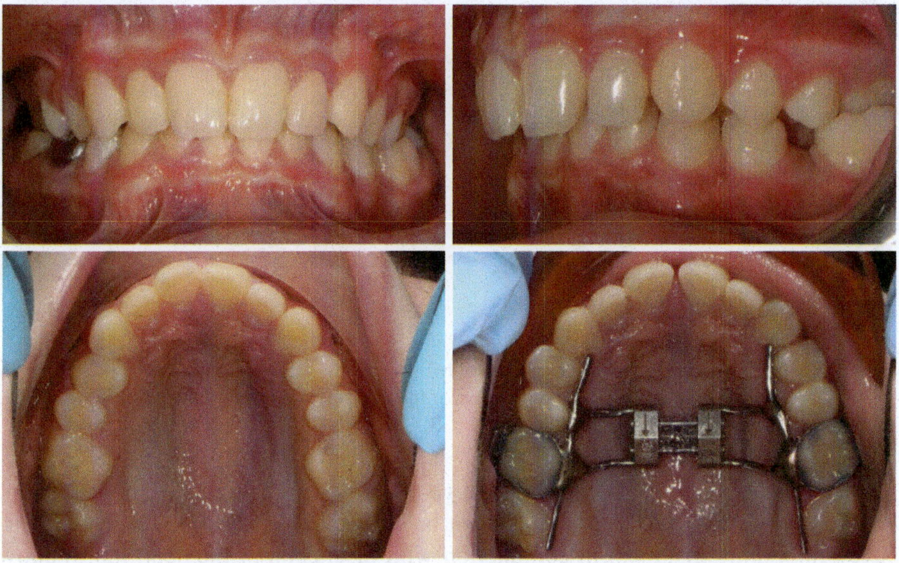

Fig. 17.11 Bilateral crossbite center and left intraoral images shown on top. Lower left showing constricted maxilla and lower right showing same maxilla after expansion

Crossbites are usually treated by using fixed or removable expansion appliances. The decision for fixed or removable is based on clinician experience, patient compliance, and the specific indications for each. The most commonly used appliances are the rapid palatal expander, activated by a screw turned by the patient, and the quad-helix, made of a series of preactivated helical springs. Expansion is optimally obtained in a growing patient with a palatal suture which has not yet fused, usually before the ages of 13–15 (Bishara and Staley 1987). Retention of expansion, usually by keeping the expansion appliance passive, for 3–6 months after active expansion, is critical due to the significant risk for relapse after transverse correction.

17.2.2.4 Anterior Crossbites

Crossbites of the anterior teeth can cause dental, occlusal, and periodontal trauma as well as abnormal mandibular growth and development. Over time patients may develop abnormal wear facets, incisal edge fractures, or chipping of teeth. Traumatic occlusal forces can result in periodontal conditions such as hypermobility, recession, and loss of alveolar bone support. Sagittal (anterior-posterior) skeletal growth may be restricted or become uneven due to an anterior crossbite, potentially leading to a skeletal Class III malocclusion. The growth potential, severity of the anterior crossbite, and skeletal pattern will determine whether the patient should be treated at this point. If the anterior crossbite is severe (i.e., includes multiple anterior teeth, a large negative overjet, or a Class III skeletal pattern with a horizontal growth tendency), it may be necessary to wait until the child has completed growth if they are not experiencing trauma or they will most likely continually outgrow the correction. An orthodontic referral for observation and possible growth modification using

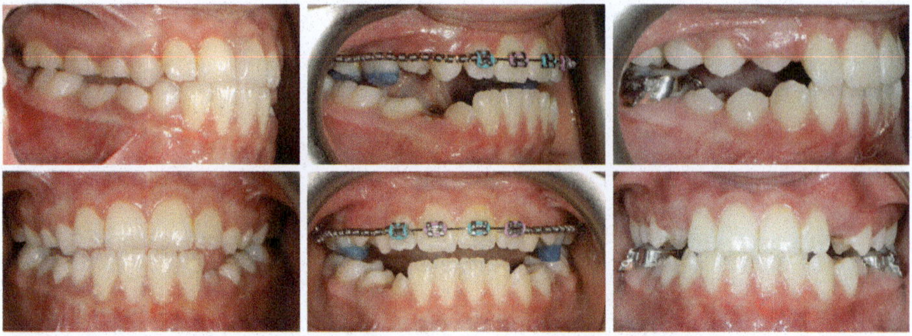

Fig. 17.12 Mild anterior crossbite with CR to MI shift. Center and right intraoral images shown before, during, and after orthodontic correction of the crossbite and associated shift. (*Left*: initial, *Center*: progress, *Right*: final)

extraoral appliances or skeletal anchorage would be appropriate in this situation. Mild to moderate anterior crossbites can be corrected with limited or comprehensive orthodontic treatment in conjunction with disclusion of the dentition to allow for anterior and posterior movement of the teeth in crossbite. (Fig. 17.12)

17.2.2.5 Parafunctional Habits

Commonly seen parafunctional habits leading to malocclusion include, but are not limited to, digit sucking, tongue thrusting, and mouth breathing. Patients with these habits will present with an anterior dental open bite, which can advance into a skeletal open bite if left untreated. It is important to keep in mind that if the malocclusion is corrected but the etiology (i.e., the parafunctional habit) is not, relapse will be inevitable and the malocclusion will reappear.

It is unknown whether tongue thrusting is an actual habit, resulting in a malocclusion, or if it is merely an adaptation to a preexisting anterior open bite. Regardless, it is necessary to control the tongue or digit habit to allow for correction and retention of the malocclusion. Appliances such as the tongue crib, tongue rake (Fig. 17.13), or bonded spurs (Fig. 17.14) can be used as an adjunct to assist in controlling the habit before, during, and/or after treatment. In some less severe cases, especially during the mixed dentition, these appliances alone can correct the anterior open bite by eliminating the habit, and comprehensive treatment can be delayed. Once corrected, retention between treatment phases should be aimed at continuing to control the habit, such as including a crib or rake embedded in a removable retainer.

A mouth breathing habit is much more complicated to treat. A restricted airway or systemic condition (ex. cerebral palsy or muscular dystrophy), causing the patient to breathe through their mouth and keep it open often, may result in an anterior open bite due to supra-eruption of the posterior teeth. A medical referral to an otolaryngologist is indicated if a limited airway is suspected. Once identified, it is best to refer these patients to an orthodontist for evaluation and provision of care.

17.2.2.6 Severe Crowding

Early identification of patients which have arch length/tooth-size discrepancies is crucial. When early loss of a deciduous tooth occurs or some space has been lost, it is important to maintain or regain the space until the patient is in the permanent dentition. About 3 mm of space per posterior quadrant can be regained through orthodontic treatment. Thus it is preferred to use a space maintainer when necessary rather than allowing space loss to occur. When patients have more than 5 mm of space loss or crowding, extraction of permanent teeth must be considered. 10 mm of crowding in an arch indicates likelihood for the need for serial extraction (Ngan et al. 2003)

Crowding in the permanent dentition cannot be directly correlated to tooth size, arch length, or spacing in the primary dentition. (Leighton 2007) While crowding in the primary dentition ensures that there will be crowding in the permanent dentition, spacing in the primary dentition does not guarantee sufficient space for all permanent teeth in the future. Table 17.1 shows the chances of crowding in the permanent dentition based on the amount of spacing in the primary dentition. Leeway space is defined as the additional space gained due to the primary molars being 2–3 mm wider than the permanent premolars. Maintenance of this space during the exfoliation of the primary molars is extremely important when crowding is suspected and will be discussed in the next section of this chapter.

17.2.2.7 Ectopic Eruption

Occasionally, teeth erupt in incorrect positions. When this occurs outside of the dental arch, they are termed ectopic. There are many reasons this occurs including severe crowding, premature loss of primary teeth, congenitally missing teeth,

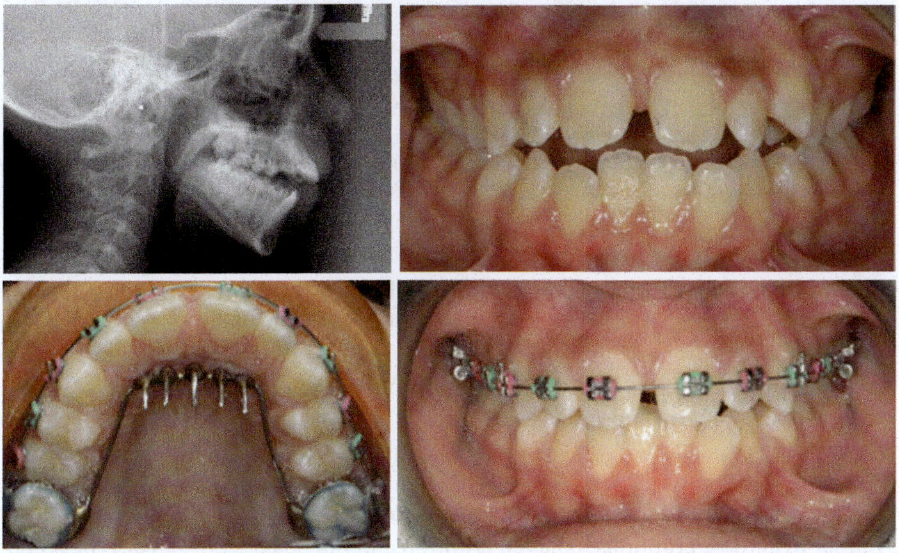

Fig. 17.13 Example of a patient with a thumb habit, vertical growth pattern, and anterior open bite. A tongue rake was used for habit cessation and the bite was closed

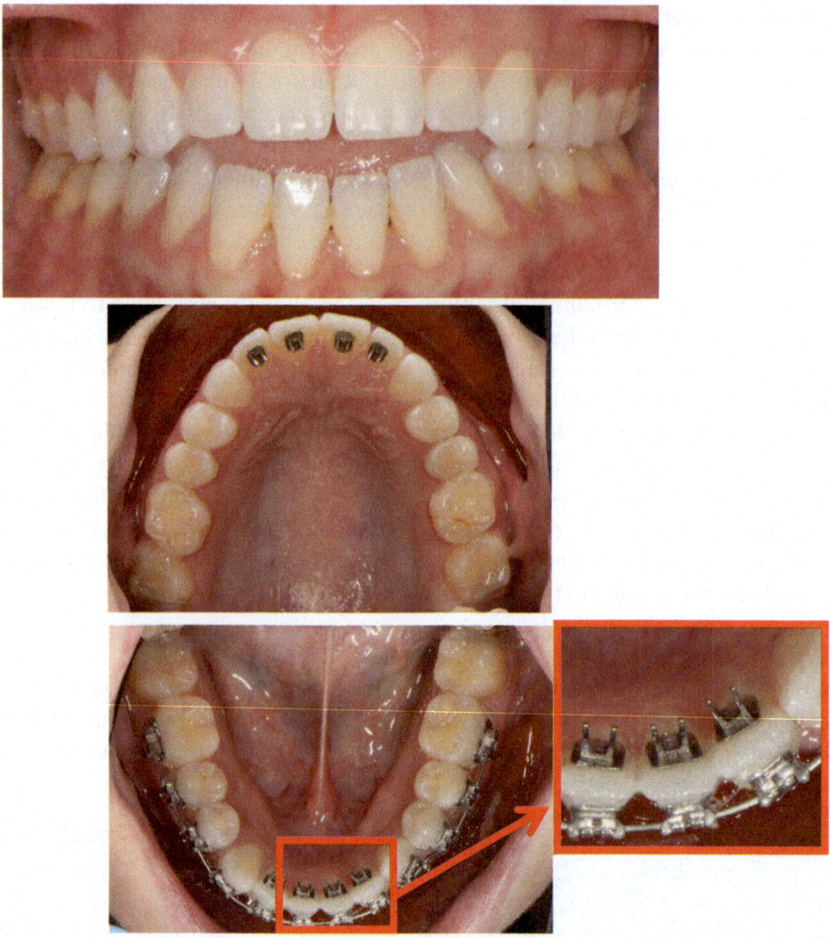

Fig. 17.14 Example of a patient with a tongue thrust habit and anterior open bite. *Top photo* shows initial presentation. Tongue spurs were bonded to the lingual of the upper and lower incisors in an effort to retrain the tongue and remove the tongue force during bite closure

misplaced permanent tooth buds, or other pathology. The potential sequelae of an ectopically erupting tooth include bony and soft tissue defects, as well as an unaesthetic appearance once erupted. These teeth need a periodontal evaluation and their prognosis should be taken into account when planning treatment, especially when trying to determine an extraction pattern. Over retained primary teeth may also be present.

17.2.2.8 Delayed Eruption and Impacted Teeth

Similar to ectopic eruptions, delayed eruption and impacted teeth can also be a consequence of space deficits, early loss of deciduous teeth, missing teeth, or incorrect position of permanent tooth buds. In addition, ankylosed primary teeth, over retained

Table 17.1 Prediction of crowding in permanent dentition based on spacing in the primary dentition (Leighton 2007)

Amount of spacing in the primary dentition	Chance of crowding in the permanent dentition (%)
<0 mm (Crowding)	100
0 mm	67
<3 mm	50
3–6 mm	20
>6 mm	0

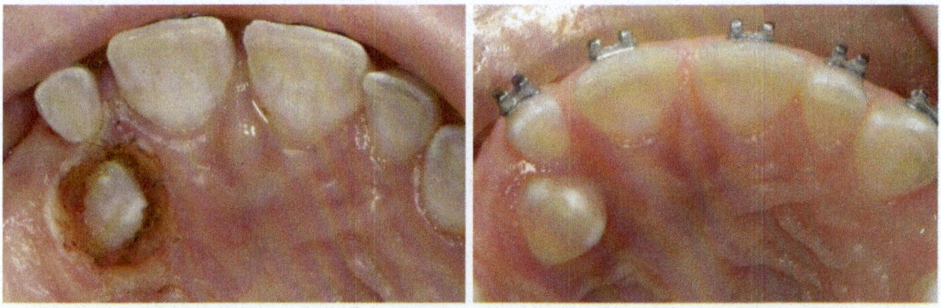

Fig. 17.15 A simple soft tissue exposure of an impacted canine followed by eruption

primary teeth, gingival fibromatosis, and tumors or cysts can also lead to impaction of permanent teeth. It is of utmost importance to monitor children on a regular basis (i.e., every 6 months to 1 year) during the transition from primary to permanent dentition. While comparing the patient's age to population norms for eruption is helpful, sequence of eruption is the most important to consider. Age of eruption will vary widely between children, but once chronological delayed tooth eruption has persisted for more than 1 year from the norm, clinicians should investigate further (Suri et al. 2004). Clinicians can also look for symmetry in eruption; if one side of the arch appears different in number of apparent teeth, radiographs should be taken to investigate further. Root length of the unerupted permanent tooth should be evaluated radiographically to evaluate development. Eruption should occur when the root has developed about two-thirds. When abnormalities are present, the clinician should rule out nutritional deficiencies, systemic conditions, genetic disorders, local conditions, and physical obstructions which could result in impaction or delayed eruption of teeth.

Besides third molars, permanent maxillary canines are the most commonly impacted teeth (Kokich 2004). Teeth can be impacted buccally, lingually, or centered over the ridge. The exact location of the tooth can be determined using a CBCT or a combination of two-dimensional radiographs. A CBCT can provide more information in regard to the location of the impacted tooth, other teeth, and important structures and can aid in the evaluation of possible root resorption. It is important to know the precise location of an impacted tooth as it will play a role in the treatment approach. In some instances, extraction of primary teeth and maintenance of space, or simple uncovering of soft and hard tissue over the impacted tooth, can be enough to promote the eruption of a delayed or impacted tooth (Fig. 17.15). Other impactions require extensive treatments, including exposure and orthodontic traction in order to erupt. After successful eruption, regardless of the approach, orthodontic treatment is usually necessary to incorporate the impacted tooth into the proper final position in the arch. Almost all cases presenting with impactions require a referral to the orthodontist as soon as it is identified.

17.2.2.9 Psychological Factors

Many elementary and middle school children are teased and bullied due to the way they look. Furthermore, a child's appearance can affect others', including teachers', perception of the child's intelligence. When this persists throughout the formative years of life, it can negatively impact a child's self-image and self-esteem. It has been shown that early orthodontic treatment can help improve self-confidence, stimulate more social interaction, and foster better opportunities (Jacobson 1979). Psychological factors are a true indication for early orthodontic intervention.

17.2.2.10 Growth Discrepancies

It may be prudent to treat severe skeletal growth discrepancies with appliances that aid in guiding growth. The ideal time to attempt this is immediately before puberty and continued throughout the growth spurt to maximize the intervention. Early treatment appliances for Class II malocclusions include headgear, bite plane, or Herbst (Fig. 17.16); facemasks, chin cups, or bone anchored maxillary protraction (BAMP) (De Clerck and Swennen 2011) can be used for Class III skeletal discrepancies. Referral for evaluation should be placed once a significant growth discrepancy is identified. While some literature indicates that the long-term results of early treatment may not be significantly different from treating later on in the adolescent stage, the decision to treat should be made by the orthodontist in conjunction with the parents (Pavlow et al. 2008; Tulloch et al. 1997).

17.2.2.11 Space Maintenance and Maintainers

During the mixed dentition phase, it may be necessary to extract primary teeth prematurely, either to relieve crowding in the erupting permanent dentition or for other dental concerns (i.e., caries, odontogenic infection, trauma, root resorption) resulting in the early loss of deciduous teeth. It is prudent to place a space maintainer in these cases to maintain the leeway space. This serves as additional space for the permanent dentition when there is an arch length deficiency. The amount of leeway space (Gianelly 1995) varies greatly in each individual, but studies report the average to be 2.2 mm (1.1 mm per side) in the maxillary arch and 4.8 mm (2.4 mm per side) in the mandible (Ngan et al. 1999). If not maintained, especially with the early loss of primary teeth, it can be lost during due to the mesial drift of the molars. A space maintainer will avoid this loss of valuable space when appropriately placed. Holding this space with simple appliances can assist in relieving or preventing crowding of the permanent dentition and can also be used to correct a discrepancy in molar classification in Class II patients.

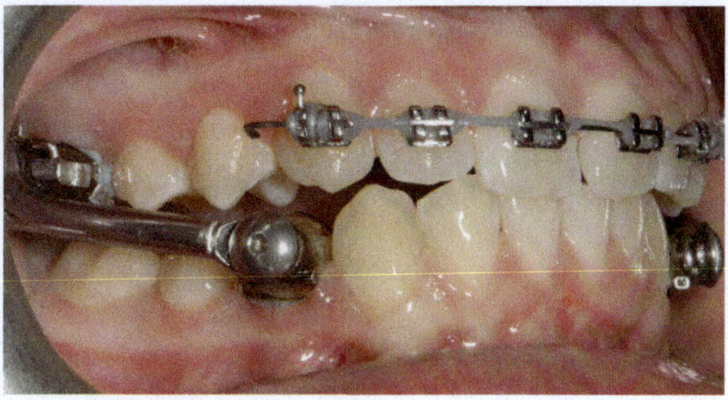

Fig. 17.16 Herbst appliance used to reduce overjet and correct A-P classification

Clinicians providing care to children should routinely and properly manage space in the primary and mixed dentitions. Once the permanent lower incisors have erupted, the clinician should measure these teeth and use either the Moyers or Tanaka-Johnston analyses to predict the amount of crowding or spacing which may develop once the permanent dentition is present. This will help the clinician determine whether a space maintainer is necessary. Indications for space maintenance include premature loss of primary molars and primary canines. Some contraindications to space maintenance are sufficient space for the permanent dentition, severe crowding resulting in little or no benefit of space preservation, and when the permanent tooth is close to eruption (within 6 months).

Many types of space maintainers exist, each indicated for particular situations. These can be fabricated in house or by a lab after bands have been sized on the specific teeth and an alginate or compound wax pickup impression has been obtained. Appliances that can be utilized in both arches include the band and loop and distal shoe appliances. The band and loop (Fig. 17.17) is a simple appliance that can be used when a unilateral primary molar has been lost prematurely. When a first primary molar is lost, the band is fitted on the second primary molar. When a second primary molar is lost, a band and loop can only be used if the first permanent molar is present to place the band on. A distal shoe is indicated when a second primary molar is lost but the permanent first molar has not yet erupted and serves to aid in the eruption of the first permanent molar into the proper position.

If tooth loss is present bilaterally, or leeway space needs to be maintained, full arch appliances can be used once the permanent first molars are present. In the maxillary arch, either a Nance holding arch or a transpalatal arch (TPA) will rigidly connect both maxillary first molars to each other (Fig. 17.18), maintaining each molar's current position. A TPA is composed of a heavy wire crossing directly across the palate soldered to the molar bands. The Nance appliance extends to the anterior palate where an acrylic button contacts the gingiva to enhance the maintaining anteroposterior position of the molars. A lower lingual holding arch (LLHA), the counterpart of a Nance or TPA, will maintain the position of the mandibular molars. (Fig. 17.19) It is constructed from a heavy wire which follows the general arch form on the lingual of the mandibular dentition and should rest anteriorly just

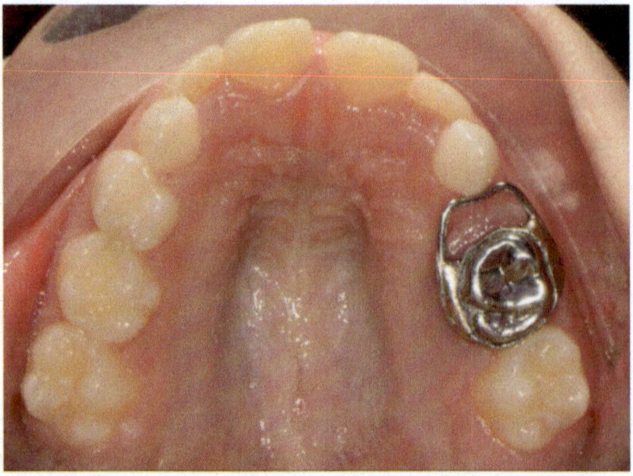

Fig. 17.17 Band and loop space maintainer

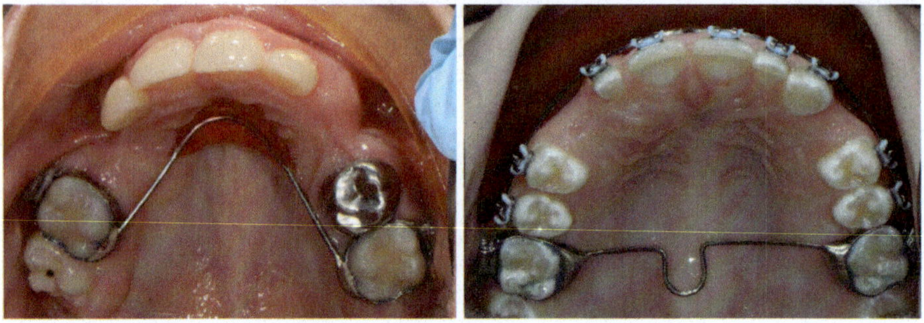

Fig. 17.18 Nance and TPA appliances as space maintainers

incisal to or at the gingival margin of the lower incisors. Side effects of this appliance are anterior displacement or flaring of the lower incisors and tipping back of the mandibular molars, both of which may or may not be desirable.

Removable appliances can also be used as an adjunct for space maintenance, regaining lost space, and small corrections of certain malocclusions during the mixed dentition. Options for removable retainers include the traditional acrylic Hawley and the thermoformed Essix retainer. A Hawley retainer can be designed with a variety of clasps which can be placed around the permanent dentition present for retention, while acrylic and clasps can be avoided in areas where teeth will be erupting in the future. Springs can be incorporated to create an active Hawley for minor tooth movements and to regain minor space loss. An Essix retainer can be fabricated to fit around the fully erupted permanent teeth after blocking out areas on the stone cast where teeth will be erupting. Both may be difficult to design, have short longevity, and necessitate frequent adjustments due to the rapid and significant dental changes occurring during this time. Furthermore, these appliances rely on compliance, have a tendency to fracture, and are lost frequently.

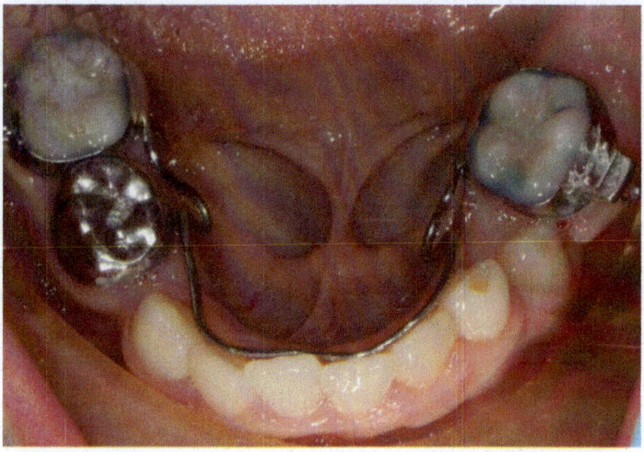

Fig. 17.19 Lower lingual holding arch space maintainer

17.3 Orthodontics for Restorative Treatment

Patients are often referred for orthodontic treatment prior to restorative treatment. The benefits include achieving:

- Proper tooth position
- Ideal spacing for restorations
- Establishment of the vertical dimension
- Direct management of the etiology of many problems that would otherwise be treated indirectly through restorative means alone

One of the main drawbacks is a long treatment time in patients that may not have desired nor expected to undergo orthodontic treatment in their adult lives. Another problem that may be encountered is a heightened risk for periodontal issues as well as general medical concerns in these patients. The patient's desires, combined with the risks and benefits, need to be considered to properly select patients for prerestorative orthodontic treatment.

Implant dentistry is becoming more common. Placing and restoring implants requires a great deal of planning to ensure that the final position of the implant is the ideal long-term location for that tooth and for the overall dentition. Practitioners that place implants know that it is important to have the sufficient mesiodistal width for the implant and the proper vertical height for the restorations. With age and tooth loss, molars and other teeth may drift into an area where a tooth was lost, and the vertical dimension may be diminished. Orthodontic treatment can ensure that the remaining natural dentition is in the proper place prior to placing implants for the best long-term outcome for the patient. Patients may require intrusion of the incisors, uprighting of molars, or simply alignment of teeth. Depending on the desired movement, these cases are some of the most challenging for orthodontists. Tooth movement requires anchorage, which is sometimes not available in a patient that has lost several posterior teeth. Additionally, uprighting molars may require either distalization of the crown or mesialization of the roots. Moving only the roots of a molar through the bone is a challenge and can present with additional difficulties when the vertical needs to be maintained. If planned in collaboration with an orthodontist, implants can be placed first and then used after a proper healing time to provide anchorage for tooth movement.

The use of mini-implants, also known as temporary anchorage devices, and miniplates has improved the ability to achieve some of these more difficult movements.(Singh et al. 2010) Mini-implants can be placed by orthodontists in their office using local anesthesia, used for a series of appointments for specific tooth movements, and then removed. They can be loaded immediately, do not osseointegrate, and have minimal risks when used properly. Their use requires planning to ensure proper space between the roots and evaluation of the anatomy to determine the best site to place it. They can be used to move teeth in all three planes of space without affecting the position of other teeth. Miniplates are used in similar ways, but are typically placed by an oral maxillofacial surgeon. The use of mini-implants and miniplates can also provide the orthodontist with an option for limited treatment. In cases requiring only single tooth movement, they can be advantageous.

Common cases requiring collaboration for the restorative dentist and the orthodontist are those with congenitally missing teeth or peg laterals. While these cases are usually more common, they require similar amounts of communication. The patient should consult with both the restorative dentist and the orthodontist prior to beginning any treatment. The orthodontist needs to understand from the restorative dentist exactly where the teeth should be to enhance the restorative outcome. Without this information, the orthodontist is moving teeth blindly. The use of wax ups and photos prior to beginning treatment are essential to ensure the best result. When creating a wax up for an orthodontist, the restorative dentist should include details about where the existing teeth should be in relation to each other and space required between roots for implants. Oftentimes, the orthodontic objectives may be limited in order to address the specific issues as defined by the restorative dentist. This is in an effort to minimize treatment time and complications for the patient.

17.4 Invisalign® for the General Dentist

A shortcoming of traditional orthodontic treatment has long been bulky and unaesthetic appliances. The recent increase in the number of adult patients seeking orthodontic treatment has led to a rise in the number of patients demanding esthetic orthodontics (Rosvall et al. 2009). Recently, modern biomaterials and fabrication processes have enabled the development of esthetic appliances, including tooth-colored brackets, lingual bracket systems, and clear aligners. The Invisalign® system has become one of the most popular and widely used approaches targeting patients' demand for esthetic treatment. Since Align Technology's conception of Invisalign® in 1997, an extraordinary number of orthodontists and general dentists have successfully treated patients of all ages. Although, limitations still exist, the Invisalign® system as a whole, including ClinCheck™, iTero™, and production facilities and methods, has been continuously evaluated and improved since its creation.

Over the years clinicians have struggled in providing full treatment with clear aligners. Most issues have been resolved through advances in materials, addition of auxiliaries, and sound clinical trials. Previously, it was necessary to obtain and send in polyvinyl siloxane impressions which were scanned to create digital models. The technician for Invisalign® would develop a setup based on the doctor's treatment requests. This setup would be reviewed by the practitioner and manual written instructions were necessary for modifications. Today, the iTero™ (and other select digital scanners), can be used to scan and send a digital model directly to Align Technology. Digital scans reduce production time by cutting out the mailing process and are more accurate with less concern for distortion. The latest updates to the ClinCheck™ software allow almost complete three-dimensional control of each individual tooth and auxiliaries. (Fig. 17.20)

Invisalign® recommends that patients wear aligners for a minimum of 22 h daily and switch to the consecutive aligner after 2 weeks (Bollen et al. 2003). Like most removable appliances, aligners provide intermittent orthodontic forces, perceived by the periodontium as light continuous forces (Nakao et al. 2007). While the forces on teeth with attachments and power ridges are greater than on teeth without, all of the forces and moments transferred to the teeth by the aligners are within the range of traditional orthodontic forces (Simon et al. 2014). Auxiliaries (i.e., traditional and optimized attachments, power ridges, precision cuts for elastic buttons and hooks, and bite ramps) and reduced activations per aligner (currently 0.15 mm to 0.33 mm) have allowed for enhanced tooth movements and expanded the clinical usefulness of the Invisalign® system. Align Technology has also improved the

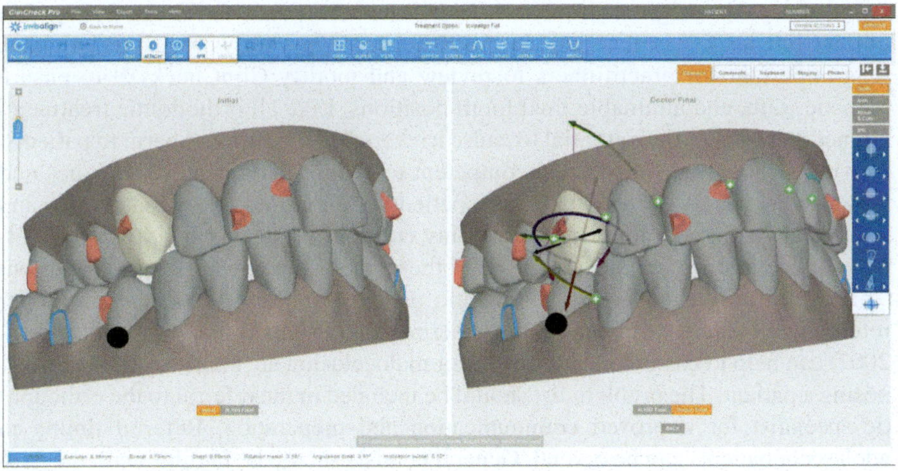

Fig. 17.20 The current ClinCheck™ Pro software still allows for visualization of the initial and predicted final occlusion but also offers the clinician almost full control of individual teeth and auxiliaries when modifying virtual setups using the 3D controls toolbar

plastic used for the aligners. The percentage of prescribed tooth movement obtained from older plastic materials was found to range from 41 to 57 %, while the latest material, SmartTrack, achieved 77 % of movements (Patel 2014; Drake et al. 2012; Chisari et al. 2014; Kravitz et al. 2009).

Practitioners should be able to discern the complexity of a case to determine if it can be treated properly with Invisalign®. Mild malocclusions and minor anterior crowding or spacing can be successfully treated by general dentists using Invisalign®. Caution suggesting or prescribing Invisalign® should be exercised when patients present with malocclusions which necessitate correction of classification, open bite, deep bite, severe crowding, or significant rotations. These cases are best treated using traditional fixed appliances or hybrid treatments (i.e., phases of both fixed and Invisalign® appliances) by an orthodontist. The most predictable movement using aligners has been found to be lingual constriction, while the most difficult movement to attain is extrusion (Kravitz et al. 2009). In general, Invisalign® cases should be treatment planned with the same orthodontic principles and goals as with fixed appliances. The only difference being the actual appliance used to achieve the same end point. General practitioners offering Invisalign® to patients should have a good understanding of what the principles of ideal occlusion are.

It is important to note that ClinCheck™ predictive models do not reflect the exact final occlusion obtained immediately after treatment with Invisalign®. It has been found that alignment, buccolingual inclinations, occlusal contacts, and occlusal relations are overestimated, especially corrections in the vertical dimension (Buschang et al. 2014; Krieger et al. 2011). A survey (Gregg 2007) conducted in 2007 reported that on average, general dentists modified ClinChecks™ 1.5 times while orthodontists usually resubmitted cases 2 times before final approval. It also found that 20 % of general dentists and 7 % of orthodontists surveyed accept the original ClinCheck™ with no modifications (Gregg 2007). The initial ClinCheck™ is generated by Align Technology's software and technicians. It is important for practitioners to review and modify ClinChecks™ to ensure realistic, safe, and attainable final tooth positions. Like all orthodontic treatment, aligner therapy has the potential to cause irreversible damage and harm to patients. Providers should be trained and competent to ensure that proper techniques and optimal care is being provided to these patients. Continuing education courses and study clubs are good opportunities to stay current on the ever-changing technology and techniques for Invisalign® and other aligner therapy systems.Conclusions

Appropriate diagnosis for orthodontic patients is important to ensure proper referral and treatment planning. The Ackerman and Profitt system (Ackerman et al. 2007) can help to ensure that all aspects of malocclusion are considered when diagnosing a patient. The problem list should be included in the referral to the orthodontic specialist for improved communication and preparation. Referral timing in adolescent patients can be crucial. General dentists should be familiar with the malocclusions presented in this chapter that need immediate referral in the primary and mixed dentitions. In adults, orthodontics can be used to improve restorative treatment outcomes. The potential for orthodontic treatment in these cases should be discussed with an orthodontic specialist. A diagnostic wax up ensures that all members of the team, including the patient, understand the goals of treatment and will help the orthodontist understand where to place the teeth to optimize restorative treatment. Invisalign® is one orthodontic appliance that many general dentists have chosen to utilize in their private practice. When treating patients with this appliance, the same diagnostic and treatment planning principles should be used to achieve ideal outcomes. Orthodontists are a part of the multidisciplinary team. Communication between the general dentist, orthodontist, and other specialists is important to ensure that the patient is well informed and that each member is playing an optimal role in the patient's treatment.

References

Ackerman JL, Proffit WR, Sarver DM, Ackerman MB, Kean MR. Pitch, roll, and yaw: describing the spatial orientation of dentofacial traits. Am J Orthod Dentofacial Orthop Off Pub Am Assoc Orthodont Const Soc Am Board Orthodont. 2007;131(3):305–10. doi:10.1016/j.ajodo.2006.05.032.

American Dental Association Council on Scientific Affairs. Dental radiographic examinations: recommendations for patient delection and limiting radiation exposure. 2012. http://www.ada.org/~/media/ADA/Member%20Center/FIles/Dental_Radiographic_Examinations_2012.ashx.

Andrews LF. The six keys to normal occlusion. Am J Orthod. 1972;62(3):296–309.

Angle EH. Classification of malocclusion. D Cosmos. 1899;41:248–64.

Asbell MB. A brief history of orthodontics. Am J Orthod Dentofacial Orthop Off Pub Am Assoc Orthodont Const Soc Am Board Orthodont. 1990;98(3):206–13. doi:10.1016/S0889-5406(05)81597-5.

Bahreman A. Early-age orthodontic treatment. Quintessence. 2013;1:1–14.

Bartzela T, Turp JC, Motschall E, Maltha JC. Medication effects on the rate of orthodontic tooth movement: a systematic literature review. Am J Orthod Dentofacial Orthop: Off Pub Am Assoc Orthodont Const Soc Am Board Orthodont. 2009;135(1):16–26. doi:10.1016/j.ajodo.2008.08.016.

Bishara SE, Staley RN. Maxillary expansion: clinical implications. Am J Orthod Dentofacial Orthop: Off Pub Am Assoc Orthodont Const Soc Am Board Orthodont. 1987;91(1):3–14.

Bollen AM, Huang G, King G, Hujoel P, Ma T. Activation time and material stiffness of sequential removable orthodontic appliances. Part 1: Ability to complete treatment. Am J Orthod Dentofacial Orthop: Off Pub Am Assoc Orthodont Const Soc Am Board Orthodont. 2003;124(5):496–501. doi:10.1016/S0889540603005766.

Bolton WA. Clinical application of a tooth-size analysis. Am J Orthod Dentofac. 1962;48(7):504. doi:10.1016/0002-9416(62)90129-X.

Buschang PH, Ross M, Shaw SG, Crosby D, Campbell PM. Predicted and actual end-of-treatment occlusion produced with aligner therapy. Angle Orthod. 2014. doi:10.2319/043014-311.1.

Cangialosi TJ, Riolo ML, Owens Jr SE, Dykhouse VJ, Moffitt AH, Grubb JE, Greco PM, English JD, James RD. The ABO discrepancy index: a measure of case complexity. Am J Orthod Dentofacial Orthop: Off Pub Am Assoc Orthodont Const Soc Am Board Orthodont. 2004;125(3):270–8. doi:10.1016/S0889540604000393.

Chen DR, McGorray SP, Dolce C, Wheeler TT. Effect of early Class II treatment on the incidence of incisor trauma. Am J Orthod Dentofacial Orthop: Off Pub Am Assoc Orthodont Const Soc Am Board Orthodont. 2011;140(4):e155–60. doi:10.1016/j.ajodo.2011.02.023.

Chisari JR, McGorray SP, Nair M, Wheeler TT. Variables affecting orthodontic tooth movement with clear aligners. Am J Orthod Dentofacial Orthop: Off Pub Am Assoc Orthodont Const Soc Am Board Orthodont. 2014;145(4 Suppl):S82–91. doi:10.1016/j.ajodo.2013.10.022.

De Clerck EE, Swennen GR. Success rate of miniplate anchorage for bone anchored maxillary protraction. Angle Orthod. 2011;81(6):1010–3. doi:10.2319/012311-47.1.

Drake CT, McGorray SP, Dolce C, Nair M, Wheeler TT. Orthodontic tooth movement with clear aligners. ISRN Dent. 2012:657973. doi:10.5402/2012/657973.

Gianelly AA. Leeway space and the resolution of crowding in the mixed dentition. Semin Orthod. 1995;1(3):188–94.

Gregg BR. A survey of Invisalign ClinCheck modifications and the types of cases treated using Invisalign: General dentists vs. orthodontists. Ann Arbor: M.S., State University of New York at Buffalo; 2007.

Jacobson A. Psychology and early orthodontic treatment. Am J Orthod. 1979;76(5):511–29.

Kokich VG. Surgical and orthodontic management of impacted maxillary canines. Am J Orthod Dentofacial Orthop: Off Pub Am Assoc Orthodont Const Soc Am Board Orthodont. 2004;126(3):278–83. doi:10.1016/S0889540604005268.

Kravitz ND, Kusnoto B, BeGole E, Obrez A, Agran B. How well does Invisalign work? A prospective clinical study evaluating the efficacy of tooth movement with Invisalign. Am J Orthod Dentofacial Orthop: Off Pub Am Assoc Orthodont Const Soc Am Board Orthodont. 2009;135(1):27–35. doi:10.1016/j.ajodo.2007.05.018.

Krieger E, Seiferth J, Saric I, Jung BA, Wehrbein H. Accuracy of Invisalign(R) treatments in the anterior tooth region. First results. J Orofac Orthop. 2011;72(2):141–9. doi:10.1007/s00056-011-0017-4.

Leighton BC. The early signs of malocclusion. Eur J Orthod. 2007;29 suppl 1:i89–95. doi:10.1093/ejo/cjl099.

Nakao K, Goto T, Gunjigake KK, Konoo T, Kobayashi S, Yamaguchi K. Intermittent force induces high RANKL expression in human periodontal ligament cells. J Dent Res. 2007;86(7):623–8.

Ngan P, Alkire RG, Fields Jr H. Management of space problems in the primary and mixed dentitions. J Am Dent Assoc. 1999;130(9):1330–9.

Ngan PW, Kao EC, Wei SH. Guidance of eruption for general practitioners. Int Dent J. 2003;53(2):100–13.

Patel ND. Effect of aligner material, duration, and force level on tooth movement. University of Florida Digital Collections. Gainesville: University of Florida; 2014.

Pavlow SS, McGorray SP, Taylor MG, Dolce C, King GJ, Wheeler TT. Effect of early treatment on stability of occlusion in patients with Class II malocclusion. Am J Orthod Dentofacial Orthop: Off Pub Am Assoc Orthodont Const Soc Am Board Orthodont. 2008;133(2):235–44. doi:10.1016/j.ajodo.2006.02.038.

Proffit WR, Fields HW, Sarver DM. Contemporary orthodontics. 5th ed. St. Louis: Mosby Elsevier; 2013.

Rosvall MD, Fields HW, Ziuchkovski J, Rosenstiel SF, Johnston WM (2009) Attractiveness, acceptability, and value of orthodontic appliances. Am J Orthod Dentofacial Orthop: Off Pub Am Assoc Orthodont Const Soc Am Board Orthodont. 135(3):276, e271–12; discussion 276–7. doi:10.1016/j.ajodo.2008.09.020.

Simon M, Keilig L, Schwarze J, Jung BA, Bourauel C. Forces and moments generated by removable thermoplastic aligners: incisor torque, premolar derotation, and molar distalization. Am J Orthod Dentofacial Orthop: Off Pub Am Assoc Orthodont Const Soc Am Board Orthodont. 2014;145(6):728–36. doi:10.1016/j.ajodo.2014.03.015.

Singh K, Deepak K, et al. Temporary anchorage devices- mini implants. Natl J Maxillofac Surg. 2010;1(1):30–4.

Steiner C. The use of cephalometrics as an aid to planning and assessing orthodontic treatment: report of a case. Am J Orthod. 1960;46(10):721–35.

Suresh M, Ratnaditya A, Kattimani VS, Karpe S. One phase versus two phase treatment in mixed dentition: a critical review. J Int Oral Health. 2015;7(8):144–7.

Suri L, Gagari E, Vastardis H. Delayed tooth eruption: pathogenesis, diagnosis, and treatment. A literature review. Am J Orthod Dentofacial Orthop: Off Pub Am Assoc Orthodont Const Soc Am Board Orthodont. 2004;126(4):432–45. doi:10.1016/S088954060400530X.

Tulloch JF, Phillips C, Koch G, Proffit WR. The effect of early intervention on skeletal pattern in Class II malocclusion: a randomized clinical trial. Am J Orthod Dentofacial Orthop: Off Pub Am Assoc Orthodont Const Soc Am Board Orthodont. 1997;111(4):391–400.

Wieslander L. Early or late cervical traction therapy of Class-Ii malocclusion in mixed dentition. Am J Orthod Dentofac. 1975;67(4):432–39. doi:10.1016/0002-9416(75)90024-X.

Implants for the General Practitioner 18

Mitch Zientz, Geraldine Weinstein, and Luiz Gonzaga

Contents

M. Zientz, DMD
Private Practice, New York, NY, USA

G. Weinstein, DDS (✉)
Department of Craniofacial Sciences, DDS University of Connecticut
School of Dental Medicine, Farmington, CT, USA
e-mail: geraldineweinstein@gmail.com

L. Gonzaga, DMD
Implant Center, University of Florida College of Dentistry, Gainesville, FL, USA

G.M. Weinstein, M.T. Zientz (eds.), *The Dental Reference Manual*,
DOI 10.1007/978-3-319-39730-6_18

Abstract

The following chapter will focus on implantology as it pertains to the general practitioner. The general practitioner is responsible for developing the restorative plan that will dictate treatment from start to finish. Oftentimes with implants, it is a team-based approach that will involve multiple specialties. For a general dentist, the standard of care is to have the ability to develop a treatment plan for a patient and discuss the option of having implants as alternatives to other dental treatments. A basic understanding of implant diagnosis and treatment planning, pre-prosthetic and surgical planning, restorative guidelines, and complications will be presented.

18.1 Implants and Osseointegration

Dental implants work by a process known as osseointegration, which occurs when bone cells attach themselves directly to the implant surface, essentially locking the implant into the bone. This process was first discovered by a Swedish researcher, Per-Ingvar Brånemark, in the 1960s. Dental implants were placed into the jaw bones by controlled surgical procedures and allowed to "osseointegrate." Osseointegration is defined as a time-dependent healing process whereby clinically asymptomatic rigid fixation of alloplastic materials is achieved and maintained in the bone during functional loading. Histologic appearance resembled a functional ankyloses with no intervention of fibrous or connective tissue between the bone and implant surface.

Implants are predominantly made of titanium, a biocompatible metal that offers strength and durability as well as a unique property of fusing directly to the bone. This process is known as osseointegration. Titanium and its alloys are the materials of choice clinically because of their superior mechanical properties and abundance in nature. The combined effect of surface energy, surface roughness, and topography on implant determines its ultimate ability to integrate into the surrounding tissue (Parithimarkalaignan and Padmanabhan 2013).

There are many different implant systems available in the market. The restorative dentist must be familiar with the choice of system, its advantages, and limitations (Table 18.1). In addition, if surgery is done by a specialist, the general dentist must

Table 18.1 Popular implant systems available in the United States have websites that contain a lot of information regarding their product choices. This is a good way for a dentist to begin the process of learning about what is out there. Some of these companies even have apps for phones that can be downloaded to assist in selecting implant parts when you are ready to order

Implant company	ISSN address
Biohorizons	http://www.biohorizons.com/professionals.aspx
Dentsply-Astra Implants	https://www.dentsply.com/en-us/implants.html
Nobel Biocare	https://www.nobelbiocare.com/us/en/home.html
Straumann	http://www.straumann.us/en/professionals/products-and-solutions/surgical-and-restorative-solutions/implants.html
Zimmer Dental	http://www.zimmerdental.com/Home/zimmerDental.aspx

communicate with the surgeon through the planning and placement of the implant. The process must be driven by the restorative end result that is desired by the general dentist and the patient. Basically, planning of the location of the final restoration and working backward as to where the implant should go. Fortunately there are many digital pathways that make this possible with computer-aided design/computer-aided manufacturing (CAD/CAM) dentistry. However we will focus on the basics of achieving this with traditional dental armamentarium. (See Chaps. 10 and 11 for information on digital pathways.) In making decisions between saving a tooth or extraction and replacement with an implant, see Chap. 6 "Restorative Considerations."

The successful outcome of any implant osseointegration is mainly dependent on the interrelationship of the various components of an equation that include the following:

- Biocompatibility of the implant material and health of the patient
- Macroscopic and microscopic nature of the implant surface and designs
- The status of the implant bed in both a health and a morphologic (bone quality) context
- The surgical technique
- The undisturbed healing phase
- Loading conditions

18.2 Diagnosis and Treatment Planning

The International Team for Implantology (ITI) has developed a formalized set of parameters to classify the nature of various implant cases, both from a surgical and restorative perspective. The guidelines were developed in a consensus in 2007. These parameters help to formulate a consistent diagnosis with regard to the degree of difficulty and can aid in case selection for any surgeon or restorative dentist. There are modifying factors that contribute to determining the final Straightforward, Advanced, Complex (SAC) classification. They are general, esthetic, surgical, and restorative modifying factors. Different factors are associated with different levels of risk. The assessment tool is available for free online: the ISSN register, http://www.iti.org/SAC-Assessment-Tool (accessed on 17 Mar 2016).

Outlined below is essential information that a general dentist requires in assessing a patient for implant consideration (Diz et al. 2013; Holzinger et al. 2014):

18.2.1 Medical Risk Assessment (Gomez-de Diego et al. 2014; Hwang and Wang 2006, 2007)

A complete and thorough medical history of the patient is necessary to access the patient's ability to tolerate the surgery and for healing after an implant is placed. In patients that have any of these contraindications mentioned below, a discussion with their physician and an experienced implant surgeon should occur.

18.2.1.1 Absolute Contraindications

1. Acute myocardial infarction
2. Cerebrovascular accident
3. Immunosuppression
4. Active treatment of malignancy
5. Bleeding issues (hemophilia, Idiopathic Thrombocytopenic Purpura (ITP))
6. Drug abuse/psychiatric illness
7. IV bisphosphonate treatment

18.2.1.2 Relative Contraindications

8. Patients taking warfarin needing multiple implants in a quadrant
9. Chronically hypertensive patients
10. Type II diabetes with poor glycemic control
11. Patients taking oral bisphosphonates longer than 5 years (without treatment modification)

18.2.1.3 Other Considerations

12. History of radiotherapy in the head and neck
13. Cardiac arrhythmias

18.2.2 Articulated Diagnostic Casts

- Good quality diagnostic casts should be obtained and mounted properly on an articulator. These casts will be duplicated later on for planning purposes (Table. 18.2).
- Training and experience will allow a practitioner to be well versed when developing a treatment plan for a patient for implants. It is critical to plan well so as not to surprise the patient with unforeseen circumstances that lead to additional expense and surgery.

Table 18.2 Items to evaluate when looking at mounted diagnostic casts

Observe	Why or what is needed
Occlusal plane	Evaluate the occlusion (bruxism or the loss of vertical dimension)
Interocclusal space (space measured between an edentulous spot where the implant is planned to the opposing tooth)	Vertically a minimum of 7 mm is recommended; 4 mm for the abutment + 2–3 mm for the restoration Horizontally (mesiodistal direction; 7–10 mm is needed to accommodate the implant abutment and restoration)
If the area for the implant is already edentulous, evaluate the width and height of the area.	Considerations for need for boney augmentation if the bone has resorbed from the area –
If the area for the implant still needs an extraction	Considerations for socket preservation when the extraction or immediate placement of the implant is done (See Chap. 15 "Oral Surgery")

Measurements are based on traditional implants available in Straumann and Dentsply-Astra

- If using traditional articulators to mount your diagnostic case, insure that you are calibrated with the laboratory to preserve the occlusal scheme. (Refer to Chap. 20 "Communicating with Dental Laboratories.")

18.2.3 Full-Mouth Radiographs and Panorex

Patients should always be treated comprehensively, addressing urgent dental issues prior to placement of implants. Periapical radiographs, bitewings, and panorex would be an initial start to evaluate possible implant sites (Figs. 18.1a and 18.2b). Oftentimes these determine the need for additional imaging (Shelley et al. 2014). The principle of as low as reasonably achievable (ALARA) should be respected in determining which radiographs are necessary for implant placement.

18.2.4 Preoperative Photographs

These are great records to keep in planning prosthodontic cases. It can also assist in treatment planning when a patient is not in the office.

18.2.5 Diagnostic Wax-Up

This is a great way to plan the restoration, use for fabrication of temporaries, and for patient acceptance. This can be accomplished the traditional way with wax and a denture tooth or digitally with CAD/CAM design programs. If this is done digitally after intraoral scanning, this would begin the digital path of planning for the implant. (See Chap. 11 "Digital Impressions") (Table 18.3).

18.2.6 CT Scan if Indicated and/or Available

The dentist doing the surgery will make this decision when planning the implant. As the general dentist in charge of the patient's well-being, insure that these CT scans are read by properly trained radiologists to insure that no pathology is missed. Proximity of the implant to be placed to the sinus walls or inferior alveolar nerve (IAN) will warrant ordering a CT scan (Bornstein et al. 2014).

18.2.7 Periodontal Status of the Patient

Patients with uncontrolled periodontal disease may not be good candidates for implant placement. Studies done by Mengel et al. have shown 83.3 % success of implants osseointegrated in a 10-year study on patients who had a history of generalized aggressive periodontitis (GAP). Similarly, a systematic review had found that the survival rates of implants in patients with GAP were in the range of 83.3–96 %

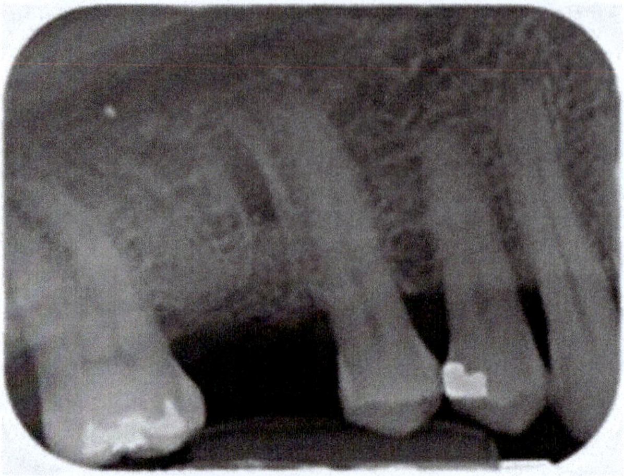

Fig. 18.1 A periapical radiograph is a screening tool to evaluate pathosis on the adjacent teeth. The periapical radiograph is a good indication of the height of the bone in the edentulous area between the teeth

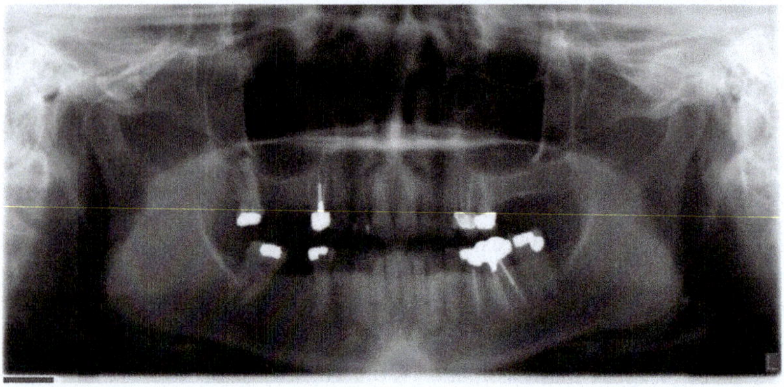

Fig. 18.2 Panoramic radiograph is for initial screening of anatomic landmarks that may alter the placement of an implant. In treatment planning of a lower implant, location of the mandibular canal and mental foramen is critical. In an upper implant, the sinus walls should be noted

Table 18.3 Critical measurements at this point

Source	What to look for
Radiographs	Vertically, the length of the implant + 2 mm (safety zone)
Diagnostic casts/ Wax-up	The implant will need 1 mm of bone circumscribing it This means that an implant with a 4-mm width will need 6 mm of bone. (Mesiodistal and buccolingual direction)

(Kim and Sung 2012). An individualized plan to control the patient's periodontal disease seems to be the key to successful implant osseointegration.

18.2.8 Patient Expectations

The patient's desire for a fixed versus a removable prosthesis and giving the patient full disclosure as to the costs and time expectations for the treatment are essential.

18.3 Planning a Single-Tooth Implant in the Posterior

- Proficiency in planning implants in the posterior should be mastered prior to attempting anterior implants for any dentist who is dealing with implants for the first time. The attention to details in order to achieve esthetic outcomes is not as complex on posteriors as they are on anterior teeth area (Buser et al. 2004). As an example is the replacement of tooth #19 with an implant (Fig. 18.3). After going through all the considerations above, the patient accepted the treatment plan.
- Proficiency and familiarity with the choice of implant system is also essential in planning for the implant. This is critical in discussions with the surgeon when referring a patient for surgery and in communicating with the dental laboratory when ordering required pieces.

18.3.1 Guided Surgery

18.3.1.1 CT- or Lab-Fabricated Guide (Guerrero et al. 2006)

The lab will fabricate your guide based on information provided by the CT/CBCT scan (Fig. 18.4). This is the safest and most predictable route for implant surgery. The location of critical structures such as the IAN and maxillary sinus is identified and considered prior to surgery. The implants are more likely to be parallel and in the ideal locations according to the restorative plan and bone. These guides are the most accurate as they provide stops in all directions such that the implant is placed in the proper location.

18.3.1.2 In-Office Guide Design

First, duplicate casts with wax and a denture tooth for a mock-up. Next, fabricate a radiographic guide using a 10-mm pin. Try in your guide to verify with a periapical film on the patient. Now fabricate your surgical guide if everything looks correct (Fig. 18.5a–e). This type of guide works but is inferior compared to the CT- or lab-fabricated guide as it does not address all the different dimensions that the implant can go. If this is made of soft plastic, it does not provide stops to prevent improper angulation and depth in placing the implant.

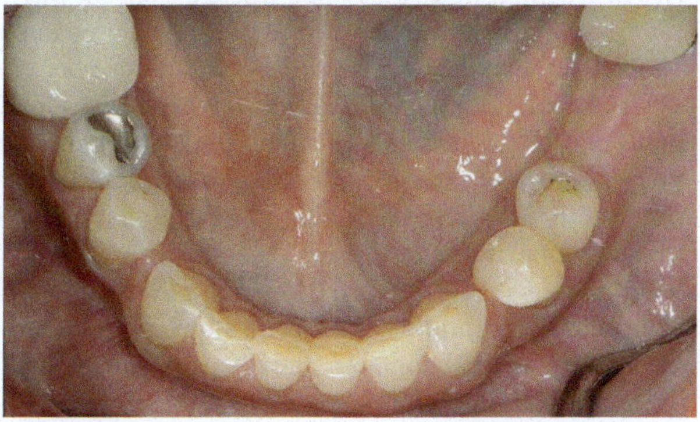

Fig. 18.3 Photograph of the mandibular arch with missing tooth #19 which we would like to replace with an implant

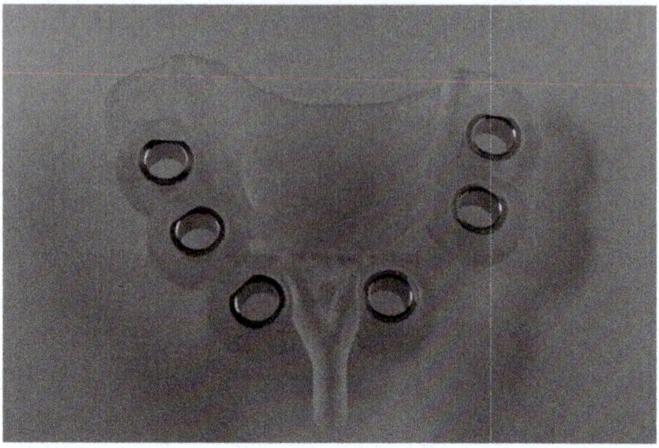

Fig. 18.4 Laboratory-fabricated surgical guide

The general dentist may or may not elect to do the surgery at this point. If the patient is being referred to a specialist for implant placement, referral with a guide is the best way to communicate to the specialist where the implant should go so that it can be restored properly. Proper training and continuing education courses should be completed prior to attempting surgical placement of implants.

A great illustration of this process can be viewed: the ISSN, https://vimeo.com/142902539 (accessed on 29 Mar 2016).

18.3.2 Ridge Preservation

Immediate implants are defined as implants placed at the same time as the tooth extraction. The literature shows similar survival rates for immediate placed implants versus healed sites, but in some cases, the immediate placement is not indicated due to infection, poor primary wound stability, or poor soft tissue. A clinician may not feel comfortable doing this modality due to the more advanced nature of immediate implants. One alternative is to graft the site with bone substitutes at the time of extraction. Many articles on this topic concluded that the addition of bone material at the time of extraction, with or without a membrane, will minimize the bone remodeling after the healing phase. (See Chap. 15 "Oral Surgery.") The clinician should learn about the different techniques and materials to educate the patient about the possible benefits of ridge preservation. This case demonstrates a situation where the patient was not financially prepared for the immediate implant treatment, and thus, ridge preservation was performed. The implant was placed 6 months after the extraction and ridge preservation (Fig. 18.6a–d).

Once healing of the implant has occurred, often 8–12 weeks after surgical placement (Fig. 18.7), an abutment is selected. There are many ways to impress the abutment (abutment-level impression) or the implant (implant-level impression). The options utilize a digital path or more traditional methods. Some implant companies are more amenable than others when using the digital pathway as scan bodies are not available for all types of implants. (See Chap. 11 "Digital Impressions.") A provisional restoration can be made at this point to preserve the integrity of the soft tissue, the proximal contacts, and the occlusion.

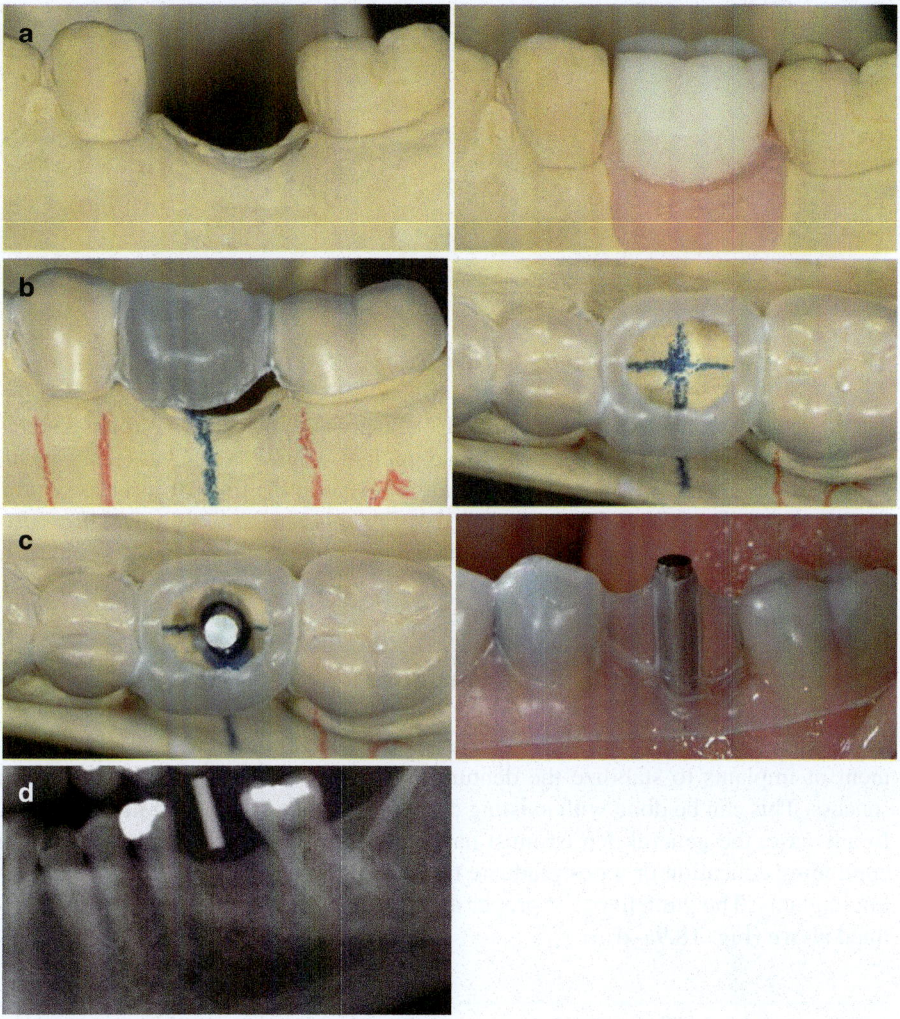

Fig. 18.5 (**a**) When using in-office guides, a wax-up can be done using denture teeth and triad material to stabilize the tooth at the correct tridimensional position, including correct occlusion and proposed gingival margin. A guide can be fabricated using the method published by Higginbottom and Wilson in 1996. (**b**) A vacuum-formed material (copyplast 1 mm) is used to create a template over the "wax-up." Lines are drawn in the cast following the adjacent root position according to the examination/initial radiography. (**c**) At this point, using a 2-mm-diameter twist drill and following the correct position, a "cast surgery" can be done, and perforation on the cast is created. A 2-mm-diameter rod is adapted to the cast and a new vacuum-formed template is done to create a radiographic guide. (**d**) The radiographic evaluation will allow the clinician to plan the best angulation of the implant to respect the adjacent roots and to plan the correct implant length to avoid the anatomic structures. (**e**) Now a sleeve guide can be fabricated to restrict the mesial/distal and buccal/lingual osteotomy, and the initial full-contour wax-up vacuum form can be use to determine the correct implant depth (vertical guide) according to the implant design. (i.e., tissue level or bone level)

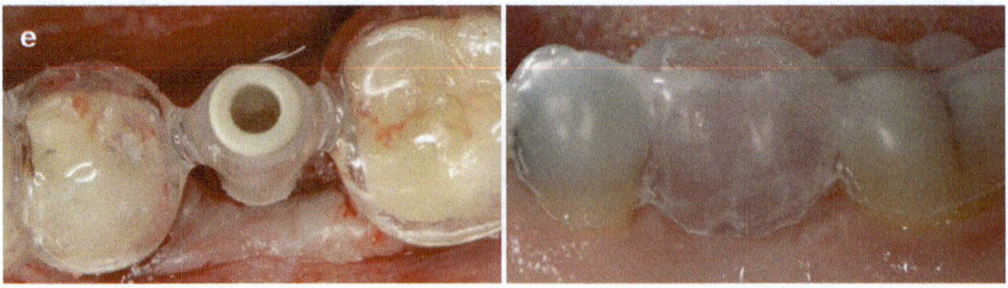

Fig. 18.5 (continued)

18.3.3 Cementation Versus Screw-In

There are many controversies regarding use of cement in placement of final restorations of implants. This is due to the fact that implant failure has been associated with the presence of excess cement that was not removed at the time of insertion of the final restoration. (Wilson 2009; AAP 2013) For this reason, a number of experienced dentists have chosen systems that utilize screw-retained restorations that avoid use of cement (Fig. 18.8a, b).

18.4 Implant Mandibular Overdenture

The standard of care in patients that have complete lower dentures is to offer placement of implants to stabilize the denture and provide the patient with long-term success. This can be done with existing dentures or when fabricating new dentures. In any case, the general dentist must have had adequate surgical training through continuing education or a postgraduate residency program prior to surgically placing implants. The guidelines for proper diagnosis and treatment planning were outlined above (Fig. 18.9a–d).

18.5 Peri-implantitis

Peri-implantitis is defined as inflammation of the soft tissue and bone around an implant. This results in the loss of bone attachment to the implant. Risk factors that lead to peri-implantitis are numerous and can be a combination of many factors (Nguyen-Hieu et al. 2012; Mengel et al. 2007):

1. History of periodontitis, dental plaque, and poor oral hygiene
2. Smoking
3. Alcohol consumption
4. Diabetes

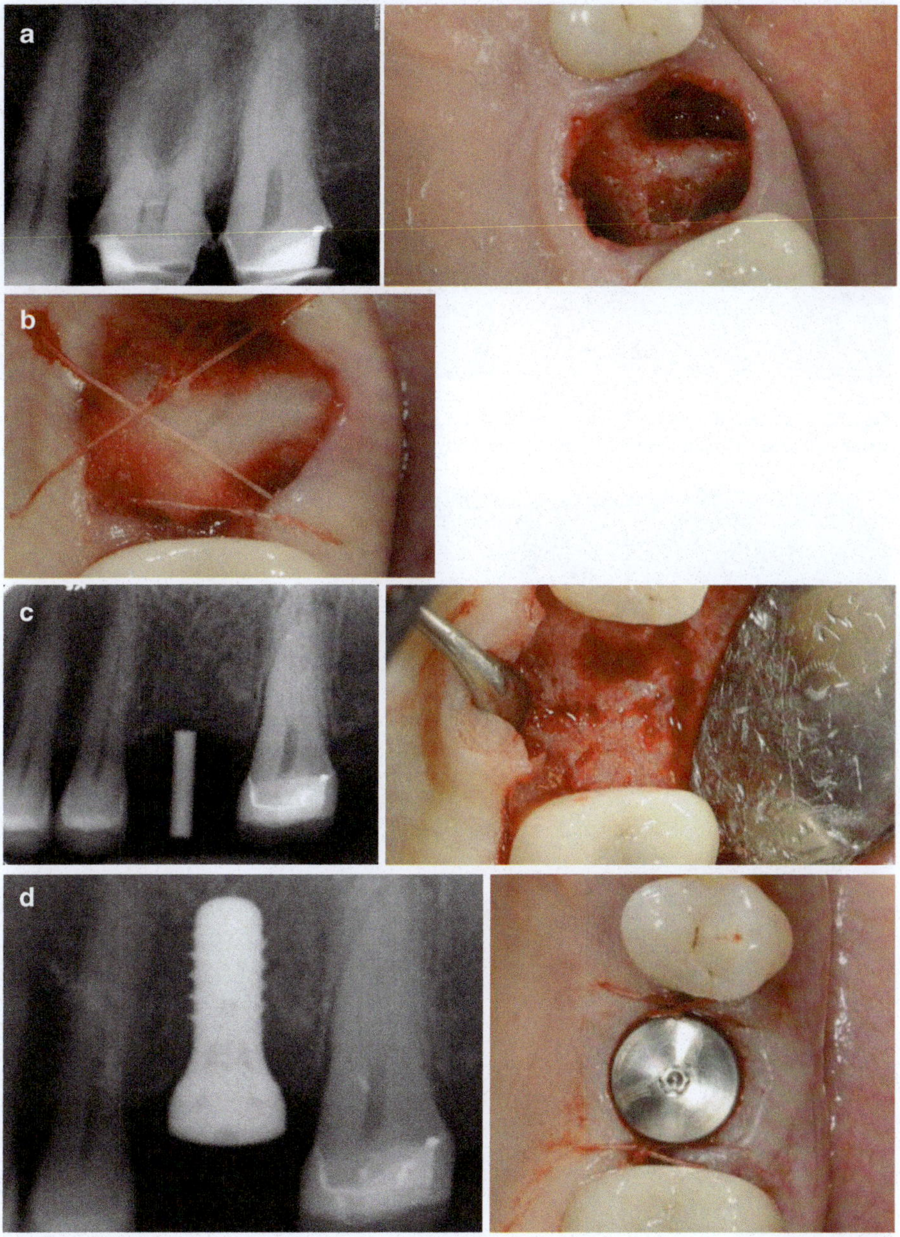

Fig. 18.6 (**a**) Tooth extracted due to a longitudinal root fracture diagnosed during an attempt to endodontically treat the tooth. (**b**) Ridge preservation done with freeze-dried bone allograft (FDBA) bone substitute and collagen membrane. (**c**) Implant placement 6 months after extraction and ridge preservation. (**d**) Postoperative radiograph and photo of the implant

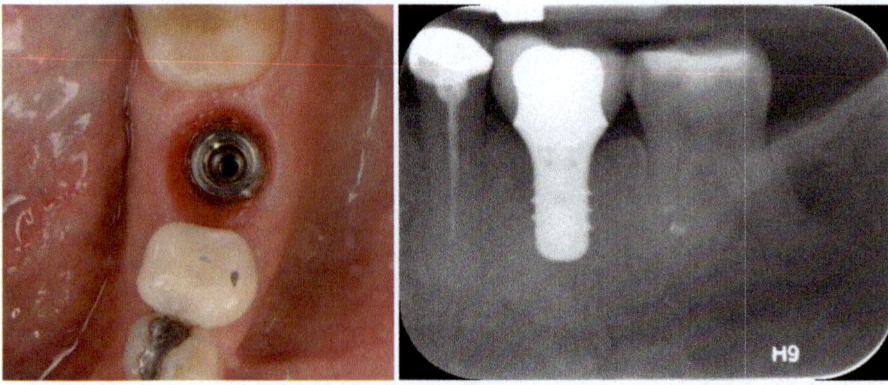

Fig. 18.7 Photo of a nicely healed implant with good gingival contour. The radiograph shows no space between the abutment and the implant body

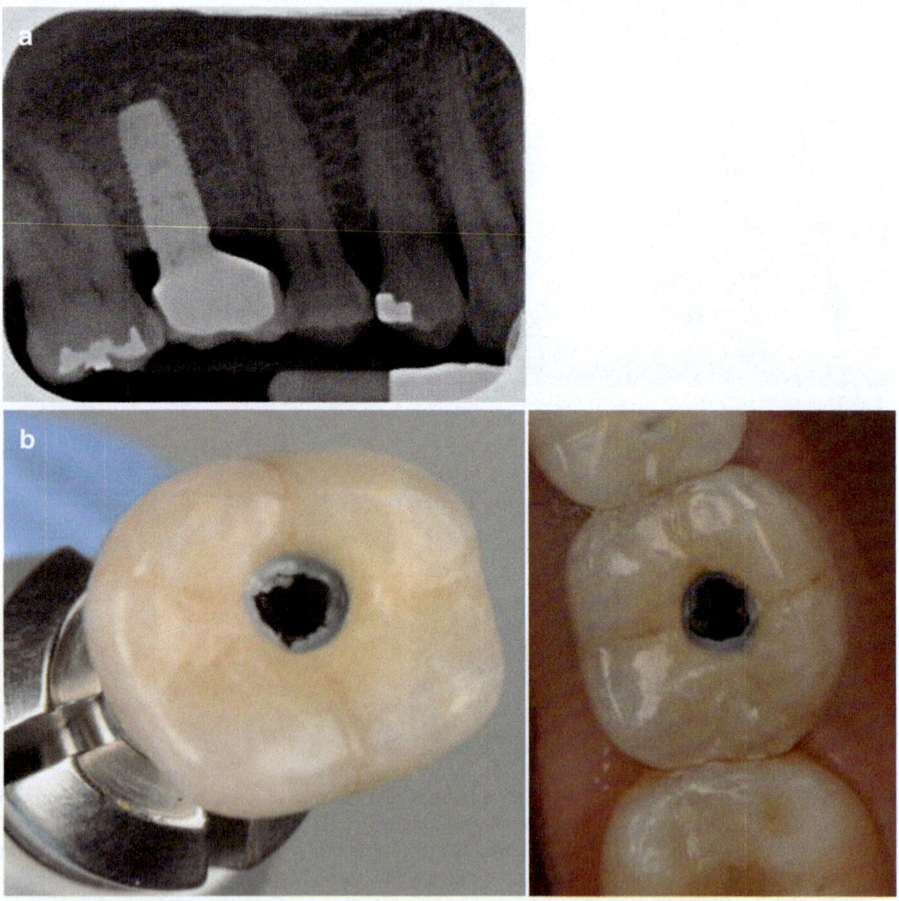

Fig. 18.8 (**a**) Radiograph of final cemented restoration confirms seating of the restoration and no excess cement present. (**b**) Screw-retained implant crown decreases the risk of leaving excess cement subgingivally

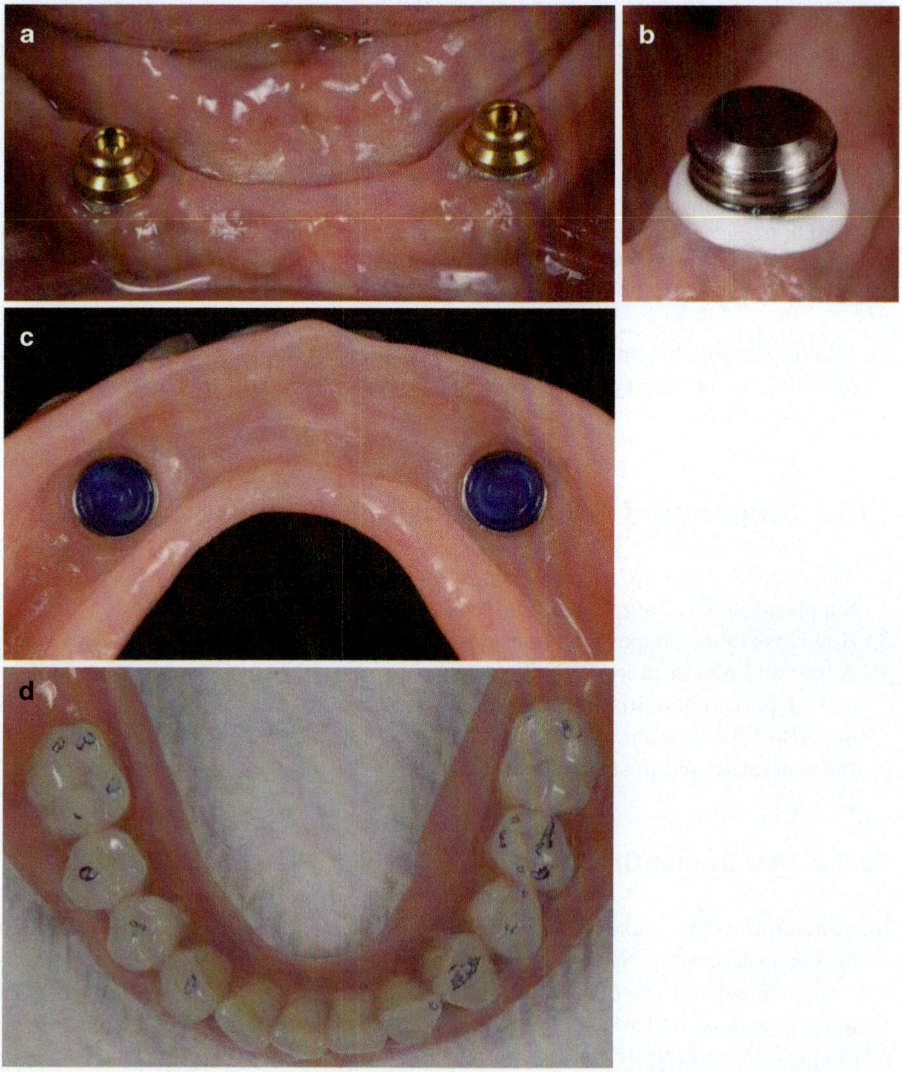

Fig. 18.9 (**a**) A minimum of two locators are needed to hold a lower complete denture. (**b**) The female attachment is on the implant body. (**c**) The male attachment is on the denture. These can be added on to existing dentures by relining the dentures. (**d**) A balanced occlusion is essential after the implant attachments are incorporated into the denture

Table 18.4 Treatments for peri-implantitis

Pocket depth + findings	Treatment recommendation
<3 mm + bleeding/pus	Oral hygiene and debridement
4–5 mm + bleeding/pus	Oral hygiene, debridement, and antiseptic therapy
>6 mm + bleeding/ pus + bone loss	Oral hygiene, local or systemic antibiotics, followed by resective or regenerative therapy

Lagervall et al. have found that there is 69 % mean success in peri-implantitis treatments. In addition, treatment of peri-implantitis has been found to be ineffective over the long term for patients with generalized periodontitis, poor oral hygiene, and plaque control. (Lagervall and Jansson 2013) Further studies are necessary to investigate the other treatment modalities that have been suggested.

Another factor that may contribute to peri-implantitis is occlusion. Although more studies are necessary to determine the predictable treatment outcomes (Elemek and Almas 2014).

18.5.1 Symptoms of Peri-implantitis (AAP 2013)

1. Deep pockets >5 mm, bleeding on probing.
2. Suppuration, swelling, and tenderness.
3. Bone loss in the shape of a crater around it as seen radiographically.
4. A loss of 2 mm or more of the bone from the marginal crest level is often indicative of peri-implantitis and can also be measured as the loss of bone from 3 threads of the implant.
5. Intraoperative and postoperative pressure.

18.5.2 Peri-implantitis Treatment (Nguyen-Hieu et al. 2012)

Identification of the cause of peri-implantitis in the patient is essential in order to control its progression. Necessary review of the patient's medical history and medical consults, where appropriate, should be considered. This is especially true in patients that have had recent diabetic diagnosis or other immune-compromising health problems (Table 18.4).

References

American Academy of Periodontology. Academy report: peri-implant mucositis and peri-implantitis: a current understanding of their diagnoses and clinical implications. Journal of Periodontology. 2013;84(4):436–43. doi: 10.1902/jop.2013.134001

Bornstein MM, Scarfe WC, Vaughn VM, Jacobs R. Cone beam computed tomography in implant dentistry: a systematic review focusing on guidelines, indications, and radiation dose risks. Int J Oral Maxillofac Implants. 2014;29:55–77.

Buser D, Martin W, Belser U. Optimizing esthetics for implant restorations in the anterior maxilla: anatomic and surgical considerations. Int J Oral Maxillofac Implants. 2004;19:43–61.

Diz P, Scully C, Sanz M. Dental implants in the medically compromised patient. J Dent. 2013;41(3):195–206.

Elemek E, Almas K. Peri-implantitis: etiology, diagnosis and treatment: an update. N Y State Dent J. 2014;80(1):26–32.

Froum SJ, Rosen PS. A proposed classification for Peri-implantitis. Int J Periodontics Restorative Dent. 2012;32(5):533–40.

Gomez de Diego R, Mang-de la Rosa M, et al. Indications and contraindications of dental implants in medically compromised patients: update. Med Oral Pathol. 2014. ISSN: http://www.ncbi.nlm.nih.gov/pmc/articles/PMC4192572/. Accessed 18 Mar 2016.

Guerrero M, Jacobs R, et al. State of the art on cone beam CT imaging for preoperative planning of implant placement. Clin Oral Invest. 2006;10:1–7.

Higginbottom FL, Wilson TG. Three-dimensional templates for placement of root-form dental implants: a technical note. Int J Oral Maxillofac Implants. 1996;11(6):787–93.

Holzinger D, et al. Effect of dental implants on bisphosphonate-related osteonecrosis of the jaws. J Oral Maxillofac Surg. 2014;72(10):1937.

Hwang D, Wang HL. Medical contraindications to implant therapy: Part I: absolute contraindications. Implant Dent. 2006;15(4):353–60.

Hwang D, Wang HL. Medical contraindications to implant therapy: Part II: relative contraindications. Implant Dent. 2007;16(1):13–23.

Kim K, Sung H. Outcomes of dental implant treatment in patients with generalized aggressive periodontitis: a systematic review. J Adv Prosthodont. 2012;4(4):210–7.

Lagervall M, Jansson LE. Treatment outcome in patients with peri-implantitis in a periodontal clinic: a retrospective study. J Periodontol. 2013;84(10):1365–73.

Mengel R, Behle M, Flores de Jacoby L. Osseointegrated implants in subjects treated for generalized aggressive periodontitis: 10-year results of a prospective, long-term cohort study. J Periodontol. 2007;78(12):2229–37.

Nguyen-Hieu T, Borghetti A, Aboudharam G. Peri-implantitis: from diagnosis to therapeutics. J Investig Clin Dent. 2012;3(2):79–94.

Parithimarkalaignan S, Padmanabhan TV. Osseointegration: an update. J Indian Prosthodont Soc. 2013;13(1):2–6. doi:10.1007/s13191-013-0252-z

Shelley AM, Glenny AM, Goodwin M, Brunton P, Horner K. Conventional radiography and cross-sectional imaging when planning dental implants in the anterior edentulous mandible to support an overdenture: a systematic review. Dentomaxillofacial Radiology. 2014;43(2):20130321.

Wilson Jr T. The positive relationship between excess cement and peri-implant disease: a prospective clinical endoscopic study. J Periodontol. 2009;80(9):1388–92.

Part III

References for Everyday Practice

The Examination, Differential Diagnosis, and Management of Toothache Pain

19

Christopher J. Spencer

Contents

Abstract

The most common reason given for dental emergencies is a toothache. This pain is usually associated with dental caries which has caused inflammation in the dental pulp and/or progressed into the periradicular region. Pulpal and periradicular diagnoses contribute to more than 90 % of reported toothache pain. Dental emergencies can be treated efficiently, and pain relief can be provided. There exists a significant subset of reported toothache pain which is not associated with caries, pulpal, or periradicular structures. Patients in this subset are reported to have experienced

C.J. Spencer, ODS
LSUHSC School of Dentistry, New Orleans, LA, USA
e-mail: cspen4@lsuhsc.edu

G.M. Weinstein, M.T. Zientz (eds.), *The Dental Reference Manual*,
DOI 10.1007/978-3-319-39730-6_19

little or no relief of their pain as they have received different dental procedures including endodontic and exodontia often without a clear diagnosis. There are three other main groups of diagnoses that need to be considered in addition to the pulpal and periradicular diagnoses: referred pain, neuropathic pain, and nonodontogenic pain. A dilemma may occur when diagnostic criteria are not well understood, the signs and symptoms are not a clear match for any diagnostic criteria, and when health-care practitioners provide treatment without a clear diagnosis.

19.1 Introduction

Reported Toothache Pain Patients often present for a dental emergency with a complaint of a toothache. Most pain in children and adults is associated with caries. If caries is left untreated, the likelihood of pain increases (Lacerda et al. 2004; Boeira et al. 2012; Ekanayake et al. 2001). Majority of the time, pain is correctly diagnosed as pain of pulpal and periradicular origin (Iqbal et al. 2007; Linn et al. 2007). The diagnoses for pulpal conditions such as symptomatic irreversible pulpitis or symptomatic apical periodontitis are well delineated and can be identified through examination, endodontic testing, and radiographic evaluation. However, there are other reasons and diagnoses that can lead patients to reporting a "toothache" even though the source of the pain is not related to the pulp or periradicular tissues.

The Difficulty in Diagnosing Pulpal Pain Even pain of pulpal origin can be difficult to diagnose and localize. If the pulp is the sole source of their pain, patients are able to localize pain to the correct tooth only 30–37.2 % of the time (McCarthy et al. 2010; Friend and Glenwright 1968). Aβ sensory neurons and to a lesser degree Aδ sensory neurons in the pulp provide localization of the pain to the central nervous system. Aβ fibers provide only 1 % of the sensory fibers within the pulp. Aδ fibers are more prevalent, present in the odontoblastic layer, extend into the dentinal tubules, and have the highest density in the pulp horns. Significant pulpal inflammation deactivates both Aβ and Aδ fibers, making it very difficult for a patient to localize the pain. The remaining sensory fibers, C fibers, are resistant to inflammation and continue to provide pain input but with no localization information. C fibers are responsible for deep aching pain and pain referral to other teeth (Bender 2000) and likely remain functional even when much of the pulp tissue is necrotic. Most endodontic testing evaluates only Aδ fibers as compared to the deeper C fibers. So pain can exist without the consistent ability to locate the source. This lack of clarity is often resolved as the inflammation extends into the periradicular tissues which are rich in mechanoreceptors (McCarthy et al. 2010) as symptomatic apical periodontitis develops. Then both the patient and the dentist are able to locate the pain as the tooth becomes sensitive to chewing and percussion testing.

Painful Pulpal and Periradicular Diagnoses There are three pulpal and periapical diagnoses that are responsible for almost all pulpal and periradicular pain.

	Symptomatic irreversible pulpitis	Symptomatic apical periodontitis	Acute apical abscess
Symptoms	Spontaneous pain, or exaggerated pain to cold or heat	Pain associated with biting, percussion or to palpation	Rapid onset of pain Spontaneous pain Severe tenderness to pressure, percussion, and palpation Pus formation, swelling of tissues
Electric pulp tester	Responsive	Responsive to no response	No response
Cold or heat	Exaggerated response	Exaggerated to no response	No response
Microbial presence	Caries or other avenue for microbial access to the pulp	Little or no microbial presence in the apical region	Microbial infection in the apical region
Radiographic findings	Likely caries or previous large restoration near the pulp chamber	Small apical radiolucency, widened periodontal ligament space, or no radiolucency	Usually a periapical radiolucency but this is not necessary for the diagnosis
Pulp status	Inflamed, incapable of healing	Irreversibly inflamed or necrotic	Necrotic
Periapical status	Normal to beginning inflammation	Inflamed	Swelling, pus, inflamed

Fig. 19.1 Diagnostic criteria for the three painful pulpal and periradicular conditions

These diagnoses are readily differentiated with appropriate understanding of the diagnostic criteria and the appropriate history, endodontic testing, and radiographic imaging (Tordik et al. 2010). Symptomatic irreversible pulpitis can provide temporary difficulty with localization as discussed in the previous paragraph but is usually readily discovered with radiographic evidence of the tooth with the large carious lesion or restoration. The diagnostic criteria are provided in Fig. 19.1 (Tordik et al. 2010).

Treatment of Pulpal and Periradicular Conditions Treatment for symptomatic irreversible pulpitis, symptomatic apical periodontitis, and acute apical abscesses usually involves treatment with the removal of the inflamed/necrotic pulp either with an endodontic procedure or extraction and only rarely require antibiotics.

19.2 Other Sources of Perceived Toothache Pain

Three Categories There are three main categories of conditions that can lead to a patient perceiving and reporting pain as coming from the tooth but are not related to caries, pulpitis, or periradicular pathology. First, chronic conditions (musculoskeletal primarily) can create nociceptive (i.e., pain impulses) pain signals that include referred pain to teeth. Second, neuropathic conditions which are nonnociceptive (pain signals are generated by the neural pathways themselves and not as result of tissue injury) can create perceived pain that can "shoot" or "stab" in an area that can include teeth, gingiva, and other oral structures. Third, there are less understood conditions that are associated with a tooth or teeth and are "nonodontogenic" in nature. The pain is perceived and centered in the tooth, but there is no detectable pulpal or periradicular pathology.

Chronic Pain's Contribution Chronic pain conditions are more likely to be associated with multiple concurrent (comorbid) diagnoses and referred pain than acute conditions. Acute conditions in one tooth may refer pain to other teeth in the posterior regions of the dentition. Diagnostic confusion from this type of pain referral is apt to be short lived since acute inflammatory conditions are usually self-limiting, will usually reveal the actual source of the pain in a few days, and will resolve upon treatment (Bender 2000). Chronic pain referral presents a more different dilemma because of the architecture of the central nervous system (CNS). Long-term pain has been shown to create changes in the CNS through an increasing ability for pain transmission to occur (plasticity) and central sensitization (sensitization of the central nervous system) which results in a significantly lowered pain thresholds and a widening of field of reported pain (Woolf 2011; Fernandez-de-las-Peñas et al. 2009). Convergence occurs from a decreasing number of neurons moving from peripheral to central. The cervical and trigeminal systems have been shown to converge into the same region of the brainstem (spinal trigeminal nucleus) creating decreasing thresholds, upregulation of pain, and pain referral (Ge et al. 2004). As an example, a cervical muscle such as the trapezius can influence pain and referral in the anterior temporalis muscle on the face. It is very understandable that this could impact patient perception. The result is that chronic pain conditions can result in consistent pain referred from a distant site to the dentition. One study reported demonstrated an 85 % incidence of pain referral for chronic orofacial pain patient during the examination. Of the same group, 11 % reported pain referred to their teeth (Wright 2000). Pain chronicity and central sensitization have significant implications for the differential diagnosis of a reported toothache.

Management of Chronic Pain Differs from Acute Pain of Tooth Origin The presentation of chronic pain and acute pain differ greatly. Therefore, the management is also very different. Acute pain is primarily monofactorial, associated with inflammation which occurs following injury, usually has a short duration, and resolves with the healing of the insult. Chronic pain is multifactorial (often presents with several diagnoses), usually not associated with inflammation, displays a long duration, and continues often after resolution of the initial injury. Acute pain occurs in the periphery, and pain is transmitted via nociceptors (pain receptors) through the afferent neurons to the brain. Chronic pain is associated with the central sensitization as described in the previous paragraph in the CNS. Treatment for acute pain is associated with supportive therapy to promote healing and, if necessary, nonsteroidal anti-inflammatories for pain relief. Chronic pain requires a management strategy that addresses each of the known contributing factors or risk factors. Each diagnosis must be included. Patient-centered care is key including patient education, self-physical therapy and self-behavioral modification, and support for coping skills. Patients need to be educated about the importance of eight hours of sleep. Interuption of sleep has been shown to negatively impact anti-pain neuro transmitters and mood. Pharmacology utilizes psychotropic medications that help re-regulate and dampen the central sensitization of the trigeminal system such as tricyclic antidepressants (Books 1). Management strategies begin with reversible approaches and escalate only as necessary. A multidisciplinary approach with other providers including clinical psychology, physical medicine (physiatrists and physical therapists), and sometimes otolaryngology or neurology is often necessary (Fricton 2014).

19.3 Myofascial Pain in the Head and Neck

Overview Myofascial pain is a chronic musculoskeletal pain condition that involves the muscles and their attachments including the masticatory or cervical regions for our discussion. Palpation of the muscles reveals painful areas of hyper contracted tissue or "taut bands" which were called "trigger points" by Dr. Janet Travell (Book 2). The quality of the pain is often dull and achy which will vary in intensity often in the moderate to severe range from day to day. The duration is usually hours to days and may be continuous for months or years. The condition is bilateral, but one side often predominates in intensity. Other chronic conditions such as headaches, fibromyalgia, sleep disturbances, depression, otalgia, and bruxism are comorbid (Fricton 2007). *The muscles of mastication likely refer pain to the dentition more than any other structures* (Ehrmann 2002).

Keys to Diagnosis During muscle palpation, the patient will report a painful muscle that duplicates the pain of the chief concern including both the local discomfort and the referral pattern – without prompting from the examiner. This duplication means that the pain descriptors are very similar (familiar) to the chief concern and the pain occurs not only at the muscle site but also at the distant referral site (i.e., the tooth or other structure). Removal of the trigger point or source of pain leading to the referral will also eliminate the pain at the distant site. Diagnostic anesthesia such as 3 % mepivacaine can be utilized to anesthetize the suspected trigger point.

Muscles That Refer to Teeth The superficial masseter, the most commonly implicated muscle, may refer pain to the ipsilateral maxillary or mandibular posterior teeth (Handa et al. 2013). Different aspects of the muscle refer to different distant sites. The superior section refers to the maxillary teeth, and the insertion or more inferior section refers pain more often to the mandibular teeth. The temporalis muscle may refer pain to the ipsilateral maxillary teeth (Wright 2000). The most anterior segment reported will refer to the anterior teeth, the middle section to the premolar teeth, and the more posterior segment to the molars. The anterior digastric muscle may refer pain to the mandibular incisors.

Imaging A panoramic survey would be utilized to rule out any gross pathology, and additional imaging would be appropriate to evaluate dental pathology.

Management This condition is usually a chronic long-term musculoskeletal condition that requires a multidisciplinary approach. The management plan needs to include the following (Fricton 2014; Romero-Reyes and Uyanik 2014):

- Patient-Centered Plan
  - Patient education about the nature of the condition and how pain referral can occur
  - Self-regulation that includes postural exercises, diaphragmatic breathing, self-behavioral modification to decrease diurnal parafunctional habits (such as clenching)
  - Self-physical therapy with stretching, thermal therapy (moist heat and ice)
  - Implement coping strategies
  - Utilize nutritional supplements such as calcium and magnesium
- Dental Orofacial Pain Plan
  - Provide patient education, appropriate referrals, needed pharmacotherapy
  - Provide occlusal guard therapy where appropriate
  - Provide trigger point injections were appropriate as part of an overall management plan
  - Provide follow-up care
- Physical Therapy
  - The therapist can provide manual therapy to stretch shortened muscles in order to mobilize greater range of motion.
  - Help train the patient to strengthen postural muscles to help stabilize core muscle groups that influence posture.
  - Provide pain relief through different modalities such as iontophoresis and tens treatments to the painful muscles.
- Pharmacotherapy
  - Tricyclic antidepressants such as amitriptyline (10–25 mg) below antidepressant dosages to help decrease central sensitization
  - Central acting muscle relaxants or antispasmodics to help with muscle tone and facilitate self-therapy and physical therapy. Baclofen 10 mg three times per day, cyclobenzaprine 10 mg at bedtime (not likely utilized with amitriptyline), or tizanidine 4 mg at bedtime are examples.
- Clinical Psychology
  - Can provide life coaching to help patients develop more effective coping strategies
  - Can teach cognitive behavioral therapy to help patient recognize thinking patterns
  - Can provide imagery, relaxation, and hypnosis strategies for patient

The goal of management is provide a comprehensive plan that includes all of the different problems and multiple diagnoses.

19.3.1 Degenerative Joint Disease (and Arthralgia) of the Temporomandibular Joint

Overview Most pain in the TM joint is of inflammatory origin from the capsule, synovial tissue, or tissues in the retrodiscal region. Osteoarthritis is often associated with orthopedic overload of forces upon the joint which is displayed on images as flattening of the condyle or other osteophytic changes. It may or may not be associated with articular disc displacement in the joint. Sharp severe pain is usually associated with function from chewing, opening wide, or clenching the teeth. The sharp pain is often intermittent but may be accompanied by a dull background pain that lasts for hours (Okeson 2007).

Keys to Diagnosis The patient will usually present a history of pain with function. Examination will reveal palpation soreness or pain directly associated with the TM joint (lateral pole, posterior lateral aspect, and load testing) as opposed to the deep masseter (in close proximity to the joint) or superficial masseter. If there is pain in both the TM joint and the masseter, an auriculotemporal block with 3 % mepivacaine may be utilized. If the pain is removed with the anesthesia, then the likelihood is great that the TM joint is the source of the pain. Auscultation of the TM joints will likely reveal moderate (or coarse) crepitus throughout most of the mandibular movements in all directions.

TM Joint Pain Referral to the Teeth Pain referral to teeth from the TM joint is infrequent. There are case reports of diagnostic confusion with third molar pain (DeAngelis et al. 2009).

Other Complications If the articular surface of a TM joint condyle degenerate rapidly, increased occlusal pressure is generated upon the second molars (or most posterior teeth). This can lead to wear, cracking, or mobility. If the condylar change is sufficiently rapid, an anterior open bite will occur.

Imaging If significant degenerative joint disease is suspected from the examination, a CBCT (cone beam computed tomography) scan would be indicated. It would require the ability to view sagittally corrected images of the TM joint condyles. The images would reveal the articular surface of the condyles and articular eminence, the intra-articular spacing between the condyle and eminence, and the position of the condyle in the glenoid fossa.

Management The management of TM joint pain relates to the pain associated with the localized inflammation within the joint itself and the decrease in range of motion. If the condition is chronic, the same principles of management apply with patient education, management of overload with occlusal splint therapy when needed, physical therapy if the range of motion is decreased, and anti-inflammatory medications (either steroid or nonsteroidal) (Okeson 2007). The most documented approach for pain management is the utilization of nonsteroidal anti-inflammatory medications such as ibuprofen, naproxen, or meloxicam (Okeson 2007; Argoff 2011). These medications all have the same pharmacotherapeutic effect with the inhibition of prostaglandin synthesis. The inter-medication differences are associated with drug potency and duration of efficacy (½ life of drug metabolism). Newer research has also differentiated different potencies in different tissues and fluids. Meloxicam is selectively absorbed in higher concentrations in synovial fluid than other NSAIDS and even greater in inflamed joints with fewer gastrointestinal side effects. Ibuprofen would usually require four dosages per day, naproxen two dosages but displays greater gastrointestinal irritation.

19.3.2 Rhinosinusitis

Overview This can be an acute or chronic condition that affects the maxillary and other sinuses. An acute rhinosinusitis is usually associated with a recent viral upper respiratory infection with a short duration of up to 4 weeks which "worsens" after an initial improvement. The patient reports a purulent nasal discharge, nasal obstruction, a feeling of fullness, and at times facial pain. Most acute episodes are viral and rarely bacterial (only .5 to 2.0 %). A chronic sinusitis is associated with nasal congestions of more than 12 weeks or four annual episodes. The chronic condition is more apt to be associated with bacterial infection but is not usually associated with pain. The chronic condition occurs with stasis or lack of clearing of the mucus in the ostiomeatal complex. Historically, sinusitis has been over diagnosed and treated with antibiotics with little efficacy (Ferguson 2014).

Keys to Diagnosis Acute rhinosinusitis must be associated with purulent discharge and with one of the following: with either nasal obstruction or facial pain or both (Ferguson 2014). If facial pain occurs but no purulent discharge is present, the condition does not match the criteria for acute rhinosinusitis. A recent or recurrent upper respiratory infection is also very likely. Unilateral pain upon palpation of the lateral wall of the maxillary sinus is often present.

Maxillary Sinus Pain Referrals to Teeth The maxillary sinus primarily refers pain to the ipsilateral maxillary 2nd premolar and the 1st maxillary molar. The maxillary 1st premolar or maxillary 2nd molars can be implicated too (Ferguson 2014).

Imaging A CBCT scan with air-fluid level opacity in the maxillary sinus would confirm the diagnosis.

Management Most rhinosinusitis is associated with a viral origin and will run its course without intervention. The patient can irrigate the ostiomeatal complex with saline solutions through sprays or nasal irrigation devices. Antibiotic therapy has historically been overutilized and should be avoided unless the condition has recurred and the purulent discharge continues. The main dental concern is to avoid unnecessary dental procedures and a likely referral to otolaryngology (Rosenfeld et al. 2015) (Fig. 19.2).

19.3.3 Sialadenitis of the Submandibular Gland

Overview Sialadenitis of the major salivary glands is associated most often with blockage by a sialolith or calcification of the major salivary duct, which occurs most commonly in the Wharton's duct of the submandibular gland. The blockage leads to salivary retention in the gland associated usually with swelling and pain. As the flow diminishes, bacteria may move into the duct toward the gland with possibility of a sialadenitis developing in the gland itself. The condition can become chronic with a decrease in pain over time (Mandel 2011).

Keys to Diagnosis The pain history will usually report pain either initiated or exacerbated with meal times. A submandibular sialadenitis will likely be reported as a deep pain near the angle of the mandible which a patient may have difficulty in localization. The salivary flow would be decreased from the affected gland. Bidigital palpation will reveal a painful submandibular gland (or occasionally a parotid gland) and possibly a sialolith in Wharton's duct if the calcification is of sufficient size.

Submandibular Gland Pain Referral to Teeth The submandibular gland may refer pain to the ipsilateral body of the mandible and the mandibular molars.

Imaging An ultrasound can now be utilized to visualize the gland and patency of the duct. CBCT or even an "old style" occlusal image would also likely image the blockage (Oliveira et al. 2014).

Management The sialolith needs to be surgically removed. Most can't be easily removed unless they are at the opening of the duct. Sialendoscopic procedures are able to view and also remove small calcifications through the duct without the removal of the submandibular gland itself (unless it has become atrophic and is the main source of the pain). This results in fewer adverse effects and a better restoration of salivary flow (Masunobu et al. 2014).

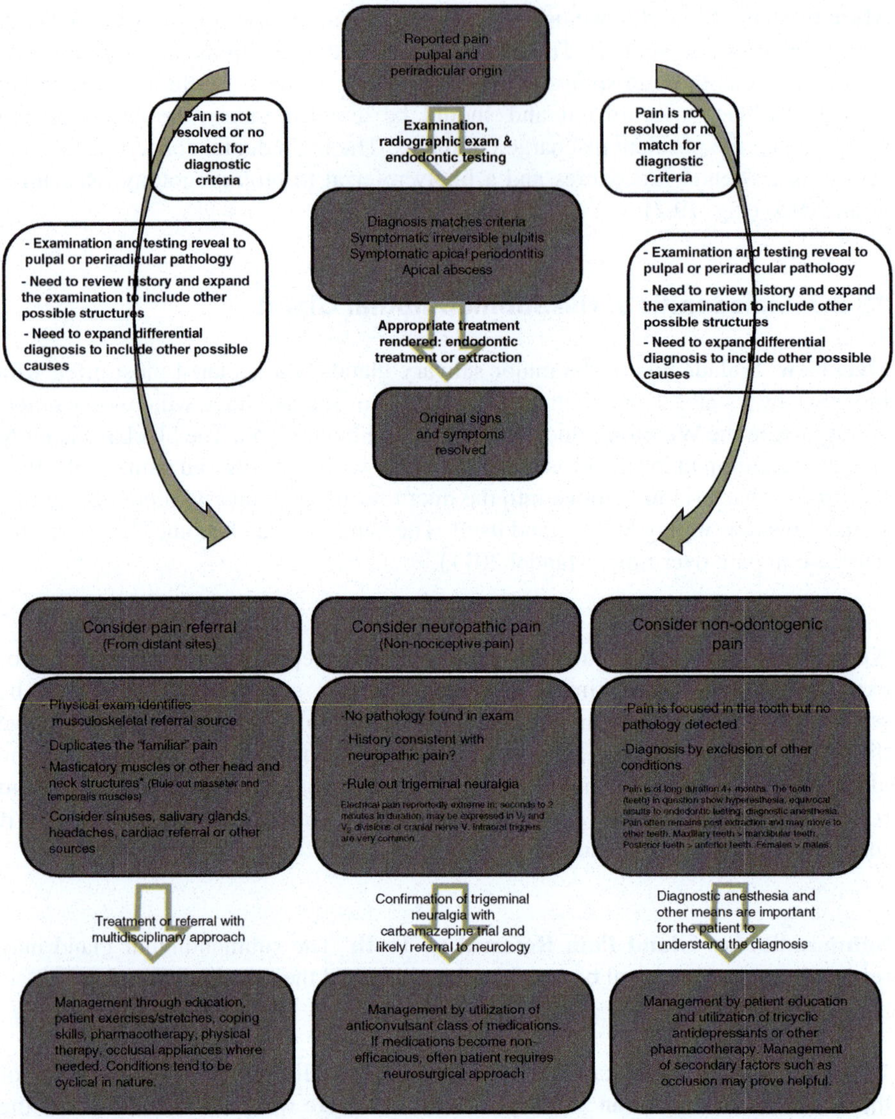

Fig. 19.2 Diagnostic flow chart for reported toothache pain. Most toothache pain follows the center pathway, but when the diagnosis doesn't fit, other conditions need to be considered

19.3.4 Ischemic Heart Disease

Overview Coronary atherosclerosis can cause a narrowing of the coronary arteries that provide blood supply to the cardiac muscle. Atherosclerotic plaques may become disrupted which initiates a reparative function with the formation of a blood clot. This further narrowed the lumen of the artery is more susceptible to an embolus that can blot it entirely. The embolus could be dislodged plaque or a thrombus (part of a blood clot that separates) that lodges in a sufficiently narrow area. The result is lack of blood supply and insufficient oxygen. This causes tissue damage and cell death if the blockage continues. The result is pain – angina pectoris – from an acute myocardial infarction. This pain is usually without a cause and will usually last longer than 15 min to hours (as opposed to angina from exertion which is increased demand with no blockage). The pain is often described as a weight or pressure. Other descriptors are burning, aching, and throbbing (Kreiner et al. 2007). The patient may report difficulty in breathing. The chest and the retrosternal regions are most frequently affected, but the pain often radiates to the throat, neck, and jaws. Significantly though, the pain can be referred to the craniofacial region both right and left including the TM joint, preauricular region, ear, and teeth. In approximately 6 % of the population, craniofacial pain may be the only symptom (Lopez-Lopez et al. 2012)

Keys to Diagnosis The pain of an acute myocardial infarction is usually accompanied by the signs and symptoms above. It is almost always bilateral as compared to pain of odontogenic origin, which is unilateral. Cardiac referral pain will almost always include a region (ear, joint, mandible, neck) – and not just a single tooth. Odontogenic pain while it may radiate to other teeth does not radiate to the chest or arms. The pain descriptors for cardiac pain are: primarily pressure and burning vs. aching and throbbing for teeth. Painful teeth pain will almost always display pathology (Kreiner et al. 2007).

Cardiac Referral to Teeth Mandibular molar teeth are usually implicated. But almost always the referral pattern will involve a region and not one specific tooth.

Imaging Adequate dental radiographs to rule out dental etiology

Management If no dental pathology is found and the signs and symptoms potentially relate to cardiac origin, the patient needs to be referred to the emergency room.

19.3.5 Neuropathic Pain

Neuropathic pain and dysfunction can arise from two types of pathological changes: demyelination and deafferentation. Multiple sclerosis is the most common condition associated with demyelination. An autoimmune response causes an inflammation and damage to the myelin sheath to nerves in the central nervous system which results in a number of signs and symptoms: numbness, loss of muscle coordination and control, weakness, blurred vision, dizziness, pain, and fatigue to mention just a few. The deterioration of neurons through the loss of the myelin sheath changes the ability to transmit information and the ability to control peripheral functions (Files et al. 2015). Guillain-Barre syndrome shows rapid demyelination which can lead muscle weakness, paralysis, and even death if motor nerves to the diaphragm muscle are severely damaged (Willison et al. 2016). Trigeminal neuralgia is the demyelinating disease (suspected) that significantly affects the masticatory system. The pain associated with these types of conditions does not arise from the normal transduction of peripheral stimulation or tissue damage that is converted to signals carried by afferent neurons to the brain and are interpreted as pain. Rather as neurons are damaged, they can generate wrong signals or aberrant information which can be interpreted as pain in a particular location even though no damage has occurred. This is "nonnociceptive" pain.

19.3.5.1 Trigeminal Neuralgia

Overview Trigeminal neuralgia is perhaps the most painful condition known to humans. It is generated in the trigeminal nerve (V cranial nerve – sensory branches) likely just as it exits the pons and before it forms the trigeminal ganglion to travel in it three divisions (ophthalmic V_1, maxillary V_2, and mandibular V_3). The exact pathology has never been proven but is thought to be a demyelination injury caused by the superior cerebellar artery (or other vascular structures) as it beats in conjunction with the blood pulsing through in close proximity to the nerve trunk (Docampo et al. 2015). The result is severe electrical stabbing pain of a duration from a few seconds to 2 min which occurs unilaterally in the maxillary or mandibular divisions (or both) of the trigeminal nerve distributions. The pain is often stimulated by a "trigger" of light touch to either extra or intraoral tissue. Following an attack, a latent pain-free period occurs in which the patient can't trigger and attack. In the clinical examination, no pathology will be found (De Siqueira et al. 2004).

Keys to Diagnosis The diagnosis is initially determined through the patient's history since there are no clinical or dental radiographic findings. If the patient matches the pain descriptors, location, duration, latency period, and no other pathology is found, the patient likely has the diagnosis of trigeminal neuralgia. Carbamazepine, 100 mg, twice a day can be utilized for a confirmation of the diagnosis by history. Literature reports at least a 70–98 % efficacy for carbamazepine within the first few doses. It is likely closer to 90 % (Sato et al. 2004). If the pain can be triggered during the examination, this will also confirm the diagnosis.

Trigeminal Pain Associated with Reported Tooth Pain Trigeminal neuralgia occurs primarily in the V_2 and V_3 divisions of the trigeminal nerve. These regions include both the maxillary and mandibular teeth. Intraoral trigger zones such as the lips, jaw, teeth, and mucosa make the presentation confusing to the patient and doctor. Patients will describe the stabbing or shooting pain that travels pointing to the structures involved. Although reported tooth pain may be involved, it is very unlikely that tooth pain would be the sole expression (De Siqueira et al. 2004).

Imaging Sufficient dental radiographs to rule out dental etiology.

Management Once the diagnosis is made, a referral to neurology is made so that anticonvulsant medications can be titrated to the correct dosage. A referral to neural surgery for an intracranial procedure may be indicated at some point since medications often lose their efficacy. The procedure with the best long-term pain relief is the microvascular decompression which entails a separation of the local vascular structures off of the trigeminal nerve. Patients and doctors are not often familiar with trigeminal neuralgia and may treat suspected teeth only to find no benefit. The real problem with trigeminal neuralgia is that it misdiagnosed or not diagnosed for extended periods of time. Many individuals receive misdirected dental and other treatment as a result. Individuals most often see a dentist first in their pursuit of treatment for their pain complaint. One study reports that this happens 82 % of the time (Von Eckardstein et al. 2014). The onset of the first incidence of this pain occurs following treatment or in conjunction with dental conditions (De Siqueira et al. 2004). This diagnostic confusion (for doctors and patients) occurs often because of signs and symptoms that overlap with other conditions. Trigeminal neuralgia is not a common condition, and many dentists are unfamiliar with its presentation. Often the initial presentation of trigeminal neuralgia is vague and does not coincide with trigeminal neuralgia criteria. There are no diagnostic tests, no imaging, or peripheral pathology that can be elucidated during the clinic exam.

19.4 Nonodontogenic Sources of Pain

The concept of nontooth toothache (nonodontogenic pain in a tooth) sounds like an oxymoron. The pain is centered in a tooth or several teeth as reported by the patient. The examination is performed, and there is no adequate pathology found to explain the pain. The pain or discomfort is very real to the patient and they often report a history of dental treatment provided to the teeth in question with no relief of the pain. In fact the pain may actually increase. There are two conditions that are quite similar that need to be considered.

19.4.1 Nonodontogenic Toothache or Persistent Dentoalveolar Pain (Previously Atypical Odontalgia)

Overview The epidemiology displays predominately females with age of greater than 40 years. This is a condition with a history of pain in a tooth for 4–6 months with an unknown etiology (Yatani et al. 2014). The quality of the pain can vary from throbbing, burning to sharp and shooting and is usually of moderate intensity. Patients have trouble localizing the pain (normal for chronic pain). Examination results for endodontic testing are ambiguous with results changing from day to day. Percussion testing, cold testing, and heat testing do not relate consistently with the pain. But the toothache remains constant. Local anesthesia for diagnostic purposes may or may not relieve the pain – or may on one occasion only to fail the next. The pain may move to other teeth – especially following extractions or endodontic treatment – but remains relatively constant in quality and intensity.

Keys to Diagnosis To diagnose this condition requires understanding the patient's history and a rigorous examination with a strong reluctance (or refusal) to treat the patient without a clear diagnosis. This condition remains unchanged with no evidence of pathology and does not respond to dental treatment but remains after extractions or other interventions. The diagnosis is often made following ineffective dental treatment but may be made earlier by astute doctors. Diagnostic anesthesia may be beneficial in not only helping to diagnose potential sources of the pain but also may provide help in communication with the patient. If diagnostic anesthesia provided does not eliminate the perceived pain, it may help the patient and doctor to consider that the believed source of the pain, "the tooth," is not the actual cause of the pain.

Teeth Affected Maxillary teeth as affected more often as compared to mandibular and posterior teeth as compared to anterior. Still any tooth could be involved in this diagnosis (Oshima et al. 2009).

Imaging Sufficient dental radiographs to rule out dental etiology

Management Since the etiology is unknown, treatment modalities have been directed at symptoms and the central sensitization that is a part of this chronic condition. The previously discussed management for chronic conditions in sections 19.2 and 19.4 applies to this condition as wellwith patient education and involvement being the most important. Amitriptyline (10–25 mg) or other tricyclic antidepressants have a reported efficacy of 60–75 % from case reports (Yatani et al. 2014). If there are parafunctional habits present, they may help lower the overall discomfort with management with an occlusal splint.

19.4.2 Phantom Tooth Pain

Overview This condition is similar to nonodontogenic toothache and may be included by some authors in the same category. The difference is that this is a pain that follows invasive treatment such as a pulpectomy (endodontic procedure) or extraction. The etiology is associated with a deafferentation injury or a severing of a neural structure (an axon) no matter how small in diameter. This is no small matter since hundreds (or more) of axons enter a single tooth in the periapical region (Abd-Elmeguid and Yu 2009). The result is a phantom pain similar to a phantom limb pain postamputation. The neural injury may induce both peripheral changes and central nervous system responses in the attempt to heal the injury. Peripherally, a neuroma may form as the axon grows in attempt to reconnect with its missing section. This can produce a stump with many projections and receptors that are very sensitive. It also often produces inflammatory changes in the tissues nearby. The central changes can produce a sensation of the missing structure still present with pain or a dysesthesia (weird sensation such as itching, ants crawling). The incidence of prolonged pain following endodontic treatment is thought to be in the 2–6 % range and coincides with the likely incidence of phantom tooth pain (Battrum and Gutmann 1996; Nixdorf et al. 2010).

Keys to Diagnosis This condition follows a dental procedure and will occur postoperatively. The challenge is to be aware of the possibility of a "phantom" pain and to include it in the differential diagnosis of post operative pain following endodontic or extraction procedures especially. It can be difficult to assess the apical region of a very complex tooth to determine whether an adequate seal has been established or whether further pathology is present. Sometimes a progression of procedures can occur on the same tooth either with no pain resolution or perhaps an exacerbation of pain. Multiple procedures associated with the same tooth or area rarely provide the desired relief from pain (Allerbring and Haegerstam 2004). Improved cone beam CT scans provide diagnostic imaging to assess both preoperative and postoperative apical regions of teeth (Venskutonis et al. 2014). Small periapical defects or radiolucencies can now be viewed that would not be visible to a periapical radiograph since they would be superimposed over tooth structure (buccal or lingual to the apex of a tooth) or hidden by more radiopaque structures such as the buccal plate of the alveolus of the mandible. Phantom tooth pain is a diagnosis by exclusion. If no pathology can be found, a reevaluation needs to be provided before retreatment or apical surgical procedures are initiated. The pain may be the result of a deafferentation nerve injury.

Teeth Involved All teeth are susceptible, but condition occurs primarily in posterior teeth (Oshima et al. 2009).

Imaging High-resolution CBCT scan or a triangulation of 3 periapical radiographs (distal, mesial, and straight angulation) to diagnose postoperative healing sites.

Management The management for phantom tooth pain is very similar to management of many chronic pain conditions. It involves patient education first. Most of the time, a deafferentation injury can't be imaged or clinically discovered (with the rare exception of a palpable neuroma that could be surgically removed). Since the likelihood of a resolution of the deafferentation injury is unlikely, pain control through neuropathic medications such as gabapentin, pregabalin, or amitriptyline may decrease the severity and symptoms of the pain to more manageable levels (Clark 2006). Medication can be applied to the mucosa associated with the specific locale of the pain through transdermal or transmucosal medications compounded by pharmacies that specialize in customizing medications for specific symptoms. These transmucosal medications are fabricated with a vehicle that carries the active medication to the site. Medications such as ketoprofen, lidocaine, amitriptyline, and gabapentin can be applied to the area with few if any systemic adverse effects. Nutritional supplements such as B complex, calcium, and magnesium can also be helpful. In the end, it is the patient who has to face this pain and suffering long term. Therefore a clinical psychology consultation may help the patient to develop more effective coping strategies.

19.5 Other Considerations

The list in this chapter is not exhaustive in conditions that influence the trigeminal sensory system and affect perceived pain in the dentition. Certain headaches including migraine (neurogenic inflammation in nerves adjacent to blood vessels in the meninges) can either refer pain to dental structures or actually occur in blood vessels outside of skull creating "mini" migraines and pain in other structures (Alonso and Nixdorf 2006). Other headaches (trigeminal autonomic cephalgias such as cluster headaches) produce neuralgiform pain similar to trigeminal neuralgia which can include teeth and alveolar structures. Brain tumors that occur in the region of the trigeminal nerves in the middle cranial fossa can refer pain to dental structures. The complexity of orofacial pain requires of the following: a complete history, the development of an understanding of the patient's chief concern, a thorough examination process including appropriate imaging, formulation of credible diagnoses, and treatment of the reported pain only when a diagnosis has been established. When a condition is not clear, ask for help.

References

Abd-Elmeguid A, Yu DC. Dental pulp neurophysiology: part 1. Clinical and diagnostic implications. J Can Dent Assoc. 2009;75(1):55–9.

Allerbring M, Haegerstam G. Chronic idiopathic orofacial pain. A long-term follow-up study. Acta Odontol Scand. 2004;62(2):66–9.

Alonso AA, Nixdorf DR. Case series of four different headache types presenting as tooth pain. J Endod. 2006;32(11):1110–3.

Argoff CE. Recent developments in the treatment of osteoarthritis with NSAIDS. Curr Med Res Opin. 2011;27(7):1315–27.

Battrum DE, Gutmann JL. Phantom tooth pain: a diagnosis of exclusion. Int Endod J. 1996;29:190–4.

Bender IB. Pulpal pain diagnosis – a review. J Endod. 2000;26(3):175–9.

Boeira GF, Correa MB, Peres KG, Peres MA, Santos IS, Matijasevich A, Barros AJ, Dmarco FF. Caries is the main cause for dental pain in childhood: finding from birth cohort. Caries Res. 2012;46(5):488–95.

Clark GT. Persistent orodental pain, atypical odontalgia, and phantom tooth pain: when are they neuropathic disorders? CDA J. 2006;34(8):599–609.

De Siqueira SR, Nóbrega JC, Valle LB, et al. Idiopathic trigeminal neuralgia: clinical aspects and dental procedures. Oral Surg Oral Med Oral Pathol Oral Radiol Endod. 2004;98:311–5.

DeAngelis AF, Chambers IG, Hall GM. Temporomandibular joint disorders in patients referred for third molar extraction. Aust Dent J. 2009;54:323–5.

Docampo J, Gonzalez N, Muňoz A, et al. Neurovascular study of the trigeminal nerve at 3 T MRI. Neuroradiol J. 2015;28(1):28–35.

Ehrmann EH. The diagnosis of referred orofacial dental pain. Aust Endod J. 2002;28(2):75–81.

Ekanayake L, Weerasekare C, Ekanayake N. Needs and demands for dental care in patients attending University Dental Hospital in Sri Lanka. Int Dent J. 2001;51(2):67–72.

Ferguson J. Rhinosinusitis in oral medicine and dentistry. Aust Dent J. 2014;59:289–95.

Fernandez-de-las-Peñas C, et al. Bilateral widespread mechanical sensitivity in women with myofascial temporomandibular disorder: evidence of impairment in central nociceptive processing. J Pain. 2009;10(11):1170–8.

Files DK, Jausurawong T, Katrajian R, Danoff R. Multiple sclerosis. Prim Care Clin Office Pract. 2015;42:159–75.

Fricton J. Myogenous temporomandibular disorders: diagnostic and management considerations. Dent Clin N Am. 2007;51:61–83.

Fricton J. Temporomandibular disorders: a human systems approach. CDA J. 2014; 42(8):523–32.

Friend LA, Glenwright HD. An experimental investigation into the localization of pain from the dental pulp. Oral Surg Oral Med Oral Pathol. 1968;25(5):765–74.

Ge HY, Wang K, Madeline P, Svensson P, Sessle BJ, Arendt-Nielsen L. Simultaneous modulation of exteroceptive suppression periods in the trapezius and temporalis muscles by experimental muscle pain. Clin Neurophysiol. 2004;115:1399–408.

Handa T, Fukuda K, Ichinohe T. Effect of combination of trigger point injection and stellate ganglion block on non-odontogenic mandibular molar pain referred from masseter muscle: a case report. Bull Tokyo Dent Coll. 2013;54(3):171–5.

Iqbal M, Kim S, Yoon F. An investigation into differential diagnosis of pulp and periapical pain: a PennEndo database study. J Endod. 2007;33(5):548–51.

Kreiner M, Okeson JP, Michelis V, et al. Craniofacial pain as the sole symptom of cardiac ischemia: a prospective multicenter study. J Am Dent Assoc. 2007;138(1):74–9.

Lacerda JT, Simioinato EM, Peres KG, Traebert J, Marcenes W. Dental pain as the reason for visiting a dentist in a Brazilian adult population. Rev Saude Publica. 2004;38(3):453–8.

Linn J, Trantor I, Teo N, Thanigaivel R, Goss AN. The differential diagnosis of toothache from other orofacial pains in clinical practice. Aust Dent J. 2007;52(1 suppl):S100–4.

Lopez-Lopez J, Adserias-Garriga MJ, Garcia-Vicente L, et al. Orofacial pain of cardiac origin, serial of clinical cases. Med Oral Patol Oral Cir Bucal. 2012;17(4):e633–7.

Mandel L. Salivary gland disorders. Dent Clin N Am. 2011;55(1):121–40.

Masunobu T, Kurioka T, Miyagawa Y, et al. Minimally invasive surgery of sialolithiasis using sialendoscopy. Auris Nasus Larynx. 2014;41(6):528–31.

McCarthy JP, McClanahan S, Hodges J, Bowles WR. Frequency of localization of the painful tooth by patients presenting for an endodontic emergency. J Endod. 2010;36(5):801–5.

Nixdorf DR, Moana-Filho EJ, Law AS, et al. Frequency of persistent tooth pain after root canal therapy: a systematic review and meta-analysis. J Endod. 2010;36(2):224–30.

Okeson J. Joint intracapsular disorders: diagnostic and nonsurgical management considerations. Dent Clin N Am. 2007;51:85–103.

Oliveira LG, Hurst ND, Magajna PW. Bedside emergency ultrasound in a case of acute parotid duct sialolithiasis. J Emerg Med. 2014;47(2):e49–51.

Oshima K, Ishii T, Ogura Y, et al. Clinical investigation of patients who develop neuropathic tooth pain after endodontic procedures. J Endod. 2009;35(7):958–61.

Romero-Reyes M, Uyanik JM. Orofacial pain management: current perspectives. J Pain Res. 2014;7:99–115.

Rosenfeld RM, Piccirillo JF, Chandrasekhar SS, et al. Clinical practice guideline (update): adult sinusitis. Otolaryngol Head Neck Surg. 2015;152(2S):S1–39.

Sato J, Saitoh T, Notani KI, et al. Diagnostic significance of carbamazepine and trigger zones in trigeminal neuralgia. Oral Surg Oral Med Oral Pathol Oral Radiol Endod. 2004;97:18–22.

Tordik PA, Webb TD, Weber CD. Pulpal and apical diagnosis. Clin Update Navl Postgrad Dental School. 2010;32(2):1–2.

Venskutonis T, Daugela P, Strazdas M, Juodzbalys G. Accuracy of digital radiography and cone beam computed tomography on periapical radiolucency detection in endodontically treated teeth. J Oral Maxillofac Res. 2014;5(2):1–7.

Von Eckardstein KL, Keil M, Rohde V. Unnecessary dental procedures as a consequence of trigeminal neuralgia. Neurosurg Rev. 2014. doi:10.1007/s10143-014-0591-1.

Willison HJ, Jacobs BC, van Doorn PA. Guillain-Barré syndrome. 2016. The Lancet Published online Feb 29, doi:10.1016/S0140-6736(16)00339-1.

Woolf CJ. Central sensitization: implications for the diagnosis and treatment of pain. Pain. 2011;152(3 Suppl):S2–15.

Wright EF. Referred craniofacial pain patterns in patients with temporomandibular disorder. J Am Dent Assoc. 2000;131(9):1307–15.

Yatani H, Komiayama O, Matsuka Y, et al. Systematic review and recommendations for nonodontogenic toothache. J Oral Rehabil. 2014;41:843–52.

Books and Chapters

Sharav Y, Benoliel L. The diagnostic process. In: Orofacial pain & headache. New York: Mosby Elsevier; 2008. p. 1–17.

Simons DG, Travell JG, Simons LS. Chapter 2. General overview. In: Travell and Simons' myofascial pain and dysfunction. The trigger point manual volume 1. Upper half of body. 2nd ed. New York: Lippincot Williams & Wilkins; 1999. p. 11–93.

Communicating with Dental Laboratories

20

Tamra Culp and Lee Culp

Contents

Abstract

Many times dentists receive restorations from the laboratory only to find that they did not meet the expectations of the dentist or patient. Unfortunately, these problems and many others are seen all too often, due to poor communication between the dentist and dental laboratory. This chapter will provide the information the dentist needs to communicate to the laboratory technicians in order to fabricate high-quality, consistent dental restorations. These protocols were developed through years of hands-on experience plus many interviews with dentists and technicians. Dentists and dental technicians share a unique relationship in that we are totally dependent on each other for success. Though we are trained and practice apart from each other, this chapter will illustrate how common tools can be used to facilitate this relationship.

T. Culp, DMD
Private Practice, Florida, CA, USA

L. Culp, CDT (✉)
CEO Sculpture Studios, Chapel Hill, NC, USA
e-mail: tculp@gmai.com

G.M. Weinstein, M.T. Zientz (eds.), *The Dental Reference Manual*,
DOI 10.1007/978-3-319-39730-6_20

20.1 The Architect-Builder Relationship

To begin, we need to define the roles and responsibilities of each half of the dentist-technician team. This relationship is similar to that of an architect and builder, where the dentist is the architect and the technician is the builder. The responsibility of the architect is to visit the building site and get a feel for the "lay of the land" or, in our case, the oral cavity. Based on this investigation, the architect creates a preliminary blueprint or treatment plan. On completion of the plan, the architect and builder meet to study the blueprint and discuss construction methods and building materials. After both sides have agreed on all phases of the construction process, a final blueprint is created, and construction is completed following the sequencing, construction methods, and fabrication materials that were decided upon by the restorative team.

For this type of relationship to work, there must be equality and mutual respect from both sides of the team. The relationship between the dentist and technician is a partnership, and great partnerships are built on a foundation of shared responsibility and an understanding of each other's abilities, strengths, and limitations. Each member of the dental restorative team can learn a tremendous amount by looking over the other's shoulders, asking questions, observing challenges, and offering solutions. By seeing through the other's eyes, both can grow through a better understanding of the total restorative process.

20.2 The Restorative Process

Initially, one must complete a thorough evaluation of the temporomandibular joint for any sign of instability, tenderness, or other discomfort. If any of these signs are noted, then diagnose and treat before continuing with a diagnostic and treatment plan. Before starting final diagnosis and treatment plan, take into account any periodontal, occlusal, orthodontic, and surgical factors that may affect the final restorative outcome. Below is a guide for prosthodontic cases to insure proper records and communication with the laboratory:

20.2.1 Step 1: Diagnostic Wax-Up

The goal of a diagnostic wax-up is to preview the approach to the final restorative outcome. This is done by the addition of wax and/or by removing from the tooth structure (stone model). Reductions to the stone model are marked in red, and wax additions are often a different color than the base stone, so all changes can be easily seen (Fig. 20.1).

20.2.2 Step 2: Preparation and Impressions

Finally, make sure you understand correct preparation design as it relates to the type of restoration you want. With the choice of materials for restorations multiplying

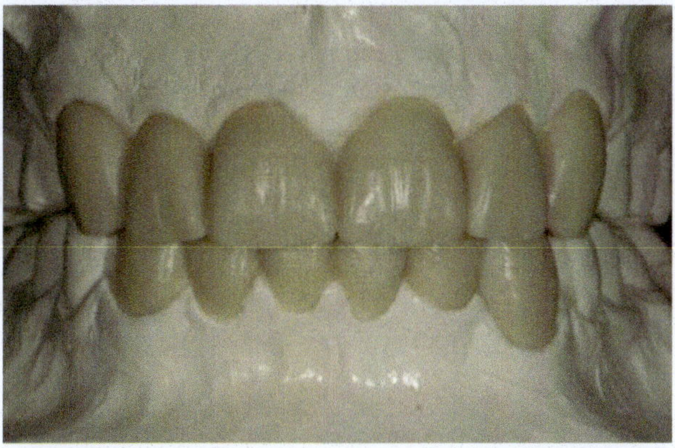

Fig. 20.1 Completed diagnostic wax-up, for maxillary and mandibular anterior restorations

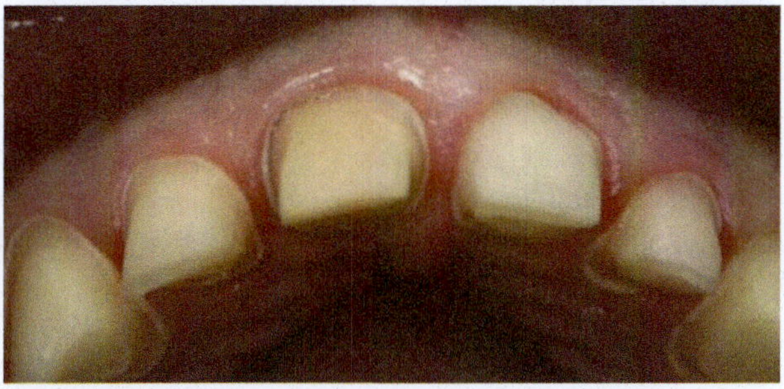

Fig. 20.2 Proper preparations for maxillary anterior all-ceramic restorations

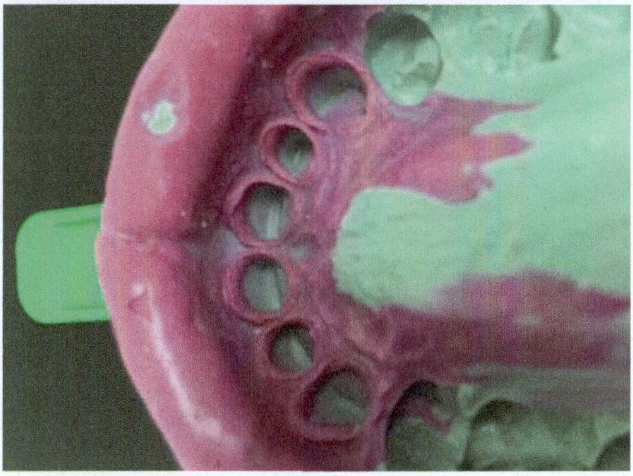

Fig. 20.3 Impression of maxillary anterior preparations, showing definite margins 360° around margin

every day, it is critical to prepare the tooth (teeth) correctly in order to allow the technician to fabricate the best possible restoration (Fig. 20.2).

Of equal importance is the accuracy of the impression. After the impression is removed, check the marginal integrity (Fig. 20.3). If you cannot see the margin 360° around the tooth, retake the impression. Never ask the laboratory to guess at a margin. Doing so leads to hard feelings and a lot of wasted time and money. The opposing model or any other models you decide to send should be of the same excellent quality as the working impression and casts. The alginate impression should be taken with the same care as the master, with the impression capturing all teeth and tissues with no pulls, tears, or voids. Opposing models should be poured in the dental office to avoid shrinkage of the alginate impression. The person responsible for pouring the alginate impression must be trained to mix high-quality die stone in a vacuum mixer to ensure a dense, bubble-free cast. "Buff" stone should not be used as it is a low-quality stone designed for denture processing. It is not designed for complex restorative dentistry.

20.2.3 Step 3: Occlusal Records

With the models completed, they must be articulated correctly. This calls for accurate occlusal records, commonly known as the bite. Choose an accurate material that won't distort. Most waxes are inappropriate because they are influenced by temperature and bend and break easily. The bite is the only reference the technician has to attain the proper maxillary-mandibular relationship, so it's important to take the time and care to ensure accuracy (Fig. 20.4).

A "facebow" is not required in all cases. However, it is advisable to use the articulator system's facebow in cases involving changes to the function and aesthetics of the anterior segment or complex posterior reconstruction.

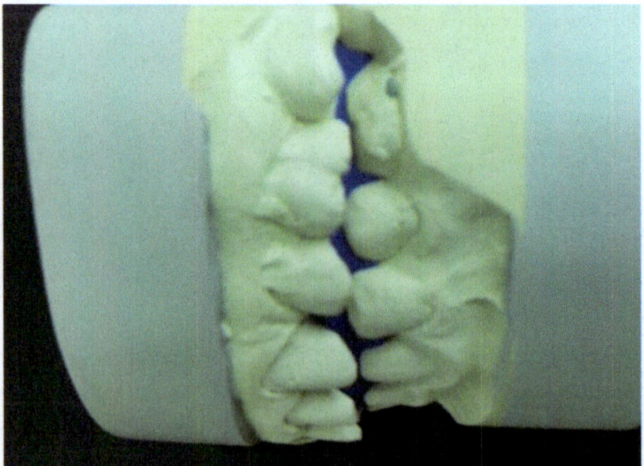

Fig. 20.4 Properly referenced maxillary and mandibular models, with trimmed interocclusal record

20.2.4 Step 4: Creating the Blueprint

What constitutes a blueprint in restorative dentistry? Several items, which can be classified as either two- or three-dimensional communications:

1. Two-dimensional communication tools include a properly filled out laboratory prescription, photos, color mapping form, or drawing for tooth shade.

   To properly communicate aesthetics, especially in the case of matching existing dentition, photos are an invaluable tool in relating shape, color, internal effects, translucency, texture, and luster (Fig. 20.5). A digital camera and some training on how to use it are a great investment. Images are not only a good communication tool; they document pre- and postoperative treatment results for patient education and marketing. If done correctly, photos become a three-dimensional communication tool. Along with visual communication should be a properly filled out laboratory prescription form. Take the time to thoroughly document the results you want so there is no question on the technician's part as to what you and your patient expect. Include all information relating to aesthetics, function, color, and patient expectations.
2. There are two ways to utilize a three-dimensional communication tool:
   A. When restoring anterior teeth, use the *approved provisional model* (Donovan and Cho 1999) (Table 20.1). To create predictable anterior restorations, two models are needed: the "approved provisional" model and the preoperative model. The approved provisional model is the blueprint from which the anterior case will be created. It dictates proper tooth length, incisal edge position, lip support, and anterior function. This model of the provisional restorations (temporaries) is vitally important for the proper creation of anterior restorations. This can be accomplished by:
   1. Completing a diagnostic wax-up and fabricating silicon putty mold of the teeth to be restored. When the final preparations are completed and the final impression is taken, the putty mold is placed in the mouth, checked for fit and trimmed if necessary. The mold is then removed and filled with your

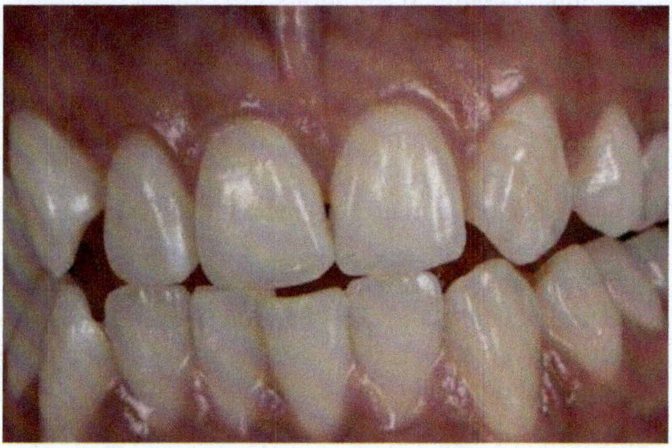

Fig. 20.5 Intraoral digital image, showing shade, color nuance, translucency, and surface texture

Table 20.1 Approved provisional model for anterior restorations

Steps	Purpose
1. Diagnostic wax-up of what your final restorations should look like	Ability to visualize where your final restorations can be and the limitations
2. Make a silicone putty matrix or clear vacuform stent of the wax-up	This is your carrier and mold for provisional material once the tooth preparations are completed
3. Fabricate your provisional restoration using the matrix above	Protects the prepared teeth and holds the occlusion until the final restorations are placed
4. Correct occlusion and all excursive movements with the provisionals cemented in place	Allows the patient proper function
5. Check for aesthetics and speech and polish. Recontour as needed and acquire patient approval for function and aesthetics	Critical step to prevent adjustments when the final restoration is returned from the laboratory
6. Take an alginate impression of the "Approved Provisionals" to send to the laboratory	This gives the laboratory a "blueprint" which can be used to make the final restorations

temporary material of choice. After the material has set, remove the mold and the temporaries. Trim, polish, and reinsert the temporaries. Check your margins, contacts, and occlusion and adjust accordingly.

2. Now comes the important part; after cementation of the temporaries, take the time to adjust them to perfection. First, check to make sure occlusion and function are correct. Insure that there is cuspid guidance and tracking of the maxillary and mandibular teeth in protrusive and lateral excursive movements. Next, check the length of the centrals, overbite and overjet, to insure that the new smile does not affect speech or the lip closure path, as it often does. Now is the time to be an artist and create a beautiful smile. Function, occlusion, and phonetics should be evaluated. The visual presentation must be examined and corrected. General tooth contours, length, size, harmony, and the balance of the smile in relation to the lips must all be verified. If all intraoral recontouring is done now, it will not be necessary in the completed final ceramic restorations.
3. When the dentist and patient are satisfied with function and aesthetics of the provisional restoration, take an impression of the "approved provisionals" and send it along with the rest of the case to the laboratory (Table 20.1).

This model, or blueprint, will be used to create these laboratory fabricated verification tools:

- Incisal edge matrix to recreate incisal edge position (overbite, overjet) of anterior teeth (Fig. 20.6)
- Soft tissue matrix to recreate soft tissue contours, to insure correct emergence profile and anatomical harmony between teeth and tissue (Fig. 20.7)

The final ceramic restorations are now created to your exact specifications using your instructions and models as the communication blueprint. Take the time to

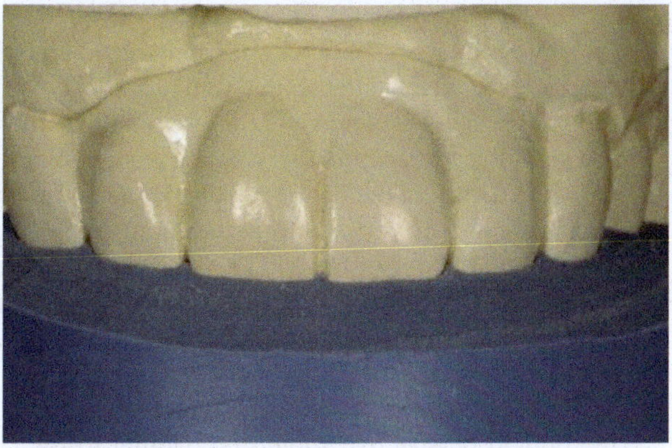

Fig. 20.6 "Approved provisional model," with incisal edge matrix for the correct incisal edge positioning (overbite, overjet) of final all-ceramic restorations

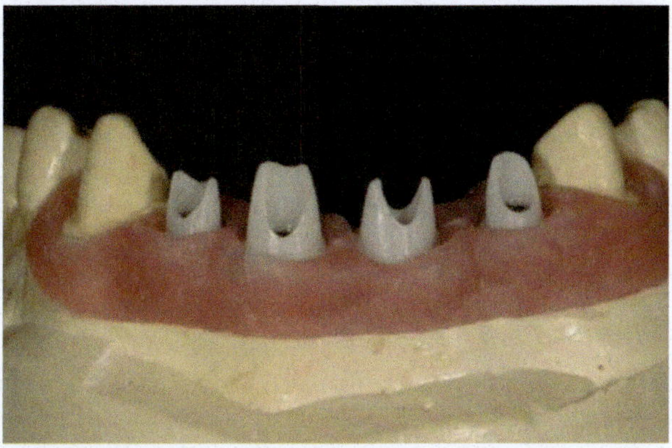

Fig. 20.7 Soft tissue matrix to recreate soft tissue contours, to insure correct emergence profile and anatomical harmony between teeth/implants and tissue

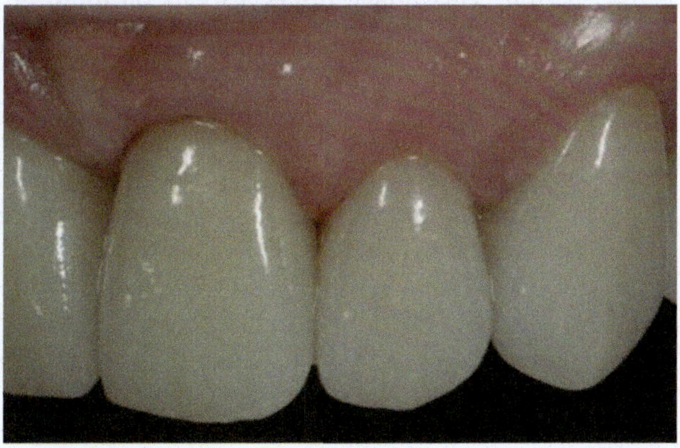

Fig. 20.8 The final ceramic restorations are now created to your exact specifications using your instructions and models as the communication blueprint (all-ceramic restorations on teeth 8–11)

accept your responsibility as oral architect and any high-quality laboratory that understands these philosophies and techniques will gratefully accept their role as builder (Fig. 20.8).

B. *Digital Photography*

Photographs or computer images are invaluable in creating a visual reference for the restorative dental team (Ahmad 2009). Photography as a communication tool was once considered a luxury item, but should now be considered standard practice in prosthetic dentistry. The introduction of simple point and shoot digital cameras offers the dentist/technician team an accurate, reproducible way to communicate all visual information that cannot be conveyed by a stone cast. Training in the use of the dentist's chosen digital camera is essential to achieve the proper settings for the most accurate images. Camera settings, the flash, and the angulation of the shot should be done correctly for the proper image to be achieved.

The photographer should insure that images are in the correct axis. Facially, the optical perspective should be parallel to the occlusal plane. Images taken above or below this plane will distort the images. Additional images from different angles should be taken from the same axis, so that the viewer does not have to reorient his visual perspective. Below are general and specific views that the dentist should include when taking a series of photographs to utilize in prosthodontic cases:

A. *General views* – there are several images that are helpful to the technician in visualizing the case to achieve predictable restorative success.
   1. *A full face shot* is an efficient way of allowing the laboratory to "meet" the patient if the dentist and laboratory are not in the same geographical location. A full face shot is also helpful in determining possible resolution of aesthetic problems including canting, reverse smile line, incisal edge relationship to the lips, and general aesthetics in relationship with the face.
   2. *A chin-to-nose photo* allows the viewer to concentrate on the lower facial view with teeth and smile, without the rest of the face becoming a distraction. This image offers a focus on tooth arrangement and the aesthetic effects of gingival architecture.
   3. *An image of the fully retracted anterior segment* allows for complete inspection of definitive tooth shape, general shade requirement, and tooth-to-tooth relationships.

B. *Specific Views* – the general views are especially helpful in the creation of a smile design restoration, but specific views are required when technicians are called upon to restore existing dentition.
   1. *A 1 to 1 image* offers additional information to establish color nuances, internal effects, and translucency patterns. This information is gathered using images in the 1 to 1–1 to 2 focal ranges. The addition of a black background enhances visual interpretation even further (Fig. 20.9).
   2. *End-to-end image* of the maxillary and mandibular anterior teeth is another view that is helpful in color and translucency communication. This image allows the laboratory technician to compare color, internal effects, and translucency patterns when several teeth are to be restored. A common mistake with this image is to allow the patient's tongue to be in contact with the linguals of the anterior teeth. The pink color of the tongue

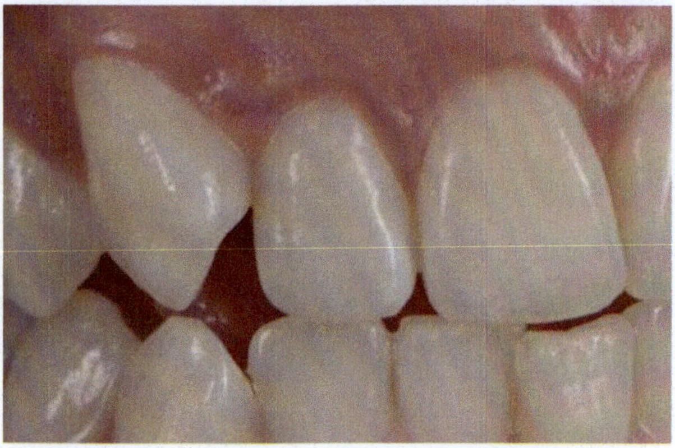

Fig. 20.9 The end-to-end view is a great way to compare the maxillary and mandibular teeth to see color and translucency

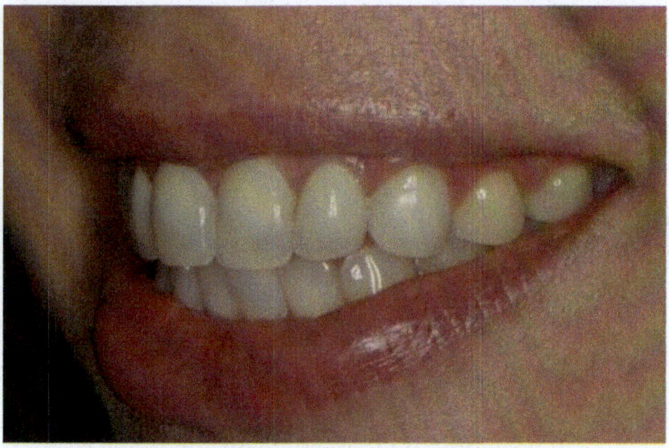

Fig 20.10 End to end view showing effect of tongue on color and translucency of teeth

will influence both the color and translucency of the teeth in the image (Fig. 20.10).

3. *An image with the tooth and the closest possible shade guide*, even though not perfect, allows the ceramist to make an educated guess as to the adjustments required to achieve a good match in general shade and value. In this image, the reference number on the shade guide must be visible. The cameras, printers, and monitors that we currently use are not capable of reproducing accurate, repeatable colors that we can use for tooth shade matching. With that established, a good image of the tooth with the shade guide provides us with invaluable color information. In addition to the external shade of the tooth, a stump shade that matches the dentin should be sent to the laboratory as well (Fig 20.11).
4. *An image taken at an angle*, so that the "flash" light reflects across the tooth surface to show minute surface texture through the use of light and shadow. Images taken 90° from the facial reproduce color and translucency well, but tend to "flatten" the facial contours and textures. The dental model and facial images help to define proper tooth form and arrangement. Shape and color are only two of the three areas that need to

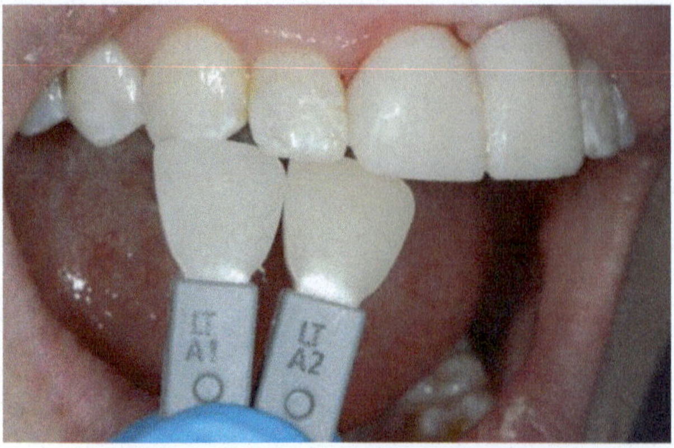

Fig. 20.11 Shade guide image showing shade reference number in black

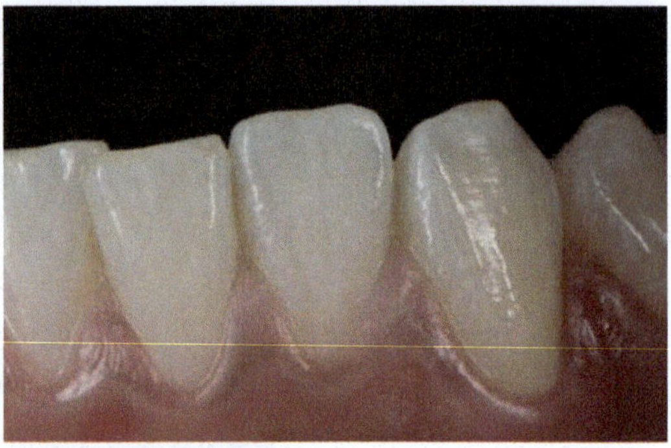

Fig. 20.12 Camera has been placed at an oblique angle to the tooth to cause shadowing so that surface texture is clearly seen

be addressed to recreate disappearing restorations. The third is the recording and reproduction of the surface texture and luster of the natural dentition (Fig. 20.12).

These images for dental photography in the past were perceived as complicated, time consuming, and expensive. With the ease of use of today's digital cameras, image communication should become part of every dentist and technician's communication toolbox.

C. Articulators

It is difficult to give specific opinions on which articulator system is best for each situation. Described below are the different articulator categories and options they offer which should be considered before purchasing a system. Basically, articulator systems are divided into two groups, Arcon and non-Arcon (Hobo et al. 1976).

1. Arcon articulators have the mechanical condyle located on the lower frame of the articulator to imitate the condyle of the natural joint. *The joint cavity imitating the natural joint fossa is part of the upper frame of the articulator. Arcon articulator copies the natural bones of the skull.*
2. *Non-Arcon articulators place the mechanical condyle on the upper part of the frame. The non-Arcon articulator is in reverse with the condyle moving in*

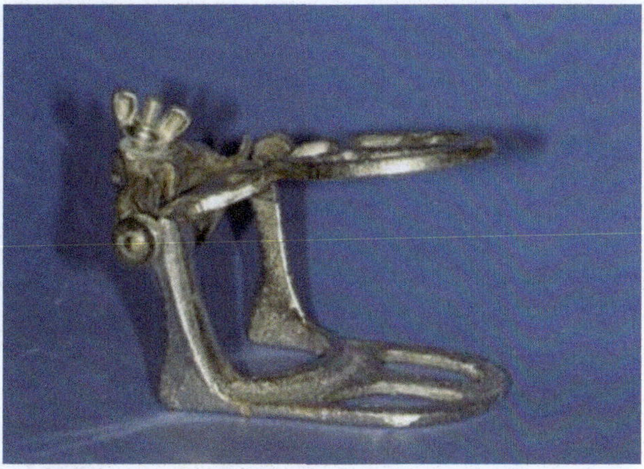

Fig. 20.13 A non-anatomical articulator

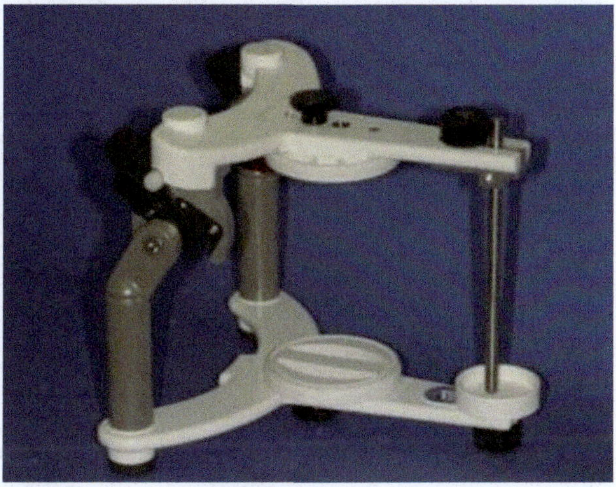

Fig. 20.14 An average value, nonadjustable articulator

the opposite direction. Non-anatomical articulators do not accurately represent anatomical movements of the mandible because of their small size (Fig. 20.13).

Non-anatomical articulators are referred to in dental slang as a "barn door hinge"; this type of articulator permits only opening and closing movements around a fixed axis. Lateral, protrusion, or retrusion movements cannot be accurately achieved. Model orientation using non-anatomical articulators is arbitrary and offers no natural relationship to the patient's temporomandibular joint (TMJ) Since no relationship to the TMJ can be established, and no excursive movements can be accurately simulated, these articulators are best suited for small single unit cases, where excursive movements can be copied from wear patterns on the remaining teeth. As a result of extensive research, anatomical articulators can very accurately replicate anatomical movements of the mandible. Within this category are three primary types:

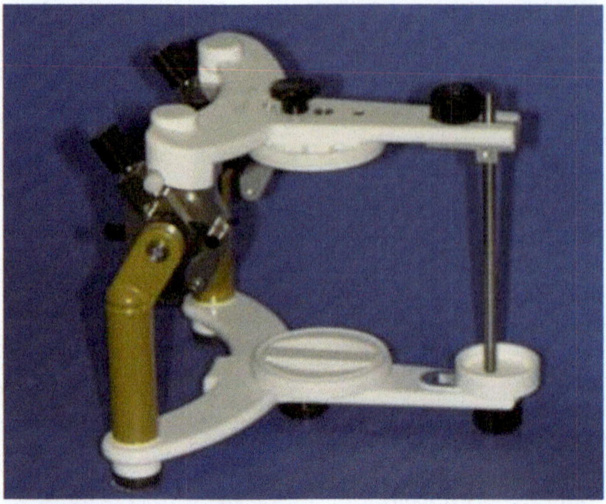

Fig. 20.15 A semi-adjustable articulator

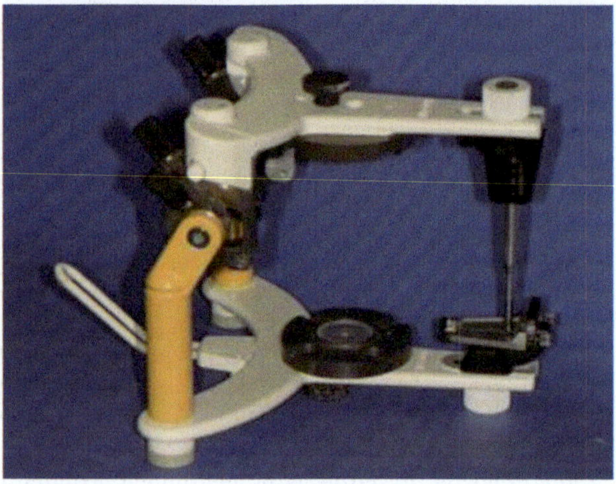

Fig. 20.16 Fully adjustable articulator

1. Nonadjustable articulator: Average value articulators are equipped with an approximate protrusive path of approximately 30°. The settings of individual patient parameters are not possible because the condyles are fixed. Model orientation is generally accomplished according to average values (Fig.20.14).
2. Semi-adjustable: Semi-adjustable articulators usually permit the transfer of individual patient parameter, such as inclination of the protrusion path and Bennett angle. Using a facebow for model orientation, a relationship to an individual patient's TMJ is possible (Fig. 20.15).
3. Fully adjustable: All of the above-mentioned settings are offered in fully adjustable models with the addition of individual adjustable settings such as intercondylar, programmable retrusion, and custom settings to duplicate exact condylar movements. Settings on fully adjustable articulators are programmed using a manual or computer-generated pantographic tracing (Fig. 20.16).

Considerations for Selection of Articulators

Aside from the mechanics, there are several other variables to take into consideration before deciding on which articulator system to purchase.

1. Price: The more complex the articulator becomes, obviously the higher the price. Generally, average value articulators range anywhere in price from $100 to $600, depending on the quality of the instrument and the accessories offered for the system. Semi-adjustable and fully adjustable articulators can range in price from $500 to more than $1500 with pantographic instrumentation costing up to $5000.
2. Ease of use: Choose an articulator that is "technician friendly." Many are excellent diagnostic tools, but do not hold up very well under the rigors of everyday use in the laboratory. A feature that is necessary in an articulation system is increased vertical height between upper and lower mounting structures. Low-vertical height systems sometimes will not allow correct facebow positioning of the model when both the upper and lower models are pinned because the upper and lower models require too much space.
3. Calibration: When dentist/technician teams choose an articulator system, calibration between articulators becomes a necessity. Calibration allows models from one articulator to be accurately transferred to another articulator. When working with dental laboratories outside your geographical area, calibration transfer allows models to be shipped without sending your articulator. Transfer becomes even easier if the system offers the option of a magnetic mounting system. Magnetic mounting systems are becoming very popular and allow quick, efficient model transfer in the laboratory and to the dentist. The choice of an articulator system is a combined effort between the technician and dentist team. Take your time to research all the systems available and choose the one(s) that will work best for your needs. The initial cost may seem expensive, but the purchase of a quality articulator system is a worthwhile investment in your future for producing high-quality dentistry.

The evolution of aesthetic, restorative dentistry in the twenty-first century continues to demand that the discerning dentist be thoroughly well-versed in form and function. To successfully emulate the human model, today's dentist must spend a great deal of time in pursuit of continuing education that trains critical decision-making for proper aesthetics and function. Knowledge of smile design principles, anatomic form for optimal function, and proper material selection all play a part in the successful resolution of the severely compromised dentition.

For a case to be fully successful, a marriage of the patient's aesthetic objectives and the dentist's functional parameters must take place. Through a series of diagnostic systems, precise data can be accurately evaluated to determine the extent of change that must take place and what alternatives are possible, *before* a restorative appointment is initiated. With all of the facts known to the patient, dentist, and laboratory technician through systematic communication, a complete treatment plan can be unveiled and a precise treatment sequence can be carried out without complication (Christensen 2009).

Once a dentist has presented the technician with the information presented above to create the ultimate in restorative dentistry, the following is a list of what a dentist can expect from the technician when the final restorations are presented for your inspection.

I. Model work:
   - All laboratory fabricated models are dense and bubble-free.
   - All models are neat and clean for possible presentation to the patient.

II. Restorations:
   - Margins should be sealed to working model dies, and verify margin on solid model, if possible.
   - Contacts should be closed with proper interproximal contours; please verify contacts on solid model, as this model will be more accurate.
   - Occlusion should be checked on articulator to verify that posterior occlusion is in proper cusp-to-fossa relationship and that anterior occlusion has proper stable holding contacts.
   - Incisal edges of anterior teeth fit properly into the incisal edge matrix.
   - Gingival emergence contours are in harmony with the soft tissue model.
   - Contours of restorations are in harmony and balance with surrounding natural dentition.
   - Surface of ceramic and/or composite restorations is properly glazed and polished with no porosity or surface roughness. Any exposed metal is polished to a high luster.
   - Shade matches appropriate shade guide, photos, or drawings.
   - All details of written prescription have been followed to detail.

20.3 The Digital Future

While it took slightly longer than anticipated to integrate into the daily practice of dentistry, the new millennium seemed to be the catalyst for change in digital dentistry, as more than ten different CAD/CAM systems have now been introduced as solutions for restorative dentistry. Refer to Chaps. 10 and 11 on Digital Dentistry.

Dentistry has cautiously welcomed this influx of technology that was promised so long ago. Based on technology adopted from aerospace, automotive, and even the watch-making industry, this technology is being accepted now due to its advantage of increased speed, accuracy, and efficiency without a compromise in quality. Today's CAD/CAM systems are being used to design and manufacture metal, alumina, and zirconia frameworks, as well as all-ceramic and composite full-contour crowns, inlays, and veneers that may be stronger, fit better, and are more aesthetic than restorations fabricated using traditional methods.

As restorative dentistry evolves into the digital world of image capture, computer design, and creation of dental restorations through robotics, our perceptions and definitions of the dental laboratory must evolve also. First, in order to fully understand this concept, we must clearly define what a laboratory is. At first thought we might say that a lab is the place that a dentist sends his or her patient's impressions, which are then processed, by that laboratory into restorations, which are sent back to the dentist for adjustment and delivery. This definition does seem to fit well with the traditional concept of a dentist-laboratory workflow. However, just as the Internet has forever changed the landscape of communication through related computer technology, the possibility to use CAD/CAM restoration files electronically has provided the catalyst for a significant change in the way we view and structure the dentist-lab relationship.

Let us imagine first that our laboratory is not a place, does not have walls, and exists only in the talents for the partners in the restorative process – the dentist and technician. The equipment we use to create the restoration may be located next to the chair, in an in-office laboratory area, or remotely or any or all of the above. Our "laboratory" is actually nothing more than a workflow, which is flexible to the degree that our abilities, access, and equipment will allow. The primary decision becomes where the handoff from one partner to another should occur. Moreover, a dentist who has the ability to optically scan intraorally for impressions and who often chooses CAD/CAM restorations as the best treatment option for their patients has enhanced freedom as to where I believe the handoff to the technician partner should occur. The lab is no longer a place; it is, to a large degree, a virtual and a fluid entity (Fig. 20.17).

In some instances, it makes sense for the dentist to work independently and to prepare, design, and finish the restoration chairside in a single visit with the obvious advantages a clinical CAD/CAM system has to offer (Fig. 20.18). These might include less complex restorations or fewer numbers of restoration for the same patient that do not require any special characterization other than perhaps stain and glaze or polish. Other times, it is advantageous to engage the services of the restorative partner, a dental technician, because he or she possesses the skill and perhaps more importantly the time to create restorations that either demand more complex characterization or can be more efficiently created in an indirect manner (Fig. 20.19a, b).

Whether using digital or conventional techniques, effective communication is a two-way street, and we are presented daily with new challenges that arise from working in the oral cavity. Keep the communication lines open and honest, always do your best, and expect no less from the laboratory. Judge all clinical and technical work by whether you would place it in your own mouth.

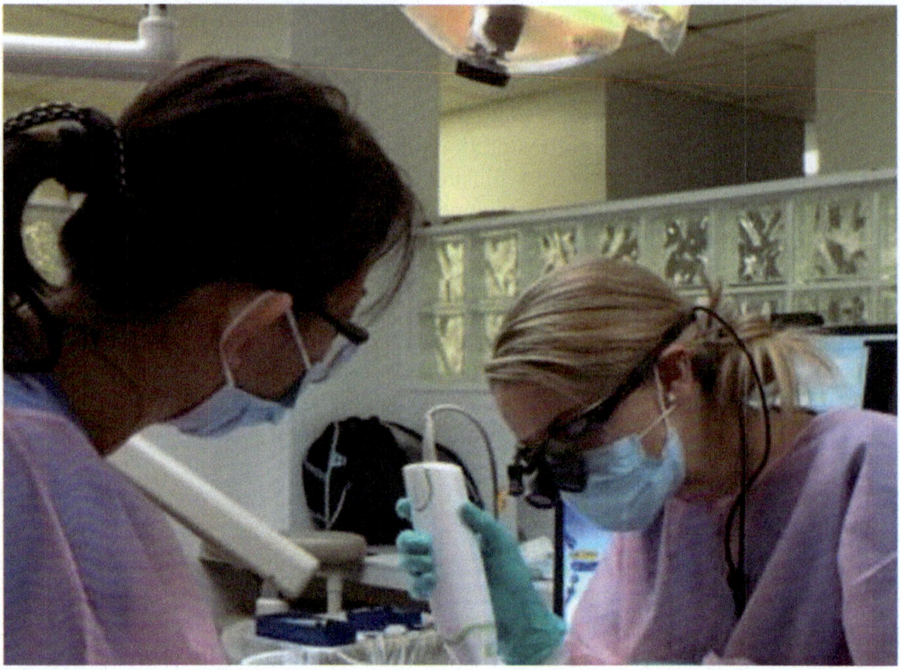

Fig. 20.17 Digital intraoral scanner (IOS)

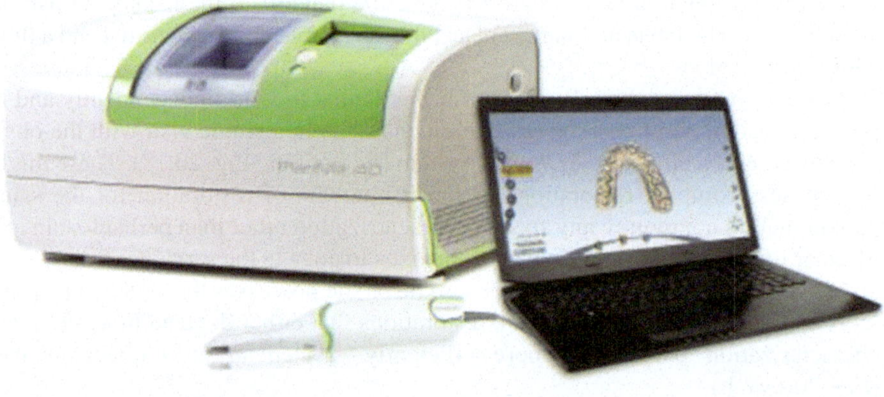

Fig. 20.18 IOS, with chairside design and milling capabilities

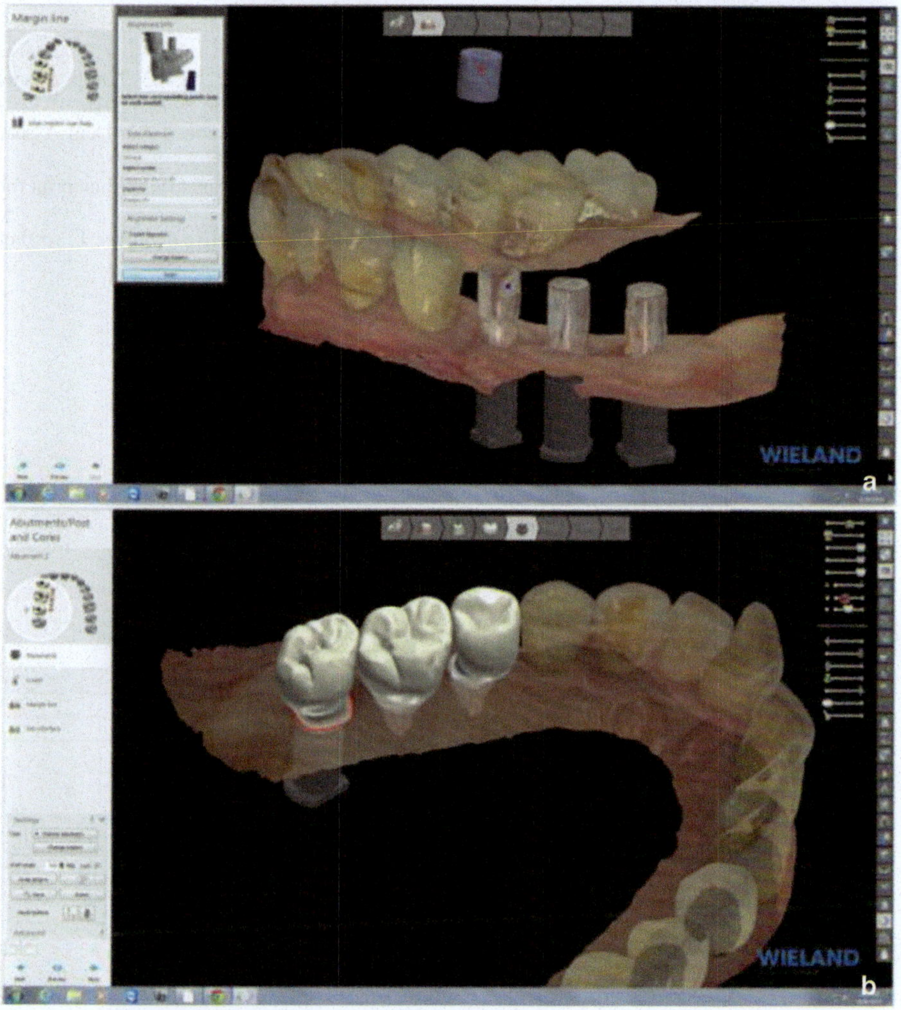

Fig. 20.19 (**a**, **b**) In the event of CAD/CAM, a dental laboratory technician designs a more complex dental restoration

References

Ahmad I. Digital dental photography part 1: an overview. Br Dent J. 2009:206:403–7. http://www.nature.com/bdj/journal/v206/n8/full/sj.bdj.2009.306.html. Accessed on: 29 Feb 2016.

Christensen G. Improving dentist-technician interaction and communication. J Am Dent Assoc. 2009;140:475–8.

Donovan TE, Cho GC. Diagnostic provisional restorations in restorative dentistry: the blueprint for success. J Can Dent Assoc. 1999;65(5):272–5.

Hobo S, Shillingburg Jr HT, Whitsett LD. Articulator selection for restorative dentistry. J Prosthet Dent. 1976;36(1):35–43.

Navigating Evidence-Based Dentistry

21

Jaana Gold and Scott L. Tomar

Contents

Abstract

Dentistry is a rapidly changing profession that requires lifelong learning. Clinicians must stay current with changing standards of clinical care. Evidence-based practice helps clinicians offer their patients the best available care by keeping up-to-date on the science of their profession. It is important to know where and how to access the evidence efficiently. This chapter gives a short introduction to the basic concepts of evidence-based dentistry and provides tutorials and sources of information for independent learning and evidence-based decision-making.

J. Gold, DDS, PhD, MPH, CPH (✉) • S.L. Tomar, DMD, DrPH
Department of Community Dentistry and Behavioral Science, AT Still University of Florida College of Dentistry, Gainesville, FL, USA
e-mail: jgold@atsu.edu

G.M. Weinstein, M.T. Zientz (eds.), *The Dental Reference Manual*,
DOI 10.1007/978-3-319-39730-6_21

21.1 How to Assess the Validity of Research and Make Informed Decisions

The American Dental Association (ADA) defines evidence-based dentistry (EBD) as "an approach to oral healthcare that requires the judicious integration of systematic assessments of clinically relevant scientific evidence, relating to the patient's oral and medical condition and history, with the dentist's clinical expertise and the patient's treatment needs and preferences." (American Dental Association 2014). EBD is described by the ADA as a patient-centered approach to treatment decisions that provides personalized dental care based on the most current scientific knowledge. The integration of the components of EBD into clinical decision-making enhances the quality and ethical delivery of clinical care.

Dentistry is a rapidly changing profession that requires lifelong learning. The technologies and methods learned in dental school rapidly become outdated as dental research continually discovers new treatment methods, materials, and procedures. Clinicians must stay current with changing standards of clinical care. Evidence-based practice helps clinicians offer their patients the best available care by keeping up-to-date on the science of their profession. It is important to know where and how to access the evidence efficiently.

Evidence-based decision-making requires efficient searching of the scientific literature and the application of the formal rules of evidence in evaluating the clinical literature. There are a few professional centers that are dedicated to developing resources to help practitioners and students to integrate clinically relevant scientific evidence into the decision-making process in clinical care. The Center for Evidence-Based Dentistry operates under the advisement of the ADA Council on Scientific Affairs (American Dental Association 2014). You can start your search for systematic reviews, critical summaries, and clinical practice guidelines on their website at http://ebd.ada.org/en/evidence/. If you cannot find the answer, you have several options to extend your search for the evidence. You can either look for other similar centers, EBD journals and organizations, or you can conduct your own EBD search. However, to conduct the efficient search of your own, you need to understand basic principles of finding and searching the evidence.

There are tutorials and resources for practitioners or students who need a basic introduction to the principles of evidence-based practice. Some of these include:

http://guides.mclibrary.duke.edu/ebmtutorial
http://medlib.bu.edu/tutorials/ebm/
http://ebd.ada.org/en/education/tutorials

21.2 Learning How to Use Databases and Literature to Find Evidence

PubMed is a database maintained by the National Library of Medicine that includes more than 25 million biomedical literature citations from MEDLINE, life science journals, and online books (approximately 200 dental journals are included). You

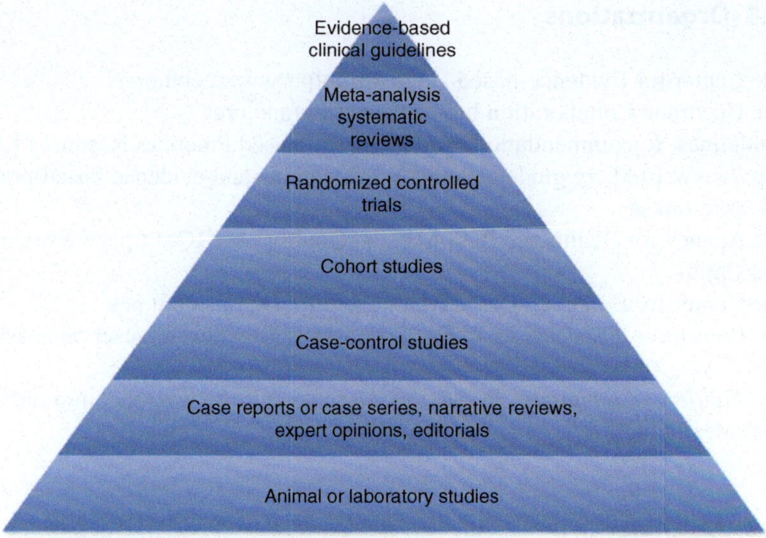

Fig. 21.1 Study types and levels of scientific evidence

can access PubMed tutorials to learn how to find the best evidence for any clinical questions by reviewing tutorials online at https://www.nlm.nih.gov/bsd/disted/pubmed.html.

To learn how to assess the literature, you need to understand the validity principles of study design and levels of evidence. The levels of evidence are typically depicted as a pyramid, with evidence-based clinical practice guidelines, meta-analyses, and systematic reviews at the apex representing the highest quality of evidence (secondary, pre-appraised, or filtered studies) (Fig. 21.1). Randomized controlled trials and observational studies, such as cohort and case-control studies, are primary, i.e., original research studies.

You should start EBD search by looking for the highest available level of evidence to answer a specific clinical question (Forrest 2016). If a clinical practice guideline or meta-analysis is not available on the topic, look next for systematic reviews without statistical synthesis, followed by individual randomized control trials, cohort studies, and so on.

Here are some of the links to learn more about EBD process:

http://www.cebm.net/study-designs/
http://www.casp-uk.net/#!appraising-the-evidence/c23r5
http://www.casp-uk.net/#!e-learning/cd70

21.3 Sources of Information

Additional resources to use to find and appraise the evidence:

21.3.1 Organizations

- The Center for Evidence-based Dentistry http://www.cebd.org/
- The Cochrane Collaboration http://www.cochrane.org/
- Guidelines, Recommendations and Evidence-based Practices Resource Links
- http://www.astdd.org/guidelines-recommendations-and-evidence-based-practices-resource-links/
- The Agency for Healthcare Research and Quality (AHRQ) http://www.ahrq.gov/index.html
- The Center for Evidence-Based Medicine http://www.cebm.net/
- *US Preventive Services Task Force* http://www.uspreventiveservicestaskforce.org/
- *The Guide to Community Preventive Services* http://www.thecommunityguide.org/index.html

21.3.2 Journals

- The Journal of Evidence-Based Dental Practice http://www.journals.elsevier.com/journal-of-evidence-based-dental-practice/
- Evidence-Based Dentistry http://www.nature.com/ebd/index.html

21.3.3 Databases

- The Cochrane Library http://www.cochranelibrary.com/
- PubMed http://www.ncbi.nlm.nih.gov/pubmed
- TRIP database http://www.tripdatabase.com/

21.3.4 Critical Appraisal Tools

- Critical Appraisal Skills Programme http://www.casp-uk.net/# Different critical appraisal tools to be used when reading literature
- Preferred Reporting Items for Systematic Reviews and Meta-Analyses http://www.prisma-statement.org/ for systematic reviews and meta-analyses

21.3.5 Other Resources

- Dental Elf http://www.thedentalelf.net/
- UTHSCSA Dental School Oral Health searchable CAT library at https://cats.uthscsa.edu/

References

American Dental Association. ADA center for evidence-based dentistry: about EBD [website]. 2014. Retrieved from http://ebd.ada.org/en/about/.

Forrest J. Evidence-based decision making: introduction and formulating good clinical questions. 2016. Retrieved from http://www.dentalcare.com/en-US/dental-education/continuing-education/ce311/ce311.aspx?ModuleName=introduction&PartID=-1&SectionID=-1.

22 Common Dental Prescriptions

Geraldine Weinstein and Fong Wong

Contents

Abstract

This chapter directs a new dental practitioner on how to write prescriptions correctly. The most common prescriptions that are necessary in a dental practice are illustrated here and their contraindications. This is meant as a guide, a proper review of the patient's medical history and medications is essential prior to considering any prescriptions. If there are any questions regarding the patient's conditions, a physician should be consulted.

My sincere gratitude to my mentor, Dr. Richard Wynn for reviewing this manuscript. It is a simplification of your work but nevertheless, I appreciate your guidance.

G. Weinstein, DDS (✉)
Department of Craniofacial Sciences, DDS University of Connecticut
School of Dental Medicine, Farmington, CT, USA
e-mail: geraldineweinstein@gmail.com

F. Wong, DMD, MS
William S. Middleton Memorial Veterans Hospital, Dental Service, Madison, WI, USA
e-mail: fongwong@mac.com

G.M. Weinstein, M.T. Zientz (eds.), *The Dental Reference Manual*,
DOI 10.1007/978-3-319-39730-6_22

22.1 Anatomy of a Prescription

The basics of what a prescription should look like are illustrated below. It is essential that there is clarity in your prescriptions so that the intended effect is obtained and there is less confusion on the pharmacist's and patient's end. The drug of choice and the available dosage should be clarified prior to writing the prescription. For instance, if it is a tablet, does it come in 200 mg or 300 mg tabs? If the drug of choice is a liquid suspension, what is the formulation that you prefer 250 mg/5 ml or something else? The instructions (*Signa* in Latin means write) are essential as well to remind patients how to use the medication and what the medication is for. In general for dentistry, refills should only be given for preventive prescriptions like fluoride or chlorhexidine rinses. Prescriptions for pain and antibiotics should not get refills so as to encourage the patients to seek treatment for the underlying problem. Most medications have generic counterparts which will give the patient/insurance some monetary savings. Precautions should be taken to prevent tampering of prescriptions. In today's electronic medical record, special paper should be utilized to print out prescriptions.

- Drug Enforcement Administration (DEA) numbers are required when prescribing narcotics. It may also be required by the pharmacy for billing certain managed care agencies. DEA numbers can be obtained online from: https://www.deadiversion.usdoj.gov/webforms/jsp/regapps/common/newAppLogin.jsp
- National Plan Identifier (NPI) number – This is a ten digit number that is utilized on claim forms submitted to payors. The number can be obtained free of charge from: http://www.apta.org/NPI/Applying/

John Doe, DMD
123 Main Street
Any town, USA
(000) 123-4321

DEA#____________ NPI#______________

Patient Name:________________ Date:__________
Patient Address:________________ Date of Birth:__________

Rx:
Name of Drug (Include dosage ie:if it comes in 200mg tabs etc)
Please dispense (Spell out the amount)

Sig: These are instructions on how to take the medication and what it is being prescribed for.

# of refills allowed?__________ Rx is gooduntil ______________

Generic Substitution Allowed: Dispense as written:

______________ ______________

Common Abbreviations Utilized in Prescription Writing There are many variations of abbreviations in writing prescriptions. One must be very cautious in using them. A few common ones to dentistry are listed in the table:

Abbreviation	Its meaning:
b.i.d. or b.d.	Means twice daily
npo	Nothing by mouth
po	By mouth
prn	As needed
q.6.h	Every 6 h, you can change the number of hours, i.e., q.8.h means every 8 h
stat	Immediately
t.i.d.	Three times daily

22.2 Antibiotics Indications

22.2.1 Precautions for All Antibiotics

- Note that all antibiotics have the potential to interfere with oral contraceptives. Patients should be advised to take additional precautions when taking antibiotics and oral contraceptives together.
- Antibiotics can cause "nuisance" diarrhea which is nonthreatening. Patient should call the prescriber before discontinuing the medication.
- In general all antibiotics have the potential of causing pseudomembranous colitis which manifests itself as severe diarrhea. The patient should be instructed to discontinue use of medication and seek treatment from their physician.
- In dentistry, antibiotic use should be limited to 7–10 days. Patients should be encouraged to seek treatment for their dental problems or return if their symptoms persist. Short term use of antibiotics will also prevent superinfections with fungal growth.

22.2.1.1 Guidelines for Antibiotic Prophylaxis

- For current guidelines on antibiotic prophylaxis for prevention of infective endocarditis, visit the American Dental Association(ADA) and the American Heart Association website at: http://www.ada.org/en/member-center/oral-health-topics/antibiotic-prophylaxis and http://www.heart.org/HEARTORG/Conditions/CongenitalHeartDefects/TheImpactofCongenitalHeartDefects/Infective-Endocarditis_UCM_307108_Article.jsp#.Vmrz1LgrK7Q.

  Cardiac Conditions for Which Prophylaxis with Antibiotics for Dental Procedures Is Recommended (AHA Guidelines Published May 2007):
  - Prosthetic heart valve
  - Previous infective endocarditis
  - Congenital heart disease (CHD)

    - Unrepaired cyanotic CHD, including palliative shunts and conduits
    - Completely repaired congenital heart defect with prosthetic material or device whether placed by surgery or by catheter intervention, during the first 6 months after the procedure (endothelialization occurs within 6 months of procedure)
    - Repaired CHD with residual defects at the site or adjacent to the site of a prosthetic patch or adjacent or prosthetic device (which inhibits endothelialization)
  - Cardiac transplant recipients who develop cardiac valvulopathy
- Patients with any of the above conditions who are scheduled to undergo a dental procedure that is at risk of bleeding should be given antibiotics prior to initiation of procedures.
- For current guidelines on antibiotic prophylaxis in patients with prosthetic joints who may be at risk of developing infections following dental procedures, the ADA is a good site as well or the American Association of Orthopedic Surgeons Guidelines.

ADA 2014 Clinical Recommendation

In general, for patients with prosthetic joint implants, prophylactic antibiotics are not recommended prior to dental procedures to prevent prosthetic joint infection. For patients with a history of complications associated with their joint replacement surgery who are undergoing dental procedures that include gingival manipulation or mucosal incision, prophylactic antibiotics should only be considered after consultation with the patient and orthopedic surgeon. To assess a patient's medical status, a complete health history is always recommended when making final decisions regarding the need for antibiotic prophylaxis.

- The most recent evidence-based guideline was published in the Journal of the American Dental Association (JADA) in 2015. This is accessible on: http://jada.ada.org/article/S0002-8177(14)00019-1/fulltext?nav=rotatorJanmain.

Antibiotic indication	First choice: non-penicillin-allergic patients	Second choice: penicillin-allergic patients	Patients unable to take oral medication
Prophylaxis for patients at risk for developing bacterial endocarditis	[a]Amoxicillin 500 mg tabs Disp: dependent on the anticipated number of appointments Sig: Take 4 tabs (2 g) an hour before dental procedure *Also available in suspensions*	[b]Clindamycin 150 mg tabs Disp: dependent on the anticipated number of appointments Sig: Take 4 (150 mg) tabs = 600 mgs; 1 h before dental procedure *Also available in suspensions*	Ampicillin 2 g IM or IV For penicillin or ampicillin-allergic patients: clindamycin (600 mg IM or IV; 1 h before dental procedure)

Antibiotic indication	First choice: non-penicillin-allergic patients	Second choice: penicillin-allergic patients	Patients unable to take oral medication
Prophylaxis for patients at risk for developing bacteremia in prosthetic joints	Amoxicillin 500 mg tabs Dispense 12 tabs Sig: Take 4 tabs(2 g) 1 h before procedure	Clindamycin 150 mg tabs Dispense 12 tabs Sig: Take 4 tablets = 600 mg an hour before procedure Note: AAOS has no official recommendation for penicillin-allergic patients, this would be a reasonable alternative	
Acute dental infections where organism is unknown	[a]Penicillin VK 500 mg tabs Disp: 21 (twenty-one) tabs Sig: Take 1 g = 2 tablets stat; followed by 500 mg q.6.h for 7 days [b]Clindamycin can also be considered depending on the severity of the infection or if no response is obtained after use of penicillin for 48 h	[b]Clindamycin 150 mg tabs Disp: 21(twenty-one) tabs Sig: Take 2 tabs = 300 mg stat; 1 tab q.6.h for 7 days	Referral to emergency room for IV antibiotics

[a]Pen VK and amoxicillin contraindications: allergy to Penicillin, hypersensitivity to cephalosporins
[b]Clindamycin contraindications: allergy to clindamycin, clindamycin notes
Most pharmacies carry clindamycin only in 150 mg tabs
Most prominent antibiotic to cause pseudomembranous colitis
Cautious use in elderly patients, patients with renal or hepatic disease or colitis

Augmentin 500 mg (500 mg amoxicillin, 125 mg clavulanic acid)
Dispense: 21 (twenty-one) tabs
Sig. 1 tab po q.8. h until gone

Note Augmentin is another option for non-penicillin-allergic patients; presence of clavulanic acid allows medication to be taken with or without meals.

22.2.1.2 Antibiotics for Upper Respiratory Tract Infections

- In patients with sinus congestion, a use of the over-the-counter decongestants would be helpful in conjunction with antibiotic use.
  Azithromycin (*Zithromax*) 250 mg tabs

Dispense 6 tabs
Sig: 2 tabs (500 mg) po on day 1; followed by 1 tab daily on days 2–5

Z-Pak
Dispense: one
Sig: Take as directed
Contraindications: Allergy to erythromycin, high dose of theophylline, taking (Claritin) loratadine or astemizole, taking cisapride (Propulsid); liver disease

- Should be taken an hour before food or 2 h after food.

22.2.1.3 Antibiotics for Periodontal Disease

Doxycycline 100 mg
Dispense: 15 (fifteen) caps
Sig. 1 cap po q 12 h until gone
Use: Periodontitis associated with *Actinobacillus actinomycetemcomitans*

Contraindications: Pregnancy and children up to 9 years (during tooth development), should not be used with renal or liver disease, decreased effectiveness when used with oral contraceptives and iron preparations or antacids

Metronidazole 250 mg (Flagyl)
Disp: 30 (thirty) tabs
Sig: 1 tab po t.i.d for 7–10 days

Use: bacterial anaerobic infections, refractory adult periodontitis, necrotizing periodontitis in immune-compromised patients

Contraindications: hypersensitivity, renal or hepatic disease, pregnancy (1st trimester), lactation, blood dyscrasias, seizures, and neuropathies

Drug interactions with alcohol, lithium, increased bleeding with warfarin, increased phenytoin levels, decreased oral contraceptive effectiveness, and interacts with many drugs used in HIV patients.

22.2.1.4 Antibiotics for Dental Implants

Use of antibiotics prior to implant surgery in healthy, low to moderate risk patients is controversial. Use of antibiotics is recommended in high-risk individuals such as patients with risk of endocarditis, immunodeficiency, or previous prosthetic instrumentation. The recommendation prior to implant placement is 2 g of Amoxicillin taken an hour before the surgery (Ata-Ali and Ata-Ali 2014). Use of antibiotics prior to surgery according to Ata-Ali's study did not affect postoperative infection.

22.3 Prescriptions

22.3.1 Antifungals

In patients that present with oral fungal infections, a thorough review of the patient's medical history is necessary to insure that the infection is not a systemic one. Systemic fungal infections should be treated in consultation with the patient's physician. Oral fungal infections are often noted in patients with dentures. This can be noted intraorally on the soft tissue of denture-bearing areas or for patients with loss of vertical dimension on the commissure of the lips. In such cases, the prosthesis should be treated as well. Patients should be advised to remove the dentures at bedtime to allow tissues to heal. When denture is inserted, apply antifungal to the denture as well as their mouth.

Nystatin Cream
Disp: 15 g tube
Sig: Apply to affected areas tid

Nystatin Ointment
Disp: 15 g tube
Sig: Apply thin coat qid to corners of mouth and/or inner surface of denture

Nystatin Pastilles (Mycostatin)
Disp: 30 (thirty) tabs
Sig: Remove denture, dissolve 1 tablet in mouth until gone, tid

- Note: Pastilles contain sucrose.

Nystatin Powder
Disp: 16 g
Sig: Sprinkle over dentures inner surface tid

For chronic angular cheilitis:

Nystatin and Triamcinolone Acetonide Ointment or Cream (Mycolog)
Disp: 30 g tube
Sig: Apply over affected area qid for 10–14 days

22.3.2 Antivirals (for Oral Herpes Simplex)

- Oral herpes simplex occurs on bound mucosal tissue. It often occurs in clusters and is precipitated by certain events.

  Viscous Xylocaine 2 %
  Disp: 100 or 450 ml
  Sig: Swish 1–2 teaspoons around mouth as needed for pain, and then spit out

  Valacyclovir (Valtrex) 500 mg
  Disp: 8 (eight tablets)

Sig: Take 4 tablets at first sign of attack and then take 4 tablets 12 h later
Note: Not to be used for HIV patients, may cause thrombocytopenia; start within 3 days of symptom onset.

- Prophylactic use of Valtrex for recurring ulcers that are precipitated by events like a dental appointment
  Valtrex 500 mg
  Disp: 8 (eight) tablets
  Sig: 1 day before and day after appointment, take 1 tab q.12.h
    Abreva (over the counter)
    Disp: 2 g
    Sig: Apply to lesion 5X daily until gone

22.3.3 Anxiolytics

A patient who is prescribed an anxiolytic should be advised not to drive after taking the medication. The medications listed below are in order of the longest acting to shortest acting anxiolytics. Pregnancy is a contraindication for these drugs. Dose limitation should be considered for elderly patients.

Valium 5 mg
4 (four) tabs
Take 1 tablet in the evening before bed and 1 tablet 1 h before your appointment

- Longest acting, half-life of 20–100 h

Ativan 1 mg
8 (eight) tabs
Take 2 tabs in the evening before bed and 2 tablets 1 h before your appointment

- Shorter acting, half-life of 12–14 h

Halcion 0.25 mg
4 (four) tablets
Take 1 tablet in the evening before bed and 1 tablet 1 h before your appointment

- Shortest acting, half-life of 2–3 h

22.3.4 Fluoride Considerations

- Fluoride supplements for children, refer to pediatric chapter for dosage

ACT Fluoride Rinse or Any Generic Fluoride Rinse (OTC)

Sig: Rinse after brushing and flossing; NPO 30 min after use twice daily

Note: inexpensive way to supplement fluoride in patients undergoing orthodontic treatment for prevention of caries. It is also effective when small decalcified areas on teeth are to be monitored for progression of caries.

Prevident Gel (Neutral Sodium Fluoride Gel)

Disp: one tube

Sig: Brush teeth with regular toothpaste and floss. Followed by brushing on Prevident for 2 min. Expectorate excess, NPO for 1 h after use

Note: In high caries rate patients, consider fabricating custom trays to apply Prevident daily.

Prevident 5000 Plus Toothpaste (Neutral Sodium Fluoride Gel)

Disp: One tube

Sig: Brush teeth with Prevident 5000 toothpaste and floss. Expectorate excess, NPO for 1 h after use

Note: In high caries rate patients, consider fabricating custom trays to apply Prevident daily.

22.3.5 Other Considerations

Rx: *chlorhexidine oral rinse 0.12 %*

Dispense one 16 oz bottle

½ oz swish and expectorate 2 times per day; NPO 30 min after use

Note: Long-term use causes staining of teeth and calculus deposit that will require scaling and root planning. Great for use for pre- or postsurgical care or control of oral flora in periodontal and high caries rate patients.

Rx: *70 ml 2 % viscous lidocaine*

200 ml Benadryl elixir (alcohol free)

200 ml Maalox

Sig: Rinse with 1–2 teaspoons for 15 s and expectorate. Use before mealtimes to alleviate pain from oral ulcers or trauma. Not advisable for children as it affects the gag reflex.

22.4 Pain Management

Pain management in each patient is unique. One should always be cognizant of the situation a patient presents with and customize the pain medication for that problem. It would be prudent to begin management with nonnarcotic, over-the-counter medication like Ibuprofens or Acetaminophens. Narcotic medication should be utilized only when use of nonnarcotics is not sufficient for controlling pain. It is recommended that no refills be given to a patient for pain medications as prolonged dental pain should be solved with treatment of the problem not through medication. This also minimizes the risk of drug abuse of the patient.

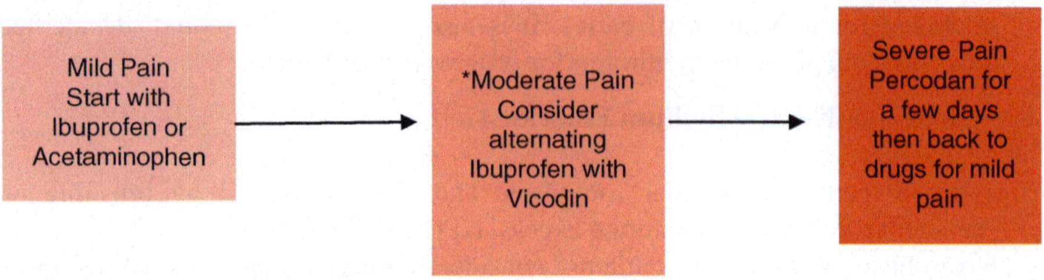

- *Use of Ibuprofen 600 mgs + Acetaminophen 325 every 6 h has been found to be more effective than Ibuprofen alone. (Menhinick)

22.4.1 Examples of Pain Rxs

Mild Pain

Ibuprofen (*Advil or Motrin* over the counter)
200–400 mg q6h
Maximum dose of 1200 mg in 24 h
Actions: Ibuprofen is anti-inflammatory, effective for muscle pain and controls swelling
Contraindications: Pregnancy, Allergies to Aspirin and other NSAIDs, GI bleeding, ulcers, corticosteroids, and Coumadin
Drug Interactions: Possible interactions with antihypertensive medications, acetaminophen and, oral anticoagulants
Or
Acetaminophen (*Tylenol or Anacin* over the counter)
325 mg Acetaminophen q6h
Maximum dose of 3 g total in 24 h (Consider Max. dose of 2 g/24 h for elderly and alcoholics.)
Contraindications: hepatic disease (alcoholics), renal disease, G6PD deficiency
Or
Naproxen sodium (*Alleve* 220 mg/tablets)
Sig. Take 2 tabs stat, 1q6-8 h
Maximum dose of 3 tablets per day
Contraindications: Allergy to aspirin; NSAIDs should not be taken together or combined with aspirin

Moderate Pain

Ibuprofen (*Advil or Motrin*; Rx strength)
Sig. 600–800 mg q6h

Maximum dose of 2400 mg in 24 h
Contraindications: See above
Drug Interactions: See above
Or/And alternating doses of Tylenol #3 or Vicodin
Tylenol #3 (contains Acetaminophen 300 mg + Codeine 30 mg)
Dispense: 18 (eighteen) tabs
Sig. 1 tab po q 4 h prn pain or 1–2 tabs po q 6 h prn pain
Maximum dose of 3 g total in 24 h (Consider Max. dose of 2 g/24 h for elderly and patients with liver disease.)
Contraindications: See Tylenol contraindications, allergies to codeine, morphine, hydrocodone, oxycodone, hepatic disease (alcoholics), renal disease, G6PD deficiency
Caution: elderly and patients with severe renal or hepatic disease
Or
Vicodin 5 (contains 300 mg Acetaminophen + 5 mg hydrocodone)
Dispense: 18 (eighteen) tabs
Sig: 1–2 tabs q6h prn pain
Maximum dose of 4 g total in 24 h (Consider Max. dose of 2 g/24 h for elderly and liver disease.)
Contraindications: See Tylenol contraindications, allergies to codeine, morphine, hydrocodone, oxycodone, hepatic disease (alcoholics), renal disease, G6PD deficiency
Caution: Elderly and patients with severe renal or hepatic disease
Or
Vicodin ES (contains 300 mg of Acetaminophen + 7.5 mg hydrocodone)
Dispense 18 (eighteen) tabs
Sig: 1 tab q6h
Maximum dose of Acetaminophen 4 g total in 24 h (Consider Max. dose of 2 g/24 h for elderly and liver disease.)
Contraindications: See Tylenol contraindications, allergies to codeine, morphine, hydrocodone, oxycodone, hepatic disease (alcoholics), renal disease, G6PD deficiency
Caution: Elderly and patients with severe renal or hepatic disease

Severe Pain

Percocet 5 (5 mg oxycodone, 325 mg acetaminophen)
12 (twelve) tabs
1 tab po q 4–6 h prn pain
Maximum dose of acetaminophen 4 g total in 24 h (Consider Max. dose of 2 g/24 h for elderly and patients with liver disease.)
Contraindications: See Tylenol contraindications, allergies to codeine, morphine, hydrocodone, oxycodone, prostatic hypertrophy, urethral stricture, head injury, increased intracranial pressure, hypothyroid, hepatic disease (alcoholics), renal disease, G6PD deficiency
Drug interactions for oxycodone:

Caution: Elderly and patients with severe renal or hepatic disease
Or
Percodan (4.5 oxycodone + 325 mg aspirin)
Dispense 12 (twelve) tabs
Sig: 1 tab q6h prn pain
Contraindications: allergy to aspirin and NSAIDs or oxycodone

Reference

Ata-Ali J, Ata-Ali F. Do Antibiotics decrease implant failure and postoperative infections? A systematic review and meta-analysis. Int J Oral Maxillofac Surg. 2014;43(1).

Further Reading

Arduino PG, Tirone F, Schiorlin E, Esposito M. Single preoperative dose of prophylactic amoxicillin versus a 2-day postoperative course in dental implant surgery: a two-centre randomized controlled trial. Eur J Oral Implantol. 2015;8(2):143–9.

Bahl R, Sandhu S, Singh K, Sahai N, Gupta M. Odontogenic infections: microbiology and management. Contemp Clin Dent. 2014;5(3):307–11.

Dar-Odeh NS, Abu-Hammad OA, Al-Omiri MK, Khraisat AS, Shehab AA. Antibiotic prescribing practices by dentists, a review. Ther Clin Risk Manag. 2010;6:301–6.

Menhinick KA, Gutmann JL, Regan JD, Taylor SE, Buschang PH. The efficacy of pain control following nonsurgical root canal treatment using ibuprofen or a combination of ibuprofen and acetaminophen in a randomized, double-blind, placebo-controlled study. Int Endod J. 2004;37(8):531–41.

Nabeel A, Najeeb S. Effects of antibiotics on dental implants: a review. J Clin Med Res. 2012;4(1):1–6.

Rubinstein E. Short antibiotic treatment courses or how short is short? Int J Antimicrob Agents. 2007;30S:S76–9.

Stewart C. Dental drug reference. University of Florida; Gainesville, Florida. 2012.

Wynn R, Meiller T, Crossley H. Drug information handbook for dentistry. 21st ed. Lexi-Comp; Hudson, Ohio. 2015–2016.

Yingling NM, Byrne BE, Hartwell GR. Antibiotic use by members of the American Association of Endodontists in the year 2000: report of a national survey. J Endod. 2002;28(5):396–404. ISNN: https://www.aae.org/uploadedfiles/publications_and_research/endodontics_colleagues_for_excellence_newsletter/ss95ecfe.pdf. Accessed on 14 Mar 2016.

Medical Considerations and Emergency Protocols

23

Mary Kuhns and Christopher Kuhns

Contents

Abstract

In setting up a dental office, an emergency action plan is necessary such that all members of the team are aware of their responsibilities. The plan would insure immediate activation of emergency medical services and basic life support for the patient. Contents of an emergency kit should be properly stocked, labeled, and kept up to date. This chapter focuses on the most common medical considerations encountered in the dental office including guidelines for reference. A comprehensive review and understanding of the patient's medical history and medications is the most important factor in preventing medical emergencies.

M. Kuhns, DMD, MS (✉)
Malcom Randall VAMC, 1601 SW Archer Rd, Gainesville, FL 32608, USA
e-mail: mary.kuhns@va.gov

C. Kuhns, DMD
Oral Surgery Department, University of Florida College of Dentistry, Gainesville, Fl 32601, USA

G.M. Weinstein, M.T. Zientz (eds.), *The Dental Reference Manual*,
DOI 10.1007/978-3-319-39730-6_23

23.1 Emergency Action Plan for the Office

- If the dental patient demonstrates clinical signs or symptoms of a medical emergency
  - Immediately stop the dental treatment.
  - Evaluate the patient.
  - Monitor the patient's vital signs and check blood glucose.
  - Provide oxygen to the patient.
  - Be prepared to provide basic life support procedures.
  - Place the patient in a comfortable position.
  - Activate the emergency medical system: Call 911 and document the time of the call.
- When emergency medical personnel arrive
  - Provide them with information about the emergency
    - Vital signs
    - Oxygen administration: time and flow rate
- Document the occurrence in the patient's dental record
  - Time emergency began
  - Dental office activities related to the emergency
  - Arrival time of emergency personnel
  - Emergency personnel medical procedures
  - Time of departure for the emergency room

23.1.1 Designation of Responsibility

Each member of the team should have a designated responsibility in the event of an emergency. Emergency cards attached to your crash cart may facilitate assignment of such duties and eliminate confusion (Fig 23.1). Proper labeling location of emergency cart, oxygen, and automated external defibrillator (AED) should be visible to everyone.

- Team Member 1
  - Call 911.
  - Stay on phone with dispatcher until told to hang up.
- Doctor
  - Confirm emergency medical call was placed.
  - Place supplemental oxygen.
  - Confirm open airway.
  - Assess breathing.
  - Check pulse, blood pressure, and respirations.
  - Initiate basic life support if indicated.
  - Administer medications if indicated.
  - Provide pertinent information to paramedics.

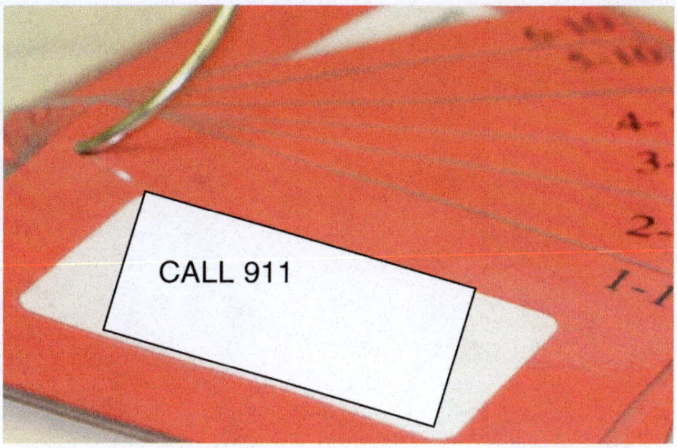

Fig. 23.1 Emergency cards (Photo credit: Dr. Joshua Yanover)

- Team Member 2
  - Get emergency kit.
  - Open emergency drug kit.
  - Draw up drugs as instructed by doctor.
- Team Member 3
  - Obtain AED.
  - Place AED pads if instructed.
  - Assist Doctor.
- Team Member 4
  - Record sequence of events: blood pressure and pulse; drugs administered including dose and time.
- Team Member 5
  - Clear room and hallways for emergency medical services (EMS) personnel
  - Wait for EMS outside, near elevator, or at point of entry
  - Take EMS to emergency scene

23.1.2 Adult Cardiopulmonary Resuscitation (CPR) (AHA 2015)

In most states, training on CPR needs renewal on a biennial basis. Each member of the dental team should be trained to do CPR and use of the automated external defibrillator (AED) (Fig.23.2). There are online training courses that can be used as refreshers on a regular basis. In addition to formal training, mock drills in the office that simulate true emergencies would be a wise decision.

In the Event of an Emergency

- Make sure environment is safe for rescuers and victim.
- Check responsiveness: no breathing or only gasping (no normal breathing), no definite pulse felt within 10 s.

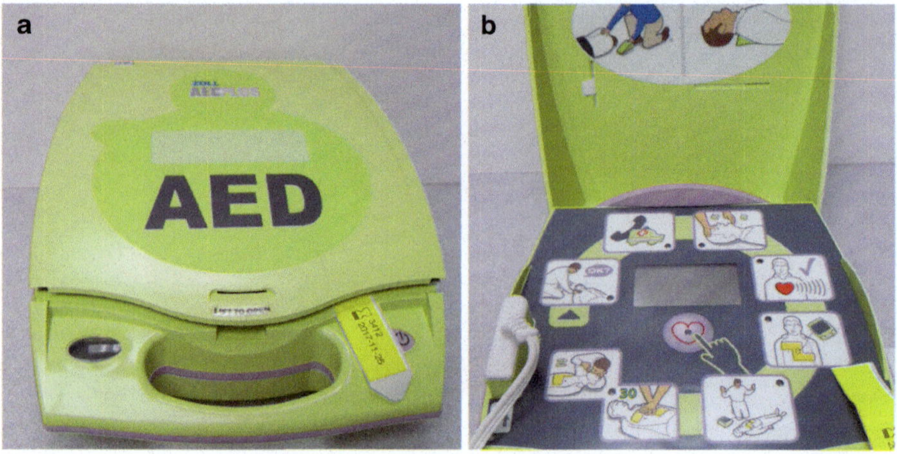

Fig. 23.2 (**a**, **b**) Use of the AED is essential when a patient is in cardiac arrest. Instructions for use are given by the voice commands that the AED is equipped with

- Activate emergency response system: Send someone to get AED and begin CPR immediately; use the AED as soon as it is available.
- Begin cycles of 30 compressions and 2 breaths at compression rate of 100–120/min; Compressions are approximately 2 in. or 5 cm in depth.
- Regardless of the cause of the cardiac arrest, the 2015 guidelines stress the need for continuous compressions with 10 breaths/min.
- Once AED arrives, turn it on, attach the pads; the AED will check if a shock is necessary and will direct you.

23.1.3 Child and Infant CPR (Infant to Puberty)

- Compression-ventilation ratio 15:2

23.2 What Should Be in Every Office's Emergency Kit? (Fig. 23.3)

The emergency medications needed in a dental office are included in Table 23.1. Use of these medications should be reviewed on a regular basis. Familiarity with the patient's medical history prior to treatment and making special arrangements are the best ways to avoid injury to the patient.

23.3 What to Ask for in a Medical Consult

- Medical condition or disease of concern including severity, stability, and how well the patient is controlled

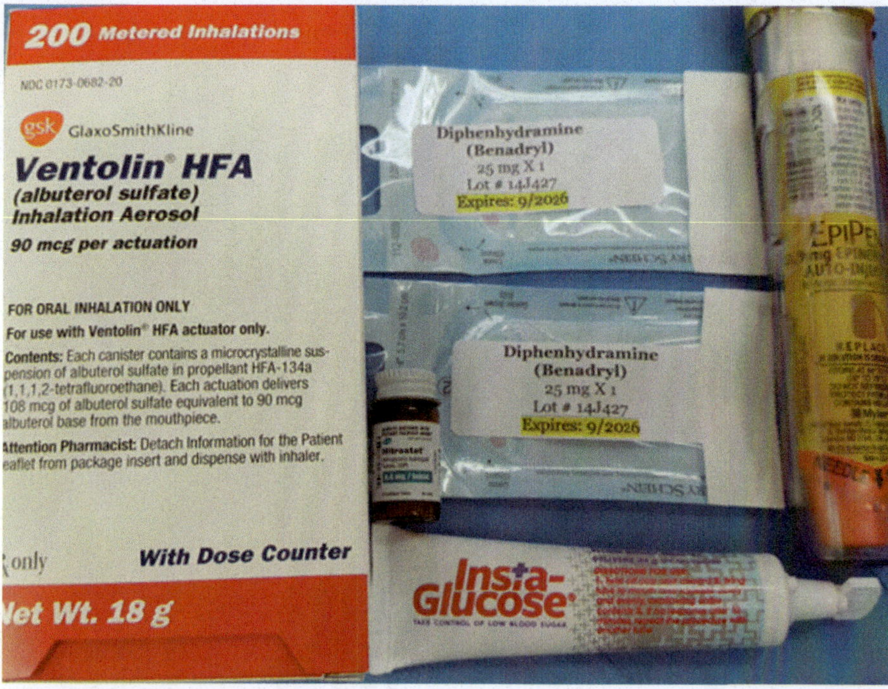

Fig. 23.3 The location of the emergency medications should be known to everyone who works at the dental practice. A designated person in the office should be in charge of checking these medications on a regular basis to insure that they are not expired

- Explanation of planned dental treatment and systemic consequences (avoid dental jargon)
  - Outline planned procedures
  - Invasiveness
  - Length of appointments
  - Surgical procedures
  - Anticipated blood loss
  - Possible complications
  - Anesthetic use – with or without epinephrine? Local or sedation?
  - Pre- and postop medications
- Request patient's most recent:
  - History and Physical (H and P)
  - Laboratory data
  - Current cardiovascular condition
  - Coagulation status
  - Status of chronic diseases
  - Use of bisphosphonates, receptor activator of nuclear factor-kB ligand (RANKL) inhibitors, etc.
  - Any other recommendations

Table 23.1 Emergency medications for a dental office

Drug name	Category	Indications	Quantity/dose	Side effects
Injectable				
Epinephrine	Allergy, anaphylaxis	Acute allergic reaction, bronchospasm	Two (2) preloaded autoinjector syringes (EpiPen) of 1:1000 epinephrine (0.3 mg per dose) for patients weighing 30 kg (66 lbs) or greater	Tachydysrhythmias; decreases placental blood flow and may induce premature labor
Diphenhydramine/Benadryl	Allergy, histamine blocker	Delayed-onset allergic reactions only involving skin	Two (2) 1 mL ampules of diphenhydramine (50 mg/mL)	Central nervous system (CNS) depression, decreased blood pressure, thickening of bronchial secretions (not for use in acute asthmatic episodes)
Non-injectable				
Oxygen	Oxygen	Respiratory distress, O_2 should be used during all medical emergencies	E cylinder with nasal cannula at 6 L	Not indicated in the treatment of hyperventilating patient but will not cause any adverse effects
Nitroglycerine	Vasodilator	Angina pectoris (chest pain)	Metered spray bottle (0.4 mg) or sublingual tablets	Headache, facial flushing, hypotension, severe hypotension in patients taking erectile dysfunction drugs
Albuterol	Bronchodilator, β2 agonist	Bronchospasm (acute asthmatic episodes), allergic reactions with bronchospasm component	1 metered-dose inhaler	Tachycardia, ventricular dysrhythmias

Drug name	Category	Indications	Quantity/dose	Side effects
Glucose source	Antihypoglycemic	Hypoglycemia secondary to diabetes mellitus or fasting hypoglycemia in the conscious patient	Orange juice, non-diet soda, Gatorade, glucose gel, icing/frosting	Not for use in patients without active gag reflex or unable to drink without assistance
Aspirin	Platelet aggregation inhibitor	Suspected myocardial infarction (MI) or unstable angina	Powdered or chewable aspirin (325 mg)	Not indicated for patients with aspirin allergy, predisposition to major hemorrhage, recent bleeding peptic ulcer

- Patient's signature authorizing the release of information, dentist's signature, dental office's address, phone number, fax number, and email address

23.3.1 Surgical Risk Assessment

No one can "clear" a patient for surgery. Being "cleared" for surgery implies there is no risk. The provider should evaluate the risks and benefits of a procedure and discuss these with the patient prior to any procedure.

23.4 Most Common Medical Conditions and the Necessary Precautions

A thorough review of the patient's medical history and a complete list of medications are necessary prior to dental treatment. These should all be noted in the patient chart. Medical consults where appropriate should be completed as well to insure safety of the patient. The following is meant as a guideline for the most common medical conditions that a patient may present with (Table 23.2).

Table 23.2 Most common medical considerations (Little 2013; Malamed 2015)

The American Society of Anesthesiologists (ASA) classification	ASA I	Normal healthy patient
	ASA II	Patient with mild systemic disease. No significant impact on daily activity; unlikely to have an impact on anesthesia and surgery (mild asthma, well-controlled hypertension (HTN))
	ASA III	Patient with significant or severe systemic disease that limits daily activity. Significant impact on daily activity; probable impact on anesthesia and surgery (hemodialysis, class 2 heart failure)
	ASA IV	Patient with severe systemic disease that is a constant threat to life or that requires intensive therapy. Serious limitation of daily activity; likely major impact on anesthesia and surgery (acute MI, respiratory failure requiring mechanical ventilation)
	ASA V	Moribund patient not expected to survive the next 24 h
Stress reduction guidelines	Normal, healthy, anxious patient (ASA 1): Recognize patient's level of anxiety Consider premedication the evening prior to the operation Consider premedication immediately before appointment Schedule morning appointments Short appointments Minimize patient's wait time Consider sedation during therapy Administer adequate pain control during therapy Follow up with postop pain and anxiety control Telephone patient later the same day that treatment was delivered Medical-risk patient (ASA 2, 3, 4): Recognize patient's degree of medical risk Consider medical consultation before dental therapy Schedule morning appointments Short appointments Monitor and record preop and postop vitals Consider sedation during therapy Administer adequate pain control during therapy Follow up with postop pain and anxiety control Telephone patient later the same day that treatment was delivered	
Cardiovascular disease	Limit dental care in patient with low metabolic equivalent	
	Emergency dental care: benefit received by intervention outweighs the risk of cardiovascular complications: pain relief, treatment of infection, hemostasis	
	Limit use of epinephrine	
	Have nitroglycerine on hand	

Blood pressure	**Classification**	**Systolic**	**Diastolic**
	Normal	<120	<80
	Prehypertension	120–139	80–89
	Stage 1 hypertension	140–159	90–99
	Stage 2 hypertension	≥160	≥100
Hypertension guidelines	Preoperative: Measure blood pressure (BP) and review health history and medications Refer/encourage patient to see physician if BP is elevated Minimize stress, consider oral sedative BP less than 180/110 and no evidence of target organ involvement (encephalopathy, MI, unstable angina), dental treatment can be provided BP greater than 180/110, defer elective dental care and refer to physician Operative: Profound local anesthesia Patients on nonselective beta blocker, limit epinephrine to 2 cartridges of 1:100,000 epinephrine Avoid epinephrine-containing retraction cord Intraoperative monitoring of BP for patients with stage 1 or higher HTN Postoperative: Make slow changes in chair position to prevent orthostatic hypotension Ensure stable vitals prior to dismissal Record pre- and postop vitals		
Allergic reactions	Clinical manifestations:		
	Type I: anaphylactic Response time: 1–30 min	Depends on portal of entry; Hives (localized cutaneous swellings), allergic rhinitis and conjunctivitis (nasal or conjunctival discharge), food allergy (bronchial asthma, hay fever, allergic gastroenteritis) Look for pruritus (itching), flushing, urticaria (rash), angioedema, rhinorrhea, wheezing, weakness, dizziness, dyspnea (difficulty breathing), dysphagia (difficulty swallowing) Timing of treatment is critical due to sudden onset and rapidly progressing and often life-threatening	
	Type II: cytotoxic Response time: minutes to hours	Necrosis Examples: pemphigus, transfusion reactions from mismatched blood type and rhesus incompatibility	
	Type III: immune complex mediated Response time: 3–8 h	Erythema, necrosis Examples: lupus erythematosus, renal glomeruli and synovial membrane	
	Type IV: cell mediated (delayed) Response time: 48–72 h	Erythema, induration Examples: tuberculosis testing, contact dermatitis, drug hypersensitivity, transplant rejection, graft-versus-host reaction	

Respiratory disorders	Asthma	*Preoperative:*
		Minimize stress
		Determine past triggers of attacks
		Have patient bring inhaler(s) to appointment
		Review all medications and potential interactions
		For moderate to severe asthmatics, consider use of inhaler prophylactically
		Operative:
		Avoid triggers
		Monitor vitals, recognize signs of difficulty breathing, tachypnea, etc.
		Sedation: N_2O or short-acting benzodiazepines. Avoid barbiturates and opiates because they may cause asthmatic events in some patients
		Be prepared to manage emergency:
		Stop care (remove rubber dam and comfortably position patient)
		Administer inhaler
		Oxygen 2–3 L/min
		Administer epinephrine if needed
		Activate EMS
		Consider referral/transport of patient
		Postoperative:
		Avoid macrolide (erythromycin) and clindamycin if patient takes theophylline (methylxanthine) as it may lead to toxicity
		Avoid aspirin, nonsteroidal anti-inflammatory drugs (NSAIDs), barbiturates and local anesthetic with sulfites (may trigger attack)
	Chronic obstructive pulmonary disease (COPD): chronic bronchitis and emphysema	Airflow limitation associated with abnormal inflammatory response of the lungs Chronic bronchitis: chronic productive cough of at least 3 months during 2 consecutive years Emphysema: abnormal permanent enlargement of the respiratory bronchioles and alveoli accompanied by the destruction of the alveolar septa Dental management: If orthopnea is present, use semi-supine position to avoid respiratory distress Consider use of pulse oximeter Limit use of local anesthetic with vasoconstrictor if patient has tachycardia or hypertension Avoid rubber dam in severely compromised patients Consider use of O_2 N_2O is contraindicated in patients with severe COPD or emphysema Avoid medications that cause respiratory depression (narcotics and barbiturates) Low-dose benzodiazepines may be used with caution if sedation is required Assess the presence of adrenal suppression and insufficiency in patients using corticosteroids Avoid macrolide (erythromycin) and clindamycin if patient takes theophylline (methylxanthine) as it may lead to toxicity

Metabolic diseases	Diabetes mellitus	Diagnostic tests: Fasting blood sugar (current control): >126 mg/dL Random plasma glucose: >200 mg/dL with symptoms (polyuria, polydipsia, unexplained weight loss) 2 h plasma glucose: >200 mg/dL following a 75 g glucose load Glycated hemoglobin (HbA1C): <7 % – good control; 7–9 % – fair control; >9 % – poor control During dental treatment: Patient should have eaten a balanced meal within the last 2 h before coming to the dental appointment Patient should have taken their medications Balanced nutritional supplement should be available if appointment lasts longer than 2 h Early morning appointments HbA1C prior to surgical therapy Consult/refer to physician if poorly controlled Consider postoperative antibiotics for surgical procedure with HbA1C >9 % Avoid aspirin and aspirin-containing medications which may increase insulin secretion and potentiate action of sulfonylurea drugs
	Adrenal gland disorders	Routine dental procedures (nonsurgical): Patients with current or past history of corticosteroids: no supplementation, obtain profound local anesthesia and postop pain control Patients on topical or inhalation corticosteroids: no supplementation Surgical procedures: Consider medical consult 25 mg hydrocortisone for minor surgical procedures, administer preoperatively the day of surgery Monitor blood pressure throughout the procedure Profound local anesthesia and postop pain control
	Thyroid disorders	Well-controlled hypothyroidism or hyperthyroidism does not require special precautions for routine or emergency dental treatment in the absence of comorbidities Undiagnosed, untreated, or poorly controlled hypothyroidism or hyperthyroidism: elective dental care should be deferred until the disease is controlled Epinephrine or other pressor amines should be avoided in untreated or poorly controlled hyperthyroidism as it can increase symptoms of tachycardia, dyspnea, and fatigue Hyperthyroid crisis: terminate dental procedure, cool patient with cold towels or ice packs, administer hydrocortisone (100–300 mg, IM or IV), monitor patient's vital signs, and be prepared to begin CPR

Gastrointestinal disease	Inflammatory bowel disease (Crohn's disease and ulcerative colitis): Most patients with IBD have intermittent attacks, with asymptomatic remissions between attacks. Elective treatment should be scheduled during periods of remission Patients may be taking corticosteroids or immunosuppressant drugs that can affect oral health and dental management Routine dental procedures do not require supplemental corticosteroids, obtain profound local anesthesia and postop pain control Major surgical procedures: consider medical consult, supplement corticosteroids, monitor blood pressure throughout the procedure, obtain profound local anesthesia and postop pain control Blood values should be obtained and reviewed for patients who take immunosuppressant drugs (methotrexate) prior to invasive procedures Postop pain control: acetaminophen with or without opioids can be used. Avoid prescribing additional opioids to patients taking these medications to manage intestinal pain
Liver disease	Common liver disorders: viral hepatitis, alcoholic liver disease Increased risk for impaired drug metabolism, significant bleeding complications Dental drugs metabolized primarily by the liver: Lidocaine Mepivicaine Prilocaine Bupivacaine Aspirin Acetaminophen Codeine Meperidine (Demerol) Ibuprofen Diazepam Barbiturates Ampicillin Tetracycline Metronidazole Vancomycin Consider antibiotic prophylaxis in patients with severe liver disease
Renal disease	*End-stage renal disease:* Consider consult Avoid elective dental treatment if poorly controlled or advanced stage Screen for bleeding disorder before surgery Monitor blood pressure closely Avoid nephrotoxic drugs Aminoglycosides Acetaminophen in high doses Acyclovir Aspirin NSAIDs Aggressively manage orofacial infections with antibiotics (dosage may need to be adjusted) *Hemodialysis patients:* Consider prophylaxis if abscess is present Avoid dental care on day of treatment (best to treat day after) Avoid blood pressure cuff and intravenous (IV) medications in arm with shunt Consider corticosteroid supplementation if indicated

Hematology	Anticoagulation guidelines	Coumadin/Warfarin: Routine dental treatment: Ensure regular monitoring every 4–6 weeks Patients on short-term therapy, consider waiting until cessation of therapy Surgical procedures: Confirm INR <3.5 within 48 h of surgery Minimize trauma Apply local hemostatic agents (Gelfoam, surgical) Place sutures if needed Place gauze with pressure (soaked with Amicar) Postoperative management: Avoid ASA, NSAIDs, use acetaminophen Control hemorrhage before dismissing patient Antibiotics may affect anticoagulation Give clear and complete postop instructions
	Sickle cell anemia	Antibiotic prophylaxis for major surgical procedures Avoid strong narcotics and high doses of salicylates. Use acetaminophen with or without small doses of codeine Use local anesthetic without epinephrine for routine dental care. For surgical procedures, use 1:100,000 epinephrine in local anesthetic. Avoid general anesthesia if hemoglobin level is below 10 g/dL Consider consult with physician before surgical procedures are performed
		Avoid barbiturates and strong narcotics; recommend sedation with midazolam Nitrous oxide should have oxygen at greater than 50 % with high flow rate and good ventilation Use pulse oximeter and maintain oxygen saturation above 95 % Treat acute infection with incision and drainage if indicated, high doses of antibiotics will help avoid a crisis Avoid dehydration If sickling crisis occurs, hospitalization is indicated
	Coagulation factor deficiencies (hemophilias, von Willebrand disease, thrombocytopenia, functional inadequacies of platelets)	Work closely with hematologist Be familiar with type and severity of disease Use block anesthesia with caution Never prescribe aspirin Protect soft tissue Surgical procedure: Prevention of anticipated bleeding Consult hematologist and describe specific treatment Obtain adequate factor replacement as needed Use antifibrinolytic agents as necessary Use local hemostatic measures Close follow up to monitor bleeding

	Leukemia and lymphoma	Patient with white blood cell count less than 2000 μL or a neutrophil count less than 500 μL should have antibiotic prophylaxis when invasive dental procedures are performed (recommend penicillin VK). Antifungal medications for oral candidiasis Mucositis should be treated with chlorhexidine rinse, bland mouth rinses, antihistamine solutions, and topical anesthetic gel
		If platelet count is less than 50,000 μL, platelet transfusion may be needed before invasive and surgical procedures. Consider medical consult Patients on radiation and chemotherapy should have medical consult to determine if cardiac damage is present Bone marrow transplant patients on cyclosporine may develop gingival hyperplasia
Immunology	Rheumatoid arthritis	Use stress reduction guidelines Allergic reactions or lichenoid reactions are possible in patients taking many medications Excessive bleeding may occur with major surgery if patients take aspirin or NSAIDs. Control with local hemostatic measures Obtain blood cell count prior to surgery on patients taking gold salts, penicillamine, antimalarials, or immunosuppressives Assess risk for adrenal suppression and insufficiency
	Systemic lupus erythematosus (SLE)	Determine diagnosis of SLE (onset, duration, severity, and organ involvement) Assess risk for adrenal suppression and insufficiency Consider antibiotic prophylaxis for patients taking cytotoxic and immunosuppressive drugs
	Organ transplants	Pretransplantation: Medical consult Consider postponing elective dental treatment Rule out dental infection sources Posttransplantation: No elective dental treatment immediately posttransplant, medical consult for emergency care At risk for oral mucosal disease and oral infections Assess risk for adrenal suppression and insufficiency Posttransplantation chronic rejection period: Only emergency treatment

Infectious disease	Human immunodeficiency virus/acquired immune deficiency syndrome (HIV/AIDS) guidelines	Oral manifestation of immunosuppression: Oral yeast infections Viral infections Periodontal problems Poor healing and bone sequestration following extractions Diagnostic tests: T cell count (CD4+) Viral load Complete blood count (CBC) with differential for platelet count and white count Dental procedures: HIV infection normal lab values, no special precautions needed Universal precautions are adequate Signs and symptoms of immunosuppression, refer to immunosuppression protocols Review medications to prevent drug interactions
Neurologic conditions	Seizure disorders	Determine nature, severity, control, and stability of disease Well-controlled seizure disorders pose no specific management problems Good pain control and anesthesia to avoid stress Stress reduction protocol Increased bleeding in patients taking valproic acid (Depakene) or carbamazepine (Tegretol) Monitor blood pressure; it may increase or decrease with the onset of a seizure Recommend consult to determine the level of control from physician Patients on anticonvulsant drugs may experience drowsiness, slow mentation, and dizziness Be prepared for occurrence of a grand mal seizure: Consider placing ligated mouth prop at the beginning of procedure Position chair in supported supine position During a seizure: Clear the area Turn patient to side (to avoid aspiration) Do not attempt to use a padded tongue blade Passively restrain After a seizure: Examine for traumatic injuries Discontinue treatment, arrange for patient transport Most seizures are self-limited but may progress to cardiac arrest, necessitating emergency treatment; call 911

	Stroke	Avoid use of metronidazole and tetracyclines in patients taking warfarin (Coumadin) because of its decreased metabolism Achieve good pain control, limit anesthetic with epinephrine to 2 carpules; avoid retraction cord with epinephrine Avoid aspirin and NSAIDs (increase postop bleeding), use acetaminophen instead
		Patients taking anticoagulant or antiplatelet therapy are at increased risk for bleeding: Aspirin ± dipyridamole (Aggrenox), clopidogrel (Plavix), abciximab (ReoPro), or ticlopidine (Ticlid) Coumadin: pretreatment international normalized ratio (INR) $\leq$ 3.5 Heparin IV: palliative emergency dental care only Heparin subcutaneous (low molecular weight), no changes required Use measures to minimize hemorrhage (atraumatic surgery, pressure, Gelfoam, suturing). Additional steps should be taken to achieve hemostasis in patients on an anticoagulant or antiplatelet therapy Monitor blood pressure and oxygen saturation throughout the procedure Only emergency dental procedures should be done within 6 months of transient ischemic attack (TIA), reversible ischemic neurologic deficit (RIND), or stroke. Recognize signs and symptoms of a stroke, provide emergency care, and activate EMS system as needed
	Parkinson's disease	Well-controlled Parkinson's disease does not pose management problems Provide good pain control No need for antibiotic prophylaxis Stress reduction protocols No bleeding problems are expected Monitor blood pressure (dopamine may cause hypotension) Consider consult with physician to establish level of control of disease Anticholinergic and dopamine agonist drugs have adverse effects of sedation, drowsiness, slow mentation, fatigue, confusion, and dizziness Tremors are usually self-limiting, but movement disturbance may interfere with dental treatment
	Alzheimer's disease or other dementias	Well-controlled Alzheimer's disease/dementia does not require change of treatment plan Patients with untreated or poorly controlled disease may have difficulty understanding commands or instructions; use stress reduction protocol Monitor blood pressure (some medications may cause hypotension) Patients on anticholinergic drugs may experience sedation, drowsiness, slow mentation, fatigue, confusion, and dizziness Discuss treatment plan and consent forms with next of kin if possible

<table>
<tr><td rowspan="5">Infective endocarditis prevention guidelines</td><td colspan="4">The American Heart Association only recommends antibiotic prophylaxis for the highest risk category which includes the following (updated April 2015):
A prosthetic heart valve or who have had a heart valve repaired with prosthetic material.
A history of endocarditis
A heart transplant with abnormal heart valve function
Certain congenital heart defects including:
Cyanotic congenital heart disease (birth defects with oxygen levels lower than normal), which has not been fully repaired, including children who have had a surgical shunts and conduits.
A congenital heart defect that has been completely repaired with prosthetic material or a device for the first six months after the repair procedure.
Repaired congenital heart disease with residual defects, such as persisting leaks or abnormal flow at or adjacent to a prosthetic patch or prosthetic device.</td></tr>
<tr><td></td><td>Antibiotic</td><td>Adults</td><td>Children</td></tr>
<tr><td>Oral</td><td>Amoxicillin</td><td>2 g</td><td>50 mg/kg</td></tr>
<tr><td>Unable to take oral medication</td><td>Ampicillin
Cefazolin or Ceftriazone</td><td>2 g IM or IV
1 g IM or IV</td><td>50 mg/kg IM or IV
50 mg/kg IM or IV</td></tr>
<tr><td>Allergic to penicillin or ampicillin (oral)</td><td>Cephalexin
Clindamycin
Azithromycin or Clarithromycin</td><td>2 g
600 mg
500 mg</td><td>50 mg/kg
20 mg/kg
15 mg/kg</td></tr>
<tr><td></td><td>Allergic to penicillin or ampicillin and unable to take oral medications</td><td>Cefazolin or Ceftriazone
Clindamycin phosphate</td><td>1 g IM or IV
600 mg IM or IV</td><td>50 mg/kg IM or IV
20 mg/kg IM or IV</td></tr>
<tr><td>Prosthetic joint antibiotic prophylaxis guidelines</td><td colspan="4">Recommendations from american academy of orthopaedic surgeons/ american dental association (AAOS/ADA) Clinical Practice Guideline (December 2012):
The practitioner might consider discontinuing the practice of routinely prescribing prophylactic antibiotics for patients with hip and knee prosthetic joint implants undergoing dental procedures
Consider prophylaxis only for "at-risk" patients
Immunocompromised/immunesuppressed
Rheumatoid arthritis
Systemic lupus
Disease-, drug-, or radiation-induced immunosuppression
Insulin-dependent diabetes
First 2 years following joint replacement
Malnourishment
Hemophilia
Suggested antibiotic prophylaxis:
Patient not allergic to penicillin: cephalexin, cefradine, or amoxicillin: 2 g orally 30 min to 1 h before the dental procedure
Patient not allergic to penicillin and unable to take oral medications: cefazolin or ampicillin: cefazolin 1 g or ampicillin 2 g intramuscularly or intravenously 30 min to 1 h before dental procedure
Patient allergic to penicillin: clindamycin 600 mg orally 30 min to 1 h before dental procedure
Patient allergic to penicillin and unable to take oral medications: clindamycin 600 mg intravenously 30 min to 1 h before the dental procedure</td></tr>
</table>

References

American Heart Association. The ISSN register. 2015. https://eccguidelines.heart.org/index.php/circulation/cpr-ecc-guidelines-2/part-1-executive-summary/. Accessed on 12 Feb 2016

Little F. The dental management of the medically compromised patient. 8th ed. St. Louis: Mosby; 2013.

Malamed SF. Medical emergencies in the dental office. 7th ed. St. Louis: Mosby; 2015.

Part IV

Pathways of a Dental Career

Private Practice

24

Annelise Ydstebo Driscoll

Contents

Abstract

Outside of choosing the dental school to attend and accumulating the associated debt load, the next most important decision for a graduating dentist is that of which career path to follow. There are many options such as the public health sector, the military sector, the nonprofit sector, the federal sector, the corporate sector, or buying and opening a dental office right out of school. This chapter will discuss the choice of the dental associate in a private practice setting as the postgraduate preferred choice. It will provide information on where associate opportunities can be found, the two classifications of associates, the expectations of both new associate and owner dentist, and review various portions of the agreement provisions for new associates. Lastly, it will provide insight into factors to consider for a successful associateship experience and resources for further knowledge.

A.Y. Driscoll, MBA, PhD
Department of Restorative Dental Sciences, University of Florida, College of Dentistry, Gainesville, FL, USA
e-mail: adriscoll@dental.ufl.edu

G.M. Weinstein, M.T. Zientz (eds.), *The Dental Reference Manual*,
DOI 10.1007/978-3-319-39730-6_24

24.1 Defining a Dental Associate

According to the American Student Dental Association (ASDA 2015), a dental associate is "a non-owner dentist who works in a dental practice." As a dental student graduates from dental school, they seek to enter the dental workforce through many different options and opportunities. With becoming a dental practice owner aside, most dental student graduates will become dental associates in various areas of the dental industry, as nonowners. It is the next phase, and entryway into beginning their careers by working on patients in "real-life" dental facilities. It can be said to also be the easiest choice as it does not increase a new dentist's debt load or financial burden. Increased debt loads through school loans, along with the need to build up their clinical skills in new settings, make the career option of a dental associate an attractive one. Working for someone else, or some other dental facility, postgraduation, can facilitate an easy transition from dental school to dental practice. Therefore, nonowner dental associates are a popular choice, as seen by a recent survey conducted by the American Dental Education Association, otherwise referred to hereafter as ADEA (ADEA 2013).

24.1.1 Two Types of Associate Classification

According to the Internal Revenue Service (IRS 2015b), there are two types of classifications for all workers (including the position of dental associate). The IRS provides specific criteria that must be followed to be classified as one of the two categories: employee or independent contractor (IRS 2015b). There are three different areas of control that are discussed further in the Role of the IRS section below that provide further assistance in determining which classification an associate dentist would, or could, be considered as.

- *Employee* associate classification:
  - As an associate employee, the associate is an employee of the dental practice, subject to the policies, protocols, benefits, and legal protections (local, state, and federal) that any other employee of the dental practice would be subjected to. The dentist owner of the practice is the employer and as such will deduct all appropriate taxes from the associate employee's paycheck and submit them to the appropriate government agencies, on behalf of all of the employees.
  - The associate dentist receives a paycheck that has had the necessary payroll taxes withheld and receives the amount that is left, post-tax. The associate dentist signs an IRS (Internal Revenue Service) W4 form on the first day of work in the dental practice and indicates whether they are taxed as a single person, married person, and how many deductions they will be taking, which ultimately affects the amount of taxes withheld from the associate's paycheck.
- *Independent contractor* associate classification
  - As an independent contractor, the associate is their own business owner, in a sense, and is considered self-employed. As such, they would be paying their own estimated payroll taxes to the appropriate government agencies throughout

various times of the year. This requires an investment of time to study the tax laws and regulations that a small business owner (as an independent contractor) would need to know to submit the appropriate type of payroll-related taxes and the correct amount to submit, as well as to which government agency.

- As a self-employed associate, the independent contractor would contract with a dental practice to provide services for a specified fee or percentage. They would complete a W9 form on the first day of work with the contracted dental practice. This would normally be detailed in a written agreement of terms. This type of associate would act independently, as opposed to being a supervised employee associate. An associate independent contractor acts as their own employer of their own business and can incorporate to protect themselves. They will and should purchase and/or provide all of the benefits for themselves, as their own employer. Therefore, they will not be protected by state and federal employment laws as an employee would be in a dental practice. The associate must make arrangements for their own insurances and benefits.

- Roles of IRS (Internal Revenue Service)
  - The IRS Form SS-8 (entitled *Determination of Worker Status for Purposes of Federal Employment Taxes and Income Tax Withholding*) (IRS 2015a) can be found online and can be completed by an associate dentist if they are not sure how they are classified as an employee or independent contractor, or if they have potentially been misclassified.
  - The IRS reviews three criteria to determine whether an individual is, or should be, classified as an employee or independent contractor in their Publication 1779 (IRS 2015b). The three criteria involve which party has ultimate control over specific aspects of behavior, financials, and relationships of the worker (associate) to the firm (dental employer/owner).
  - *Behavioral control examples:* (A) The independent contractor associate controls the work environment and services performed, their work schedule, and their work is generally unsupervised as they are their own business entity. They are autonomous, independent, and usually supply their own labor, such as dental assistants, laptop with dental software or individual patient charts separate from the practice's patient charts, and bring their own supplies to perform their work. (B) The employee associate is usually supervised and does not have autonomy in the work environment or with their schedule, may be given training and direction, and is provided all equipment, tools, and supplies needed to perform their work as a supervised employee of the dental practice by the practice owner/employer (IRS 2015b).
  - *Financial control examples:* (A) The independent contractor associate pays/supplies their own equipment used to perform dental services. Additionally, they pay or supply the materials, consumables, and tools used to provide their dental services to patients. They also determine their fee schedules and get paid directly from patients, and in many instances, lease or rent the space they provide their dental services in. (B) The employee associate generally does not determine the fees, nor collects the fees for services provided, nor pays for any material costs to provide the services to patients, including lab fees (IRS 2015b).

  - *Relationship between the worker to the firm examples*: (A) An independent contractor associate/worker would not receive benefits from the dental practice such as sick days, vacation days, insurance benefits, and would have a direct relationship with the customer/patient. The independent contractor associate/worker would be able to terminate the relationship with the firm/dental practice without penalty and would be able to advertise themselves as independent contractor associates without interference or geographic limitations from the firm/dental practice. (B) The employee associate/worker would be entitled to receive the benefits as the other employees of the firm/dental practice do and would need to give notice of leave, or termination, according to the terms in the written agreement. The employee associate/worker would generally have other staff members that would establish the initial contact with the customer/patient, gather information, schedule an appointment, etc. directly, before the employee associate meets or sees the customer/patient. Once again, the relational autonomy of the associate/worker with the firm/dental practice would become part of the consideration of how to properly classify the associate as either an employee or independent contractor (IRS 2015b).
- Role of the Department of Labor: While the IRS oversees the classification of workers, the Department of Labor (DOL 2016) oversees how workers get compensated and whether or not they are considered salaried, hourly, and/or exempt from overtime pay. This is regulated through the DOL's Wage and Hour Division (DOL 2016) and only relates to associates as employees of a dental practice. It does not oversee independent contractors' compensation unless they were incorrectly misclassified as an independent contractor when they met the criteria for, and should have been classified as, an associate employee.
- Misclassifying employees can be a costly mistake, therefore, careful consideration and abidance to the criteria for employee or independent contractor, as regulated by the IRS, is necessary to avoid an adverse event such as an audit or complaint response.
- Role of state dental practice act
  - Each state has its own dental practice act with laws and rules that govern dentistry within the state. Dentist associates, whether employees or independent contractors, must read and abide by the rules and regulations of the Board of Dentistry of the respective state they are practicing dentistry in. It is important for all dentists, especially those just beginning their careers, to understand the laws and rules governing dentistry for the state(s) they plan on practicing dentistry in, *before* they begin practicing (Driscoll 2014).

24.2 Seeking Out Associateships

A 2013a, b, c, d, e ADEA Survey Study of Dental School Seniors (ADEA 2013a) indicated that the top three reasons for pursuing dentistry as a career were:

1. Control of work schedule
2. Service to others
3. Self-employment

Since control of work schedule and self-employment refer to the eventuality of private practice ownership, this would lead us to believe that a dentist associate in this sector is the preference of graduating seniors. This can further be substantiated by viewing the average debt of graduating dental students in 2013 for all schools as $215,145 (ADEA 2013b). The survey indicated that 49.9 % of the 2013 graduating dental seniors stated their perceptions of preparedness for practice administration as underprepared (ADEA, 2013c), which would make the learning experience gained through a dental associate position within a private practice valuable. This, then, supports the survey's findings of 50.5 % of graduating dental seniors' immediate plans upon graduation, intended to become employed as a private practice dentist (ADEA 2013d). The dental associate in the private practice setting appears to be a valuable and intended career choice, according to the respondents. Potentially, it could be said to be the most attractive choice for 67.8 % of the respondents in the ADEA survey (ADEA 2013e); as the associate dentist in private practice.

24.2.1 Where to Find Associate Opportunities

- Dental school vendor representative liaison
  - Each dental school has relationships with dental supply vendors. In many cases, there are representatives from the dental supply vendors whose job is to be the liaison between the senior graduating dental students and senior dentist owners within the surrounding communities (who are looking for new dental associates). These dental school vendor representative liaisons can be of great service, usually at no charge to the graduating dental student, in facilitating introductions to senior dentists in private practices looking for new associates (Pritchett 2015).
- Dental school associate placement service
  - Many dental schools have an associate matching program or associate placement service that is provided to senior dental students and/or residents at no charge. There may be a link to their dental school's website for senior owner dentists to upload their information as to what they are looking for or what they can offer new dental associates. The site may also allow graduating senior dental students to upload their own information on what type of practice they're looking for and geographic areas of preference (UFCD 2015).
- Local, state, national dental society/association meetings, and newsletters
  - There are two main national dental organizations that list associateship positions within their magazines and/or newsletters; the American Dental Association and the Academy of General Dentistry. As a member of either or both, one can view the listed positions open seeking dental associates and

contact the senior owner dentist looking for a new associate in their private practice (Driscoll 2014).
  - From a state perspective, each state within the United States of America has a state dental organization that also publishes newsletters which contain listed positions for new associateships. Membership in a state dental association would allow the receipt of the publications with listed associateships offered.
  - Locally, there are regions, such as counties or affiliate regions, within each state, that are organized as dental societies. They also send out publications where associateship opportunities are listed. Membership in local dental societies would allow the access to the listed associateships offered and chances to network with prospective dental owners (ADA 2007).
- Dental networking alumni associations
  - There are affiliations, networking events, and activities that take place in person where there may be an ability to create relationships that lead to associateship opportunities. These can be held at annual conferences, state or regional dental meetings, and "alumni association and friends" meetings and their offered annual events. Dental school alumni associations are advantageous places to network as the dental philosophies are more likely to be aligned, coming from the same dental school. There may be chapters of alumni all over the country which would be advantageous for a young potential associate to join and network in.
  - Networking opportunities at pro bono events such as Mission of Mercy, Dentistry from the Heart, Give Kids a Smile, and Smile Train are also opportunities to build relationships and network with dentists that may know of other dentists who are looking for like-minded associates.
  - Take advantage of every opportunity to network within the surrounding areas in which there is a desire to practice as an associate. Introduce yourself to all dentists at events to facilitate and utilize the benefits of a networking opportunity.
- Websites
  - There are dental-specific websites that may list dental associateship opportunities in private practice, group practice, and corporate practice settings as well. They can be found at:
  - www.indeed.com by populating the "what" field with dentist and the "where" field with the practice location of choice (Indeed 2015).
  - www.dentalpost.net and viewing the post a job or find a job section (Dental Post, Inc. 2015)
  - www.ziprecruiter.com which pulls resumes/CVs from over 100 job websites (ZipRecruiter 2015)
  - www.dentalworkers.com which also pulls resumes/CVs from an array of websites (Dentalworkers.net 2015)
  - www.monster.com which is a long-standing, traditional job posting site (Monster Worldwide 2015)
  - www.careerbuilder.com which is also a long-standing, traditional job posting site (Careerbuilder, LLC. 2015)
  - www.dentaljobs.net and register free to post your CV or view open positions (Dentaljobs.Net 2015)

- Proactive approaches (Driscoll 2014)
  - Create a cover letter of introduction which highlights all of the strengths, both clinically and professionally, that the associate has, as well as what the associate will be able to bring (of value) to the practice. Example: family, friends, and established community of patients to bring to the practice that the associate works in. Include in the cover letter a trajectory of what future continuing education coursework/skills are of interest in the continued seeking of "life-long learning."
  - Create an updated and competitive curriculum vitae (CV) or resume that highlights clinical expertise, areas of focus (infant oral health, implants, CAD/CAM, etc.), plus the procedures the associate is particularly proficient in and enjoys performing, as well as professional network memberships. Include all of the continuing education courses and electives attended, seminars, conferences, and meetings.
  - Send out the cover letters and CVs/resumes to any and all dental practices within the different regions that the associate is interested in practicing. Follow up with phone calls to the owner dentists of each practice to try to facilitate a phone conversation if there is interest in bringing an associate on board.
  - If no interest currently exists currently, but may in the future, resend an updated cover letter of introduction plus an updated CV/resume a few months later to stay on the forefront of the minds of the dentist that the associate is a proactive professional.
  - When visiting new towns or areas of interest to practice in, the associate can also stop in and visit the dental practices and introduce themselves to the staff. Seeing if the dentist is available for a personal introduction is another proactive way to continue to reach out and facilitate opportunities and relationships that may not have been available before. It is recommended to bring copies of CVs and Resumes on hand when traveling for this purpose alone.
  - Keeping both a hard paper copy as well as a digital copy of an associate's cover letter and CV/resume to proactively send out can send a message to an owner dentist that the associate is confident, organized, personal (yet professional), and proactive. All of those characteristics may be viewed as favorable to the recipients and can make an associate stand out from others wanting a position but not taking a proactive approach.

24.3 Expectations of Associateships

There are very different expectations that can be seen between new associates and senior dentists. It is important to understand the expectations of both parties to create the best possibility of the success of the associateship (Pace 2015). Open, clear, fair, and transparent communication is needed, along with an understanding of the different expectations both parties have, prior to entering into any associateship agreement (Dulde 2012). Since all associateships eventually end (through death, disability, buy-in, buyout, termination, or leave of position), it is worthwhile to discuss not just the initial expectations of both parties but the short-term and long-term goals and expectations for both, as soon as possible. This will assist in creating a "best fit" for the new associate as well as the senior dentist. If the agreements or arrangements made in the documented contract lack transparency and fairness to both parties, then the associateship will almost certainly become problematic. This will then tend to lead to the likelihood of the associateship failing.

- *Why Associateships Fail*, by Roger Levin – according to Roger Levin of the Levin Group (Levin 2002):
- "The primary reason Associateships do not work…the practice is unprepared for the Associate….(who) is brought into a chaotic practice…stressed by a high volume of patients or lack of clear systems." That being said, it is worthwhile to consider that there may be different expectations of new associates versus senior dentists' expectations, therefore, it is important to discuss them early on to avoid a negative experience for either party.
- Expectations of a new associate (Driscoll 2014)
  - The senior dentist has adequately planned and prepared for taking on an associate.
  - The dental practice has enough new patients and sufficient patient base to keep a new associate busy and productive.
  - The patient flow shows that clear systems are in place for how the practice operates.
  - The dental practice is financially stable and has been growing steadily for some documented periods of time to necessitate the addition of an associate.
  - The compensation structure is specific, quantified, and clearly communicated to the associate in the written agreement, so the associate can count on a clear income which pays their monthly expenses and debt load.
  - New associates enjoy being mentored. There may be a desire or a capability for the senior dentist to mentor the new associate, where needed and/or desired.
  - The new associate will be marketed to both the staff and to patients and introductions facilitated by the senior dentist.
  - There is sufficient growth potential for the new associate and stability of the work hours as well as compensation and incentives.
  - There is sufficient staffing levels in the practice to assist, schedule, bill, etc. for services provided by the new associate.
  - Work-life balance may be an important expectation of new associates.
  - The potential for buy-in into the practice may be a desire of an associate.
  - Some associates do not want to buy in and would prefer to be employees only, for prolonged periods of time, without taking on the additional debt and responsibility of ownership.
- Expectations of senior dentist/dentist owner (Driscoll 2014)
  - The associate will bring/add value to the practice and will develop a patient pool on their own or bring patients with them to the practice from the associate's networks, family, friends, or community.
  - The associate will be able to work independently, autonomously, and confidently, with some capability to consult with the senior dentist on more complex cases.

- The associate has clinical proficiency and experience that translates into the production of quality dental procedures of varying types, able to be performed thoroughly and confidently.
- The associate will market themselves through becoming entrenched into the surrounding community to increase patient referrals to the practice.
- The associate will keep up with skills and trends through the taking of continuing education courses that enhance the services offered to patients of the practice.
- The associate is willing to accept or become contracted with insurance companies.
- There may be a desire from the senior dentist for the associate to buy into or buy-out the dental practice with the senior dentist continuing to work at the practice.
- The senior dentist may want the associate to begin part time and build up their patient base to work full time without having to fully commit to a specified compensation growth structure.

24.4 Reviewing Contracts for Associateships

All associateships, regardless of their classification, should be clearly and specifically stated in writing to clarify the agreement between the parties. While some basic components of associateship agreements are discussed below, they do not represent all of the components of an associateship agreement (ADA 2007). Agreements will vary based on classification and state laws/rules/regulations plus the state's dental practice act.

- Basic sections of an associate agreement or contract:
  - *Parties:* Who the agreement includes and relates to, such as the associate, the dental practice, the legal entity, or the organization or others that are entering into the written agreement (ADA 2007).
  - *Term:* The term of the agreement to include the effective date, the start date, the end date, or the instant renewal of the agreement after the initial term ends (ADA 2007).
  - *Classification:* This usually indicates the classification of the associate as employee and the dental practice or senior dentist or dental facility as the employer or the associate independent contractor and the dental entity it is working with (not for) (IRS 2015a).
  - *Timeframes:* This area can include the trial period length, the associate time frame length of time, and the frame of time that the associate potentially phases in, or transitions, as a buyer into the practice (Driscoll 2014).
  - *Compensation structure and methodology:* This section usually outlines how the associate will be paid/compensated, what benefits may be provided (for associate employees only), when the associate will get paid, and how their compensation will be calculated. Some of the compensation structures are to be paid on a percentage of dental services provided to patients (otherwise known as production), to be paid on a percentage of dental services collected/paid for by patients/insurance (otherwise known as collections), to be paid a daily fee regardless of what amount of dental services are performed, to be paid a set

annual salary, or to be paid a draw against future earnings. For independent contractors, this section will highlight how much the associate will pay the practice for the use of their space/lease and overhead expenses, and/or a percentage of collected production collected by the independent contractor that will be paid to the dental practice, and at what interval of time (Driscoll 2014).

- *Work schedule:* This section usually includes an outline of the proposed schedule of days, times, hours, and hours per week of work that the employee associate will be expected to be at the dental practice providing dental services. This section would be minimal and would outline what days/times the independent contractor will be at the practice to provide services, but is decided and outlined by the independent contractor (IRS 2015b).
- *Expense Allocation:* This section usually discussed what percentage of overhead expenses and lease/rent which will be paid by the associate independent contractor to the dental practice and any other expenses the associate independent contractor may be asked to pay for providing dental services to the patients within the dental practice (e.g., utilities, staff leasing, etc.). Associate employees do not pay for work-related expenses, similar to other practice employees who would not pay for work-related expenses (IRS 2015).
- *Patient Base Allocation:* Here there is a discussion of how new and existing patients will be allocated between the new associate and senior dentist or other associates in the practice. If the new associate employee will be providing hygiene checks for other dentists, it may be specified here. If the new associate employee will be expected to contract with insurance companies to see the insured patients, then it would likely be clarified here. If there is an agreement that the new associate employee will be seeing only emergency patients, or a percentage of new patients, it might be stated here in this section. If the associate independent contractor is expected to generate and build their own patient base up on their own, then it would be stated in this section. Other new patients allocated to an independent contractor associate would be known as referrals from the senior dentist, as independent contractors are their own small businesses and separate legal entities (Dulde 2012).
- *Buy-in or buyout potential:* This area may discuss the possibility of the future of the relationship with the associate and whether there is a potential for a percentage buy-in into the dental practice or a full buyout of the senior dentist's ownership. There may also be included in this section, language on what may happen if the dental practice is sold while the associate is working there and whether or not the associate would have the first opportunity to buy it; and, if not interested, then have the "right of first refusal" to buy the dental practice. It may discuss what will happen regarding the transfer of ownership and how the agreement is handled, assigned, or voided, if that occurs (Fryer and Norton 2013).
- *Termination of Agreement:* This is where the reasons for termination of the agreement are stated, including reasons and time frames for which the associate employee dentist may be terminated, or the independent contractor agreement may be terminated. It also should discuss whether or not the agreement terminates automatically or is automatically renewed unless otherwise stated in writing by either party. There may be penalties or monetary losses that the associate may have to incur if they leave the dental practice, or end the

working relationship, without abiding by the agreed terms for termination. This should be a very clearly stated and understood section that should be read carefully to avoid any costly errors made by associates; whether employees or independent contractors (Driscoll 2014).

- Restrictive covenants, nonsolicitation, noncompete, and confidentiality clauses
- These are designed to prevent employee associates from working for direct competing dental practices in the same area, as well as limit the capability of an employee associate to solicit staff to work for them at other dental practices during or after they have worked for one dental practice. These covenants and clauses avoid conflict of interest and loss of patients or staff, if and when an associate dentist works for, and then leaves, a dental practice, to work for another dental practice. A restrictive covenant and noncompete clause may place a specific geographic limitation that an associate cannot work within at another dental practice and for what period of time. An example might be 3–5 miles from the existing practice that they currently work for. It may also state that the geographic limitation can be in effect for up to 1–3 years, for example, after the employee associate leaves the existing dental practice to work elsewhere. A nonsolicitation clause may limit or prevent the employee associate from enticing or taking patients, staff, vendors, or specialists away from the existing dental practice the employee associate works with after they separate from the existing dental practice. A confidentiality clause prevents the associate from discussing or disclosing to others any of the trade secrets, operational policies, financial processes, or protected information about the dental practice or its patients, staff, processes, procedures, to anyone outside of the dental practice (Driscoll 2014).
  - *Independent contractors* – There are generally no restrictive covenants nor noncompete clauses here in these agreements because the independent contractor is its own business entity and should be able to choose their customers (dental practices) without limitations, to sustain financial viability of their independent business. Independent contractors have the capability to be autonomous and may take the customer base/patient base that they have served, with them when they leave the dental practice they are contracted with. In other words, they have ownership of their patients' dental charts to take with them when they terminate the agreement. Independent contractors are generally subject to abiding by the restrictions set forth in confidentiality agreements. This is a very important distinction that should be carefully assessed, understood, and abided by for senior dentist owners, as stated within the IRS classifications for independent contractors.
  - *Employees* – There are generally restrictive covenants placed on associate employees, as well as noncompete clauses with limitations clearly stated. As an associate employee of a dental practice, the senior dental practice owner may place limitations on where the employee can work during and after the associate works for the dental practice. There may be limitations on how far away the employee may work, in miles, and for what specified period of time the restrictions and limitations may be in force. These are particularly common in associate employee agreements where the associate employee is working part time in a dental practice. While they are also likely in effect for associate employees working full time in a dental office, they are designed to

protect the region in which the dentist employer's practice is from losing patients and staff who follow an associate employee to a new position elsewhere. The customer base/patient base seen by associate employees generally remain with the senior dentist and dental practice if/when the associate employee leaves that practice. In other words, they do not have ownership of their patients' dental charts to take with them when they terminate the agreement. Associate employees are subject to abiding by the restrictions set forth in confidentiality agreements.

- Abiding by state, federal, and dental practice act statutes, laws, and regulations
  - All associates are expected to know, and abide by, the laws, rules, statutes, and regulations regarding dentistry that arise from the state and federal agencies, as well as the dental practice act within the associate's state they are practicing dentistry in. It is strongly recommended that associates familiarize themselves thoroughly with these, prior to beginning any work as a dentist.
- Legal review of associate agreement or contract prior to signing
  - Regardless of whether an associate dentist will become an associate employee or an associate independent contractor, they should have a comprehensively written agreement that is signed, which clearly outlines all agreed upon terms for the working relationship. The written associate agreement should then be reviewed by an appropriate attorney to ensure legal compliance with the various legal entities that oversee dentistry. The type of attorney that has experience in dental contract law would likely be the most familiar with the state's dental practice act, the IRS, and the DOL's legal requirements as well as have the interests of the associate at heart to ensure that the agreement is legally compliant, fair, transparent, clear, and equitable. It is extremely unusual (and strongly discouraged) to form such an important agreement, not document it, nor have an attorney who can advise on the significant negative ramifications of such an ill-advised undertaking. Therefore, it is always advisable to have a clearly written, compliant legal agreement that is reviewed by the appropriately skilled and trained attorney who represents the best interests of the associate. Attorneys specializing in healthcare or employment law specifically for the dental field, are usually well-versed in the state's dental practice act, as well as state and federal laws applying to dentistry (Driscoll 2014).

24.5 Recommendations for Successful Associateships: Pearls for Private Practice

- "Business person/owner first; clinician second: the paradigm shift"
  - The new associate often thinks of themselves as clinicians only and not a business person. However, according to the data, the ultimate goal of new associates is to own their own private practice eventually. Therefore, shifting the mindset of the associate to one where there is a desire to learn the business side of dentistry becomes critical. A dental practice is a small business first and foremost. As such, dentists wanting to own their own dental practices must become entrepreneurial in their thinking and actions.

Setting goals for themselves, as well as for the practice, and the staff to achieve, gives everyone a strong sense of purpose and fosters teamwork in the process of achieving the goals. The dentist sets the goals and charts the path and then inspires the team to achieve them. This requires acquiring not just additional clinical skills to keep up with clinical trends and offerings to patients but to keep up with the business knowledge as well, to grow in profitability. Profitability plays an important role in reducing stress and learning how the business side of the practice works and impacts the ability of the practice to be profitable. Therefore, a mind shift is needed to one that embraces the lifelong learning of business management and entrepreneurialism and all that it encompasses.

- Introducing, integrating, and marketing the new associate
  - Onboarding, otherwise known as the process of bringing someone on board as a new team member in a work setting, can be particularly successful for new associates if certain processes are followed. The introduction of the new associate into the dental practice can be completed by posting information and photos on the practice's social media, sending letters of introduction to the patients of the practice, and adding the associate's information on to the website as well as placing marketing material on the new associate in the reception room. Additionally, holding an open house night at the dental practice where patients can stop by and meet the new associate can be beneficial for the introduction process of onboarding. Posting a welcome in the local newspapers for the new associate lets the community know about the addition of a new dentist. In completing all of these steps, the dental practice and senior dentist facilitates a much easier entry process and shows support for the new dental associate to staff, patients, and the community as a whole. These contribute to a much more positive onboarding experience for the new associate, as well as to the staff, patients, and community.
  - Marketing and advertising guidelines and regulations should be followed by the state's dental practice act, in legally marketing the new associate in a compliant manner. As the new associate is ultimately responsible for knowing how they can and cannot be legally marketed, it would benefit them greatly to become familiar with the state's dental statutes prior to the first marketing campaign beginning, to avoid a negative outcome arising out of non-compliance to the state's dental practice act.
- Leadership and communication
  - New associates as well as senior dentists are the foundational leaders within a dental practice. Their leadership can be established and viewed through positive communication or negative communication. Leadership and communication go hand in hand as an integral aspect of how the staff perceives the dental leaders in the practice. Staff management, and its success or failure, can be associated with the type of leadership and communication exhibited in the dental practice. While professionalism is taught in dental school curriculum, entrepreneurial leadership and interpersonal communication skills are likely not; however, they are highly valued skills to possess. It is strongly recommended that new associates become educated on leadership and understanding the correlations with good

communication and good outcomes with patients and staff. The impact on the quality of life and stress, as well as staff relations and retention, can make a day enjoyable or miserable, based on a dentist's leadership and communication skills used on a daily basis.

- Practice management education
  - The successful dentist practice owner is one who recognizes the need to understand how to manage all aspects of the dental practice. This includes staff management, operational management, financial and expense management, budgetary management, marketing and reputation management, legal compliance management, and planning for the future. All of this involves advanced education in practice management. It is a critical component, and some say 50 % of the financial success of a practice, which dentists often overlook. It is strongly recommended that dentists become lifelong learners of not just the clinical aspect of the practice but the business aspect of the practice. It will be a decision that pays off in many ways throughout a dentist's career. Good leadership, staff management, and operational management all lead to an increase in the overall value, and valuation, of a dental practice, as well.
- Recommended reading
  - *Business Basics for Dentists*, by David O. Willis, Wiley-Blackwell Publishing, 2013
  - *Associateships: A Guide for Owners and Prospective Associates,* American Dental Association, 2007

References

American Dental Education Association (ADEA), ADEA Survey of Dental School Seniors, 2013 Graduating Class, Pg5, Table 5: seniors' reasons for pursuing dentistry as a career, by percentage of total 2013 respondents. Accessed on 31 Dec 2015 from www.adea.org/surveys…reports/dental-school-seniors-2013-tables.aspx.

American Dental Education Association (ADEA), ADEA Survey of Dental School Seniors, 2013 Graduating Class, Pg8, Table 8. Average amount of educational indebtedness* of graduating dental students by all schools combined and by type of school, 1990 and 1996–2013. Accessed on 31 Dec 2015 from www.adea.org/surveys…reports/dental-school-seniors-2013-tables.aspx.

American Dental Education Association (ADEA), ADEA Survey of Dental School Seniors, 2013 Graduating Class, Pg17, Table 17. Seniors' perceptions of preparedness for practice in selected areas of education and training, by percentage of total. Accessed on 31 Dec 2015 from www.adea.org/surveys…reports/dental-school-seniors-2013-tables.aspx.

American Dental Education Association (ADEA), ADEA Survey of Dental School Seniors, 2013 Graduating Class, Pg20, Table 19. Seniors' immediate plans upon graduation by intended employment status, by percentage of total respondents for 2013. Accessed on 31 Dec 2015 from www.adea.org/surveys…reports/dental-school-seniors-2013-tables.aspx.

American Dental Education Association (ADEA), ADEA Survey of Dental School Seniors, 2013 Graduating Class, Pg21, Table 20. Intended types of private practice by intended employment status, by percent of graduates with immediate plans to enter private practice for 2013.

Accessed on 31 Dec 2015 from www.adea.org/surveys…reports/dental-school-seniors-2013-tables.aspx.
American Dental Association (ADA). Associateships: a guide for owners and prospective associates. 2007, Published by the American Dental Association, Chicago, Illinois.
American Student Dental Association (ASDA). What is a dental associateship? Member Resources; Life After Dental School, 2015. Accessed on 31 Dec 2015 from www.asdanet.org/postdoc/associateship.aspx.
Career Builder, LLC., accessed on 12/31/2015 at www.careerbuilder.com.
DentalJobs.Net, accessed on 12/31/2015 at www.dentaljobs.net.
Dentalworkers.Net, accessed on 12/31/2015 at www.dentalworkers.com.
Dental Post, Inc., accessed on 12/31/2015 at www.dentalpost.net.
Department of Labor (DOL), Wage and Hour Division (WHD), Final Rule: Overtime; Defining and Delimiting the Exemptions for Executive, Administrative, Professional and Outside Sales and Computer Employees Under the Fair Labor Standards Act, accessed on 10/31/2016 at https://www.dol.gov/WHD/overtime/final2016/.
Driscoll, AY. Associateships: negotiating win-win agreements. American Dental Education Association, 12 Feb 2014, Virtual School Fair, Audio-Assisted Power Point Presentation.
Dulde R. Four critical questions for evaluating an associateship. Journal of the American Student Dental Association, Mouth, Volume 32, Issue 2, Summer 2012. Accessed on 31 Dec 2015 from http://www.studentdoctor.net/2012/10/four-critical-questions-for-evaluating-an-associateship/.
Indeed, Inc., accessed on 12/31/2015 at www.indeed.com.
Internal Revenue Service (IRS), Publication Form SS-8, Determination of Worker Status for Purposes of Federal Employment Taxes and Income Tax Withholding, 2015. Accessed on 31 Dec 2015 from www.irs.gov/pub/irs-pdf/fss8.pdf.
Internal Revenue Service (IRS). Publication 1779, Independent Contractor or Employee? 2015. Accessed on 31 Dec 2015 from www.irs.gov/pub/irs-pdf/p1779.pdf.
Fryer M and Norton C. Prepare for your first experience in contract negotiation, American Student Dental Association, ASDA News, Pg6, Pg14, December 2013. Accessed on 31 Dec 2015 from http://editiondigital.net/publication/frame.php?i=187432&p=6.
Levin RP. Why some associateships fail, dental economics. Vol. 92, Issue 6, June 1, 2002. Retrieved from: www.dentaleconomics.com/articles/print/volume-92/issue-6/departments/practice-success/why-some-associateships-fail.html.
Monster Worldwide, accessed on 12/31/2015 at www.monster.com.
Pace M. Perfect match: choosing the right associate for your practice., April 30, 2015, DrBicuspid.com. Accessed on 31 Dec 2015 from www.drbicuspid.com/index.aspx?sec=ser&sub=def&pag=dis&ItemID=317771.
Pritchett C. Patterson Dental School Liaison for University of Florida College of Dentistry. Personal conversation conducted on 31 Dec 2015.
University of Florida College of Dentistry (UFCD). Senior Associate Matching Program, find an associate: associate matching, website http://dental.ufl.edu/alumni-giving/alumni-resources/find-an-associate/accessed on 31 Dec 2015.
Willis DO. Business basics for dentists. Chichester/West Sussex: Wiley–Blackwell; 2013, John Wiley & Sons, Inc. Publishing, Hoboken, New Jersey.
ZipRecruiter, accessed on 12/31/2015 at www.ziprecruiter.com.

The President's Dentist

25

Boyd Robinson

Abstract

Someone asked me once, "Why dentistry?" This caused me to think about what brought me to the desire to become a dentist. I was hoping it would be some bright moment in my life or a "life changing" moment until my mom showed me my eighth grade autobiography. I had written about how I wanted to become a dentist and how that would be the foundation for my life. A role model in my life, my family dentist influenced my desire for dentistry. I had some rough appointments with dentists growing up until I became a patient of Dr. Webster. He was all that I thought I wanted to be and he opened up my curiosity for the field of dentistry. I wanted to be that type of person, someone who, through a profession, could care for others with compassion and integrity.

I didn't really think much about a dental career through high school but when I started college I was pre-dental all the way. I majored in biology and minored in chemistry to prepare myself for dental school. At times I drifted in my education but kept my goal in mind and continued to do well enough to be accepted into dental school. I felt very fortunate to be able to attend the University of the Pacific School of Dentistry (UOP) in San Francisco, California. It was here at UOP that the foundations were laid for my dental career. Now, after close to 40 years of dental practice – serving my country and teaching – I can truly say that I thank God for leading me down this road called dentistry. The road I took had many different stops, some not the usual for a dental career, but all very rewarding and fulfilling (Fig. 25.1).

B. Robinson, DDS, MED
University of Florida College of Dentistry, Gainesville, FL, USA
e-mail: BROBINSON@dental.ufl.edu

G.M. Weinstein, M.T. Zientz (eds.), *The Dental Reference Manual*,
DOI 10.1007/978-3-319-39730-6_25

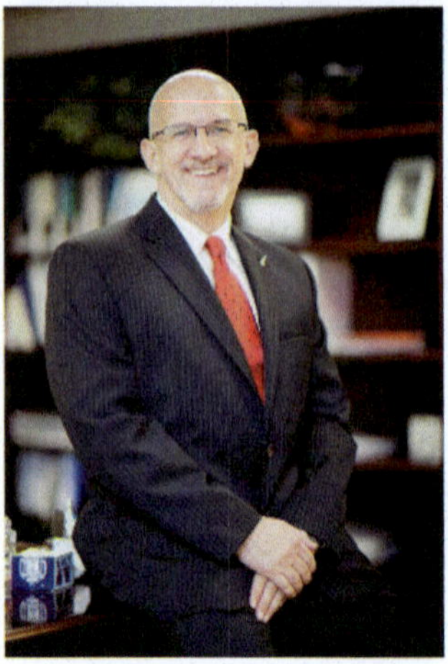

Fig. 25.1 Boyd Robinson, DDS, M.Ed

It started with saying "I will" as I took the oath of office to become a member of the US Navy. I am sure I didn't really understand all that would be required of me as I entered the Navy upon dental school graduation. I knew I would be able to practice dentistry and provide healthcare but I was not ready for strong emotional ties that develop for the men and women who give their lives to protect our freedom.

My career started in a small clinic at the Naval Air Station, Lemoore, California. I was able to perform all disciplines of dentistry at this clinic, which I am sure developed my interest in staying a general dentist. During dental school, I did not know exactly what specialty I wanted to pursue and I was glad for the general practice provided me at Lemoore. It solidified my desire to maintain and develop as a general dentist.

My naval career started to develop and I was stationed with the Marines and went on deployment with them out of Kaneohe Bay, Hawaii. The deployment was what is called a WestPac (Western Pacific) and we did operations in Japan and Australia. I learned a lot about the Marine Corp from this experience and could really appreciate what they do, how hard they work, and the sacrifices they go through to protect our country. I also learned that visiting the dentist was not one of their favorite things to do which helped me to develop a very patient-centered practice – one that made them comfortable in my chair and one that would let them know how much I care.

The Navy also gave me the opportunity for training. I was selected for a 2-year comprehensive dentistry residency. This came after I had been practicing for about 6 years. It came at the perfect time for me professionally and I was able to increase my healthcare and dental knowledge by a huge degree. From this experience I developed my philosophy on total dental care. It also gave me an opportunity to provide "state-of-the-art" dental care and to be able to decide where these modalities fit into a treatment plan. It served me well as I was assigned to several clinics, one where I was the sole provider of care. I had a

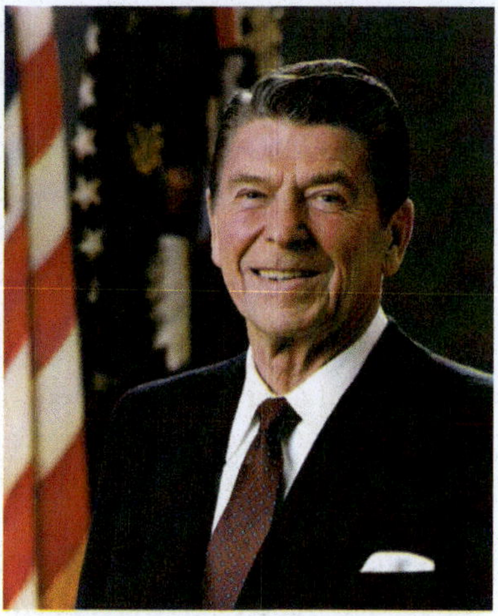

Fig. 25.2 President Ronald Reagan – US president from 1981 to 89

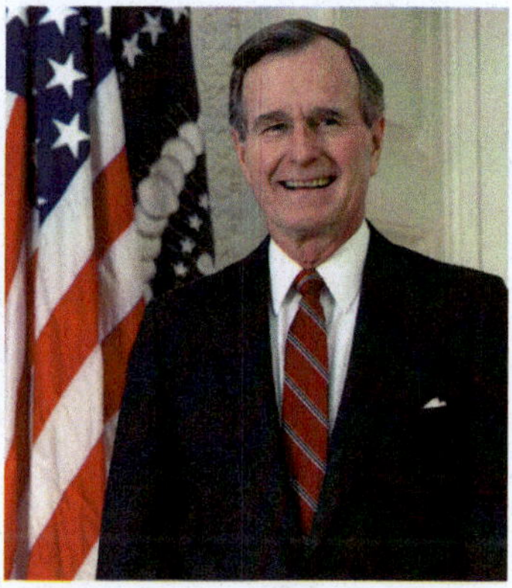

Fig. 25.3 George H.W. Bush, Sr. – US president from 2001 to 2009

very good military service reputation by that time and was known for my excellent dental practice. This lead to one of the greatest assignments anyone could have.

I was selected to be the dentist to the president of the United States. The assignment brought me to Bethesda, Maryland, where I served as the dentist to two presidents, Ronald Reagan and George H.W. Bush (Figs. 25.2 and 25.3). I provided total dental care to the president and his family. At that time I also worked on any military personnel assigned to the White House as well as those assigned to Camp David. The caliber of individuals I worked on was outstanding. It always amazed me how appreciative they all were of the care I provided. It was an honor and a privilege to be around these great men. When I was not working at the White House or Camp David, I was teaching residents at the Naval Postgraduate Dental School at the Naval Hospital. This began my desire to give back to dentistry through teaching. I loved the time I spent with the residents, especially being able to impart to them some of my knowledge of dentistry and patient care.

My naval career ended on a great note. I was selected as commanding officer of the Naval Dental Center Northeast, at Newport, Rhode Island. Even here I was able to impart my love of dentistry to the men and women under my command. The command had nine clinics in seven states in the Northeast. I was able to provide dental care at each clinic and work with different dental assistants and dentists. My hope was that they would see, through me, how important the care we provide is to our patients. Retirement after 26 years was a big change but a good one.

The road after retirement took me back to one of my loves, teaching dentistry. I was fortunate enough to be hired at the University Of Florida College Of Dentistry. At UF I was able to both practice dentistry and teach it. Teaching was my passion as it allowed me to spend time with the dental students. The students always amazed me at their desire to learn and to give back. My desire was to impart to them my love for dentistry and to give them help in developing their dental philosophy and skills. I was fortunate to be named interim dean prior to my retirement. I accepted the position so that I could help the college move to a place where molding and developing young dentists was job one. If I helped to do this at UF, my dental career was a success (Fig.25.4).

If I was talking to predental or dental students or young practicing dentists, my story would be the same. What a great road the profession of dentistry has for you. The road may have many curves in it but stay true to yourself and the profession of dentistry. Enjoy each day you are able to practice and be with patients. Also remember you have more influence than you think. There may be an eighth grade boy or girl in your practice that is watching. How you handle yourself and how you practice will make a difference. At the end of the day, it is the person in the mirror that you really are accountable to.

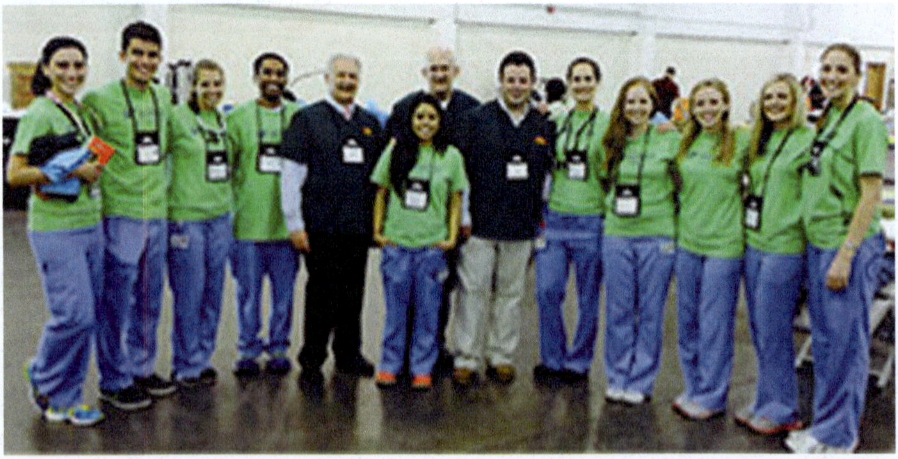

Fig. 25.4 Dr. Robinson with other faculty and students in a 2014 event in Florida providing care to those in need

On Building a Dental School

26

Margaret B. Wilson

Contents

Abstract

Louis Pasteur said: "Chance favors only the prepared mind." Throughout my life, I've been fortunate to encounter opportunities that I never could have imagined. Growing up in Virginia, there was never any doubt that I would go to college. My parents, James and Elizabeth Button, were raised during the Great Depression and had an indefatigable work ethic and a staunch commitment to ensuring that my brothers and I had every opportunity for formal education. At our mother's funeral,

M.B. Wilson, DDS, MBA
Vice Dean, Associate Dean for Student Affairs, Clinical Professor,
Department of General Dentistry, East Carolina University School of Dental Medicine,
Greenville, NC, USA
e-mail: WILSONMAR@ecu.edu

G.M. Weinstein, M.T. Zientz (eds.), *The Dental Reference Manual*,
DOI 10.1007/978-3-319-39730-6_26

my brother David spoke eloquently about how he, my brother Gilbert (Gibby), and I went to college and graduate and professional school on Elizabeth C. Button scholarships, as our mother worked outside of the home so that she could guarantee that her children had the educational opportunities she did not have. Growing up we would have never imagined I would be involved in building a new dental school.

26.1 Choosing Dentistry

I graduated from David Lipscomb College (now Lipscomb University) in Nashville, Tennessee, in 1977, with a Bachelor of Science degree in Chemistry. I chose Lipscomb because it is a Christian college and reported a very high rate of graduates' acceptance into professional school. As a college student, I wasn't sure what was next for me and considered a number of graduate and professional school options. One afternoon, the chair of the Department of Chemistry, Dr. John T. Netterville, asked me a question that at the time seemed totally random. He asked me, "Maggie, did you know that 70 % of the dentists in the Soviet Union are women?" I replied that I did not know that, and from that point forward, for the next several weeks, every time I encountered Dr. Netterville, he asked me the same question. It became a sort of a joke between us, and eventually, after having a serious conversation with him, I began to consider dentistry as a career choice. My older brother Dr. Gilbert L. Button had graduated from the Medical College of Virginia School of Dentistry in 1973, and I had previously ruled out dentistry because I did not want to enter the same profession as my brother (Fig. 26.1).

Attending the Medical College of Virginia School of Dentistry was a wonderful experience for me, and in retrospect it was transformative as well. It was challenging academically, but I was blessed to be part of a cohesive class of 110 students (Only 20 of us were women!), many of whom became like family. My brother had completed a 3-year stint in the US Army Dental Corps and had returned as a faculty member at the dental school. While there were some disadvantages to being "Gibby's little sister," there were advantages as well. I had strong family support in Richmond, and I was able to get to know some of the faculty and staff on a more personal level. I had the opportunity to serve as a student member of the Admissions Committee, working with Dr. Marshall Brownstein.

As dental school graduation approached, I was considering a number of options, including private practice and the US Army. At that time, in the early 1980s, general dentistry residency programs weren't as numerous as they are today. In the spring before graduation, one of our dental school faculty members, Dr. John Svirsky, asked me whether I had firm postgraduation plans. I replied that I had not, and he advised that the University of Maryland Hospital had contacted him regarding an available position in their General Practice Residency (GPR) program. I visited the program and was offered a position. Spending a year in the GPR provided rich opportunities to care for medically compromised patients and to work alongside other health professionals in the hospital setting in providing patient care. I gained invaluable experience in managing complex patients, learning from attending

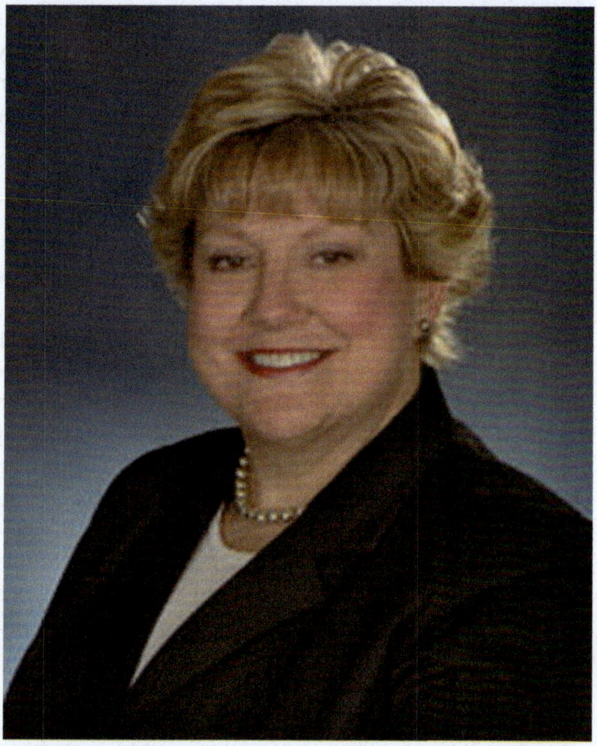

Fig. 26.1 Margaret B. Wilson, DDS, MBA

faculty and from my co-residents. As residents, we also had the opportunity to do some teaching in the dental school, and we interacted with dental students as they completed their hospital dentistry rotations. Dr. John Hasler, Associate Dean for Clinical and Hospital Affairs, led our resident seminars. As the residency program was drawing to an end, Dr. Hasler asked several of us residents whether we would be interested in a new faculty position in a pilot clinical program at the University of Maryland dental school. I declined this opportunity because my fiancé (now my husband of 34 years) was in Richmond.

Guy and I were married in late July 1982, and I began working in private practice in Fredericksburg Virginia and volunteering as a clinical faculty member at the Medical College of Virginia School of Dentistry. As the practice in Fredericksburg became busier, I transitioned to full time and regretfully had to discontinue my teaching activities. I practiced in Fredericksburg for 4 years, learning valuable lessons about how thriving practices function and the role of the dentist as a leader of the dental team and a leader within the community.

In 1986, I made the transition to a position at the University of Maryland at College Park in the Student Health Center, where I served as Director of Dental Services. We had a four-chair dental clinic and provided comprehensive care and emergency services for university students, with an emphasis on health promotion. Our clinic served as a rotation site for senior dental student externships and clerkships. Because we saw a lot of patients who needed endodontics, we established a program for postgraduate endodontics residents from the University of Maryland School of Dentistry to also rotate through our clinic. By virtue of these student and resident rotations, I had a faculty appointment at the dental school and had opportunities to periodically attend meetings at the dental school in Baltimore.

26.2 Entry into Full-Time Academia

While at the University of Maryland at College Park, I completed a Master of Business Administration at the University of Maryland School of Business in 1990. At the same time, I accepted a full-time position at the University of Maryland School of Dentistry (then called the Baltimore College of Dental Surgery) as one of the General Practice (GP) Managers in the newly established General Practice Program. This program was conceived and developed by Dr. John Hasler, whom I had known from my residency program, and Dean Errol Reese. Seven of us were hired as GP Managers, and we were each responsible for all operational aspects of our assigned group practice of third- and fourth-year dental students. As general dentists, we interfaced closely with the other general dentistry and specialty faculty, to ensure that our students received well-rounded educational experiences while providing comprehensive care for the patients. We provided clinical coverage for the students and served as their mentors and advisors.

Three years later, an administrative position – Assistant Dean for Admissions and Student Affairs – became available at the dental school. Because of the numbers of interested and qualified internal candidates, Dean Richard Ranney determined that the search would be internal. There were a number of highly qualified faculty members who applied for this position, including several who had been engaged in student-related activities and had served as members of the Admissions Committee. Given the caliber and many years of experience of the faculty who had publicly declared their interest in the position, I was reluctant to even apply for the position, given my relative youth and brief tenure at the dental school. However, with strong encouragement from several mentors and from my husband, I did apply and was fortunate enough to be selected for the position. During this time, I also had the opportunity to begin participating in the students' ethics curriculum, working with Dr. James T. Rule, author of *Ethical Questions in Dentistry*. When Dr. Rule retired, I was asked to assume responsibility for coordinating this important aspect of the curriculum. For the next 14 years, I served in various administrative capacities, with responsibilities for student affairs, admissions, and for 2 years, academic affairs. I had the opportunity to work with two Deans – Dr. Ranney and Dr. Christian Stohler.

26.3 Time of Transition

In the spring of 2008, I decided to step away from administrative responsibilities and returned to full-time clinical teaching. Collaborating with other key faculty partners, we piloted the General Practice Simulation (GPS) project in one section of the predoctoral clinics. This shift in focus allowed me to get back in touch with my clinical side and reignited my passion for clinical teaching and patient care. After about a year, as the GPS was moving forward, I learned about professional opportunities at the East Carolina University School of Dental Medicine (School of Dentistry at that time). Dr. James Hupp, who had been the chair of Oral and Maxillofacial Surgery for a number of years at University of Maryland, had gone on to be the Dean of the University of Mississippi School of Dental Medicine and had recently been appointed as Dean at East Carolina University (ECU). I applied for the position of Associate Dean for Student Affairs and, after a lengthy search process, was offered the position.

My husband Guy was absolutely thrilled (as was I!) with this opportunity and was unquestioningly supportive of our relocating to Greenville, North Carolina, knowing full well that it could prove difficult for him to find employment options in his area of expertise, financial management of manufacturing companies. We were also aware that while the commitment to establish the dental school at ECU was unwavering, there were significant budgetary concerns within the state of North Carolina that could impact the timeline or even the establishment of the school. However, the opportunity to help start a new school – one with such a clear, concise mission – was incredible, and we made the decision to embrace the opportunity. We moved to Greenville in November 2009, and Guy began his job exploration. After 9 months of searching, he ultimately accepted a position as Chief Financial Officer for a newly established manufacturing facility in Oxford, North Carolina. We were now both working with our respective "start-ups."

26.4 Early History of the East Carolina University School of Dental Medicine

Established as the School of Dentistry at East Carolina University (ECU) by the North Carolina legislature in 2007, the School of Dental Medicine (SoDM), located in Greenville, North Carolina, is the second dental school in the state of North Carolina. In considering the establishment of a second dental school, state policy makers were extremely concerned about the overall shortage of dentists in North Carolina as well as an unequal distribution of dentists across the state. North Carolina currently ranks 47th in the 50 United States, with respect to dentist-to-population ratios, and is the fifth fastest growing state in the county and the tenth most populated.

Geography matters in North Carolina. There is a rural–urban divide within the population. Approximately half of the state's population lives in the 15 urban counties, while the other half of the population is spread among the 85 rural counties. Of North Carolina's 100 counties, 79 qualify as federally designated health professional shortage areas, and 3 counties (all in the eastern region of the state) do not have a single dentist.[1]

[1] North Carolina Institute of Medicine. 2005 North Carolina Oral Health Summit Access to Dental Care: summit Proceedings and Action Plan. Durham, NC: October 2005.

In choosing ECU as the parent institution for the new dental school, legislators noted ECU's demonstrated capacity to meet the health-care needs of the state and region through its medical school and colleges of nursing and allied health. ECU's Brody School of Medicine was established in 1977, in order "…to increase the supply of primary care physicians to serve the state, to improve health status of citizens in eastern North Carolina, and to enhance the access of minority and disadvantaged students to a medical education."[2]

The plan to establish the new dental school at ECU was created under a joint agreement with the University of North Carolina (UNC), Chapel Hill, which also included an increase in enrollment for the existing public dental school at that institution. The plan included the establishment of ECU, with a class size of 50, and a future planned increase in UNC's class size from 80 to 100, substantially increasing the opportunities for dental training in North Carolina.

Dr. Greg Chadwick was the very first person to join ECU in 2005 to begin to develop the plan for the school and initially served as Associate Vice Chancellor for Oral Health. A practicing endodontist who had initially practiced general dentistry in community dental clinics in underserved areas of North Carolina, Dr. Chadwick's perspective gained from his roles as President of the North Carolina Dental Society, and the American Dental Association uniquely prepared him to lead in the further development and implementation of the plan for the school.

Dr. Chadwick had hired Dr. Todd Watkins in the spring 2008 and tasked him with developing an innovative curriculum model for the School of Dental Medicine. Dr. Watkins' background in curriculum and informatics uniquely qualified him for this undertaking. He had served as the primary architect for two other dental schools' curricula and had consulted with many medical and dental schools and other health profession schools related to curriculum development, assessment, and use of educational technology. Dr. Watkins' charge was to develop a curriculum that would prepare the students to meet the vision and mission of the school and would culminate in the students spending a large portion of their fourth year providing care in the Community Service Learning Centers (CSLCs).

26.5 The ECU Model

The vision and mission of the ECU School of Dental Medicine are clear and consistent with the school's founding principles. The school's vision – "Improving the health and quality of life of all North Carolinians by creating leaders with a passion to care for the underserved and by leading the nation in community-based, service learning oral health education" – encapsulates its commitment to the people of North Carolina. Further amplifying the vision, the school's mission is to:

- Prepare leaders with outstanding clinical skills, an ethical bearing, sound judgment, and a passion to serve.

[2] http://www.ecu.edu/cs-dhs/med/abtHistory.cfm.

- Provide educational opportunities for academically qualified North Carolinians from historically underrepresented groups, disadvantaged backgrounds, and underserved areas.
- Provide and enhance oral health services for underserved North Carolinians through implementation of community-oriented service learning and inter-professional collaborations.
- Foster a learning environment where collaboration, creativity, diversity, and professionalism are embraced.
- Influence future clinical practice and dental education through research, innovation, and discovery.

This vision and mission fully align with our parent institution, which has a motto of *servire*, to serve. Consistent with our mission, admission to the ECU School of Dental Medicine is limited to residents of North Carolina.

The ECU School of Dental Medicine was the first *public* dental school in the United States established in the past 40 years with an emphasis on serving the oral health-care needs of rural America. The ECU model focuses on the education of primary care dentists to provide dental care and leadership within communities of need across the state of North Carolina. Students spend their first three years on the Greenville campus of ECU, participating in a wide range of educational activities, including didactic, small group discussion and preclinical laboratory and simulation activities, and caring for patients in a brand-new, state-of-the-art educational and patient care facility, Ledyard E. Ross Hall. In sharp contrast, fourth-year students spend the majority of their time providing care for patients in the Community Service Learning Centers (CSLCs), constructed using state funds and located in rural and underserved regions in the state.

From 2012 until 2016, ECU has established a network of eight CSLCs, each functioning as a "branch office" of the dental school. The CSLC Directors are full-time dental faculty, hired by the school. Each of the school's eight CSLCs is an ECU built, owned, and operated 7,700 square foot, 16-operatory dental clinic. A full-time Director and a second part- or full-time dentist, both of whom are School of Dental Medicine faculty, a business manager, two dental hygienists, and a team of dental assistants and administrative support professionals, staff each CSLC. Two Advanced Education in General Dentistry (AEGD) residents complete their residency year at each CSLC, and fourth-year dental students spend more than half of their senior year on three-week CSLC rotations. The AEGD residents and students treat patients alongside the faculty who also provide direct patient care, enabling the students and residents to work in an actual care delivery system. The students' opportunity to work with all members of the dental team on a daily basis allows them to appreciate the key roles in dental practice, while enabling the students to see six or more patients per day.

The CSLCs provide much needed oral health-care services within the communities where they are located, while providing patient care experiences for the residents, and fourth-year students within the very communities we anticipate they will ultimately be practicing. CSLC faculty, staff, students, and residents also engage in

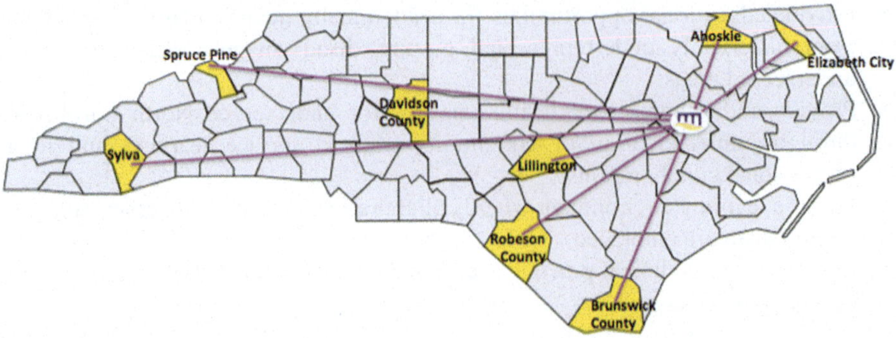

Fig. 26.2 Locations of ECU School of Dental Medicine Community Service Learning Centers

community outreach activities, with a particular emphasis on promoting oral health and encouraging young people within the communities to develop and pursue educational goals. Since most of the CSLC staff members come from the communities themselves and since the CSLC Directors, faculty, residents, and students become part of the community, the CSLCs also play a vital role in economic development, with an estimated annual impact in excess of $1 million per year, per CSLC (Fig. 26.2).

26.6 Curriculum Development

Dr. Watkins' approach to curriculum development followed Steven Covey's "Begin with the end in mind." The vision of the School of Dental Medicine – to educate leaders who will practice as primary care dentists in communities of need across the state of North Carolina – drove the curriculum development. The educational model calls for fourth-year students to spend much of their fourth year providing care for patients at the CSLCs. The CSLCs are located in communities of need – the same types of communities where we prepare them to practice.

Dr. Watkins developed a unique curriculum model where the first three years of the curriculum is compressed so that fourth-year students are prepared with the knowledge, skills, and abilities to practice alongside faculty in an actual care delivery system. The curriculum utilizes a systems-based approach to the basic sciences, utilizing problem-based and case-based approaches to facilitate the students' development of problem-solving skills and supported by the innovative use of technology. Themes rather than discrete traditional courses define the curriculum, allowing for integration of curriculum content. Since many people in underserved and rural areas are medically complex, the students' understanding of clinical medicine is essential. The curriculum exposes students to the challenges of serving patients who face an array of barriers that limit their access to health care, facilitating their understanding of public health, health disparities, and cultural competence. Since many of our graduates will be solo practitioners in these rural and underserved communities, early patient care activities and robust clinical experiences in the Ross Hall and at the CSLC's provide the students with the skills and abilities to provide a wide scope of services within their communities.

26.7 Joining the ECU School of Dental Medicine

Helping to start a dental school has proven to be simultaneously invigorating, challenging, rewarding, and occasionally terrifying. All of us who have joined the School of Dental Medicine as faculty, staff, students, and residents are united behind our common mission of improving the oral health of people across the state North Carolina. Attempting to recount the immense growth and accomplishments that have occurred over the past six-plus years is somewhat daunting, particularly since many of our undertakings occurred simultaneously, rather than as discrete, sequential events.

When I first joined the ECU School of Dental Medicine in November 2009, Dr. Hupp was serving as Dean, Dr. Chadwick was serving as Assistant Dean for Extramural Activities and Planning, and Dr. Todd Watkins had been appointed as the first faculty member. The school had three administrative support staff, and I was the seventh member of the team. Dr. Chadwick's primary responsibilities focused on identifying the sites for the school's planned network of CSLCs. In identifying potential regions for the location of CSLCs, many factors received careful consideration, including demographic factors (e.g., population, dentist-to-population ratios, percent Medicaid eligible), economic factors, and geographic characteristics.

Our temporary offices were housed in the Laupus Health Sciences Library while the module building for our long-term temporary office was being assembled. Our first "ribbon cutting" took place when we moved into Lakeside Annex #7 and was the first of many ribbon cuttings and firsts that have taken place since those earliest days. The groundbreaking for the school's building on the Health Sciences campus had occurred on February 8, 2008, but at that time, no construction activity had yet begun.

26.8 Recruiting and Admitting the Inaugural Class

One of my first orders of business was to begin building a student affairs team. We hired a Director of Admissions, Mr. Lamont Lowery, and an administrative support associate. Our target was to recruit, admit, and enroll a class of 50 students for matriculation in the fall of 2011. While I knew what a dental admissions operation was supposed to look like, developing the system in the context of a brand-new school presented unique challenges. Fortunately, supportive colleagues from the American Dental Education Association – Dr. Anne Wells and Ms. Chonte James – were extremely helpful, as were the members of our growing School of Dental Medicine team. And while some of the dentists in the practicing community were skeptical regarding the need for another dental school in North Carolina, we were blessed to have a strong network of support from many other dentists in our community, the North Carolina Dental Society and the Old North State Dental Society.

During 1 week every spring, the colleges and universities in North Carolina collaborate to host a series of health professions career fairs across the state, to facilitate the recruitment efforts of graduate and professional schools. Mr. Lowery and I had already begun networking with the pre-health advisors in North Carolina, and we were pleased to have the opportunity to visit the campuses of many of the larger colleges and universities in North Carolina. We began accepting applications for admission in June of 2010, for matriculation in the fall of 2011.

Knowing the high cost of dental education, even in a state such as North Carolina, which has a strong commitment to providing high-quality, affordable education, we determined that we needed to seek external resources for scholarships for students. We submitted an application through the US Health Resources Services & Administration (HRSA) for funds to support scholarships for students who aligned with the mission of our school, which aligns with the goals of HRSA. We were fortunate to receive funding for our project Creating Opportunities in Dental Education (CODE), which provided scholarships for students from disadvantaged, minority, and rural background who aspire to practice general dentistry in North Carolina. The CODE project provided $17,000 per year for 4 years, for ten recipients in the inaugural class and ten recipients in the following year's entering class.

26.9 Accreditation

During this same time, the school completed the initial self-study report for the Doctor of Dental Medicine (DMD) program and submitted the self-study report and supporting documents to the Commission on Dental Accreditation (CODA). CODA accreditation requires a series of accreditation site visits. The first site visit occurs prior to the enrollment of the inaugural class. The second site visit takes place at the end of the inaugural class's second year, and the third site visit occurs just before the inaugural class graduates. Each of the three site visits requires that the institution undergo and document an extremely thorough self-study, with emphasis on providing documentation to support compliance with comprehensive array of accreditation standards. After the submission and review of the self-study documents, a site visit team of peers in dental education visits the school to verify the findings and information provided in the self-study documents. At the conclusion of the site visit, the team submits a report to the Commission on Dental Accreditation, and the Commission makes the final determination. Providing that each of these three site visits goes well, the school then moves on the customary 7-year accreditation site visit interval.

Our first CODA site visit occurred in the fall of 2010, and we received the official notification of our initial accreditation status in early February 2011. CODA permits new dental schools to initiate the admissions process, interviewing students for admission and even making tentative offers of admission, with the offers contingent on the school receiving initial accreditation. We followed the custom of other dental schools in making our first round of offers on December 1, 2010, but had to clearly

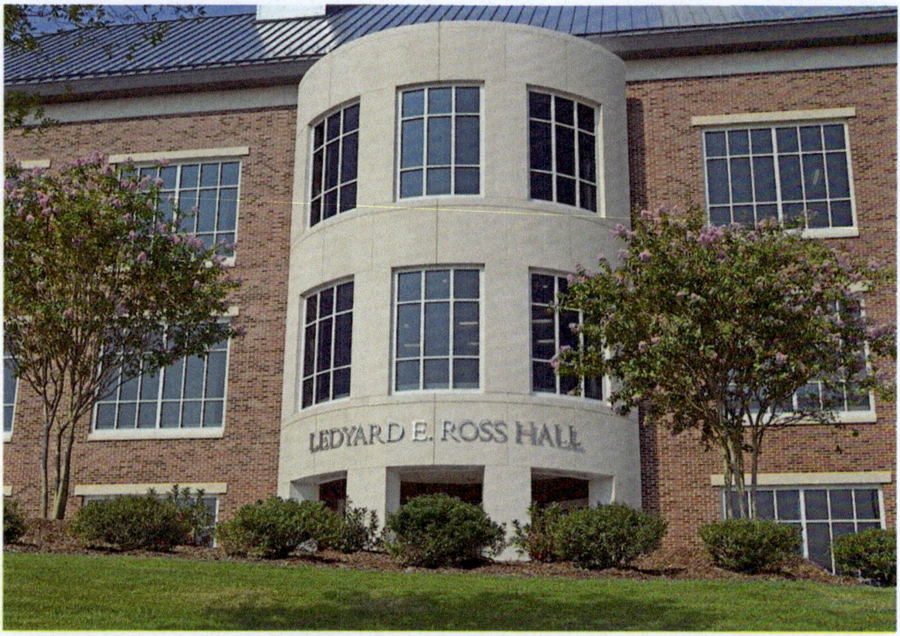

Fig. 26.3 ECU dental school building was named after Dr. Ledyard Ross, a prominent Orthodontist in Greenville, North Carolina

explain to the students that the offer was contingent on our official notification of preliminary accreditation, which we anticipated receiving in early February. Within the context of the financial challenges being faced by the university and the state, as well as the accreditation contingency, the students who accepted our first offers of admission were courageous and were fully committed to the mission of our school.

Construction on the dental school building began in the summer of 2010. ECU had received a generous gift from a Greenville, North Carolina, orthodontist, philanthropist, and businessman, Dr. Ledyard E. Ross, and the new dental school building was to be named in his honor. The ceremonial topping off celebration for the Ross Hall took place on July 16, 2011, as we were preparing for the matriculation of our inaugural class (Fig. 26.3).

26.10 The Inaugural Class

August 16, 2011, marked the first day of orientation. Fifty-two talented young people, all North Carolina residents and all committed to the mission of our new school, began their journey as the ECU School of Dental Medicine's inaugural class. On that same day, the Dean of the school resigned. For our brand-new students at a brand-new school, the announcement of this decision was unimaginable. We met with the students immediately, reassuring them that while this change was extremely unsettling, the University's commitment to their education, and to the people of North

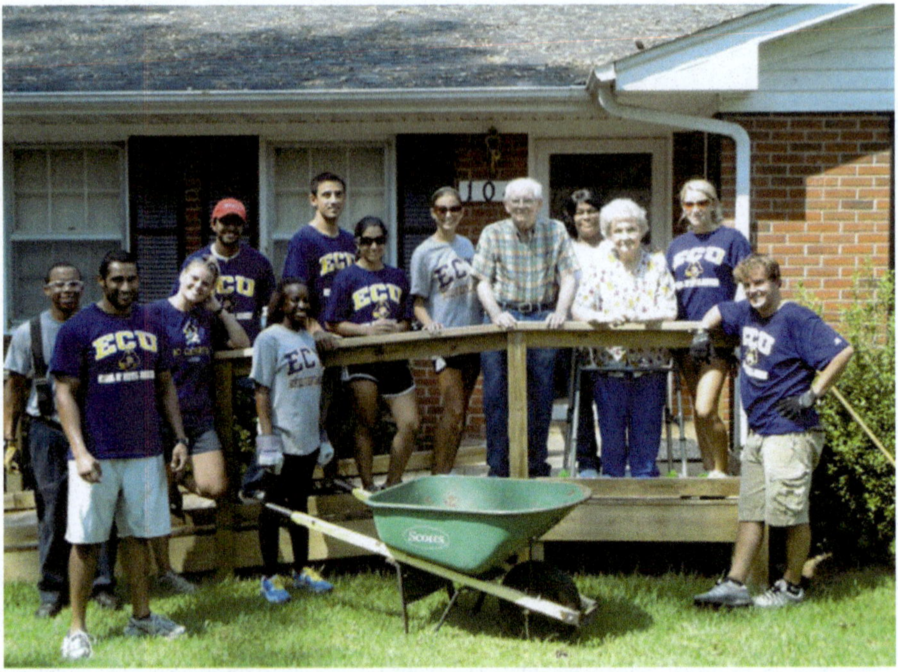

Fig. 26.4 Inaugural Class at ECU assisting during Hurricane Irene in 2011

Carolina, was unwavering. We continued to reiterate this message and provide support for the students individually and collectively amidst the swirling rumors and press activity on our campus. Thankfully, much of that activity subsided within several days, although the impact of the administrative change continued. Dr. Hupp remains on faculty as a Professor of Oral and Maxillofacial Surgery and continues to play an active role in the students' education and development of clinical skills.

Classes began the next week. Faculty and administrative offices were housed in modular buildings in the Lakeside Annex, adjacent to Laupus Lake on ECU's Health Sciences campus. Our students' classes and labs were held in the Brody Medical Sciences building. Colleagues in the Brody School of Medicine were gracious in allowing us to utilize one of their lecture halls, which we remodeled and outfitted with our new technology, and an open lab space, which we equipped as our simulation lab.

Hurricane Irene hit North Carolina on August 26 and 27, 2011. Eastern North Carolina was hit especially hard, and as a result, the ECU campus was closed for a day, and classes were cancelled for a second day. I clearly recall being contacted by one of our students, asking whether we would mind if the students put on their ECU School of Dental Medicine t-shirts and went around the Greenville area to help area residents with clean up. Of course we did not mind! In fact, this initial act, by more than half of the inaugural class, underscored for us that we had selected precisely the right students. They were already demonstrating their extreme commitment to serving others (Fig. 26.4)!

Our inaugural class spent their entire first year in classes and labs in the Brody building. In September 2011, Dr. Greg Chadwick was named Interim Dean of the school. He was named permanent Dean a year later, in September 2012. Construction on the Ross Hall continued, and we began "the big move" into the Ross Hall in the fall of 2012.

Our new home is a 188,000 square foot facility that includes 133 dental chairs (125 for general dentistry, three pediatric dental benches, three oral surgery chairs, one bariatric chair, and one DentalEz Air Glide chair), a 56-station clinical simulation suite, a 56-station preclinical technique lab, two learning halls, and numerous conference rooms. The clinics are outfitted with state-of-the-art equipment, including operating microscopes, digital radiography and imaging, and designated space for faculty practice, Special Needs Clinic, and clinical research. The School of Dental Medicine's robust technological infrastructure network allows for live broadcasts between all CSLC conference rooms, both learning halls and most conference rooms in the Ross Hall.

26.11 Simultaneous Construction, Accreditation, Ribbon Cuttings, and Ongoing Dental School Operations

In addition to constructing the Ross Hall, the School of Dental Medicine had begun constructing its first Community Service Learning Center (CSLC), located in Ahoskie, North Carolina. The construction began in the late summer of 2011, and the CSLC opened in August 2012. The Ahoskie opening meant so much to the regional community and was indeed a celebration. You can imagine the pride of the people in the area to have a branch of the ECU School of Dental Medicine in their hometown (Fig. 26.5)!

Also in 2012, construction on our second CSLC began in Elizabeth City. In August of that year, we admitted our second cohort of students and were allowed partial occupancy of the Ross Hall, so that we could access our learning halls and seminar rooms while the construction was continuing in the other areas of the school. We moved into the rest of the three floors of Ross Hall in mid-September 2012 but were unable to use the simulation lab for a number of weeks, as the lab was being disassembled from its temporary location in the Brody building and reassembled in Ross Hall. The fourth floor of Ross Hall was shelled-in space at that time. Over the course of the next several months, we encountered a number of construction challenges, and one of the most vexing was the shattering of the glass dividers between the clinic operatories in the Comprehensive Care clinic. The lower part of the partitions is made of wood, with glass above. Apparently the "periodontal ligament-like" interface between the wood and the glass did not allow for expansion and contraction of the wood, leading to shattering of glass (Fig. 26.6). For some of us, this shattering of glass – which was ultimately resolved – remains a symbol of some of the challenges we have faced and overcome. We have an unwavering commitment to our mission. We were able to get the glass problem resolved, and our inaugural class students began treating patients in the Ross Hall clinics in the spring of 2013, their second year in the DMD program. Our CSLC Elizabeth City was completed, and residents and faculty began seeing patients in April 2013.

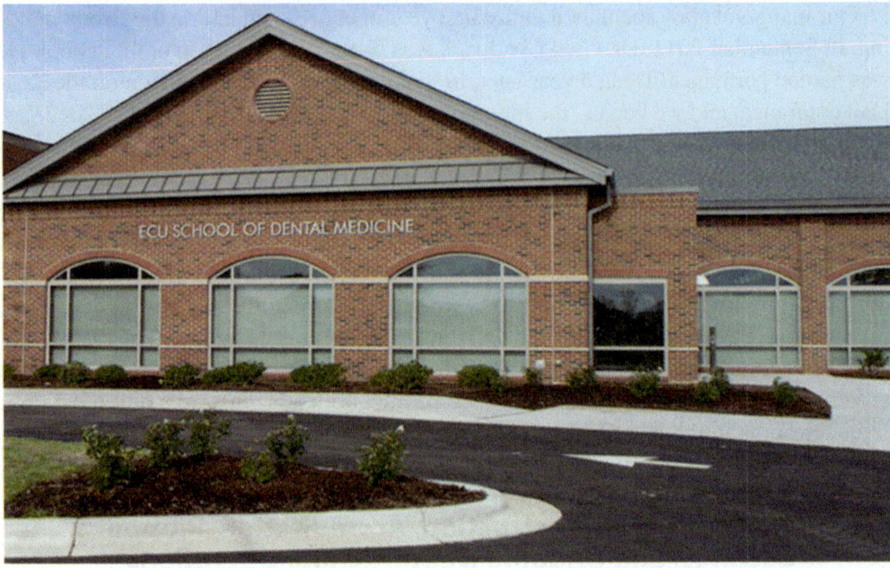

Fig. 26.5 Community Service Learning Center in Ahoskie, North Carolina, is one of the eight centers that houses fourth-year dental students and provides care for patients that live in the area

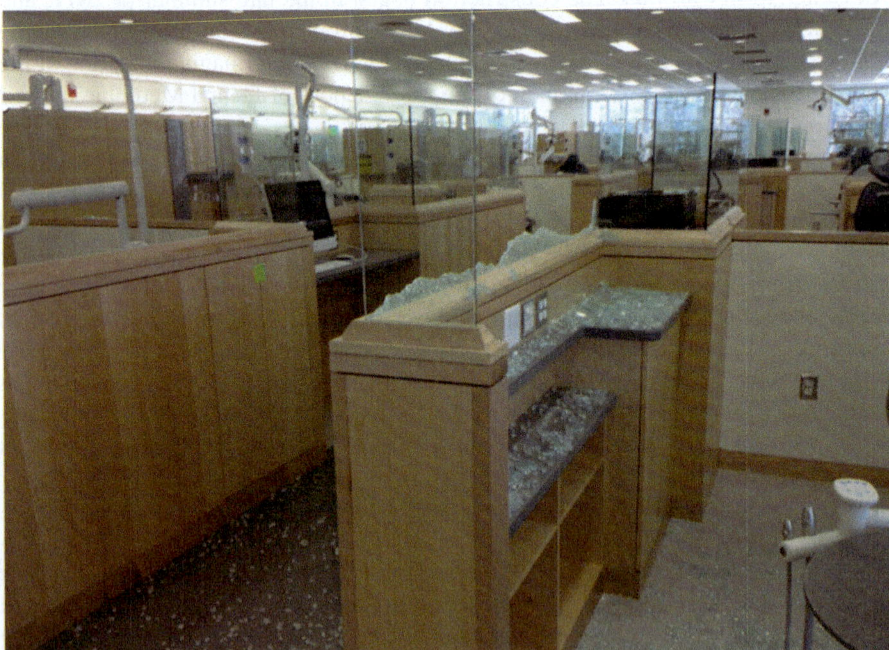

Fig. 26.6 Comprehensive Care clinic operatories at ECU, showing early shattering of glass dividers

At the same time that the Ross Hall construction was nearing completion and we were moving into our new building, and opening CSLC Ahoskie and beginning construction on CSLC Elizabeth City, we began preparations for our second CODA site visit for the DMD program scheduled for May 2013, at the end of the second year for the inaugural class. This site visit placed particular emphasis on our curriculum in the first two years of the DMD program. The integration of our curriculum made certain aspects of the accreditation process somewhat challenging, in that the accreditation standards were developed based on a more traditional curriculum approach. Dr. Watkins, Dr. Chadwick, and others expended a substantial amount of effort describing our curriculum approach, and the accreditation process went smoothly.

During the summer 2013, the School of Dental Medicine rolled out our Preparing Tomorrow's Dentists program, a two and one-half-day program developed to meet the surging interest in the dentistry. The pipeline program was funded through the American Dental Education Association from the Robert Wood Johnson Foundation in 2013–2014. For the 2013 project, ECU dental school partnered with the North Carolina Agricultural and Technical State University and the Old North State Dental Society (the state component of the traditionally African–American National Dental Association). In 2014, the partnership expanded to also include the University of North Carolina – Pembroke, to extend outreach to students who are members of the Lumbee Indian tribe. To date, 127 students have participated in the Preparing Tomorrow's Dentists pipeline program, and an additional 100 have participated in the Preparing Tomorrow's Dentists professional development workshop. Nine program participants are enrolled in the School of Dental Medicine, and an additional five program participants will matriculate in August 2016. At least six other program participants have matriculated to other dental schools. It is incredibly rewarding to have the opportunity to meet young people at the beginning of their college careers (or even earlier!) and work with them as they pursue their dream of becoming a dentist.

Our third class matriculated in the fall of 2013, and during the 2013–2014 academic year, we opened CSLC Lillington (February 2014) and CSLC Sylva (May 2014). Up until the spring of 2014, only the CSLC Directors, faculty dentists, and residents staffed the CSLCs that had opened, since the dental students had not yet reached their fourth-year planned "deployment" to the centers. In planning for fourth-year students to spend 8-week rotations in rural communities, identifying appropriate housing for the students was a critical process. When I had first interviewed for my position and asked who was responsible for locating the housing for the students on their CSLC rotations, the response was, "You are!"

Understanding the importance of the housing aspect of the rotation, and the challenges that we would likely encounter in rural areas, I assured the students that they would not be asked to stay anywhere that I would not stay. Fortunately, North Carolina has a very strong Area Health Education Center (AHEC) network across the state, and our AHEC partners have provided much support in this endeavor. Each CSLC location is unique, and there are different housing opportunities and challenges in each location. Our goal was to find housing that was safe, clean, and convenient.

26.12 CSLC Rotations, CODA, and Our First Graduation

Our inaugural students began their CSLC rotations in May 2014. The students looked forward to their rotations with great anticipation, and their experiences did not disappoint them. They readily acclimated to their roles in a group practice-type setting and as members of the community where they were living. They provided care for underserved patients and gained confidence in their clinical abilities and their patient management skills.

At the same time that our inaugural students were beginning their fourth-year CSLC experiences, we began preparing for our third CODA site visit, which was scheduled for March 2015. This site visit would particularly focus on our students' clinical experiences in Ross Hall and at the CSLCs. In February of 2014, Dr. Chadwick had asked me to assume the responsibilities of Vice Dean for the School of Dental Medicine, along with retaining my role as Associate Dean for Student Affairs. As part of my new role, I chaired the CODA Steering Committee. Again, the integration of our curriculum and our community service learning model made certain aspects of the accreditation process somewhat challenging, in that the accreditation standards were developed based on a more traditional curriculum approach. However, our faculty, module and course directors, chairs, and deans collaborated to compile a self-study document that described the intricate features of our DMD program.

We had to approach the CODA site visit with a degree of "out-of-the-box" thinking, since we knew that our site visitors had the customary two and one-half days to visit our school, and knowing that our school at that time had four fully functioning branch offices across the state. We leaned heavily on our School of Dental Medicine's Information Technology team to support this endeavor. For example, one of the key features of the CODA site visit is a lunchtime open forum meeting with all of the students in the program. Our students were not all in Ross Hall and not even all in Greenville. Some of our fourth-year students were at the CSLC sites across the state. With our technological infrastructure, we were readily able to video teleconference (VTC) between the four CSLCs where our students were on rotation and the learning halls in Ross Hall. In addition, one of the site visitors was at our Elizabeth City CSLC, and she, too, was able to participate in the discussion via VTC. And to top it all off, our Director of Student Services, Ms. Emily Craven, arranged the lunches for all participants – in Greenville and at the sites in Ahoskie, Elizabeth City, Lillington, and Sylva!

The entire site visit team needed to visit one of our CSLCs, so we made arrangements for them to visit CSLC Ahoskie, our closest location and most mature site (Fig. 26.7). Even though Ahoskie was only a little more than an hour away from Greenville, we knew that we could not afford to lose that commuting time in our tightly packed schedule. Again, our "out-of-the-box" thinking kicked in, and we decided to take our site visitors on a bus up to Ahoskie and discuss one of the accreditation standards, Standard 4, on the bus. Fortunately we were able to use one of the very plush Athletic Department buses, and we loaded up our site visitors and the faculty, administrators, staff, and students who were part of Standard 4 and took

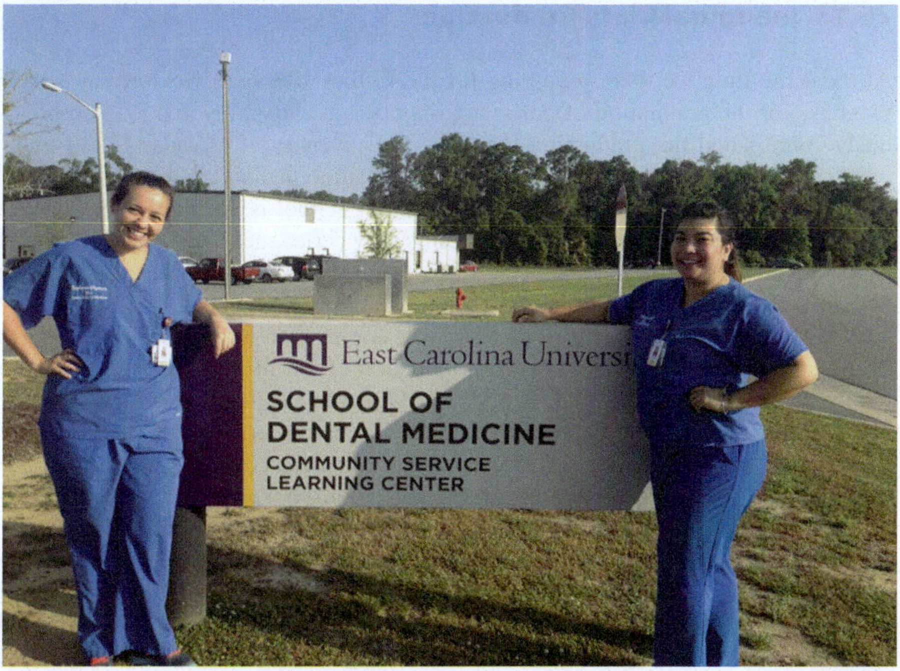

Fig. 26.7 Drs. Stephanie Chapman and Sheena Neil at CSLC Ahoskie

off for Ahoskie. Although in a very nontraditional setting for a review of an accreditation standard, we were able to have a productive discussion. We arrived in Ahoskie, and the site visitors were able to tour the CSLC and meet with the faculty, staff, residents, and students. For the return trip to Greenville, we wanted to allow the site-visiting team to have the bus to themselves so that they could hold their executive session, so we engaged a second ECU bus (a transit bus!) to transport the staff, students, and faculty back to Greenville. Overall our site visit went well, and we are pretty sure that the "road trip" to Ahoskie was a first for CODA! Our school is now on a 7-year accreditation cycle.

We opened CSLC Robeson in February 2015, CSLC Davidson in March 2015, and CSLC Spruce Pine in April 2015. Each one of these CSLC openings generated a tremendous amount of enthusiasm in the local communities. Since each academic program within a dental school must be accredited by CODA, we also have had to complete the accreditation process for our Advanced Education in General Dentistry (AEGD) program. And since our educational model calls for two AEGD residents to be assigned to each of the CSLCs for their residency year, each of our eight CSLCs sites has undergone (or will undergo) an individual accreditation self-study and CODA site visit. From 2012 until 2016, ECU has built and opened eight CSLCs. The eighth CSLC, in Brunswick County, opened in March 2016. We remain in "accreditation mode!"

26.13 Inaugural Class Graduation

At the same time we were preparing for the CODA site visit, we were also busy planning for the graduation of our inaugural class in early May 2015. I had previously coordinated the graduation activities at University of Maryland, so I knew what graduation was supposed to look like. Graduation planning is a huge undertaking, and planning graduation activities for a new school is an even more massive undertaking. Working together with our university colleagues and School of Dental Medicine faculty, staff, and students, we planned a week of graduation celebration activities, establishing traditions and customs for our new school.

The first three days of our graduation week 2015 activities included the North Carolina Dental Society's Signing Day, induction of our first alumni members into our newly established Beta Eta Chapter of the Omicron Kappa Upsilon Dental Honor Society, and a graduate recognition breakfast. On that Friday, May 8, the School of Dental Medicine participated in ECU's commencement ceremony, an impressive ceremony at the university's Dowdy–Ficklen Stadium. It was truly a moment, hearing our Dean, Dr. Greg Chadwick, proudly say: "For the first time in ECU's history, on behalf of the faculty of the School of Dental Medicine, I proudly present the inaugural class for the Doctor of Dental Medicine degree…." The following day we held our School of Dental Medicine convocation ceremony where we further affirmed and celebrated our graduates and their hard work, personal and financial investment, and unwavering commitment to their profession (Fig. 26.8). The inaugural class played an undeniable role in helping to build and shape our school.

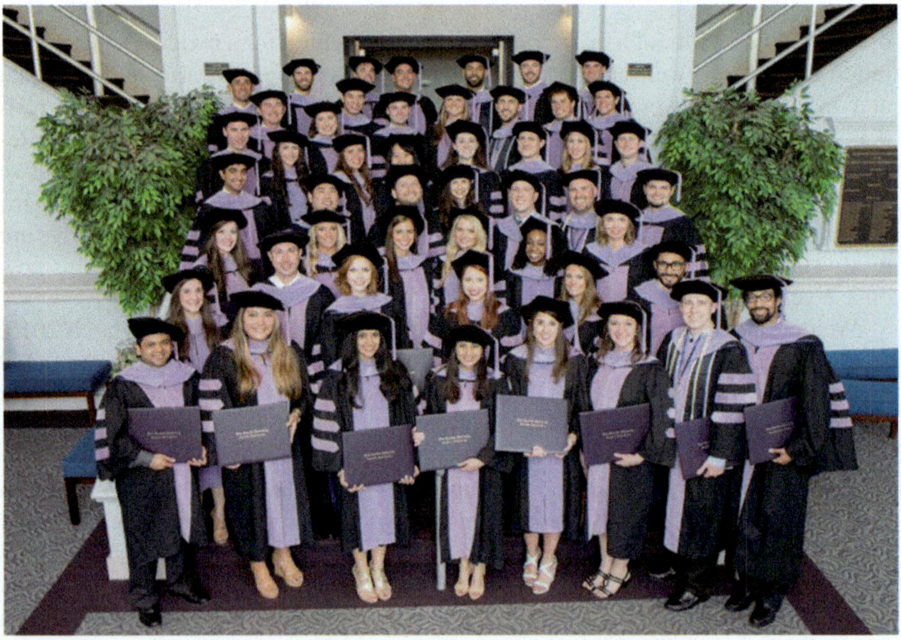

Fig. 26.8 Inaugural Class of ECU School of Dental Medicine, May 2015

Our inaugural class of 50 graduates has already begun fulfilling the mission of the ECU School of Dental Medicine. They established an endowment of a patient care fund with an initial class gift in excess of $30,000 in contributions and pledges from every single student in the class. This endowment will provide funding for care for patients who would not otherwise be able to afford treatment.

26.14 Continuing Our Mission

While the graduation of our inaugural class was a huge milestone in the history of our school, we continue to experience the enthusiasm for our mission that initially drew us to the ECU School of Dental Medicine. When people ask us about our greatest accomplishment, the response is easy: We are keeping our promises to the people of North Carolina.

In Pursuit of Dentistry from Zimbabwe! 27

Criswell Tafadzwa Gandi

Abstract

As a young boy in Zimbabwe, I developed an inquisitive mind early on in life. This, coupled with the fact that I was the only son in a family of five, made me a very unique child. I grew up and learned to love and love with a passion. I made up my mind to become a doctor while still in fourth grade, although I did not know what kind of a doctor. The journey would take me through many trying times in my life, but ultimately fulfillment of a dream.

When I was in grade six, my uncle came back from the United States and, soon after, began practicing as an orthodontist. The whole family was invited to the official opening of his practice. As I walked around the building, seeing the high-tech equipment, I fell in love with orthodontics, and I determined to become and orthodontist.

Since I was coming from a humble background, I knew my only hope was in enrolling at the University of Zimbabwe, the only university in Zimbabwe that offers dentistry even today. The University of Zimbabwe, College of Health Sciences, established the Department of Dentistry in 1997. As the school of Dentistry was still in its infancy, the number of students enrolled each year would be very limited (the largest group since the school started was 25). It follows that competition was very tough for one to be accepted in the school as a dental student (Fig.27.1).

I worked very hard from my early years of high school as I fought viciously against all odds to keep my dream alive. After the first two years of high school,

C.T. Gandi, BDS
University of Zimbabwe, Harare, Zimbabwe
e-mail: tafigand@yahoo.com

G.M. Weinstein, M.T. Zientz (eds.), *The Dental Reference Manual*,
DOI 10.1007/978-3-319-39730-6_27

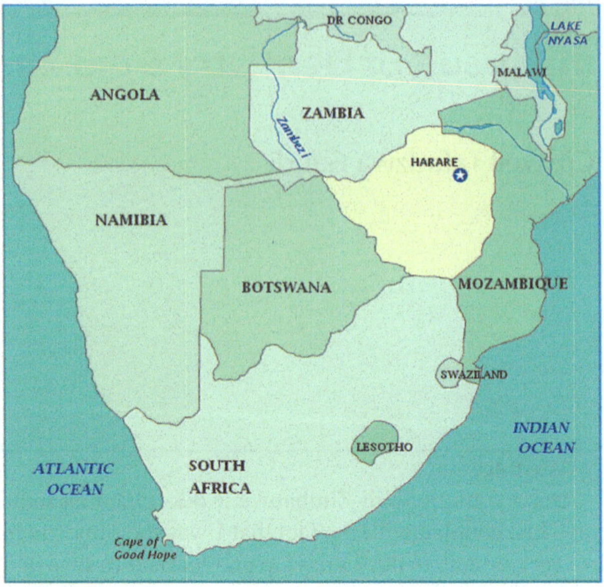

Fig. 27.1 Harare, Zimbabwe

we were screened based on our results. I was delighted to be in the first class as it was the only class in the school, of the 13 classes in my stream, to offer science subjects. I was accepted at St. Ignatius College for my advanced level studies, one of the most prestigious schools in the nation, after coming first in my school in my ordinary level results. I enjoyed Biology so much and I would spend a lot of time studying the subject. My skills in scientific reasoning and application improved much. Chemistry and Mathematics taught me to be thorough and exact. I finished my A level with merits in all my three subjects and got accepted at University of Zimbabwe for Dentistry. This was just the beginning of a long journey.

My father passed away in 2002 when I was still in the middle of my schooling. He was the sole breadwinner of the family. His loss had a double impact on me, financially and emotionally. Life as I knew it drastically changed, inevitably changing for the worst. It was an emotionally trying time for us as a family and I particularly, since I was the only boy in the family, and I was very close to my father. He was more of a friend. My school life was affected to some extent, but I received so much support from my sisters and my extended family at large. The financial challenges were compounded by the economic meltdown that the country at large was going through during that time.

University life was an experience that I can never and would not want to forget. It brought so much joy along with sorrows and pain. My background robbed me of the opportunity to freely express myself in fluent English. This impacted on me during my early life at the university. I realized that I may not be as fluent but I could understand concepts and apply them. That was my fortress. As long as I could prove myself, then I had nothing to fear. My uncle brought me textbooks to use, and that really helped me to study a lot and establish a strong foundation in basic sciences, which proved critical in my later years of practice.

For every first year student, finding accommodation on campus was a high priority. It meant only a short walk to lecture theaters and meals that were provided three times a day. To a mature student who was well focused, being in residence meant more time available for studying. I was unfortunate to be out of residence when I first enrolled. I would spend about 3 hours daily commuting to and from school! After finishing lectures at the end of the day, I couldn't use the library as I had to commute back home. I would get home each day exhausted from lectures and waiting in long queues to get transport. After several weeks had gone by, I realized that my situation was pathetic but not hopeless. I went to see the vice-chancellor of the university, the man who was at the helm of university administration, only second to the principal, who was none other than the state president. It was not without a fight that I passed through the first and second secretaries, prior to meeting the third and final secretary to his office. Although I was not allowed to see the vice-chancellor, I managed to get to talk to the pro-vice-chancellor. We had a long talk and finally he wrote a letter to the accommodation officer for me to be allocated a room. Later that day I had residence on campus. It made life much easier and enjoyable too.

The transition from high school to university was so drastic. This taught me to realize that in life, what may appear to be a disappointment may actually turn out to be an opportunity to realize one's greatness in an area they may not have ever imagined themselves in. I also learned that parents should not force their children to follow career paths the children are not passionate about. Even if one had intelligence, it doesn't follow that he/she has to become a doctor. Parents should allow their children to follow their dreams. The best they can do is to advise them and encourage them, but never impose on them what to become in life. When choosing a career, one's choice should be driven by passion, never by financial gains or the prestige associated with it. In any field, one's passion and diligence will get you through difficult times.

Now, being born in a fairly large family where I was the only son with four sisters, I can say I was mildly "spoiled," which is somehow a usual occurrence in a typical African family. I had the attention of the whole family, as the eldest and only son of my parents and also the only brother my sisters had. My siblings and I grew up with very good ties to each other and to our parents. We had our fights, but we loved each other so much. This is still true even today, with all of my sisters now married off. These ties went a long way in teaching me good interpersonal skills. I remember in the evenings we would sit and chat and laugh as a family. Family time was so precious to every one of us. Importance of good interaction with people was engraved in me at a very tender age. Now as a young man at the university, the lessons I learned as a child proved to be vital. I quickly made good friends both in class and at church. This strong support network proved indispensable to me during my college years.

The School of Dentistry in Zimbabwe had its inception in 1997 with seven students. As it was still a small department within the College of Health Sciences, dental students would be part of the medical class from first to third year, covering all basic sciences together. The two groups would then split at the end of third year, as dental students began on their journey of becoming dental professionals. Both medicine and dentistry were 5-year courses. At the end of each academic year, we would write final exams. These were barrier exams which when failed would mean a student repeating a whole year. The system was tough and although we would complain then, we are thankful now for having gone through such a grilling process. It turned us into resilient practitioners who are also competitive regionally and internationally. The system was like a tightly knitted net that was so impervious, meant to prevent passage of unsuitable and unripe professionals.

When I embarked on my fourth year, which was my first year of actual dental classes, I was eager to go. I had this insatiable hunger for dental knowledge. I remember telling my friend one day that I was reading everything and anything in dentistry as I would soon be a professional in my field in whom people will place their confidence in. I wanted to be able to answer any question about dental issues. That gave me a head start in my studies. Fourth year was mainly lectures and seminars, with very little exposure to clinical work much later in the year. I couldn't wait to be in the final year. The main drawback we faced as dental students was in finding patients to meet clinical requirements to sit for final year exams. We had so many patients for oral and maxillofacial surgery and pathology, but very little for restorative dentistry and prosthodontics. This was mainly attributed to the middle class to low class patient clientele that our clinic attracted. Our patients could not afford most restorative and prosthodontic treatment. As resources were limited, the clinic had very little equipment and few instruments for prosthodontic cases. Despite the challenges we faced as a school, we focused on what was available to us and what we could do to empower ourselves as future professionals. One dentist, Dr. Maisva, once told me to focus on what was available to me, to be good in doing a simple procedure as an extraction as good as one can get. Diligence in little things taught me diligence in even greater responsibilities.

Dental school came along with its own challenges. I remember struggling with using indirect vision in restorative procedures as we had no prior training on manikins. I remember one supervisor passing a disheartening comment to me during a procedure on a patient. One of my friends, Dr Mapanzure, cried one day as she recalled the comments that the same supervisor had passed on her. We strengthened each other and soldiered on in our quest for knowledge. In February 2012, we sat for our 7-day-long final year examinations. The period seemed never to end. At last we had reached the end of our journey as dental students. I was humbled to receive the Colgate Palmolive and Zimbabwe Dental Association Best Student in Restorative Dentistry awards.

I went on to work as a government dental officer at four different centers in Harare during my 1-year internship. As a young dentist, I had so many colleagues in the profession already. This was because as a student, I would visit dental practices around town and get to talk to the practitioners or shadow them. I attached myself as a mentee to one of my supervisors, Dr Djordjevic, from dental school. I would go and just watch him, learn how he conversed with patients, how he did certain procedures, and how he handled conflicts. I learned so much in such a short period. I finished my compulsory 1 year in government and resigned. I began working part time at two places in town, while I continued with my mentorship. My mentor later allowed me to see some of his patients under his watchful eye. It was easy for me to translate academic knowledge into practical skill as I studied a lot along with shadowing experienced practitioners.

My uncle and aunt encouraged me to look for a short course abroad to go and experience first-world dentistry and equip myself with other essential skills I had failed to acquire as a student, all expenses on their account. For that, I am forever grateful. I applied for a 1-year internship at the University of Florida in restorative dentistry. The road to getting accepted in the program was not without its hiccups. I had to process so much paperwork for an entire 6-week period. The process was demanding, both financially and emotionally. After sending documents back and forth, I still was not yet certain of going to Florida until I went for my visa application. Fortunately, I got my visa and in 5 days I was airborne to Florida (Fig.27.2). My desire to excel in dentistry had finally found an opportunity to express itself. I always had a deep desire to offer patient-focused care, and that was soon to be fulfilled.

The transition from Zimbabwe to Florida was filled with excitement and anxiety at the same time. I had two mentors that were assigned to me, Dr. Spencer and Dr. Fernandez. They both went out of their way to accommodate me and teach me. My curriculum was tailor-made to meet my needs. My main focus was in restorative dentistry, although I also spent time in several departments as well. I had preclinical training and soon after I was allowed to see patients. I would spend long hours in the lab working on my dentoform as I had not had the chance to in my former training. I soon gained respect with my fellow students and faculty. Resources were available and I grabbed every opportunity to sharpen my clinical skills. I would visit faculty and listen to every wise word they said. I observed the systems that the school had in place, and I adopted or modified them to suit my future practice back in Zimbabwe.

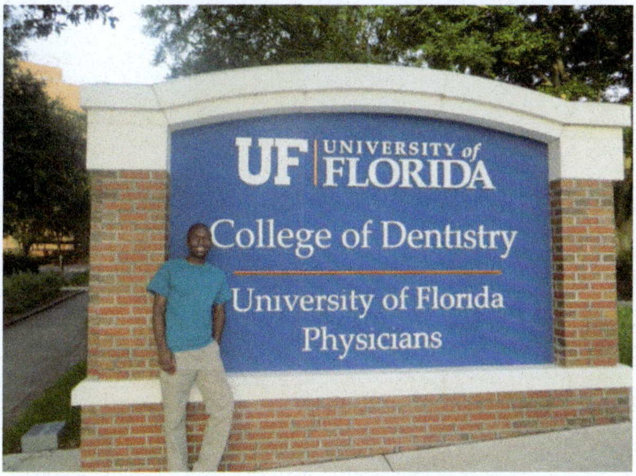

Fig. 27.2 Dr. Gandi spent a year as a fellow at the University of Florida, College of Dentistry

Some of the patients that were assigned to me did not appreciate my expertise. I had to humble myself and do my best to impress my patients. With time, my patients liked me so much and my schedule slowly became hectic while I tried to accommodate many of my patients. It was heartbreaking to leave my Florida family after almost a year of staying there in 2014.

I soon rejoined Dr. Djordjevic at his practice after returning to Zimbabwe. In November 2014, I joined the University of Zimbabwe as faculty in restorative dentistry. I felt an obligation to give back to aspiring dentists. I enjoyed sharing information with my students, and I tried to give them both academic and practical training in the courses that I taught. I feel personal satisfaction from teaching students.

In August 2015, I started my private practice in Harare while maintaining my attachment with the University. Juggling the two has been the best experience of my life. Teaching encourages one to keep abreast with current developments in the field and keeps one's skills sharp. On the other hand, the satisfaction that comes from running a private practice is unmeasurable. It also comes from growing the practice, retaining patients, putting systems in place that are specific to meet your goals, and seeing the smile on your patient's face. Personally, I would say that the greatest favor of being a dentist is not in acquiring wealth, or establishing a renowned name in the field of dentistry, but is in hearing the simple words from your patient, "Thank you, Tatenda" (Fig. 27.3a–c).

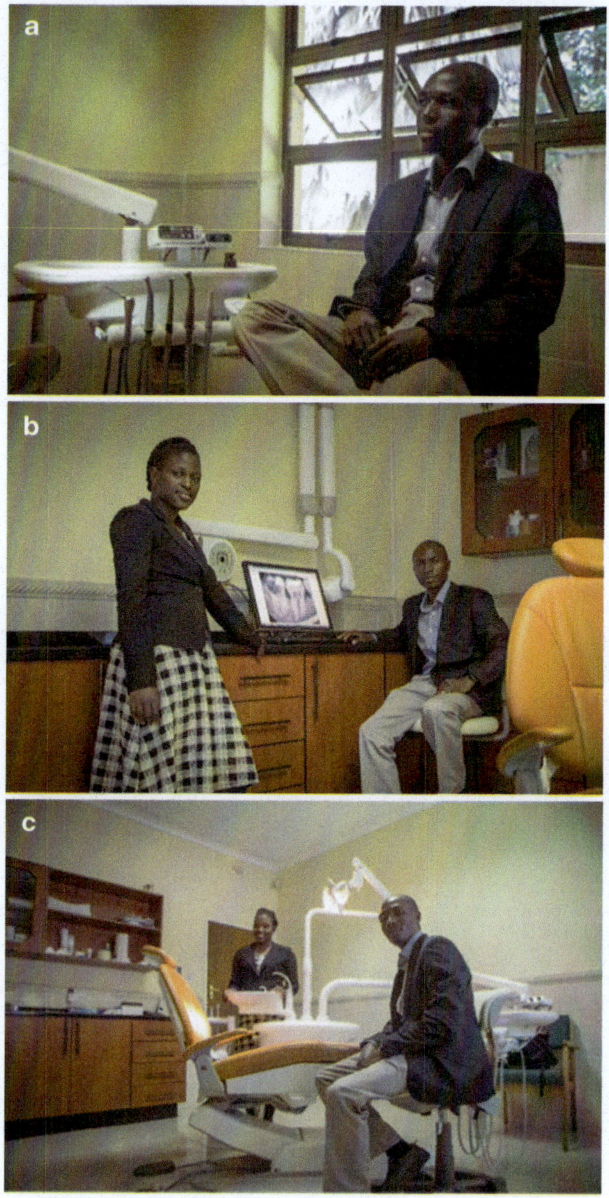

Fig. 27.3 (**a–c**) Dr. Gandi and his dream come true, a private practice to call his own in Harare, Zimbabwe

Index

G.M. Weinstein, M.T. Zientz (eds.), *The Dental Reference Manual*,
DOI 10.1007/978-3-319-39730-6

The manufacturer's authorised representative in the EU is Springer Nature Customer Service Centre GmbH, Europaplatz 3, 69115 Heidelberg, Germany. If you have any concerns regarding our products, please contact ProductSafety@springernature.com

Printed and bound by CPI Group (UK) Ltd, Croydon, CR0 4YY
28/09/2026
02224063-0001